ULTRASOUND
for Primary Care

ULTRASOUND
for Primary Care

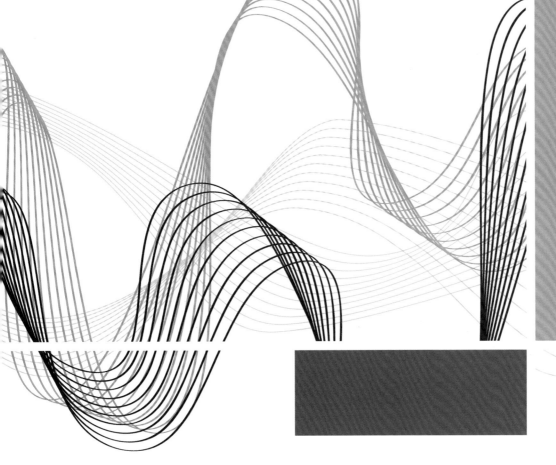

Paul Bornemann, MD, RMSK, RPVI

Associate Professor
Family and Preventive Medicine
University of South Carolina School of Medicine
Program Director
Family Medicine Residency
Prisma Health—Midlands
Columbia, South Carolina

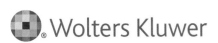 Wolters Kluwer

Philadelphia · Baltimore · New York · London
Buenos Aires · Hong Kong · Sydney · Tokyo

Executive Editor: Sharon Zinner
Senior Development Editor: Ashley Fischer
Senior Editorial Coordinator: Lindsay Ries
Marketing Manager: Phyllis Hitner
Production Project Manager: Sadie Buckallew
Design Coordinator: Stephen Druding
Manufacturing Coordinator: Beth Welsh
Prepress Vendor: S4Carlisle Publishing Services

9 8 7 6 5 4 3 2 1

Printed in China

Library of Congress Cataloging-in-Publication Data

Names: Bornemann, Paul, author.
Title: Ultrasound for primary care / Paul Bornemann.
Description: First edition. | Philadelphia : Wolters Kluwer, [2021] |
   Includes bibliographical references and index.
Identifiers: LCCN 2020016700 | ISBN 9781496366986 (paperback)
Subjects: MESH: Ultrasonography—methods | Point-of-Care Testing | Primary
   Health Care
Classification: LCC RC78.7.U4 | NLM WN 208 | DDC 616.07/543—dc23
LC record available at https://lccn.loc.gov/2020016700

DEDICATION

To my children, Danyel, Kathryn, Sebastian, Taylor, and my wife, Gina.
You are the world to me.

CONTRIBUTORS

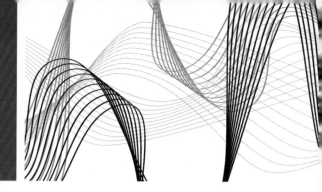

Naushad Amin, MD, FAAFP
Assistant Professor
Department of Family Medicine
University of Central Florida (UCF)
College of Medicine (COM)
Orlando, Florida

Cesar S. Arguelles, MD
Assistant Professor
Family and Community Medicine
Southern Illinois University School of Medicine
Quincy, Illinois

Keith R. Barron, MD, FACP
Clinical Assistant Professor
Department of Internal Medicine
University of South Carolina
School of Medicine
Prisma Health Midlands
Columbia, South Carolina

Kevin Bergman, MD
Assistant Clinical Professor
Department of Family and Community Medicine
UCSF School of Medicine
San Francisco, California
Co-Director, Ultrasound and Global Health Programs
Emergency Department, Family Medicine
Contra Costa Family Medicine Residency
Martinez, California

F. Laura Bertani, MD
Family Medicine Physician
Department of Clinical Medicine
Mee Memorial Hospital
King City, California
Hospitalist
Sound Physicians Hospitalist Program
Natividad
Salinas, California

Keisha Bonhomme Ellis, MD
Associate Clinical Professor
Department of Outpatient
Augusta University/University of Georgia Partnership

Endocrinologist
PAR Community Care Clinic
Piedmont Athens Regional Medical Center
Athens, Georgia

Gina Bornemann, MMIS, MS

Paul Bornemann, MD, RMSK, RPVI
Associate Professor
Family and Preventive Medicine
University of South Carolina School of Medicine
Program Director
Family Medicine Residency
Prisma Health—Midlands
Columbia, South Carolina

Caroline Brandon, MD
Assistant Professor of Emergency Medicine
Department of Emergency Medicine
Keck School of Medicine of USC
Assistant Professor
Emergency Department
LAC+USC Medical Center
Los Angeles, California

Androuw Carrasco, MD
Physician Family Medicine
Valleywise Health Medical Center
Phoenix, Arizona

Lauren Castleberry, MD, FACOG
Assistant Professor, Obstetrics and Gynaecology
University of South Carolina School of Medicine
Attending Physician, Obstetrics and Gynaecology
Prisma Health, Richland Hospital
Columbia, South Carolina
Attending Physician, Obstetrics and Gynaecology
Lexington Medical Center
West Columbia, South Carolina

Carol Choe, MD
Physician
Critical Care Medicine
Lexington Medical Center
West Columbia, South Carolina

William Chotas, MD
Department of Pediatrics
Commonwealth Healthcare Corporation
Saipan, Northern Mariana Islands

Holly Beth Crellin, MD
Family Medicine Physician
Department of Primary Care
Martin Army Community Hospital
Fort Benning, Georgia

James M. Daniels, MD, MPH, RMSK
Professor
Family and Community Medicine and Orthopedic Surgery
Southern Illinois University School of Medicine
Quincy, Illinois

Darien B. Davda, MD
Academic Hospital Internist
Prisma Health Upstate Hospitalists Service
Hospitalist
Department of Internal Medicine
Prisma Health Upstate
Greenville, South Carolina

Alexei O. DeCastro, MD
Associate Professor
Department of Family Medicine
Medical University of South Carolina
Charleston, South Carolina

Daniel P. Dewey, MD
Staff Physician Ultrasound Director
Emergency Department
M Health Fairview Northland Hospital
Princeton, Minnesota

John Doughton, MD
Assistant Professor
Department of Family Medicine
University of North Carolina
Chapel Hill, North Carolina

Matthew Fentress, MD, MSc, DTM&H
Assistant Professor
Family and Community Medicine
University of California, Davis
Sacramento, California

Melissa Ferguson, MD
Core Faculty
Contra Costa Family Medicine Residency Program
Affiliated with UCSF
Physician
Department of Family Medicine and Hospital Medicine
Contra Costa Regional Medical Center
Martinez, California

Matthew Fitzpatrick, MBBS

David Flick, MD
Clinical Preceptor
Department of Primary Care
University of Colorado Denver School of Medicine
Aurora, Colorado
Family Physician
Department of Primary Care
Evans Army Community Hospital
Fort Carson, Colorado

Mohamed Gad, MD, MPH(c)
Resident Physician
Department of Internal Medicine
Cleveland Clinic
Cleveland, Ohio

Francis M. Goldshmid, MD, FAAFP
Assistant Professor
Department of Community and Family Medicine
University of Missouri at Kansas City, School of Medicine
Kansas City, Missouri

Mark H. Greenberg, MD, FACR, RMSK, RhMSUS
Associate Professor of Medicine
Chief, Musculoskeletal Ultrasound in Rheumatology
Department of Internal Medicine, Rheumatology Division
University of South Carolina School of Medicine
Columbia, South Carolina

Robert Haddad, RDCS, RVT
Director of Ultrasound Education
Ultrasound Institute
University of South Carolina School of Medicine
Columbia, South Carolina

Claire Hartung, MD
Resident Physician
Department of Family Medicine
UCSF
San Francisco, California
Contra Costa Regional Medical Center
Martinez, California

Wynn Traylor Harvey, II, MD
Resident Physician
Department of Family Medicine
Prisma Health USC
Columbia, South Carolina

Benjamin J. F. Huntley, MD, FAAFP
Assistant Professor
Obstetrics and Gynecology, Family Medicine
McGovern Medical School–UT Health
Medical Director Family Medicine OB Clerkship and OB Fellowship
Obstetrics and Gynecology
Memorial Hermann Southwest
Houston, Texas

Erin S. L. Huntley, DO
Maternal Fetal Medicine Fellow
Maternal Fetal Medicine, Obstetrics and Gynecology
McGovern Medical School–UT Health
Physician
Memorial Hermann Hospital–Texas Medical Center
Maternal Fetal Medicine, Obstetrics and Gynecology
Houston, Texas

Aaron C. Jannings, MD
Squadron Surgeon
2nd Cavalry Regiment
United States Army
APO, Armed Forces Europe

Neil Jayasekera, MD
Associate Clinical Professor
Department of Family and Community Medicine
UCSF School of Medicine
San Francisco, California
Family and Emergency Medicine, Advanced Faculty
Contra Costa Family Medicine Residency Program
Contra Costa Regional Medical Center
Martinez, California

Patrick F. Jenkins, III, MD, CAQSM
Physician
Family and Sports Medicine
Piedmont Physicians Group
Conyers, Georgia

Dae Hyoun (David) Jeong, MD
Assistant Professor
Department of Family and Community Medicine
School of Medicine
Southern Illinois University
Director, Sports and Musculoskeletal Medicine
Director, Point-of-Care, Ultrasound Program
Department of Family and Community Medicine
Southern Illinois University for family Medicine
Springfield, Illinois

Kendra Johnson, MD
Family Physician
Hopi Health Care Center
Polacca, Arizona

Tarina Lee Kang, MD, MHA, FACEP
Associate Professor
Department of Emergency Medicine
University of Southern California
Medical Director
Evaluation and Treatment Clinic
Keck Hospital, Obstetrics and Gynaecology
Los Angeles, California

Andrew Kim, MD
Staff Physician
Department of Hospitalist Medicine
Emory Decatur Hospital
Decatur, Georgia

Esther Kim, MD

Nicholas Adam Kohles, MD
Faculty
Department of Family Medicine
Tripler Army Medical Center
Honolulu, Hawaii

Charisse W. Kwan, MD, FRCPC
Director, Point of Care Ultrasound Program
Division of Emergency Medicine
Sickkids Hospital
Assistant Professor
Department of Pediatrics
University of Toronto
Toronto, Ontario, Canada

Joseph C. Lai, DO
Physician
Department of Family Medicine
Atrium Health
Rock Hill, South Carolina

Jennifer S. Lee, DO, MPH
Assistant Professor
Department of Family Medicine
Wright State University Boonshoft School of Medicine
Fairborn, Ohio

Nicholas LeFevre, MD
Assistant Professor
Department of Family Medicine
TCU and UNTHSC School of Medicine
Faculty Physician
Department of Family and Community Medicine
John Peter Smith Hospital
Fort Worth, Texas

Margaret R. Lewis, MD
Associate Professor
Department of Emergency Medicine
Atrium Health Carolinas Medical Center
Charlotte, North Carolina

Michael Marchetti, DO
Director of Sports Medicine
Family and Sports Medicine Core Faculty
Eastern Connecticut Health Network Family Medicine
Residency Program
Manchester Memorial Hospital
Manchester, Connecticut

Sofia Markee, DO, MS
PGY-3
Department of Pediatrics
USC/Palmetto Health Children's Hospital
Columbia, South Carolina

Brooke Hollins McAdams, MD
Assistant Professor of Medicine
Director, Endocrine Fellowship Program
Division of Endocrinology,
Diabetes & Metabolism
Department of Internal Medicine
University of South Carolina School of Medicine
Clinical Endocrinologist
Prisma Health-Midlands Hospital
Columbia, South Carolina

Erica Miller-Spears, MS, PA-C, ATC, RMSK
Assistant Professor
Department of Family and Community Medicine
Southern Illinois University School of Medicine
Quincy, Illinois

Alex Mroszczyk-McDonald, MD, CAQSM, FAAFP
Family and Sports Medicine Physician
Department of Family Medicine
Kaiser Permanente Fontana
Fontana, California

Michael J. Murphy, MD, CAQSM
Primary Care Sports Medicine
Camden Bone & Joint, LLC
Attending Physician
Department of Surgery
Kershaw Health Medical Center
Camden, South Carolina

Tenley E. Murphy, MD, FAAFP, CAQSM
Team Physician
Athletics
Clemson University
Clemson, South Carolina
Attending
Department of Orthopedics
Prisma Health Blue Ridge Orthopedics
Seneca, South Carolina

Francisco I. Norman, PA-C, MPAS, RGR
Physician Assistant
Department of Critical Care Medicine
Orlando Regional Medical Center
Orlando, Florida

Duncan Norton, MD
Assistant Professor of Pediatrics
Department of Pediatrics
University of South Carolina Columbia Campus
Pediatric Hospitalist
Department of Pediatrics
Prisma Health Children's Hospital–Midlands
Columbia, South Carolina

Jennifer Madeline Owen, MD
Alumni
Contra Costa Family Medicine Residency
Martinez, California

Casey Parker, MBBS, DCH, FRACGP
District Medical Officer
Broome Hospital
Broome, West Australia

Joshua R. Pfent, MD
Volunteer Clinical Professor
Department of Family and Community Medicine
UC Davis School of Medicine
Sacramento, California
Physician
Department of Family Medicine
Tahoe Forest Hospital
Truckee, California

Mena Ramos, MD
Clinical Faculty
Department of Emergency Medicine
Contra Costa Family Medicine Residency Program
Attending Physician
Department of Emergency Medicine
Contra Costa Regional Medical Center
Martinez, California

Victor V. Rao, MBBS, DMRD, RDMS (APCA)
Ex-Director of Ultrasound Education
USC School of Medicine
Columbia, South Carolina
Manager, Global Clinical Content and POCUS Education
POCUS Academy
Rockville, Maryland

Julian Reese, DO
Pulmonary and Critical Care Fellow
Pulmonary and Critical Care
University of South Carolina School of Medicine
Prisma Health
Columbia, South Carolina

Jason Reinking, MD
Medical Director
Lifelong TRUST Clinic
Oakland, California

John Rocco MacMillan Rodney, MD, FAAFP, RDMS
Associate Professor
Department of Family Medicine
Medicos Clinica Camellia
Memphis, Tennessee

William MacMillan Rodney, MD, FAAFP, FACEP
Professor
Department of Family Medicine and Obstetrics
Meharry Medical College
Nashville, Tennessee
William Carey Osteopathic College of Medicine
Hattiesburg, Mississippi

Jilian R. Sansbury, MD, FACP
Associate Program Director
Department of Medicine
Graduate Medical Education
Grand Strand Medical Center
Myrtle Beach, South Carolina

Linda M. Savage, AS
Sports Medicine Fellowship Coordinator
Department of Family and Community Medicine
Southern Illinois University School of Medicine
Quincy, Illinois

David Schrift, MD, RDMS
Assistant Professor of Clinical Internal Medicine
Division of Pulmonary and Critical Care Medicine
Department of Internal Medicine
University of South Carolina School of Medicine
Prisma Health-Midlands
Columbia, South Carolina

Zachary B. Self, MD, FAAFP
Ultrasound Director
Ventura Global Health Fellowship
Ventura County Medical Center Family Medicine Residency
Ventura, California
Founder and Medical Director
Point of Care Ultrasound
Ajkun Pa Le Qatinimit—Clinica Medica Cristian
Santo Tomás La Unión, Guatemala

Mark E. Shaffer, MD
Assistant Professor
Department of Family and Preventive Medicine
University of South Carolina School of Medicine
Columbia, South Carolina
Medical Director
John A Martin Primary Health Care Center
Winnsboro, South Carolina

Naman Shah, MD, PhD
Resident Physician
Department of Family Medicine
Contra Costa Regional Medical Center
Martinez, California

Andrew W. Shannon, MD, MPH
Assistant Professor
Department of Emergency Medicine
University of Florida College of Medicine
Fellowship Director
Advanced Emergency Medicine Ultrasound
Department of Emergency Medicine
UF Health Jacksonville
Jacksonville, Florida

Joy Shen-Wagner, MD, FAAFP
Assistant Professor
Department of Family Medicine
University of South Carolina School of Medicine–Greenville
Director of Family Medicine Point of Care Ultrasound
Department of Family Medicine
Greenville Memorial Hospital Prisma Health
Greenville, South Carolina

Peter James Snelling, BSc, MBBS (Hons), MPHTM, GCHS, CCPU, FRACP, FACEM
Senior Lecturer
School of Medicine
Griffith University
Staff Specialist, Paediatric Emergency Physician
Department of Emergency Medicine
Gold Coast University Hospital
Southport, Australia

Aun Woon (Cindy) Soon, MD, FAAP, FRACP
Pediatric Emergency Physician
Emergency Department
Flinders Medical Centre
Bedford Park, South Australia, Australia

Joshua N. Splinter, MD
Private Practice Physician
Department of Family Medicine
UT Health Athens
Athens, Texas

Erin Stratta, MD
POCUS Project Coordinator
Médecins Sans Frontières International
Doctors Without Borders
New York, New York

Vivek S. Tayal, MD
Professor
Chief, Ultrasound Division
Department of Emergency Medicine
Atrium Health Carolinas Medical Center
Charlotte, North Carolina

Jock Taylor, MD
Clinical Instructor
Department of Orthopedics
Primary Care Sports Medicine
University Hospitals
Cleveland, Ohio

Elana Thau, MD
Postgraduate Trainee
Department of Pediatric and Emergency Medicine
University of Toronto
Academic Fellow
Emergency Department
The Hospital for Sick Children
Toronto, Ontario, Canada

Sergio Urcuyo, MD
Residency Faculty
Contra Costa Family Medicine Residency
Contra Costa Regional Medical Center
Hospital Medical Director
Departments of Hospital Medicine and Critical Care
Contra Costa Regional Medical Center
Martinez, California

Maria G. Valdez, MD, RDMS
Clinical Instructor
Department of Family Medicine
University of Washington
Seattle, Washington
Core Faculty
Department of Family Medicine
Madigan Army Medical Center
Joint Base Lewis-McChord, Washington

Andrew D. Vaughan, MD
Assistant Clinical Professor of Family Medicine
Associate Director of Family Medicine Ultrasound Education
University of South Carolina School of Medicine
Director of Undergraduate Education
Family and Preventative Medicine
Prisma Health Midlands
Columbia, South Carolina

Michael Wagner, MD, FACP, RDMS
Assistant Professor
Internal Medicine
University of South Carolina School of Medicine
Director of Internal Medicine Ultrasound
Internal Medicine
Prisma Health
Greenville, South Carolina

Gary Paul Willers, II, DO
Site Coordinator, Community Preceptor
Department of Family Medicine
Texas A&M University College of Medicine Family Medicine
Residency Program
Bryan, Texas
Chief of Staff, Medical Director of Obstetrics
Department of Family Medicine and Obstetrics
Cuero Regional Hospital
Cuero, Texas

Brandon Williamson, MD
Associate Program Director, Texas A&M Family Medicine
Residency
Clinical Assistant Professor
Primary Care and Population Health
Texas A&M Health Science Center
Bryan, Texas

Ximena Wortsman, MD
Adjunct Professor
Department of Dermatology
University of Chile
Pontifical Catholic University of Chile
Institute for Diagnostic Imaging and Research of the Skin
and Soft Tissues—IDIEP
Santiago, Chile

Nicole T. Yedlinsky, MD, CAQSM, FAAFP, RMSK
Assistant Professor
Department of Family Medicine and Community Health
University of Kansas Medical Center
Kansas City, Kansas

PREFACE

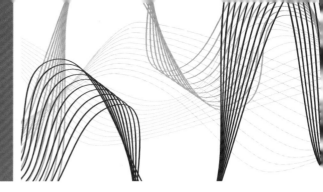

The first medical use of ultrasound is often attributed to the Austrian neurologist Karl Dussik, who, in 1942, used it to peer into the brains of patients in an effort to diagnose tumors. In the following decades, early adopters used ultrasound to image gallbladders, hearts, and fetuses. However, early medical ultrasound devices were large, immobile, and very expensive. This relegated the use of ultrasound to the few researchers and specialists who had access to this equipment. As technology improved, ultrasounds shrunk from the size of rooms to devices that could be placed on a wheeled cart. This newfound mobility allowed for the development of the concept of Point-of-Care Ultrasonography. Point-of-care ultrasound, or POCUS as it is often called, refers to limited and specific ultrasound protocols performed at the bedside by the provider caring for a patient. The protocols usually answer a specific question that helps guide treatment and can be performed after a relatively brief training period. This is in distinction from consultative, comprehensive, or formal ultrasound examinations that are performed by sonographers and interpreted by specialists with specific residency or fellowship training.

Some of the first published accounts of POCUS were by family physicians in the late 1980s and early 1990s.[1-3] Family physicians were caring for pregnant women and incorporating the newly available ultrasound technology into their clinics. However, unlike specialist colleagues who were charged with caring for a single organ, family physicians cared for the entire patient. So, if they were looking at the pregnant patient's abdomen, why not use the ultrasound to look at the gallbladder of the patient with suspected biliary colic? It just made sense. However, the concept didn't catch on widely. It wasn't until the mid-1990s when POCUS was incorporated into trauma management through the Focused Abdominal Sonography in Trauma (FAST) protocol that it really started to catch on with a much larger audience.

The FAST protocol was developed to visualize intra-abdominal hemorrhage in unstable patients with blunt abdominal trauma. It allowed emergency physicians to forego the invasive diagnostic peritoneal lavage, which was previously the standard. The initial protocol started with images of the abdomen, but it wasn't long before additional pictures of the heart and lungs were incorporated, expanding the territory of the POCUS examination. This was a turning point for the POCUS movement. Now that ultrasound was standard for trauma assessment, machines were readily available in emergency rooms, and emergency physicians were becoming more and more comfortable with their use. Emergency physicians found more applications for POCUS and started collecting multitudes of data on how it could be used effectively in the form of focused protocols that required only limited amounts of training. During this same time frame, physicians were starting to use POCUS to guide procedures such as central line insertions and data accumulated on how ultrasound could improve safety and reduce complications.

From that point forward, POCUS spread from emergency medicine to other specialties that cared for acutely ill patients, including hospitalists and critical care physicians. It was a natural fit, as many of the emergency applications carried over nicely. However, POCUS remained elusive in the largest group of care providers, those in the field of primary care. It was not until only the recent past few years that this has started to change. The mid-2010s saw an inflection point with a rapidly increasing interest in POCUS in primary care providers.

It seems there are three main reasons for this change. The first was the aforementioned data accruing over the feasibility and benefits of POCUS in diagnostic protocols and procedure guidance accumulating in the emergency medicine literature. The second was the fact that since its initial introduction into a medical school curriculum in 2006, more and more medical schools were adopting integrated ultrasound curricula.[4] This meant that medical students were graduating medical school with comfort and skills in POCUS and naturally wanting to continue to develop this skillset through their residency training in primary care specialties. The final reason was the rapid advancements in pocket ultrasound technology. Ultrasounds were becoming smaller and much less expansive. This put them very reasonably in the gasp of all primary care providers.

Although many primary care providers are now learning to use POCUS in their practices, most of the applications for its use are still derived from the first experiences with acutely ill patients. Although these applications will often apply to patients seen in primary care, as they may often be acutely ill, there is a whole other area that has yet to be explored. The potential for POCUS to be used in chronic disease management and preventive care is one of the most exciting possibilities for the future as primary care physicians begin to incorporate POCUS into their practices. This is the role that I envision for *Ultrasound in Primary Care*.

Ultrasound in Primary Care is organized by chapters that focus on common questions that arise in the primary care clinic. Each question is followed by a clinical vignette that illustrates a common scenario. Then the book gives evidence for how each of these questions can be answered at the bedside using POCUS. Evidence is summarized in a way that will be familiar to many primary care providers, the Strength-of-Recommendation Taxonomy utilized by the American Academy of Family Physicians.[5] Each chapter then goes into illustrated step-by-step instructions on how to perform the protocol. Additionally, a patient management section, including an easy-to-follow algorithm, walks through how the ultrasound findings

can be used to plan for the care of the patient in the clinic. Pearls and pitfalls are then included. Pearls are expert-level tips and tricks that help the reader more easily perform the examination. Pitfalls are common mistakes that beginners are especially prone to making. Advice on how to avoid these are also included. Finally, information on billing and coding is provided for each chapter. In addition to the clinical question chapters, there are eight procedure chapters that go through detailed instructions on how to use ultrasound to guide clinic procedures. Information on evidence and billing is included for these chapters, as well.

I am a firm believer that POCUS has the potential to improve the quality of care in a cost-efficient manner. Most of the chapters in this book give examples of how ultrasound can be used to answer a question in lieu of more expensive imaging such as CT or MRI. Additionally, the book offers examples of how patients may be triaged in the clinic, decreasing the number of patients who need to be referred to the emergency room or for specialist care. This is all very important in this age of low-quality, high-expense care. It is my hope that this book not only serves to educate primary care providers on how to use POCUS in their practices but also inspires them to think outside the box and to develop new and exciting uses. Though we are still in the early stages of this journey, it is one filled with hope and excitement, and one that I look forward to continuing with you.

References

1. Rodney WM, Deutchman ME, Hartman KJ, Hahn RG. Obstetric ultrasound by family physicians. *J Fam Pract*. 1992;34(2):186-194.
2. Hahn RG, Davies TC, Rodney WM. Diagnostic ultrasound in general practice. *Fam Pract*. 1988;5(2):129-135.
3. Deutchman ME, Connor P, Hahn RG, Rodney WM. Maternal gallbladder assessment during obstetric ultrasound: results, significance, and technique. *J Fam Pract*. 1994;39(1):33-37.
4. Hoppmann R, Cook T, Hunt P, et al. Ultrasound in medical education: a vertical curriculum at the University of South Carolina School of Medicine. *J S C Med Assoc*. 2006;102(10):330-334.
5. The strength-of-recommendation taxonomy. https://www.aafp.org/dam/AAFP/documents/journals/afp/sortdef07.pdf. Accessed 27 October, 2019.

CONTENTS

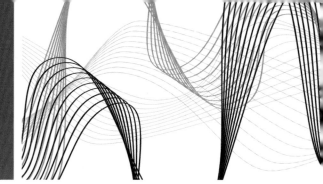

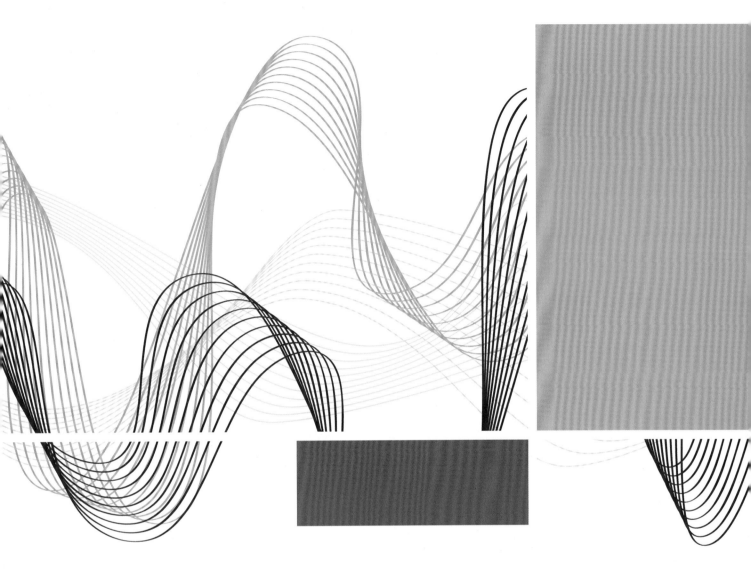

PART **I**

INTRODUCTION

Ultrasound Basics: Physics, Transducers, Conventions, Terminology, and Artifacts

Victor V. Rao, MBBS, DMRD, RDMS (APCA) and Robert Haddad, RDCS, RVT

BASIC ULTRASOUND PHYSICS

Ultrasound physics is a vast subject, but fortunately for most practical purposes in the point-of-care ultrasound (POCUS) setting, a basic knowledge of the ultrasound physics should be sufficient in a majority of the clinical scenarios. The underlying physics will have an impact on why a specific transducer would be ideal for a particular ultrasound examination or how to adjust the ultrasound system parameters to produce optimal images including deciding how to problem-solve artifacts.

What is Ultrasound

Ultrasound is a sound wave. Just like the sound we hear, it needs a medium in which to travel. The medium could be a solid, liquid, or gas. The reason it is classified as ultrasound is because it is beyond the hearing range of humans. We can only hear sound in the range of 20 Hz to 20 kHz and we progressively lose hearing ability as we age at a rate of about 1 Hz a day under normal circumstances.

Ultrasound is a form of energy, and it travels as a longitudinal pressure wave. The best way to experience the sound pressure wave would be to stand close to and in front of a large woofer that is playing loud music with enhanced bass settings. Observe the woofer diaphragm motion. As it moves back and forth, the air is compressed and decompressed. You can even feel the pressure wave on your hand if placed near the woofer diaphragm. That is precisely how an ultrasound wave moves through any medium, by producing alternating compression and rarefaction (or decompression) zones through the medium. Ultrasound waves have a specific frequency and wavelength.

Frequency

Frequency refers to the number of waves or cycles per second. The unit of frequency is Hertz. Each wave has a zone of positive compression (represented by the crest) and a zone of negative compression or rarefaction (represented by a trough). **Figures 1-1 and 1-2** show an example of a wave traveling through a medium at four cycles per second or 4 Hz.

It is important to note that there is a trade-off when it comes to selecting the ideal frequency of ultrasound to use for different applications. High-frequency transducers provide high-resolution images but with limited depth of penetration—usually only up to around 6 cm. This limits their use to more superficial structures. On the other hand, low-frequency transducers provide more depth, up to 30 cm, but the image is of lower quality.

How Does An Ultrasound Imaging Device Work?

Although knowledge of the intricacies of an ultrasound system is not essential to scanning, it is important to have a basic idea of the process by which the placement of a transducer on the body leads to the creation of an ultrasound image on the display.

As shown in **Figure 1-3**, there are eight main components to an ultrasound system. They are:

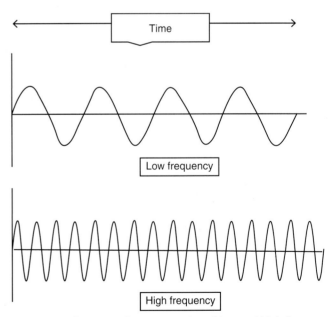

FIGURE 1-2. A diagrammatic representation of low- and high-frequency waves. Note that the wavelength (length of the wave) decreases as the frequency increases. In diagnostic ultrasound, low-frequency range would be in the range of 1.5 to 5.0 MHz. The high-frequency range would be approximately in the range of 7.0 to 20.0 MHz. 1 MHz = 1 million cycles per second.

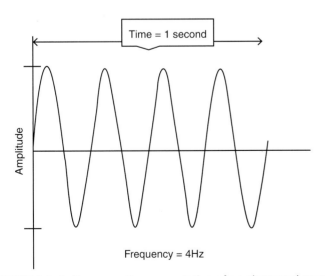

FIGURE 1-1. A diagrammatic representation of an ultrasound wave with a frequency of 4 Hz.

Information flow through an ultrasound system

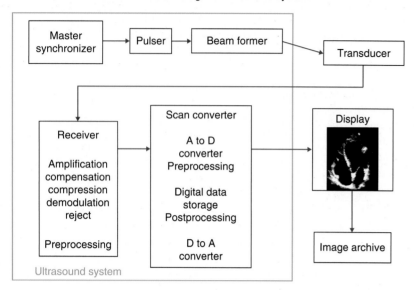

FIGURE 1-3. A representation of how the data are collected and flow from the transducer to the ultrasound receiver and scan converter and then processed to display an image on the monitor. Adapted from Edelman SK. *Understanding Ultrasound Physics*. 3rd ed. Woodland, TX: ESP, Inc.; 2004:542.

1. Master synchronizer
2. Transducer
3. Pulser
4. Beamformer
5. Receiver
6. Scan converter
7. Display
8. Storage

The master synchronizer is responsible for communication with all the individual parts of the ultrasound system. It times and organizes the functions of each component to make them operate as a single unit. The transducer converts electrical energy into acoustic energy during transmission and then reconverts the returning acoustic energy from different areas of the body into electrical energy.

The pulser works by controlling the electrical signals sent to each of the elements in the transducer. It is responsible for controlling the pulse repetition frequency, pulse repetition period, and pulse amplitude. Pulse repetition frequency is the number of pulses that occur in 1 second. Pulse repetition period is the time from the start of one pulse to the start of the next pulse. It includes the time that the crystal is vibrating and producing sound and the time the crystal is dormant and is listening to the returning pulses. Pulse amplitude is the distance between the average value and the peak value of a pulse. The pulser works in conjunction with the beamformer to create a specific firing pattern for a transducer.

The receiver is associated with processing the returning electronic signals from the transducer and processing them for the display. The scan converter helps convert analog signals to digital signals and vice versa between the transducer and the display.

The monitor displays the ultrasound imaging data. The system may also have speakers to produce audible sound during spectral Doppler mode. Storage can be a variety of media devices used to archive the ultrasound data produced by the equipment permanently. On modern ultrasound systems, data can be stored on the internal hard drive of the ultrasound device or a USB flash drive, digital thermal printer, film, writable discs using an external

DVD writer or even transferred to an electronic medical record (EMR) system. You may discuss the options available with the device vendor.

ULTRASOUND TRANSDUCERS

The terms "transducer" and "probe" are often used interchangeably. The transducer is the component of the ultrasound that is held in the hand of the operator and used to obtain images by being placed on the patient. There are different types of ultrasound transducers available for various applications. However, the modern transducers now available in the market are much better and more versatile as compared to those available a couple of decades ago. The newer transducers are multifrequency transducers with a frequency range that in some ultrasound systems can be adjusted by the user during scanning within the bandwidth range of that transducer.

Curvilinear Sequential Array Transducer

The curvilinear or convex ultrasound transducer is perhaps the most widely used transducer in ultrasound imaging. It is made up of multiple sound-producing elements aligned in a curved array. Each element pulses in sequence. It has a large convex footprint and a wide field of view and is the transducer of choice for scanning the abdomen and female pelvic organs and for obstetric examinations. Other uses include some limited chest ultrasound and even extremity ultrasound when the region of interest is deeper and beyond the range of a high-frequency linear transducer. See **Figure 1-4**.

Linear Sequential Array Transducer

The linear array transducer is also made up of an array of elements, but they are arranged linearly as opposed to the curvilinear array. As with the curvilinear, it also has elements that pulse in sequence. It produces high-frequency waves and is commonly used to scan superficial structures. It yields high-resolution images and is the transducer of choice for imaging soft tissue, the musculoskeletal system, peripheral vessels, and carotid artery, to name a few. The image resolution is superior to the curvilinear low-frequency

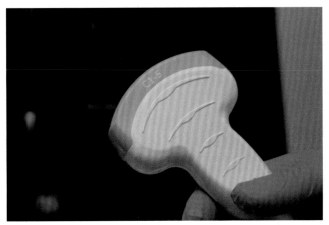

FIGURE 1-4. A typical low-frequency curvilinear transducer recommended for abdomen and ob-gyn scans and some chest applications.

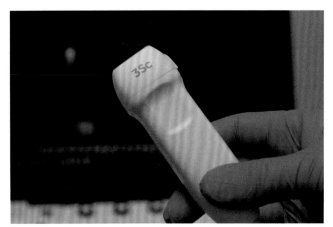

FIGURE 1-6. A typical phased array sector transducer recommended for echocardiography.

transducer; however, there is one serious disadvantage with this transducer. Most high-frequency linear transducers cannot be used to scan images beyond 4.0 to 6.0 cm from the point of contact on the body. See **Figure 1-5**.

Phased Array Transducer

The phased array transducer is made up of only a few sound-producing elements that pulse together in different phases and thus shoot an ultrasound beam in different directions across the field of view to make up an ultrasound image. It has a small footprint with a wide field of view, which allows the user to use a relatively small window to view and display a large structure without any obstruction of the ultrasound beam. It is also able to function at very high frame rates, which is especially useful for imaging moving structures. It is a low-frequency transducer with good tissue penetration. Given these characteristics, the phased array transducer is ideal for transthoracic echocardiography. It can also be used to scan other deep structures in the abdomen or pelvis, but the resolution will be lower than a sequential array probe of the same frequency. Being a low-frequency transducer, it should not be used to image superficial structures because the image resolution in the near field will be very low. See **Figure 1-6**.

MODES OF ULTRASOUND

The commercially available ultrasound systems in the market may offer other modes of ultrasound in addition to the B-mode ultrasound. At the very least, every ultrasound will be capable of producing B-mode images. The other common modes of ultrasound are discussed in the section that follows.

B-Mode/2D Mode

The B-mode is also referred to as 2D mode in some newer ultrasound systems. This mode generates a two-dimensional black and white image of the structure being scanned. The image is composed of pixels that are tightly packed together to form a smooth looking ultrasound image. If you magnify the image significantly, you will be able to see the individual pixels in the image. Each pixel has a certain shade of gray, black, or white color demonstrable in the grayscale depending upon how reflective or echogenic the structure is that is being represented on the display. B-mode is most effective when the angle of insonation (the angle at which the wave hits its target) is closest to 90°. See **Figure 1-7**.

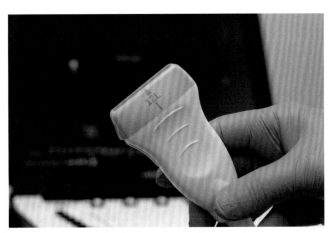

FIGURE 1-5. A typical high-frequency linear transducer.

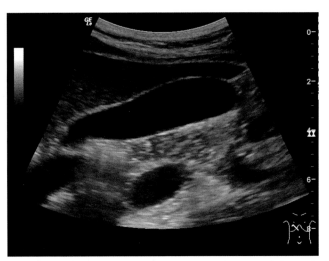

FIGURE 1-7. B-mode mid-longitudinal view of a normal distended gallbladder.

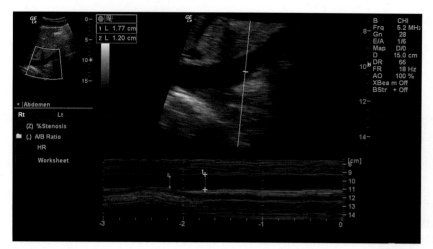

FIGURE 1-8. M-mode tracing obtained through the desired level in the inferior vena cava. Note that there is a B-mode image above the M-mode tracing. The M-mode spike is seen in the B-mode image as a white line. The M-mode tracing represents the pixels along the spike (Y-axis) over time (X-axis). The cursor location can be moved by the user to obtain the M-mode tracing at the desired region of interest.

M-Mode

The M-mode is also known as the motionscape mode. It displays one-dimensional information that is obtained along the M-mode line (or spike) in relation to time. The X-axis represents time in seconds, and the Y-axis represents pixels captured along the M-mode cursor. It is helpful to document any structure in the body that shows linear motion. For example, in echocardiography, it can show the motion of the valves of the heart and the ventricle walls. It could also be used to document motion of the inferior vena cava (IVC) wall with respiration, in which we observe, document, and measure the IVC diameter variability with respiration as shown in **Figure 1-8**.

Doppler Mode

The Doppler mode is very helpful in detecting movement or flow by using the measurements of the Doppler shift of the ultrasound waves. Doppler is most accurate when the angle of insonation is parallel to the flow being measured.

There are three main types of Doppler modes that are commonly available in most laptop ultrasound systems. They are:
A. Color Doppler
B. Power Doppler
C. Spectral Doppler

Color Doppler

Color Doppler is useful to determine if flow is present in a certain region and the direction in a semiquantitative manner. Any motion detected is represented with a red or blue color depending on the direction of motion in the region being interrogated in relation to the direction of the color Doppler ultrasound beam. During color Doppler mode, a color Doppler box that can be repositioned using the trackball or the mouse is superimposed on a B-mode image. See **Figure 1-9**.

Power Doppler

Power Doppler is similar to color Doppler but is more ideal for detecting flow in low-flow conditions. It is very sensitive to low levels of flow and is minimally affected by the angle of insonation. It is often used to detect increased flow in an inflamed tendon or in cellulitis or to determine if there is perfusion in the testis in the case of suspected torsion. Power Doppler does not provide directional information and thus a shade of one color (usually orange) is used. The color provides information about the overall amount of flow in an area but not the direction. See **Figure 1-10**.

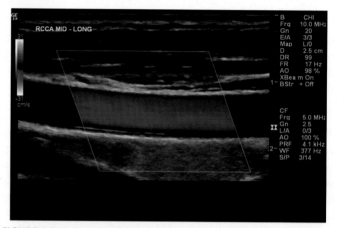

FIGURE 1-9. Color Doppler display showing a normal color display in the lumen of the common carotid artery. Note the legend on the left side. The red and yellow colors represent flow toward the transducer and the blue and light blue colors represent flow away from the transducer. Also note that the frequencies of the B-mode and color Doppler are different as seen on the right side.

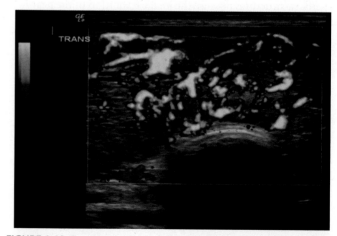

FIGURE 1-10. Transverse view of the thyroid gland obtained through the isthmus and a portion of the right lobe. The power Doppler shows evidence of increased vascularity in the thyroid tissue as indicated by the red and yellow colors. This was a case of Graves' disease. Note the legend on the left. Note that there is no blue color as seen in color Doppler mode, as power Doppler does not include information on direction of flow.

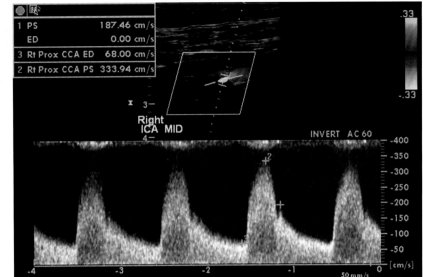

FIGURE 1-11. Increased peak systolic (PS) velocity seen and also spectral broadening seen in the midsegment of the internal carotid artery (ICA). The findings are consistent with a stenosis in the ICA causing hemodynamic changes. Also note that the system automatically calculated the PS velocity and the end diastolic (ED) velocity, which were incorrect. The correct PS and ED were 333.94 and 68.00 cm/s, respectively, which were measured manually by the user.

Spectral Doppler

Spectral Doppler provides quantitative information on the flow measured at a certain location. It is mapped as a spectrum of flow velocities on the Y-axis against time on the X-axis. Two variations are pulsed and continuous wave Doppler. Pulsed wave measures flow at a specific location, whereas continuous wave measures it additively along a line in the vertical plane. The quantitative measurements provided by spectral Doppler can be useful to determine and grade the degree of stenosis present in a blood vessel or across a heart valve. See **Figure 1-11**.

ULTRASOUND SYSTEM CONSOLE

The POCUS systems available nowadays vary a lot in the buttons, knobs, and functions that are available. Some newer pocket ultrasound devices have much fewer buttons and knobs. However, every system will have some basic controls and functions such as

B-mode imaging (by default), depth control, overall gain control, basic linear distance measurement, and image/video storage. See **Figure 1-12**.

ULTRASOUND—OTHER CONTROLS AND FUNCTIONS

The function of the knobs and buttons of the ultrasound device can vary a lot depending upon the make and model of the device. Some may have many controls available, whereas some pocket ultrasound devices may only have a handful of buttons and functions. The most common functions and controls are noted in the section that follows.

Gain

The gain control allows the user to make the whole image brighter or darker. The aim should be to have an optimal image with fluid being represented as black (anechoic). See **Figure 1-13**.

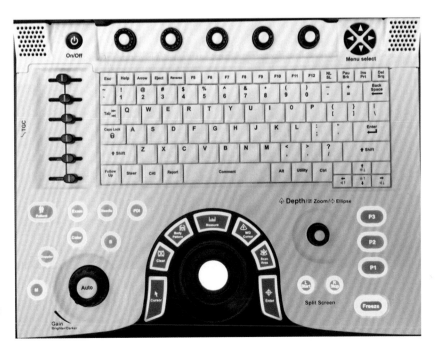

FIGURE 1-12. A laptop ultrasound system console. Laptop ultrasound systems will have an alphanumeric keyboard and some additional buttons and knobs and a port to connect the ultrasound transducer.

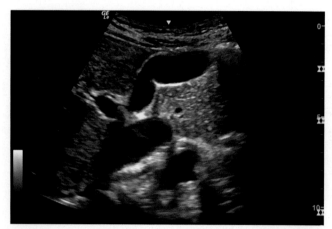

FIGURE 1-13. An optimal ultrasound image of the liver and gallbladder, with the liver showing normal homogeneous echotexture and the blood vessels, lumen and bile in the gallbladder are seen as anechoic regions on the ultrasound image.

When the gain is excessive, the whole image looks brighter than normal. See **Figures 1-14 and 1-15** for an example of the gain set too high.

Depth

The depth control is crucial. If the depth is set too deep, the structure or organ may look much smaller and can increase the chances of missing a lesion and may also lead to significant measurement errors. If the depth is set too shallow, a deeper structure will not be visible at all. See **Figures 1-16 to 1-18** for parasternal long-axis (PLAX) views of the heart obtained with different depth settings.

ULTRASOUND B-MODE/2D MODE IMAGING TERMINOLOGY

Because the ultrasound system processor processes ultrasound waves reflected off different tissue interfaces or medium, the ultrasound image is described based upon how reflective the tissue or medium is relative to the surrounding structures.

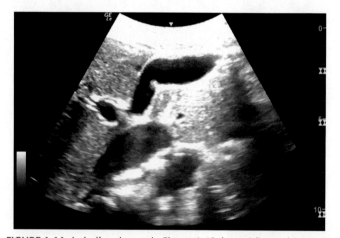

FIGURE 1-14. A similar view as in Figure 1-13, but with very high gain settings. The whole image looks very bright. A pathologic finding if located in the bright areas could very easily be missed if the gain is set too high.

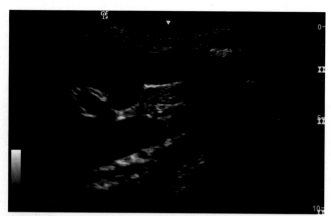

FIGURE 1-15. An ultrasound image obtained with low gain settings. The whole image looks very dark and structures and anatomic details are unrecognizable. A pathologic finding can easily be missed in the dark areas because of incorrect gain settings.

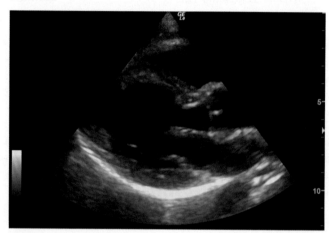

FIGURE 1-16. Ultrasound image obtained with appropriate depth settings.

Hyperechoic

The term "hyperechoic" describes anything that is highly reflective inside the body and appears to be brighter on the ultrasound monitor. In general, bone, calcifications, air, foreign body, and calculi tend to be hyperechoic. However, sometimes the region or structure in the

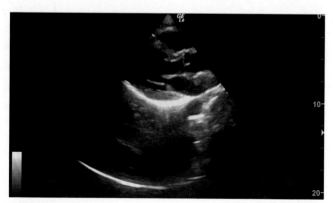

FIGURE 1-17. Parasternal long-axis view of the heart with depth setting too high. The heart view only occupies a small portion of the screen and appears much smaller as compared to the image in Figure 1-16 and a significant portion of the screen space is wasted.

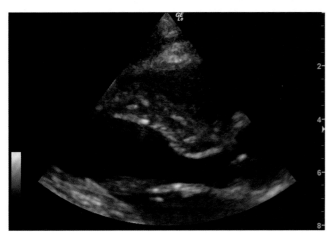

FIGURE 1-18. Parasternal long-axis view taken with depth setting too low. The left atrium is not completely visualized. The pericardium and posterior leaflet of the mitral valve are not visible. This can be corrected by simply adjusting to a deeper depth setting to include the structures of interest and having a 1 to 2 cm zone included beyond the structures of interest.

body may not be as reflective as a bone; it could be relatively brighter as compared to the surrounding structures. So, the term "hyperechoic" could be used to describe such a lesion. See **Figure 1-19**.

Hypoechoic

The term "hypoechoic" describes anything that is less reflective inside the body and appears to be relatively darker as compared to the surrounding structures and appears gray but not black on the ultrasound monitor. See **Figure 1-20**.

Anechoic

The term "anechoic" describes anything in the body that does not produce any echoes. Anechoic generally suggests that the region contains some form of fluid. Normal anechoic fluid could be urine in the urinary bladder or bile in the gallbladder or even blood in the blood vessel lumen or the heart chambers. Common examples of abnormal anechoic would be ascites in the abdominal cavity or pleural effusion. See **Figure 1-21**.

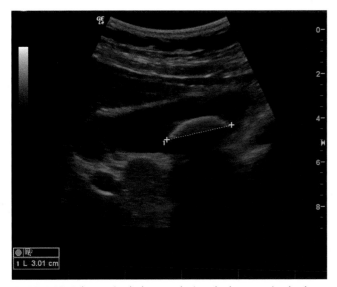

FIGURE 1-19. A large single hyperechoic calculus seen in the lumen of the gallbladder.

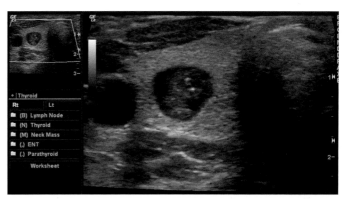

FIGURE 1-20. A nodule is seen in the thyroid with a hypoechoic solid area in the center and anechoic area surrounding it.

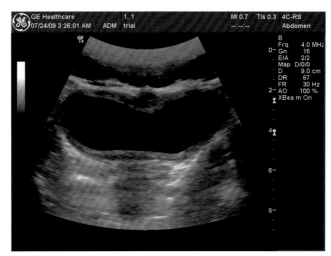

FIGURE 1-21. The urine in the center of this bladder image is anechoic as almost no ultrasound is reflected back from it.

Isoechoic

Isoechoic describes any structure within the body that has the same echogenic property as the structure or structures around it. A good example would be an anechoic mass in the liver. That would make it difficult to detect the mass in the liver, as it will tend to blend in with the normal liver parenchyma. See **Figure 1-22**.

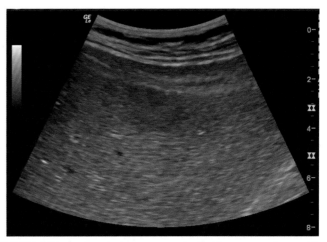

FIGURE 1-22. An isoechoic mass seen in the liver parenchyma. The mass is barely visible on ultrasound and seems to blend with the surrounding normal liver parenchyma.

ULTRASOUND ARTIFACTS

Most ultrasound images will have some form of ultrasound imaging artifacts. Artifacts are images that appear on the display but that do not represent true physical structures. Artifacts are caused by a violation of the assumptions of ultrasound physics, equipment malfunction or design, and/or operator error. It is important to recognize the different artifacts and their causes.

B-Mode Artifacts

Some common ultrasound artifacts that may be encountered during B-mode imaging are:

Acoustic Shadow

When an ultrasound wave encounters a structure that possesses extremely high reflective properties, the entire beam is reflected to the transducer with no sound moving beyond the border. This creates an acoustic shadow in the region immediately distal to the reflector. Common examples of structures producing an acoustic shadow are calculus in the gallbladder, kidney, or bladder and bone. Bowel gas also causes shadowing, but it is not a clean shadow and is referred to as a "dirty shadow." See **Figure 1-23**.

Acoustic Enhancement

This artifact is visually the opposite of acoustic shadowing. When an ultrasound wave passes through tissue, attenuation of the wave occurs. Attenuation is the weakening of a sound wave's intensity, power, and amplitude. Acoustic enhancement occurs when an ultrasound beam travels through a fluid medium with low attenuation properties. This results in the ultrasound beam being attenuated less than in the surrounding tissue. A bright or hyperechoic zone immediately posterior to the fluid-filled medium is created. This useful artifact helps us to confirm the fluid nature of some deeper lesions that may not appear to be anechoic. See **Figure 1-24**.

Reverberation Artifact

In the presence of two hyperechoic structures, the echoes get trapped between the two and bounce back and forth, creating multiple, equally spaced lines in the shape of a ladder or Venetian blind. A great example is "A-lines" seen during lung ultrasound. See **Figure 1-25**.

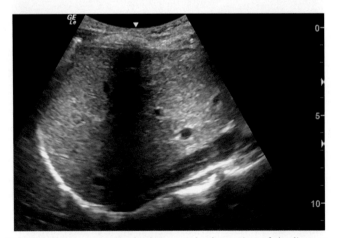

FIGURE 1-23. An acoustic shadow seen in the region of the liver parenchyma that was produced by a rib.

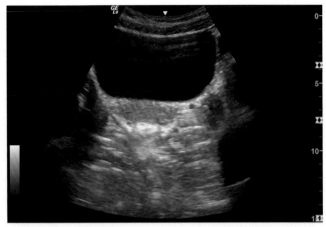

FIGURE 1-24. An acoustic enhancement artifact posterior to the bladder. The region behind the posterior wall of the bladder appears hyperechoic (brighter) as compared to the area surrounding it at the same depth level from the skin surface.

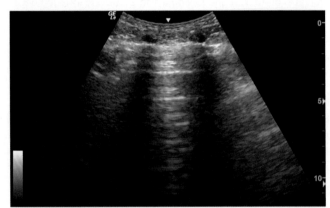

FIGURE 1-25. A-lines are seen while performing lung ultrasound that simply suggest the presence of air in the chest cavity. A-lines are a good example of reverberation artifact.

Ring Down Artifact

This artifact is also known as the comet tail artifact, and it appears as an echogenic zone directed downward from the top of an image toward the bottom. It is thought to occur secondary to a mechanism similar to reverberation. It is commonly seen when imaging structures such as prosthetic cardiac valve and a needle during an ultrasound-guided procedure. See **Figure 1-26**.

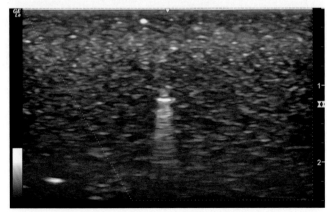

FIGURE 1-26. Ring down artifact seen while performing an ultrasound-guided procedure.

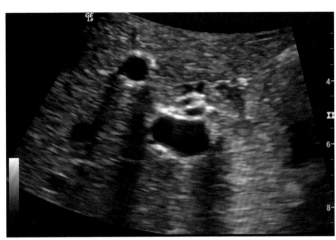

FIGURE 1-27. Edge shadow artifact seen arising from the edges of the portal veins while scanning the liver.

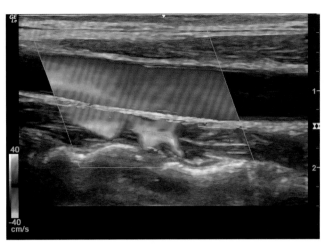

FIGURE 1-29. Color bleeding artifact. Note the color Doppler signal that is seen below the lower wall of the blood vessel.

Edge Shadow Artifact

This artifact is common at the edge of a circular structure. It appears as a hypoechoic line that is parallel to the beam and is caused by beam diverging from its original path as it hits the wall of the circular structure. It occurs secondary to refraction of the ultrasound wave. See **Figure 1-27**.

Mirror Image Artifact

In the presence of a strong reflector, a mirror image of the structure may be formed on the other side of the reflector and is deeper and equidistant from the reflector. This happens when the ultrasound beam strikes a structure obliquely, resulting in a duplicate copy of the reflector alongside the original. See **Figure 1-28**.

Color Doppler Artifacts

Color Bleeding

This happens when the equipment is unable to distinguish low-magnitude Doppler shifts associated with moving anatomy from those arising from red blood cell movement. This creates the appearance of color flash or "ghosting," which looks as if the color is bleeding outside the vessel. This can be easily fixed by adjusting

the wall filter, whereby low velocities such as tissue motion will be removed from the Doppler spectrum. Additionally, the color gain can be reduced and thus the overall sensitivity of the ultrasound device to detecting color flow will be reduced. See **Figure 1-29**.

Aliasing

Aliasing occurs when the Doppler signal is so high that it goes off the scale of the current Doppler settings. It will then alias back down to the lower end of the scale. This can be seen during very high flow states, such as blood traveling through a stenosis, or when the Doppler settings are inappropriate. Aliasing can occur with color or spectral Doppler. The pulse repetition frequency and thus the overall scale of the Doppler measurements can be adjusted. If aliasing is an issue, the pulse repetition frequency should be turned up. On the other hand, if low-flow needs to be measured, it may not be accurately picked up if the pulse repetition frequency is set too high. See **Figure 1-30**.

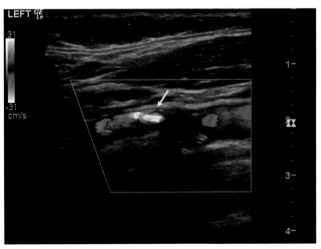

FIGURE 1-30. Aliasing artifact. Note the area of high-velocity flow to the left of the stenotic area in this artery (yellow arrow). The color changes from red to yellow as flow increases in velocity from the periphery of the artery to the center of flow. As the velocity increases outside of the Doppler scale range, it appears as blue, because of aliasing.

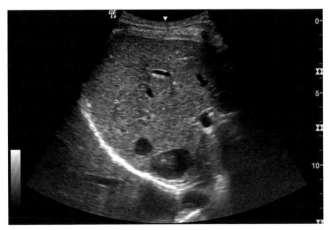

FIGURE 1-28. Mirror image artifact seen while scanning the right lobe of the liver. The liver-like structure is also seen above the diaphragm.

ULTRASOUND SAFETY

When using an ultrasound machine, it is essential to be familiar with the ALARA (As Low As Reasonably Achievable) principle. Overall, ultrasound is very safe and there is no record of injury occurring from Food and Drug Administration (FDA)-approved diagnostic ultrasounds in humans. However, there are still some theoretical concerns, especially with susceptible tissue such as in retina or the human embryo. It, therefore, remains the responsibility of the user to minimize transducer dwell time to avoid exposing the patient to unnecessary prolonged exposure to ultrasound energy. Thus, it is important not to use ultrasound any more than medically necessary or to keep exposure to the patient as low as reasonably achievable.

CHAPTER 2

Point-of-Care Ultrasound Billing and Credentialing

Francisco I. Norman, PA-C, MPAS, RGR and Paul Bornemann, MD, RMSK, RPVI

A FORMALIZED ULTRASOUND PRACTICE PRESENCE

Any practitioner who is interested in incorporating point-of-care ultrasound (POCUS) into their practice will at some point come to the question, "What do I need to do to become competent in POCUS?" Perhaps it is best to answer this question by first defining competency. The American College of Emergency Physicians (ACEP) defines ultrasound *competency* as the ability to recognize indications and contraindications for ultrasound, obtain ultrasound images, interpret the images, and then integrate the findings into patient management.[1]

Furthermore, there are several terms used to describe methods for proving competency. These can be for an individual or group and come from external or internal organizations.

Accreditation is given by an outside organization to an institution, practice, or facility. Generally, it is an affirmation that those systems have met certain criteria including:

1. Interpreting physicians meet relevant ultrasound training guidelines, case volume requirements, and continuing ultrasound education;
2. Sonographers are or will become appropriately certified by a specific date;
3. Ultrasound equipment is adequately maintained;
4. Safeguards are in place to protect patients and staff and ensure infection control measures;
5. Ultrasound examinations and reports meet or exceed accepted guidelines for content, timelines, and record retention; and
6. There is regular monitoring for quality assurance.

Certification is given by an outside organization to an individual practitioner. Generally, it is an affirmation that the practitioner has met specific requirements and has the knowledge, skills, and abilities to perform within a professional area. Most ultrasound-related certifications will include requirements such as:

1. A certain number of hours of training or educational experience that can be in the form of graduate medical education (GME) or continuing medical education (CME)
2. A certain number of ultrasound examinations be performed or interpreted under supervision
3. Verification of clinical skills, which usually entails a letter from an instructor or certified peer attesting to competency
4. "Successful completion of a certification examination" to decrease confusion with an ultrasound examination versus written/performance test

Credentialing is the process of confirming the qualifications of a medical professional and is performed internally by a medical institution, practice, or facility. Frequently, a credentialing specialist or electronic service will obtain background information that is then reviewed by a credentialing committee. It may include granting and reviewing specific clinical privileges and medical staff membership.

Privileging is the process where a local authority grants a clinician, who is competent to perform a specific procedure or action, permission to perform a said procedure within the facility. Privileging is based on the experience and education of the clinician. Requirements for privileging are determined internally but may follow the recommendations set forth by organizations like ACEP, the American Academy of Family Practice (AAFP), and the Society of Point of Care Ultrasound (SPOCUS). Recommendations on pathways to competency are detailed in the next section of this chapter.

BECOMING COMPETENT WITH POINT-OF-CARE ULTRASOUND

It is generally well-accepted that ultrasound competency is developed through a process that involves knowledge building through a didactic experience and skills development through supervised hands-on training.[2,3]

The didactic training may be achieved by enrolling in an on-location educational workshop, through online training (many of which are free), or even by partnering with a mentor who can teach the basics. Whichever method is employed, the education should focus on the ultrasound applications that the learner wishes to perform and should include basic ultrasound physics and equipment operation—a term often called "knobology."

After the initial didactic learning, the supervised hands-on training should begin. During this phase of training, the learner will focus on performing educational ultrasound examinations. An *educational ultrasound examination* is one that is performed by a provider who is still learning ultrasound. This is in contrast to a *clinical ultrasound examination* that is performed with the intent to aid in diagnosing or treating a patient. Clinical ultrasound examinations are further divided into diagnostic ultrasound examinations and procedural ultrasound examinations. *Diagnostic ultrasound examinations* are performed or interpreted by an experienced POCUS provider or a medical specialist. Diagnostic ultrasound examinations performed by sonographers with medical specialists' interpretation are often also referred to as formal or *consultative ultrasound examinations*. When bedside ultrasound is utilized to guide a procedure, the ultrasound is termed a *procedural ultrasound examination*.

Clinical decisions should not be made based on findings of educational ultrasounds unless first confirmed with diagnostic testing or performed under the direct supervision of an experienced provider. Patients should provide informed, verbal consent before they are subjected to an educational ultrasound. They should be informed that it is for education only and that they will not be informed of the results, although if anything concerning is found, an experienced provider should be notified. They can help make the decision if further diagnostic testing or treatment is warranted based on the abnormal educational ultrasound examination.

Educational ultrasound examinations can be accomplished by several methods:

1. Supervised scanning, where an ultrasound experienced clinician "looks over the shoulder of the learner." Recent technology may

allow for this method to be used remotely, as some manufacturers have placed a camera on the ultrasound machine and the software allows a remote viewer to "screen share" in real time.

2. Confirmatory tests of choice, where the learner performs an educational ultrasound examination but confirms the results with a secondary test that meets the accepted standard of care. This can be a diagnostic ultrasound or a different imaging modality.

3. Clinical outcomes can also be used. For example, if a skin infection has clinical characteristics of an abscess, the learner may perform an educational ultrasound examination and confirm the abscess by draining the fluid collection.

Although no minimum number of scans in any application will guarantee competency for every learner, there are recommended ranges of scans in which competency appears to develop.

ACEP, which first published the competency-based "Emergency Medicine Guidelines" in 2001, has had a great deal of success in safely implementing bedside ultrasound education into clinical practice. ACEP recommends that a minimum of 25 to 50 scans are needed to develop competency for each specific diagnostic application. A minimum of 150 to 300 is recommended for global competency in POCUS. For ultrasound guidance of procedures that a provider already has competency to perform without guidance, the number of supervised examinations required is less. It is recommended that 5 to 10 of these scans be supervised.[1]

Societies like the AAFP and SPOCUS mirrored the ACEP competency-based model by creating and endorsing similar recommendations. The AAFP Recommended Curriculum Guidelines for Family Medicine Residents and The Guidelines for Point of Care Ultrasound in Clinical Practice both mirror the recommendations in the ACEP guidelines.[2,4]

Practicing clinicians who have attained competency through the above-described method or clinicians who gained equivalent ultrasound education in medical school, residency, or fellowship can start to integrate ultrasound into their practice, as well as document the findings in the medical record (MR) and bill for the ultrasound procedure.

REIMBURSEMENT

Successful billing and reimbursement for ultrasound services provided can help sustain a practice and allow for a practice to grow. Billing for all diagnostic ultrasound examinations, whether consultative or point-of-care, are treated in the same manner utilizing current procedural terminology (CPT) codes.

CPT codes are specific to corresponding anatomic regions and not necessarily the examination being performed. For example, the Extended Focused Assessment with Sonography in Trauma (eFAST) is a commonly performed POCUS examination that involves scanning the abdomen, heart, and thorax for signs of trauma (see Chapter 50). However, there is no CPT code specifically for the eFAST examination. The correct coding would include the CPT codes for "limited cardiac," "limited abdomen," and "limited thoracic" examinations.

Every CPT code is assigned a relative value unit (RVU). The RVU is a constant and independent of where the examination is performed (ie, clinic vs hospital), who performs the ultrasound (ie, POCUS clinician vs sonographer), who interprets the ultrasound (POCUS clinician vs radiologist), or the type of ultrasound machine (cart based vs pocket sized).

The Centers for Medicare and Medicaid Services (CMS) has no specific requirements for whom can be paid for diagnostic CPT codes. They need only be a licensed provider, including physician assistants (PAs) and nurse practitioners (NPs), with a National Provider Identification (NPI) number. PAs and NPs are typically reimbursed at 85% of the physician's fee schedule.[5]

Although Medicare and Medicaid follow the rules of CMS, other private payers may have their own rules. This may also include regional Medicare Administrative Contractors (MACs). It is recommended to check with individual private payers and MACs for local coverage determinations.

Complete and Limited Ultrasound Examinations

Complete ultrasound studies require the evaluation of every structure within the anatomic region. For example, the CPT 76700 code is a complete abdominal ultrasound and would require evaluation of the liver, gallbladder, common bile duct, pancreas, spleen, kidneys, aorta, and inferior vena cava (IVC). Because the goal of bedside ultrasound is to answer a specific clinical question, focused or limited studies are more commonly used. Limited ultrasounds are defined as an ultrasound study where any subset of the components of a complete study is met. Often this will only include a single image.

For example, if the clinical question is "Does the Patient Have Cholecystitis?" the clinician would perform an ultrasound of the gallbladder and common bile duct. The spleen, pancreas, aorta, IVC, and kidneys are not likely to be relevant. Therefore, the correct CPT code is 76705 "limited ultrasound of the abdomen," because all the items for a complete abdominal study were not included.

Professional and Technical Components

The fees paid for each diagnostic CPT code are broken down to a professional and technical component. The professional component is meant to reimburse for the interpretation of the study and creation of a report in the chart. The technical component is meant to reimburse for the cost of the ultrasound machine and the sonographer to perform the study. The professional component is coded by adding a -26 modifier to the CPT code. A -TC modifier is added to the CPT code to denote the technical component. In general, the technical component will account for about two-thirds to three-fourths of the total CPT code fee (**Figure 2-1**).

Because most POCUS examinations will be performed and interpreted by a provider who also owns the equipment, generally the global CPT code is appropriate, and it does not need to be further broken down into the professional and technical component. However, it should be noted that CMS will not reimburse a technical component to a provider performing an ultrasound in a facility that shares a Medicare ID number with the hospital. Thus, when performing a POCUS ultrasound in the hospital, emergency room, or a hospital-based outpatient clinic, CMS will only reimburse the technical component to the hospital. Even if the hospital owns the ultrasound, the fraction of the technical component that is meant to cover the sonographer is still being performed by the provider. In order to recuperate this portion, a contract or some other arrangement would need to be worked out between the provider and the hospital.

The fees paid for procedural ultrasound examinations are not divided into a professional and technical component. The entire CPT code reimburses for the professional services, which usually

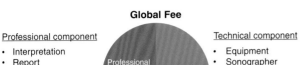

Global Fee

Professional component
• Interpretation
• Report
• -26 Modifier

Professional component

Technical component

Technical component
• Equipment
• Sonographer
  • Image acquisition and storage
  • Preliminary report
• Overhead
• -TC Modifier

FIGURE 2-1. Diagnostic current procedural terminology code reimbursement.

include the ultrasound and the procedure being performed. As with most procedural CPT codes, there is a separate facility fee that can be reimbursed by a hospital if the procedure is performed in the hospital or a hospital-owned clinic. Using a common procedure, arthrocentesis of the knee joint without ultrasound guidance, the CPT code 20610 for "Arthrocentesis, aspiration and/or injection; major joint or bursa **without** ultrasound guidance" was reimbursed US $61.92 per the 2016 Medicare national average. Arthrocentesis of the knee joint **with** ultrasound guidance, the CPT code 20611 for "Arthrocentesis, aspiration and/or injection; major joint or bursa **with** ultrasound guidance" was reimbursed US $92.88 per the 2016 Medicare national average. The approximately US $30 difference in reimbursement between the two codes is meant to cover the ultrasound component. Some procedures do not have CPT codes that include ultrasound guidance. For these procedures, the CPT code for the procedure can be used in conjunction with a separate diagnostic CPT code—76942, "Ultrasonic guidance for needle placement." CPT 76942 is itself a diagnostic CPT and thus is subdivided into a professional and technical component. The professional component reimburses US $34.04.

In most instances, a diagnostic and procedural guidance ultrasound examination cannot be reimbursed if performed at the same visit. However, "If a diagnostic ultrasound study identifies a previously unknown abnormality that requires a therapeutic procedure with ultrasound guidance at the same patient encounter; both the diagnostic ultrasound and ultrasound guidance procedure codes may be reported separately."[6] For example, if a suspected joint effusion of the knee is evaluated by POCUS in the office, it may be coded with CPT 76882, "limited diagnostic ultrasound of the extremities." If an effusion is found and an aspiration is indicated, then the provider may also bill for 20611 for "Arthrocentesis, aspiration and/or injection; major joint or bursa with ultrasound guidance."

Billing Documentation

There are several points of documentation required to bill for any diagnostic ultrasound CPT code. These are required regardless if it is a consultative ultrasound or ultrasound performed at the point-of-care.

1. An order must be placed in the MR.
2. There should be documentation attesting to the indication and a medical necessity for the examination.
3. A written report should be placed in the MR and it must be separately identifiable from any other records. The interpretive report should include:
   a. Date and time of examination
   b. Name and MR number of the patient
   c. Patient age, date of birth, and sex
   d. Name of the person who performed and/or interpreted the study and clinical findings
   e. Indication for the study, the scope (complete vs. limited), and if this is a repeat study by the same provider, repeat by a different provider, or reduced level of service
   f. Impression (including when a study is nondiagnostic) and differential diagnosis, as well as the need for follow-on examinations and incidental findings
4. Ultrasound images must be stored for archive.

Procedural guidance ultrasounds, which have a CPT code that includes the procedure and ultrasound guidance, only require a procedure note that includes mention that it was performed under ultrasound guidance. At least one ultrasound image is required to be stored for archive. It does not necessarily need to include imaging of the needle in the target or otherwise, except for vascular access (CPT 76937), which does require "concurrent real time ultrasound visualization of vascular needle entry, with permanent recording."

Other than CPT 76937, there are no specific requirements of which images must be saved or even how many should be saved for each diagnostic CPT code. Neither are there requirements for how images should be saved. Common methods employed for image archiving range from a sophisticated system-wide Picture Archiving and Communication System (PACS), to web and cloud-based software, as well as saving images to local drives, or even printing images and placing the image in the MR. However, images must be retrievable if records are requested from the patient or another provider or in the case of an audit by a third-party payer. The Federal Code of Regulations requires hospitals save images for 5 years.[7] Local jurisdictions may require MR retention up to 30 years. Check your local requirements at https://www.ordermedicalrecords.com/wp-content/uploads/2012/09/Retention-of-Health-Information.pdf.

ULTRASOUND MACHINE PURCHASE

Deciding on which ultrasound equipment to invest in can be a daunting task especially when first starting to incorporate POCUS into a clinical practice. There are many different options to consider and rapid advances in technology ensure that new options are constantly being added to the equation. There are wide ranges in the sizes of devices, from pocket-sized to cart-based machines. Increasing improvement in image quality and functional capabilities also increase along this spectrum. The number and type of transducers are also an important consideration and the types needed will depend on the examinations that a practice will plan to perform.

Other considerations include warranty and software packages that support various applications. Given the number of choices, providers considering purchase of a new equipment should make the effort to work with different models and manufacturers at workshops and should take advantage of the manufacturers' willingness to loan systems to practices for a "test drive." Whatever the type of equipment that is chosen, there are no limitations on what types of ultrasound devices can be used for billing. Pocket- and cart-based equipment are considered equal in this regard.

The cost of equipment is also variable, and most venders now offer different types of financial arrangements for acquisition of equipment ranging from upfront purchasing, financing, leasing, or renting. This can range in cost from over US $100,000 for upfront purchase of a top-of-the-line cart-based unit with multiple transducers to only a few hundred dollars a month for leasing or renting a pocket-sized device. It is important to consider that the cost of ultrasound equipment is a business expense and can be deducted from federal income taxes. Even equipment that is leased out over a period of years can be eligible for a deduction for depreciation of value over the life of the equipment and can be done as a lump sum at the time of purchase or averaged out yearly over the expected life of the equipment.[8]

Given all these considerations, a simple business model for a provider to first consider learning and incorporating POCUS in their practice is suggested as follows:

1. Purchase a small device that is portable and inexpensive on a month-to-month basis.
2. Plan to use this device to guide a procedure that the provider is already comfortable performing, such as joint arthrocentesis. This will help defray the monthly cost of the equipment while giving the provider increased experience with the equipment.
3. Practice new applications of diagnostic ultrasound examinations by performing educational examinations on patients in the practice. These opportunities will arise frequently when consultative examinations are ordered.
4. Once competency is developed in these new applications, and the provider feels comfortable replacing some of the consultative examinations with POCUS examination, then the provider can expand their billing to include the new application.

5. Once enough revenue is generated by expanding the applications that are billed for, additional equipment can be invested, such as a new type of transducer. This in turn will expand the opportunity to learn new applications and grow.

References

1. American College of Emergency Physicians. Policy Statements—Ultrasound guidelines: emergency, point-of-care, and clinical ultrasound guidelines in medicine. June 2016.
2. American Academy of Family Physicians. Recommended curriculum guidelines for family medicine residents. Point of care ultrasound. https://www.aafp.org/dam/AAFP/documents/medical_education_residency/program_directors/Reprint290D_POCUS.pdf. Accessed January 1, 2019.
3. Tayal V, Blaivas M, Mandavia D, et al. Ultrasound guidelines: emergency, point-of-care and clinical ultrasound guidelines in medicine. *Ann Emerg Med.* 2017;69(5):e27-e54.
4. Spocus. Guidelines for point of care ultrasound utilization in clinical practice. https://spocus.org/Practice-Guidelines. Accessed January 1, 2019.
5. American Academy of Physician Assistants. Third-party reimbursement for PAs. https://www.aapa.org/wp-content/uploads/2017/01/Third_party_payment_2017_FINAL.pdf. Accessed January 1, 2019.
6. National Correct Coding Initiative. Radiology section, IX-21. https://www.cms.gov/Medicare/Coding/NationalCorrectCodInitEd/Downloads/2017-NCCI-Correspondence-Manual.pdf. Revised April 1, 2017. Accessed February 20, 2020.
7. Govinfo. Title 42—Public Health. Chapter IV—Centers for Medicare & Medicaid Services, Department of Health and Human Services (Continued). Subchapter G—Standards and certification. Part 482—Conditions of participation for hospitals. http://www.gpo.gov/fdsys/granule/CFR-2011-title42-vol5/CFR-2011-title42-vol5-sec482-26/content-detail.html. Accessed January 1, 2019.
8. Internal Revenue Service. Publication 946 (2018), how to depreciate property. https://www.irs.gov/publications/p946. Accessed January 1, 2019.

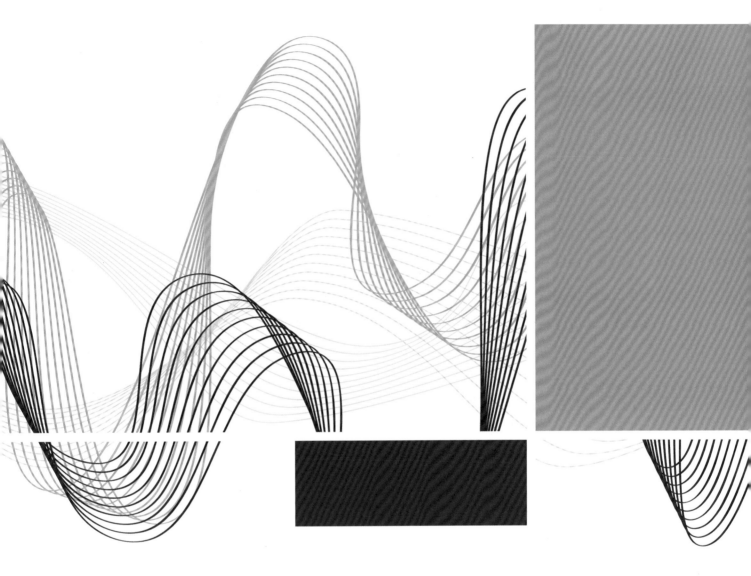

PART 2

ANSWERING CLINICAL QUESTIONS

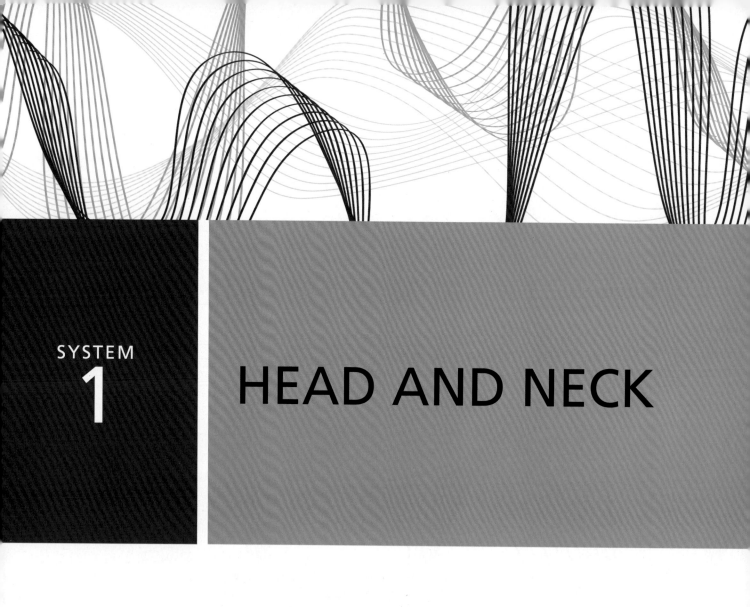

SYSTEM
1

HEAD AND NECK

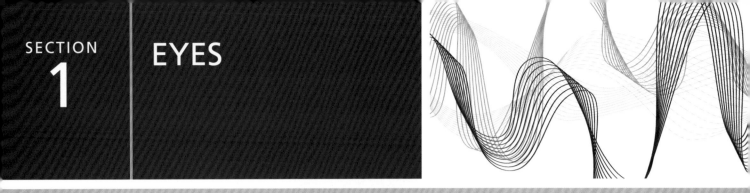

CHAPTER
3

Is the Patient's Intracranial Pressure Elevated?

James M. Daniels, MD, MPH, RMSK, Erica Miller-Spears, MS, PA-C, ATC, RMSK, and Linda M. Savage, AS

● Clinical Vignette

A 45-year-old man makes an urgent visit to your rural clinic, presenting with new-onset headache and visual changes off and on for the past 2 weeks. His headaches are associated with nausea and photophobia. They began after he bumped his head at work. He denied loss of consciousness. The patient has a history of hypertension that is controlled with Lisinopril 20 mg/d and hydrochlorothiazide 12.5 mg/d. He does not use alcohol, tobacco, or recreational drugs and is otherwise in excellent health. His vital signs are normal. His physical examination, including a detailed neurologic examination, is normal. However, he cannot tolerate a fundoscopic examination. Because of photophobia, is this patient's intracranial pressure elevated?

LITERATURE REVIEW

In 2002, Blaivas[1] published the first article that described the use of bedside ultrasonography to evaluate patients with ocular symptoms. This technology has been particularly useful in evaluating the eye. Much serious pathology occurs in the posterior aspect of the eye, ie, posterior chamber, retina, and optic nerve. Conditions that occur in the anterior aspect of the eye, ie, corneal abrasion, hyphema, and iritis, are more easily diagnosed by nonophthalmologists, whereas conditions occurring in the posterior part of the eye are more challenging to evaluate.

The evaluation of the intracranial pressure (ICP) can be difficult in a noncooperative patient. The examination of the eye with point-of-care ultrasound (POCUS) is relatively straightforward, and a number of studies have shown that primary care providers (nonophthalmologists/radiologists) can accurately scan the eye after 5 to 10 monitored studies.[2-4]

A discussion about the anatomy of the eye is necessary to be able to properly scan and understand its pathology. **Figure 3-1**[3-7] illustrates the anatomy and its appearance on the ultrasound screen.

The eye is surrounded by the bony orbit of the skull. It sits in a membranous sac, termed the tenon capsule. It is attached to those bony structures by the corneoscleral junction and the extraocular muscles and tendons.[7] The iris, lens, and anterior chamber are easily identified at the top of the scan.[8] The optic nerve enters the posterior part of the eye (bottom of scan) from a medial direction. It is not exactly centered in the posterior of the eye. The nerve is surrounded by the optic nerve sheath (ONS). This sheath is continuous with all three layers of the dura. The dura then blends into the outer layer of the eye itself so that the optic nerve is bathed in spinal fluid. When the ICP rises, so does the pressure inside the ONS, and it dilates. Other ways to measure the ONS pressure include computed tomography (CT), magnetic resonance imaging (MRI) measurements and measurement of opening pressure during a spinal tap.[3-5,7]

The ONS diameter (ONSD) varies throughout its course, averaging 3.65 mm at deeper depths to almost 6 mm at other locations.[9-11] There are other variables that may affect the ONSD, such as ethnicity,[12,13] age,[10] and even activities performed by the patient.[14-16] When the ICP is very high or the condition is chronic, there can be changes noted on the optic disc itself.[2] See **Figure 3-2**. There is now general agreement in the literature that ONSD should be measured at 3 mm proximal to where the nerve enters the eye.[3,4,9-11,17-19]

A systematic review from 2011 found that sonographic measurement of ONSD had a sensitivity of 0.90 and specificity of 0.85.[20] This was further corroborated by a meta-analysis from 2018, which found that sonographic measurement of ONSD may be a potentially useful technique for assessing intracranial hypertension when invasive monitoring methods are not available.[21] However, they did caution that further, high-quality studies were needed to confirm this.

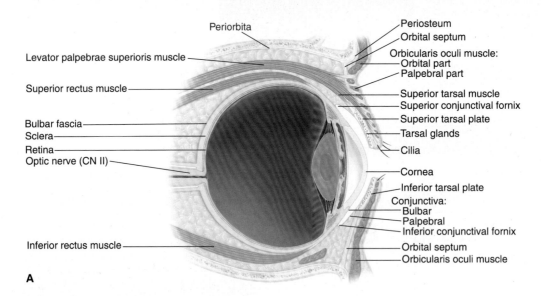

Periorbita

Levator palpebrae superioris muscle

Superior rectus muscle

Bulbar fascia
Sclera
Retina
Optic nerve (CN II)

Inferior rectus muscle

Periosteum
Orbital septum
Orbicularis oculi muscle:
Orbital part
Palpebral part
Superior tarsal muscle
Superior conjunctival fornix
Superior tarsal plate
Tarsal glands
Cilia
Cornea
Inferior tarsal plate
Conjunctiva:
Bulbar
Palpebral
Inferior conjunctival fornix
Orbital septum
Orbicularis oculi muscle

A

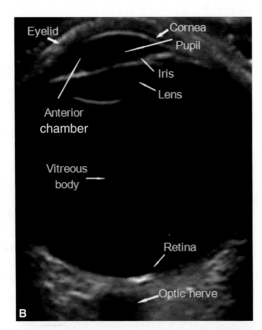

Eyelid
Cornea
Pupil
Iris
Lens
Anterior chamber
Vitreous body
Retina
Optic nerve

B

FIGURE 3-1. A, A medical illustration shows the important structures necessary to identify when measuring the optic nerve sheath diameter (ONSD). B, The photo shows a scan of the eye. The important points are: (1) the scan has to include the lens or the retina (preferably both) to ensure that a proper "slice" is being evaluated; (2) most authorities agree that the ONSD should be measured 3 mm posterior (inferior on illustration) from its entry into the globe; and (3) always measure the outside diameter of the ONSD and take the average of two measurements.[3-7]

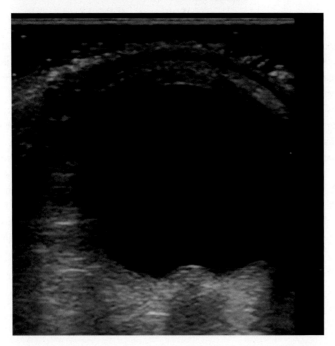

FIGURE 3-2. Papilledema can be seen on ocular ultrasound, represented by a bulging of the optic disc into the orbit. It is a late finding when intracranial pressure (ICP) is elevated. Additionally, it is not pathognomonic for increased ICP as other conditions, such as optic neuritis, can cause it. Image courtesy of Thomas Cook, MD.

TABLE 3-1	Recommendations for Use of Point-of-Care Ultrasound in Clinical Practice		
Recommendation		Rating	References
Nonophthalmologists can easily be trained to accurately measure the optic nerve sheath diameter (ONSD)		A	3-6, 10, 18
The measurement of the ONSD should be read at 3 mm from where it enters the eye		A	2, 4, 6, 9, 17, 19, 22

A = consistent, good-quality patient-oriented evidence; B = inconsistent or limited-quality patient-oriented evidence; C = consensus, disease-oriented evidence, usual practice, expert opinion, or case series. For information about the SORT evidence rating system, go to http://www.aafp.org/afpsort.

PERFORMING THE SCAN [3-8,18]

1. Place the patient in supine position with their eyes closed. Use the high-frequency (7.5-10.0 MHz), linear array ultrasound probe. Use the ocular preset if one is available, otherwise turn the output power down to the lowest effective level. Do not utilize Doppler mode. The retina is sensitive to acoustic output. Use the least possible energy to obtain an acceptable scan. Ask the patient to close both eyes. Instruct the patient to look straight ahead. Place copious amounts of ultrasound gel over the closed eye. This thick layer of gel allows for easy scanning without putting pressure on the eye. Additionally, a Tegaderm can be placed over the closed eye before applying gel, taking care to eliminate air bubbles.

2. Hold the transducer between the index finger and the thumb much like you would hold a pen. Rest your ring, small finger, and hypothenar eminence on the patient's bony orbit. This allows easy control of the probe without placing pressure on the eye. See **Figure 3-3**.

3. Place the probe in the center of the eye in a transverse plane. The gel allows the transducer to "float," while toggling, to get the best view of the ONS (**Figure 3-4**). Repeat these maneuvers in

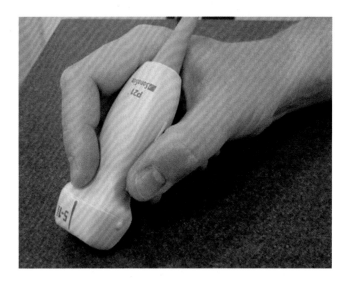

FIGURE 3-3. The "pencil grip" to hold the probe that allows control of the probe without putting too much pressure on the eye.

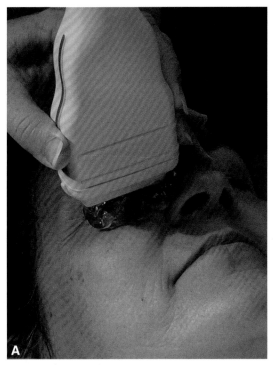
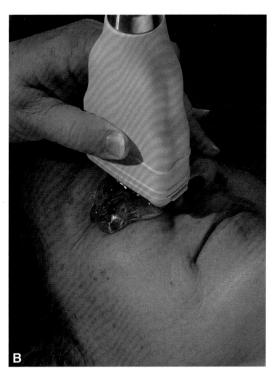

FIGURE 3-4. How to float (A) and toggle (B) the probe to obtain an optimal picture.

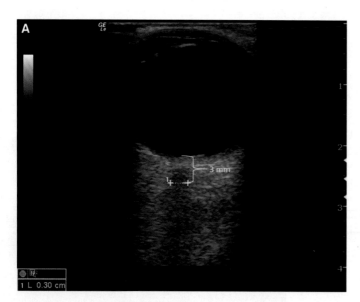

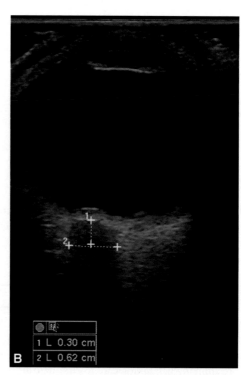

FIGURE 3-5. Eye scan with measurements of optic nerve sheath (ONS) at 3 mm. A, Normal measurement of 3 mm. B, Abnormal measurement of 6.2 mm. Images courtesy of Thomas Cook, MD.

the sagittal plane. Always orient the probe so that the indicator is pointing to the head or to the right.

4. Adjust the gain to get the clearest image of the ONS. Next, set the depth so the image takes up most of the screen. The lens should be at the top of the screen and the ONS at the bottom. This ensures that a full "cut" is being imaged and not an angled view that may affect the measurement.

5. Take care to "freeze" the clearest image of the ONS possible, then measure 3 mm from its entry into the eye. Use the "caliper" setting to measure the width of the ONS in both transverse and sagittal plane, then average them (**Figure 3-5**).

PATIENT MANAGEMENT

On a semi-cooperative patient, this scan is easily performed. The findings of the scan should never overrule the clinical findings and suspicions. The test is very helpful if the measurement is over 6.2 mm as it indicates increased cranial pressure or if it is at or below 3 mm diameter. Measurements in the middle are not that useful (Table 3-2).

This scan is most useful to confirm clear clinical impressions, ie, patient with suspected brain bleed and ONSD estimate of 6.5 or a person with an intact neurologic examination after a minor injury and an ONSD estimate of 3 mm. The majority of patients will need a CT scan to confirm or rule out the diagnosis, but the ultrasound evaluation of the eye can help determine the urgency of action. **Figure 3-6** demonstrates an algorithm for POCUS scanning of the eye.

TABLE 3-2	Normal Values for Optic Nerve Sheath Diameter Measured 3 mm From Its Entrance Into the Eye
≤5.0	Adults over 15 y
≤4.5 mm	Children 1-15 y
≤4.0 mm	Infants less than 1 y

PEARLS AND PITFALLS[7]

Pearls

- If the ONS or the optic disc cannot be seen, be suspicious of an intraocular bleed or ruptured globe.
- Minimize the amount of pressure you place on the globe by using copious amounts of gel and resting your hand on the bony prominence of the orbit.
- The optic nerve is not at the center of the eye and angulating the beam nasally may help to center the ONS.

Pitfalls

- The scan must include the lens or iris or the ONSD may be off-axis and could be underestimated.
- If the patient is overly agitated and will not cooperate (won't open eye or thrashes head, etc.), this technique should not be attempted.
- This technique is contraindicated if the patient has a ruptured globe.

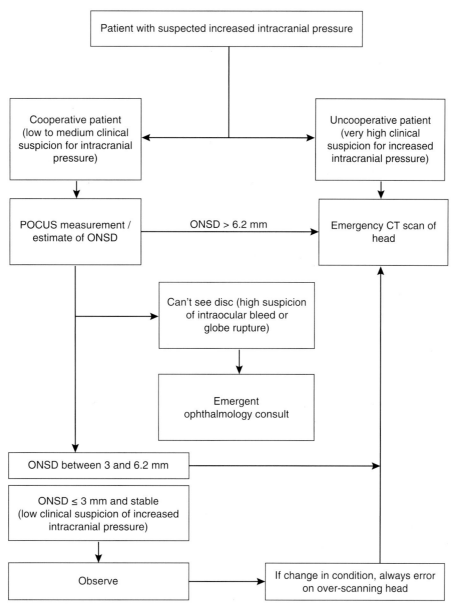

FIGURE 3-6. Algorithm for patient with suspected increased intracranial pressure. ONSD, ONS diameter.

BILLING

CPT Code	Description	Global Payment	Professional Component	Technical Component
76512	Ophthalmic ultrasound diagnostic; B-scan (with or without superimposed nonquantitative A-scan)	$93.81	$53.71	$40.10

CPT codes and average national reimbursement for Medicare in 2016. Payment data are from https://www.cms.gov/apps/physician-fee-schedule/search/search-criteria.aspx. See Chapter 2 for details on ultrasound billing.

References

1. Blaivas M. Bedside emergency department ultrasonography in the evaluation of ocular pathology. *Acad Emerg Med.* 2000;7:947-950.
2. Teismann N, Lenaghan P, Nolan R, et al. Point-of-care ocular ultrasound to detect optic disc swelling. *Acad Emerg Med.* 2013;20(9):920-925.
3. Gottlieb M, Bailitz J. Can ocular ultrasonography be used to assess intracranial pressure? *Ann Emerg Med.* 2016;68(3):349-351.
4. Kilker BA, Holst JM, Hoffmann B. Bedside ocular ultrasound in the emergency department. *Eur J Emerg Med.* 2014;21(4):246-253.
5. Adhikari SR. Small parts—ocular ultrasound. In Hoffman B, ed. *Ultrasound Guide for Emergency Physicians: An Introduction.* https://www.acep.org/sonoguide/smparts_ocular.html. Accessed August 6, 2019.
6. Weingart S. Optic nerve sheath ultrasound for detecting increased intracranial pressure (ICP). EMCrit Blog. http://emcrit.org/blogpost/optic-nerve-sheath-ultrasound-for-detecting-increased-icp/. Published July 24, 2012. Accessed November 14, 2016.

7. Roque PJ, Hatch N, Barr L, Wu TS. Bedside ocular ultrasound. *Crit Care Clin.* 2014;30:227-241.

8. Jeong DH, Chitturi S. Eye (Ocular). In: Daniels JM, Hoppmann RA, eds. *Practical Point-of-Care Medical Ultrasound.* New York, NY: Springer; 2016:141-154.

9. Vaiman M, Gottlieb P, Bekerman I. Quantitative relations between the eyeball, the optic nerve, and the optic canal important for intracranial pressure monitoring. *Head Face Med.* 2014;10:32.

10. Hassen GW, Bruck I, Donahue J, et al. Accuracy of optic nerve sheath diameter measurement by emergency physicians using bedside ultrasound. *J Emerg Med.* 2015;48(4):450-457.

11. Vaiman M, Abuita R, Bekerman I. Optic nerve sheath diameters in healthy adults measured by computer tomography. *Int J Ophthalmol.* 2015;8(6):1240-1244.

12. Chen H, Ding GS, Zhawo YC, et al. Ultrasound measurement of optic nerve diameter and optic nerve sheath diameter in healthy Chinese adults. *BMC Neurol.* 2015;15:106.

13. Wang L, Feng L, Yao Y, et al. Optimal optic nerve sheath diameter threshold for the identification of elevated opening pressure on lumbar puncture in a Chinese population. *PLoS One.* 2015;10(2):e0117939.

14. Lochner P, Falla M, Brigo F, et al. Ultrasonography of the optic nerve sheath diameter for diagnosis and monitoring of acute mountain sickness: a systematic review. *High Alt Med Biol.* 2015;16(3):195-203.

15. Sutherland AI, Morris DS, Owen CG, et al. Optic nerve sheath diameter, intracranial pressure and acute mountain sickness on Mount Everest: a longitudinal cohort study. *Br J Sports Med.* 2008;42(3):183-188.

16. Mehrpour M, Shams-Hossenini NS, Rezaali S. Effect of scuba-diving on optic nerve and sheath diameters. *Med J Islam Repub Iran.* 2014;28:89.

17. Soldatos T, Chatzimichail K, Papathanasiou M, Gouliamos A. Optic nerve sonography: a new window for the non-invasive evaluation of intracranial pressure in brain injury. *Emerg Med J.* 2009;26(9):630-634.

18. Hightower S, Chin EJ, Heiner JD. Detection of increased intracranial pressure by ultrasound. *J Spec Oper Med.* 2012;12:19-22.

19. Shirodkar CG, Munta K, Rao SM, Mahesh MU. Correlation of measurement of optic nerve sheath diameter using ultrasound with magnetic resonance imaging. *Indian J Crit Care Med.* 2015;19(9):466-470.

20. Dubourg J, Javouhey E, Geeraerts T, Messerer M, Kassai B. Ultrasonography of optic nerve sheath diameter for detection of raised intracranial pressure: a systematic review and meta-analysis. *Intensive Care Med.* 2011;37(7):1059-1068. doi:10.1007/s00134-011-2224-2.

21. Robba C, Santori G, Czosnyka M, et al. Optic nerve sheath diameter measured sonographically as non-invasive estimator of intracranial pressure: a systematic review and meta-analysis. *Intensive Care Med.* 2018;44(8):1284-1294. doi:10.1007/s00134-018-5305-7.

22. Lee SU, Jeon JP, Lee H, et al. Optic nerve sheath diameter threshold by ocular ultrasonography for detection of increased intracranial pressure in Korean adult patients with brain lesions. *Medicine* 2016;95(41):e5061. https://www.ncbi.nlm.nih.gov/pmc/articles/PMC5072948/. Accessed November 14, 2018.

Does the Patient Have a Retinal or Vitreous Detachment?

Dae Hyoun (David) Jeong, MD, James M. Daniels, MD, MPH, RMSK, and Cesar S. Arguelles, MD

● Clinical Vignette

A 58-year-old man with a past medical history of hypertension and hyperlipidemia presents to your clinic with a vision change in his right eye that started yesterday afternoon and has been progressively worsening. The patient describes the vision change as if a curtain was coming up over his eye and is now affecting his central vision. The patient states that he noticed flashing lights and floaters in his left eye starting 4 days ago. Mr. M denies eye pain, double vision, halos, or watery eyes. He has no history of recent trauma or surgery in his eyes. He has been compliant on hypertension medications but recently his blood pressure has been somewhat elevated. His family history is significant for macular degeneration (father) and cataract (mother). He takes amlodipine, simvastatin, and omega-3. External eye examination is negative. Visual acuity is 20/20 on the left eye and 20/40 on the right eye (baseline visual acuity: 20/20 on each eye). Visual field examination reveals extensive nasal field loss on the right eye and normal field on the left eye. Does the patient have a retinal or vitreous detachment?

LITERATURE REVIEW

Ocular complaints represent between 2% and 3% of emergency department visits and they require rapid assessment and treatment.[1,2] The acute onset of flashes and floaters is a common complaint in older adults. This is usually caused by posterior vitreous detachment (PVD).[3] PVD is usually benign, but can have a 10% to 15% risk of progressing to a retinal tear.[4] Retinal tears can progress to a full retinal detachment (RD), a true emergency that can lead to permanent blindness. RD occurs when the neurosensory layer of the retina separates from the underlying retinal pigment epithelium.[5]

Point-of-care ocular ultrasound can be performed accurately by nonophthalmologists and does not require extensive training

or experience. A recent systematic review revealed that bedside ocular sonography had sensitivity and specificity for RD ranging from 97% to 100% and 83% to 100%, respectively.[2] Another large retrospective study confirmed that a similar level of accuracy was obtainable in inexperienced sonographers. After only a 30-minute lecture followed by a supervised hands-on scanning session using models, the providers could accurately and consistently identify RD.[6] Indirect fundoscopic examination is challenging for nonophthalmologists to perform. This is especially true when pupillary dilation is not possible. However, there may be instances where fundoscopy can be impossible for even experienced ophthalmologists such as in patients with cataract, occluded pupils, or vitreous hemorrhage. Ultrasound is very effective in these cases.[7,8] See Table 4-1.

PERFORMING THE SCAN

Ultrasound Machine and Setting

The eye is vulnerable to thermal and mechanical hazard because the lens, aqueous, and vitreous humor do not have any cooling blood supply. An ophthalmic setting or a lower power preset (ie, thyroid, small part setting) should be selected for the sonographic eye examination, as they emit less energy that could damage the eye. The depth should be adequately adjusted to visualize all the structures of the globe including the optic nerve, and the gain should be set appropriately to create a hypoechoic posterior chamber. If the gain is set too high, it can cause small artifacts that may lead the examiner to overcall pathology. If gain is set too low, the examiner can miss subtle pathology. In addition, the lowest power setting possible should be used to avoid potential damage to the eye. The Doppler setting should never be used in this setting because of the amount of energy exposed to the eye.

Transducer

The eye is best visualized with high-frequency probe that is suitable for scanning superficial structures. High-frequency (7.5-10 MHz or higher frequency range) linear array transducer with small footprint is used. See Figure 4-1.

TABLE 4-1 Recommendations for Use of Point-of-Care Ultrasound in Clinical Practice		
Recommendation	Evidence Rating	References
Ocular point-of-care ultrasound has high accuracy in detecting retinal detachment.	A	1, 2
Nonophthalmic ultrasound equipment is highly accurate for excluding and detecting retinal detachment or other retinal disorders in patients with opaque media.	B	7, 8
Nonophthalmologists can accurately perform ocular ultrasound with minimal amount of training.	B	1, 6
Ultrasound can help differentiate between retinal detachment and posterior vitreous detachment.	C	9, 10

A = consistent, good-quality patient-oriented evidence; B = inconsistent or limited-quality patient-oriented evidence; C = consensus, disease-oriented evidence, usual practice, expert opinion, or case series. For information about the SORT evidence rating system, go to http://www.aafp.org/afpsort.

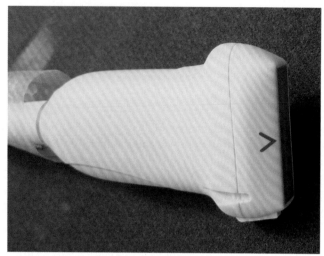

FIGURE 4-1. High-frequency linear array.

Gel Application

The gel for an ocular ultrasound examination does not need to be sterile. However, sterile gel is less irritating to the eye. Alternatively, you may place a piece of Tegaderm (transparent film dressing) to the closed eyelid before applying the gel, but make sure to remove all air bubbles trapped beneath the film to avoid production of the artifact. See **Figure 4-2**.

Any pressure to the globe could cause discomfort or potentially damage the eye. A copious amount of water-soluble ultrasound gel should be applied to cover the entire eyelid after the eyes are closed. Filling the eye orbit with gel after the eyelid is closed allows the probe to "float" over the eye without putting direct pressure on the globe. See **Figure 4-3**.

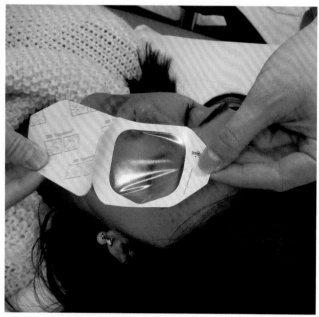

FIGURE 4-2. Applying Tegaderm on the eye.

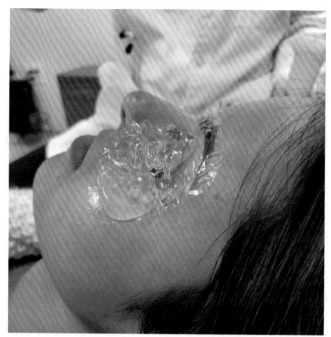

FIGURE 4-3. Applying copious gel on the Tegaderm.

Transducer Placement and Scanning Technique

The transducer needs to be stabilized by holding the probe like a pen with the thumb, index, and middle finger. This allows the examiner to rest his or her hand on the maxilla and bridge of the patient's nose. This technique also is less fatiguing to the examiner. There are two views of ocular ultrasound examination: transverse view (the pointer toward patient's right) displayed in **Figure 4-4** and ▶ **Video 4-1** and longitudinal view (the pointer toward patient's head) that can be seen in **Figure 4-5** and ▶ **Video 4-2**.

When scanning in both planes, sweep the transducer from up and down in transverse plane and side to side in longitudinal plane; tilt and fan the transducer for thorough evaluation. A dynamic scan should be performed by asking the patient to move his or her eyes slowly up and down and side to side in all four directions while the eyelid is closed. See **Figure 4-6**.

Look for Pathology

RD appears as a hyperechoic floating membrane in the vitreous body that is usually firmly attached to the retina at the optic nerve head and the ora serrata and will not cross the midline of the posterior chamber. Complete RD has a V-shape because of the attachment at the optic nerve, but detachments may appear as a linear hyperechoic floating structure. PVD will appear similar to an RD with a hyperechoic membrane but it will cross the midline and not have an attachment at the optic nerve. Vitreous hemorrhage has a semi-mobile appearance with eye movements that mimic swaying seaweed showing a wave-like aftermovement.[9,10]

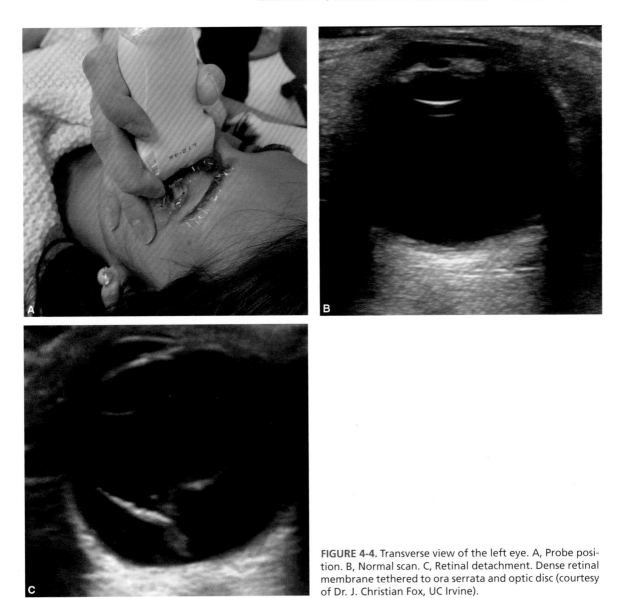

FIGURE 4-4. Transverse view of the left eye. A, Probe position. B, Normal scan. C, Retinal detachment. Dense retinal membrane tethered to ora serrata and optic disc (courtesy of Dr. J. Christian Fox, UC Irvine).

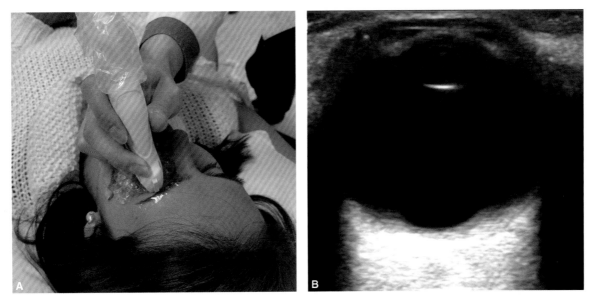

FIGURE 4-5. Longitudinal view of the left eye. A, Probe position. B, Normal scan.

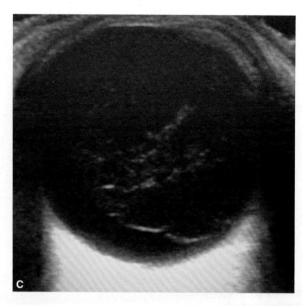

FIGURE 4-5. (*continued*) C, Posterior vitreous detachment with vitreous hemorrhage. Less dense membrane compared to retinal detachment (courtesy of Dr. J. Christian Fox, UC Irvine).

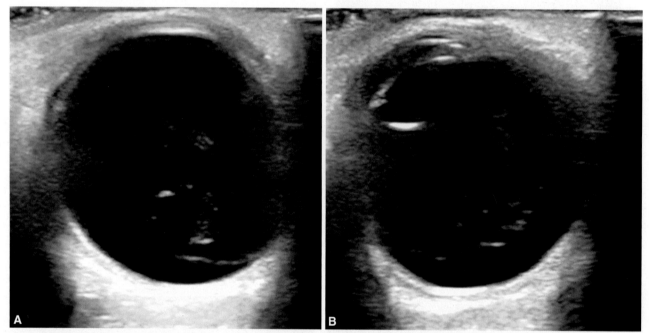

FIGURE 4-6. Dynamic scan with side-to-side eye movement. Note swaying seaweed movement of vitreous hemorrhage. A, Eye movement toward right side (courtesy of Dr. J. Christian Fox, UC Irvine). B, Eye movement toward left side (courtesy of Dr. J. Christian Fox, UC Irvine).

PATIENT MANAGEMENT

All patients with a recent onset of RD confirmed by ultrasound or symptoms suggesting RD (decreased visual acuity or visual field defect) should be referred to an ophthalmologist the same day.[3-5] There is no general consensus on how soon patients with PVD, without decreased acuity or distortion of vision, should be referred, but it should be within days because of the high risk of retinal tears or earlier if symptoms get worse or a defect of visual field develops.[3,4] Vitreous hemorrhage is a surgical emergency that needs emergent same-day referral to an ophthalmologist if an RD, retinal tear, intraocular tumor, or neovascularization of the iris is detected on the ultrasound scan.[11] See **Figure 4-7**.

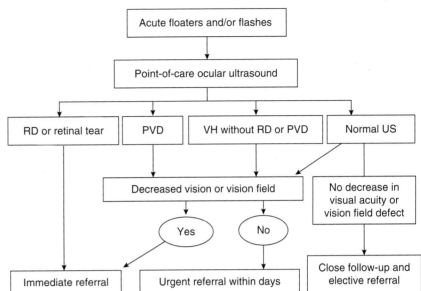

FIGURE 4-7. Algorithm describing the use of point-of-care ultrasound in a primary care setting when evaluating a patient with a possible retinal tear. PVD, posterior vitreous detachment; RD, retinal detachment; US, ultrasound; VH, vitreous hemorrhage.

PART 2

PEARLS AND PITFALLS

Pearls

- Use sterile gel with or without Tegaderm on the closed eyelid. Tegaderm may prevent eye irritation if the patient inadvertently opens their eye with the gel in place.
- It can be very difficult to distinguish between vitreous hemorrhage, RD, and PVD with ocular ultrasound. The posterior surface of the PVD is less dense than the retina, which fades when the ultrasound gain is decreased. Vitreous hemorrhage is also less dense than RD and moves rapidly in a staccato motion with ocular movement. The retina is dense

and stiffer, so it has a slower movement when the patient is asked to move their eye.[9,10,12]

Pitfalls

- A small vitreous hemorrhage may not be detected with normal gain setting. Increasing the gain and having the patient move their eyes in all four directions may help identify these lesions, which allows detection of swaying seaweed aftermovement.
- Retinal tears can be quite small and more difficult to locate than a true detachment.[13]

BILLING

Code	Description	Professional Component	Facility Fee
76512	Ophthalmic ultrasound B-scan with nonquantitative A-scan	$93.81	$93.81

CPT codes and average national reimbursement for Medicare in 2016. Payment data are from https://www.cms.gov/apps/physician-fee-schedule/search/search-criteria.aspx. See Chapter 2 for details on ultrasound billing.

References

1. Jacobsen B, Lahham S, Lahham S, et al. Retrospective review of ocular point-of-care ultrasound for detection of retinal detachment. *West J Emerg Med.* 2016;17(2):196-200.
2. Vrablik ME, Snead GR, Minnigan HJ, Kirschner JM, Emmett TW, Seupaul RA. The diagnostic accuracy of bedside ocular ultrasonography for the diagnosis of retinal detachment: a systematic review and meta-analysis. *Ann Emerg Med.* 2015;65(2):199-203.
3. Hollands H, Johnson D, Brox AC, Almeida D, Simel DL, Sharma S. Acute-onset floaters and flashes; is this patient at risk for retinal detachment? *JAMA.* 2009;302(20):2243-2249.
4. Kang HK, Luff AJ. Management of retinal detachment; a guide for non-ophthalmologist. *BMJ.* 2008;336:1235-1240.
5. Gelston CD. Common eye emergencies. *Am Fam Physician.* 2013;88(8):515-519.
6. Shinar Z, Chan L, Orlinsky M. Use of ocular ultrasound for the evaluation of retinal detachment. *J Emerg Med.* 2011;40(1):53-57.
7. Kongsap P, Kongsap N. Use of non-ophthalmic ultrasound for evaluation of retinal detachment in patients with opaque media. *Asian J Ophthalmol.* 2011;12:208-210.
8. Sen KK, Parihar J, Saini M, Moorthy RS. Conventional B-mode ultrasonography for evaluation of retinal disorders. *Med J Armed Forces India.* 2003;59(4):310-312.
9. Kilker BA, Holst JM, Hoffmann B. Bedside ocular ultrasound in the emergency department. *Eur J Emerg Med.* 2014;21(4):246-253.
10. Schott ML, Pierog JE, Williams SR. Pitfalls in the use of ocular ultrasound for evaluation of acute vision loss. *J Emerg Med.* 2013;44(6):1136-1139.
11. Rajesh P, Dheeresh K, Safarulla MA, Hussain S. Vitreous hemorrhage. *Kerala J Ophthalmol.* 2011;23(3):192-195.
12. Frasure SE, Saul T, Lewiss RE. Bedside ultrasound diagnosis of vitreous hemorrhage and traumatic lens dislocation. *Am J Emerg Med.* 2013;31:1002.e1-1002.e2.
13. Brod RD, Lightman DA, Packer AJ, Saras HP. Correlation between vitreous pigment granules and retinal breaks in eyes with acute posterior vitreous detachment. *Ophthalmology.* 1991;98:1366-1369.

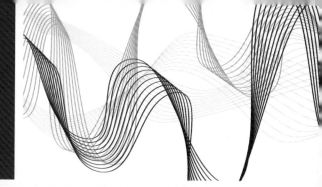

CHAPTER 5

Does This Thyroid Nodule Need to Be Biopsied?

Brooke Hollins McAdams, MD and Keisha Bonhomme Ellis, MD

● Clinical Vignette

A 57-year-old woman presents to her primary care physician for hospital follow-up, after receiving treatment following a motor vehicle accident. Computed tomography of the head and neck was done to rule out injury; imaging revealed a thyroid incidentaloma. The patient has no significant family history for thyroid cancer and no compressive symptoms. Does this thyroid nodule need to be biopsied?

LITERATURE REVIEW

A thyroid nodule is an abnormal growth of thyroid cells that form a sonographically distinct lesion within normal thyroid parenchyma. General practitioners are faced with the increasingly common clinical scenario of these usually asymptomatic thyroid nodules, because of the widespread use of diagnostic studies. Although palpable nodules are only detected at a prevalence of approximately 3% to 7% in iodine-sufficient areas on routine physical examination, they are being found at increasingly higher rates given the exponential use of medical imaging.[1,2] In contrast to the relatively low prevalence seen on palpation, clinically inapparent thyroid nodules are detected on high-resolution ultrasound (US) in 20% to 75% of the general population, with higher frequencies among females and the elderly.[3,4] Increased detection of these nonpalpable nodules has subsequently amplified the number of biopsies, and this has resulted in a surge in the diagnosis and treatment of thyroid malignancies, specifically papillary thyroid microcarcinomas.[5,6]

Ninety percent of all thyroid malignancies are differentiated thyroid cancer, with the vast majority being a papillary variant.[7] A large Minnesota-based population study noted a doubling in the incidence of thyroid cancer from 2000 to 2012, when compared to the decade prior; this was attributed to the detection of clinically occult nodules on imaging.[8] At this rate, it has been estimated that papillary thyroid carcinoma (PTC) will be the third most common cancer in American females of any age by 2019 behind only breast and lung cancer, respectively, costing roughly 20 billion dollars in treatment and follow-up.[9]

Because of the substantial increase in thyroid nodule detection, many national societies and practicing endocrinologists have become concerned with the possibility of overdiagnosis and overtreatment of clinically insignificant PTCs. Long-term observational studies have seen comparable survival rates for monitored verse surgically treated papillary microcarcinomas, suggesting that it is not only safe but also cost-effective to clinically follow small thyroid nodules lacking suspicious US findings.[10-12]

Despite the increase in the detection of PTC, the overwhelming majority of thyroid incidentalomas return benign, with cancer being present in only 4.0% to 6.5% of thyroid nodules.[13,14] Therefore, distinguishing between the few clinically significant malignant nodules and the vast majority of benign nodules is important to avoid unnecessary biopsies and surgical procedures. With some clinical controversy surrounding management of these increasingly prevalent thyroid lesions, many practitioners find themselves asking, "does this thyroid nodule need to be biopsied?"

TABLE 5-1	Recommendations for Use of Point-of-Care Ultrasound in Clinical Practice		
Recommendation		**Rating**	**References**
Thyroid ultrasound and survey of cervical lymph nodes should be obtained in known or suspected thyroid nodules.		A	15-18, 21
FNA is the procedure of choice in assessment of thyroid nodules		A	15, 18-21

A = consistent, good-quality patient-oriented evidence; B = inconsistent or limited-quality patient-oriented evidence; C = consensus, disease-oriented evidence, usual practice, expert opinion, or case series. For information about the SORT evidence rating system, go to http://www.aafp.org/afpsort.

PERFORMING THE SCAN

1. **Preparation and equipment.** The study should be labeled with patient identifiers and examination date. Remove any necklaces or other accessories on the neck. Ask the patient to lay supine with their neck extended; this can be accomplished by placing a pillow or pad under the patient's shoulder blades and asking them to

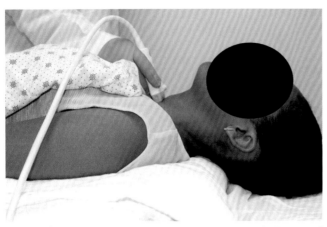

FIGURE 5-1. Patient positioning for thyroid ultrasound. The use of a small pillow allows gentle hyperextension of the neck.

tilt their head back allowing it to rest on the table (**Figure 5-1**). This position may be uncomfortable but should not be painful. Use a linear array transducer with a mean frequency between 10 and 14 MHz. Obese patients may require a transducer with a lower frequency. Of note, there are several ways to grip the probe (ie, like a pencil, a paint brush); choose a method that

will allow you to tilt/fan the transducer forward and backward easily. If necessary to steady the image, rest your forearm/hand gently on the patient's chest.

2. **Locate and identify important structures of the thyroid gland.** The thyroid gland consistent of two lobes flanking both sides of the trachea, connected in the midline of the anterior neck by the isthmus, and resides mostly in the center of level 6 (**Figure 5-2**). Locate the gland by palpating just inferior to the cricoid cartilage and holding the distal phalanx of each thumb in the shape of a V. Once located, apply a liberal amount of US acoustic gel on the transducer probe and place at the junction of the V (the isthmus), with the transducer's marker pointed toward the patient's right shoulder. This probe position will give the transverse view of the thyroid gland (**Figure 5-3**).

Normal thyroid parenchyma has a uniformed, medium-level echogenic texture. The air-filled trachea will appear as a black half circle posteromedial to the isthmus, with a characteristic reverberation artifact in the center. Surrounding the thyroid are a pair of three muscle groups appearing as hypoechoic bands. These are the strap muscles: sternothyroid, sternohyoid, and omohyoid. The sternocleidomastoid muscles are anterolateral, and the longus colli muscles are posterolateral. The carotid sheath and internal jugular (IJ) are lateral to the gland on either side; the IJ can be distinguished from the carotid by its compressibility. These large vessels can

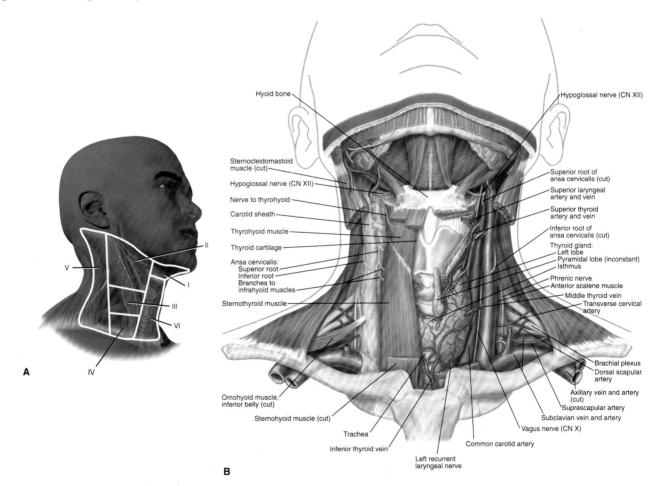

FIGURE 5-2. A, Levels of the neck. Reprinted with permission from Ferris R, Myers E, eds. *Master Techniques in Otolaryngology - Head and Neck Surgery: Head and Neck Surgery: Volume 2*. Philadelphia, PA: Wolters Kluwer Health/Lippincott Williams & Wilkins; 2013. Figure 2.1b.. **B,** Thyroid gland anatomy. Reprinted with permission from Pansky B, Gest TR. *Lippincott Concise Illustrated Anatomy: Volume 3*. Philadelphia, PA: Wolters Kluwer Health/Lippincott Williams & Wilkins; 2013. Figure 1.13c.

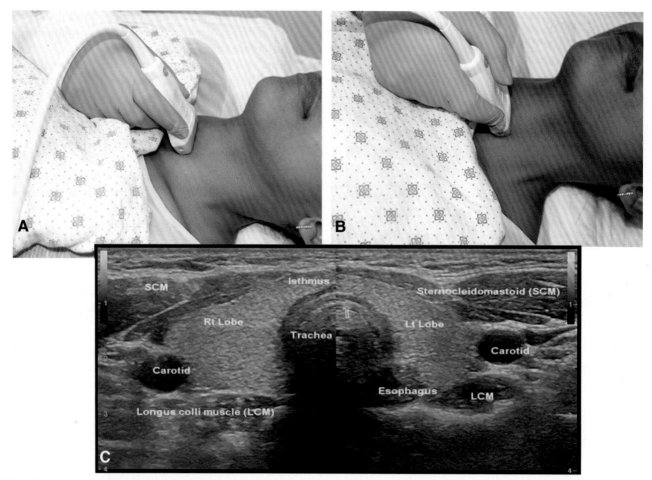

FIGURE 5-3. Transducer probe position for transverse view (A, B). Normal anatomy of the thyroid gland in transverse (C). Trachea reverberation artifact (yellow arrow, C).

sometimes be confused for cystic nodules; however, they are easily recognized on Doppler flow. The esophagus can be seen adjacent to the trachea on the left.

3. **Measure thyroid gland.** Next measure the thyroid gland in both the transverse and longitudinal (sagittal) planes. For a complete thyroid examination, one would measure all three portions (superior, mid, inferior) of both lobes in three dimensions (width, depth, and length). However, for the sake of time, often the three dimensions are only recorded at the largest portion of the gland, usually the midpole. The width of a lobe is measured

in the transverse view, from the lateral aspects of the trachea to the lateral border of the thyroid lobe, whereas the depth is the anteroposterior (AP) measurement (**Figure 5-4**). Length is measured in the longitudinal plane by turning the transducer marker toward the patient's head (**Figure 5-5**). The dimensions of a normal sized gland are roughly 2 cm in width, 2 cm in depth, and 4 to 6 cm in length, with the isthmus measuring less than 0.5 cm.[15]

4. **Document and describe any thyroid nodules.** Following general measurements of the thyroid gland, scroll through each

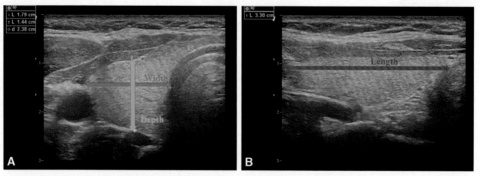

FIGURE 5-4. Thyroid lobe width (transverse) and depth (anteroposterior) measurements (A). Lobe length measurement (B).

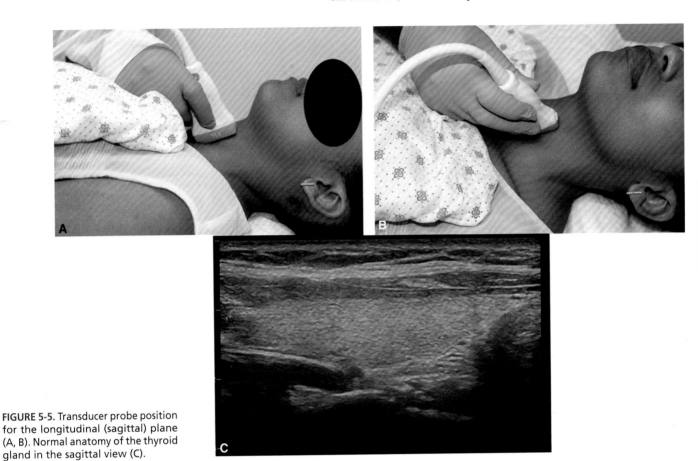

FIGURE 5-5. Transducer probe position for the longitudinal (sagittal) plane (A, B). Normal anatomy of the thyroid gland in the sagittal view (C).

lobe slowly searching for nodules. If discovered, the following characteristics should be recorded and compared to any previous images if available.

- Location—Report if the nodule is in the superior, mid, or inferior lobe of either the right or left thyroid. Occasionally, a nodule will be located in the isthmus.
- Size—Make an effort to measure in a manner that is easy to replicate. Consistently take measurements in AP and perpendicular planes (**Figure 5-6**). This will allow one to compare measurements on serial US. It is important to measure in all three dimensions, as 1 cm in any direction is the usual cutoff for biopsy requirements.
- Shape—Note if the nodule is taller than wide, or lobulated. A ratio of AP/transverse diameter greater than 1.0 implies an increase malignancy risk (**Figure 5-7**).[16]
- Number—Patients may have multiple nodules present. Focus on dominate nodules greater than 1 to 1.5 cm and any nodule (regardless of size) with worrisome features (**Table 5-3**).

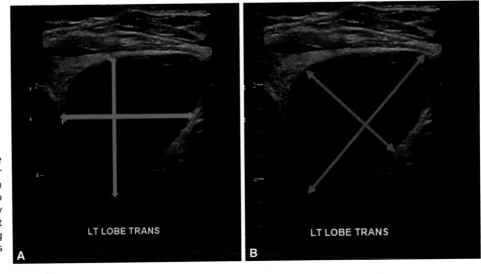

FIGURE 5-6. Measuring a thyroid nodule in the anteroposterior and perpendicular planes (A) allows for easy comparison on serial ultrasounds. Another method is to measure the greatest dimension in any direction (B); while this may be difficult to replicate, if there is previous imaging available for comparison, this method is useful for following growth over time.

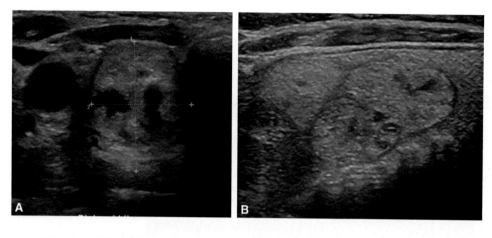

FIGURE 5-7. Taller-than-wide nodule (A). Lobulated nodule (B).

- Margins—Note if the margins are well-defined, irregular, or infiltrative. Irregular, poorly defined margins are associated with increased risk of malignancy. Regular margins with a characteristic halo sign infers a benign nodule (**Figure 5-8**).
- Consistency/Echogenicity—Record if the nodule is isoechoic (same echogenicity as thyroid tissue), hypoechoic (darker), or hyperechoic (brighter) (**Figure 5-9**).
- Composition—Record the degree of cystic changes in the nodule. Note cystic, mixed, spongiform, or solid features (**Figure 5-10**). Simple cysts will appear anechoic with posterior acoustic enhancement and are benign. Colloid cysts may contain an artifact known as a comet-tail (an echogenic focus with posterior acoustic reverberation because of microcrystals or colloid degeneration). Spongiform nodules appear as honeycomb-like lesions with small pockets of cystic areas; these are also usually benign. The more solid the nodule, the higher the risk of malignancy.

- Calcification—Look for any hyperechoic, calcified areas. Microcalcifications (<1 mm) are associated with psammoma bodies and imply an increased risk of malignancy, whereas larger macrocalcifications (>2 mm) are usually not. Eggshell (rim) calcifications are a benign feature if present along the entire peripheral rim; however, if there is focal discontinuity of the eggshell, there is an increased risk (**Figure 5-11**).[17]
- Vascularity—Use color Doppler to note the absence or presence of blood flow of the nodule. Absent or peripheral vascular flow is associated with benign nodules, whereas intranodular vascularity conveys increased risk (**Figure 5-12**).

PATIENT MANAGEMENT

The exclusion of malignancy is the primary consideration when evaluating a newly discovered thyroid nodule, and the initial assessment should include a detailed history and physical to establish risk factors. Physicians should enquire about a family history of thyroid

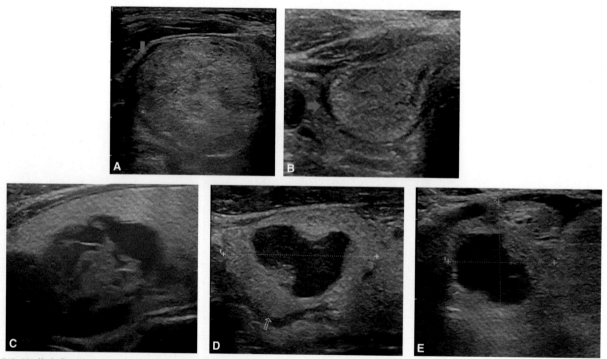

FIGURE 5-8. Well-defined margins with halo sign present (blue arrow A, B). Irregular boarders and those with interrupted/incomplete halo signs (yellow arrow) are at increased risk of malignancy (C-E).

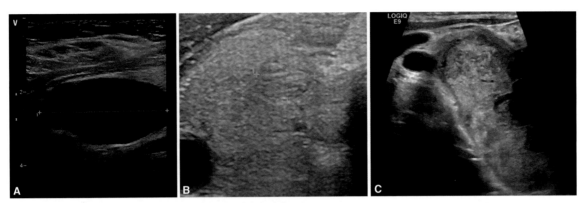

FIGURE 5-9. Hyperechoic (A), isoechoic (B), and hypoechoic (C) nodules.

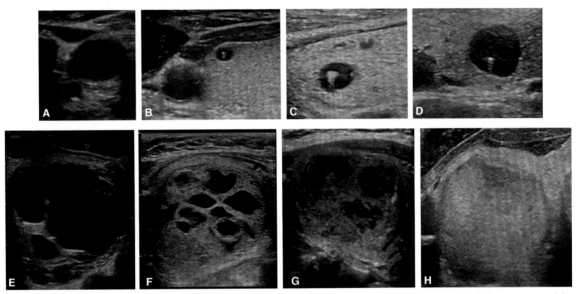

FIGURE 5-10. Simple cyst (A). Colloid cyst with characteristic comet-tail artifact (B-D). Cystic nodule with solid component (E). Spongiform nodule (F). Solid nodule with central necrosis (G). Solid, isoechoic nodule (H).

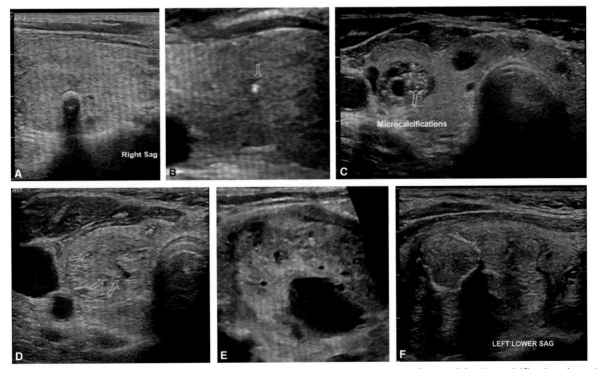

FIGURE 5-11. Benign eggshell calcification with an acoustic shadowing (A). Benign macrocalcification (B). Microcalcifications in nodules that returned malignant (C-E). Malignant nodule with focal discontinuity of an eggshell calcified rim (F), the note posterior shadowing.

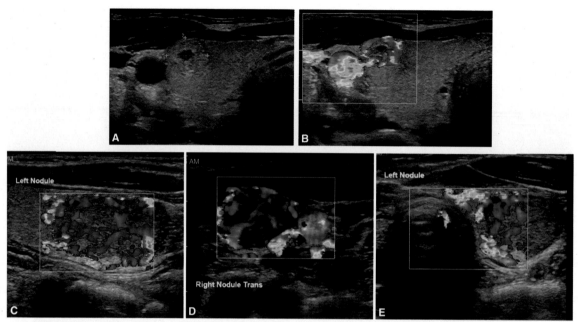

FIGURE 5-12. Before and after Doppler flow imaging of a benign nodule with peripheral vascularity (A, B). Malignant nodules with abnormal central/intranodular vascularity (C-E).

disease or other endocrine disorders, including multiple endocrine neoplasia type 2 (MEN2). Patients should also be questioned on any previous irradiation to the head or neck during childhood, or total body irradiation as done for bone marrow transplants. One should keep in mind that there is a higher rate of thyroid cancer in a bimodal age distribution, with it being more common in the presence of a nodule during childhood and advanced age (Table 5-2).[18]

Most thyroid nodules will be asymptomatic; if symptoms are present, it is important to assess if the lesion appeared rapidly or had a more gradual onset. Benign nodules usually grow slowly over the course of several years, whereas progressive growth during weeks to months is more suggestive of aggressive malignancies, such as primary lymphoma of the thyroid, anaplastic or medullary thyroid carcinoma.[19,20]

TABLE 5-2	Clinical Factors Suggesting Increased Risk of Thyroid Malignancy
Family history of thyroid cancer, MEN 2	
Head/neck or whole-body irradiation	
Adolescent <15 or elderly >70	
Firm or hard nodule	
Fixed nodule	
Rapid growth of nodule	
Dysphagia, dyspnea, or dysphonia	

MEN 2, multiple endocrine neoplasia type 2.

Data from Haugen BR, Alexander EK, Bible KC, et al. 2015 American Thyroid Association Management Guidelines for Adult Patients with Thyroid Nodules and Differentiated Thyroid Cancer: The American Thyroid Association Guidelines Task Force on Thyroid Nodules and Differentiated Thyroid Cancer. *Thyroid.* 2016;26(1):1-133; AACE/AME Task Force On Thyroid Nodules; Gharib H, Papini E. American Association of Clinical Endocrinologists and Association Medical Endocrinologist Medical Guidelines for Clinical Practice for the Diagnosis and Management of Thyroid Nodules—2016 Update. *Endocr Pract.* 2016;22(1):1-60; Campanella P, Ianni F, Rota CA, Corsello SM, Pontecorvi A. Quantification of cancer risk of each clinical and ultrasonographic suspicious feature of thyroid nodules: a systematic review and meta-analysis. *Eur J Endocrinol.* 2014;170(5):203-211.

Once a thyroid nodule has been identified, one must rule out a hyperfunctioning adenoma. Thyrotropin, more commonly called thyroid-stimulating hormone (TSH), should always be measured in the presence of a thyroid nodule. Suppressed levels of TSH are associated with a decreased probability of cancer, whereas elevated levels imply a statistically increased risk of malignancy in the presence of a thyroid nodule.[20,21] If subclinical or overt hyperthyroidism is present, further evaluation and treatment are required, often in the form of a thyroid uptake and scan. "Hot" or hyperfunctioning nodules need no cytologic evaluation; however, "cold" nodules on thyroid uptake and scan should undergo biopsy as they do pose an increased risk.[15,20,22]

Following a detailed history and evaluation of thyroid biochemical function, a high-resolution thyroid US should be performed to assess the nodule's characteristics, including the dimensions, content, changes to the surrounding thyroid architecture, and the presence of suspicious lymph nodes that may be in both the central and lateral compartments. It is a combination of sonographic features and nodule size that is used to stratify the risk of malignancy and thus guide fine needle aspiration (FNA) decision-making.[23,24] A higher risk of malignancy is inferred if the nodule demonstrates any of the following: solid composition, hypoechogenicity, height greater than width, microcalcifications, irregular boards, or central vascularization (Table 5-3).[18] The presence of two or more suspicious US criteria greatly increases the risk of malignancy.[25]

There are several proposed US classification systems; however, the most commonly used in the United States are the American Association of Clinical Endocrinologists (AACE) and American Thyroid Association (ATA) classifications (Table 5-4). There is increasing popularity for the American College of Radiology Thyroid Imaging Reporting and Data System (ACR TI-RADS); however, the majority of endocrinologists still heavily favor the AACE and ATA US classification systems. In general, all nodules over 1.0 cm should be evaluated. If the nodule is mostly cystic or spongiform, it is low risk and can be monitored, as the risk of malignancy is less than 5% (Figure 5-13). More solid, isoechoic nodules are considered

| TABLE 5-3 | Ultrasound Features of Benign Versus Malignant Nodules |

Benign	Malignant
Simple cyst or spongiform appearance	Solid
Peripheral vascularity	Intramodular vascularity
Well-defined margins	Irregular or lobulated margins
Regular "eggshell" calcifications along the periphery	Microcalcifications
Round	Taller than wide (AP > TR in the transverse plane)
Isoechoic	Hypoechogenicity (compared to strap muscles)

Abbreviations: AP, anteroposterior; TR, transverse.

Data from Haugen BR, Alexander EK, Bible KC, et al. 2015 American Thyroid Association Management Guidelines for Adult Patients with Thyroid Nodules and Differentiated Thyroid Cancer: The American Thyroid Association Guidelines Task Force on Thyroid Nodules and Differentiated Thyroid Cancer. *Thyroid.* 2016;26(1):1-133; AACE/AME Task Force On Thyroid Nodules; Gharib H, Papini E. American Association of Clinical Endocrinologists and Association Medical Endocrinologist Medical Guidelines for Clinical Practice for the Diagnosis and Management of Thyroid Nodules—2016 Update. *Endocr Pract.* 2016;22(1):1-60; Baskin HJ, Duick DS, Levine RA. *Thyroid Ultrasound and Ultrasound-Guided FNA.* New York, NY: Springer; 2013.

| TABLE 5-4 | Comparison of Thyroid Nodule Ultrasound Classification Systems (Expected Risk of Malignancy) |

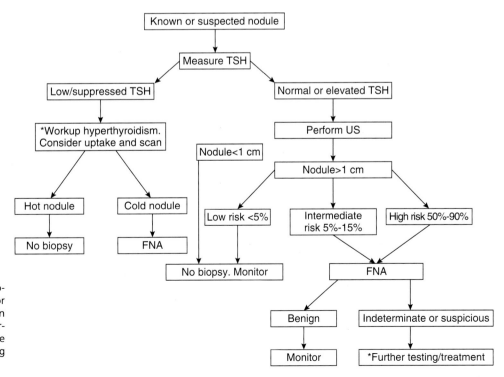

Benign US Features

FNA

Suspicious US Features

AACE

Low-risk lesion: Cystic or mostly cystic nodules. Spongiform. Halo present (1%-5%)

Intermediate risk: Slightly hypoechoic when compared to thyroid tissue. Ovoid to round shape. Ill-defined margins (5%-15%)

High risk: At least one of the following: Hypoechogenicity compared to prethyroid muscles, irregular or lobulated margins, microcalcifications, taller-than-wide shape (AP > TR), extrathyroidal growth, pathologic adenopathy (50%-90%)

ATA

Benign: Purely cystic (<1%)

Very low suspicion: Spongiform (<3%)

Low suspicion: Iso- or hyperechoic solid nodule without worrisome features (5%-10%)

Intermediate suspicion: Hypoechoic solid, with smooth margins without worrisome features (10%-24%)

High suspicion: Solid hypoechoic with one or more of the following: Irregular/infiltrative/microlobulated margins, microcalcifications, taller-than-wide shape. Rim calcifications, extrathyroidal extension (>70%-90%)

Abbreviations: AACE, American Association of Clinical Endocrinologists; AP, anteroposterior; ATA, American Thyroid Association; FNA, fine needle aspiration; TR, transverse; US, ultrasound.

Adapted from 2015 ATA Management Guidelines for Adult Patients with Thyroid Nodules and Differentiated Thyroid Carcinoma. 2016 AACE Clinical Practice Guideline, for the Diagnosis and Management of Thyroid.

FIGURE 5-13. Thyroid nodule biopsy algorithm. *Consider endocrinology consult for workup and treatment of hyperfunction nodules, or lesions that return indeterminate or suspicious on FNA. FNA, fine needle aspiration; TSH, thyroid-stimulating hormone; US, ultrasound.

PART 2

an intermediate risk of 5% to 15% for malignancy; nodules in this category should only undergo FNA if 1.0 to 1.5 cm or larger. High-risk lesions are those with marked hypoechogenicity and at least one worrisome feature (taller than wide, microcalcifications, etc.); FNA is highly recommended as risk of malignancy is as high as 90%.[15,22]

FNA is a safe, well-tolerated procedure that is most commonly performed by endocrinologists or interventional radiologists (see Chapter 58). If cytology returns benign, then low-risk nodules can be followed clinically, whereas sonographically intermediate and high-risk lesions can be monitored with thyroid US at 24 and 12 months, respectively. Repeat FNA for nodules with benign cytology if a subsequent US discovers at least a 20% increase in two dimensions, or greater than 50% increase in volume.[15,22] Consult endocrinology if FNA cytology results as indeterminate or suspicious, as many factors including molecular markers, risk of recurrence, and histology must be considered when developing a treatment strategy.

PEARLS AND PITFALLS

Pearls

- If a nodule is only seen in one plane then it is probably a pseudo-nodule, and FNA is not warranted.
- When encountering nodules that extend downward into the mediastinum, have the patient briefly further hyperextend their neck and angle the transducer inferiorly.
- Make use of dual imaging for nodules too large to measure on a single screen (**Figure 5-14**).
- The thyroid is a highly vascular gland. Locating vessels with a combination of color and pulse wave Doppler can be helpful when planning FNA (**Figure 5-15**).
- When assessing blood flow, try to have a portion of the trachea in the Doppler view. If there is any flow being measured in the air-filled trachea, then Doppler sensitivity is set to high and needs to be decreased until no activity is seen there. This will ensure that Doppler sensitivity is set so that normal thyroid tissue will not display increased vascularity.

Pitfalls

- Do not confuse poorly defined margins (difficult to visualize) with irregular margins, which have a clearly visible demarcation from the thyroid parenchyma but are asymmetrical.
- Do not mistake the esophagus for a nodule. It can be differentiated by peristaltic movement when the patient is asked to swallow (**Figure 5-16**).
- The diffusely heterogeneous thyroid glands seen in Hashimoto thyroiditis and Graves' disease may contain focal fibrous regions or echogenic septa that can be confused as lesions (**Figure 5-17**). Simply turn the probe to the sagittal view; if lesion is no longer visualized then pseudo-nodule is confirmed.
- Be sure to apply adequate pressure in order to properly visualize deeper lesions.
- Parathyroid adenomas can masquerade as thyroid lesions (**Figure 5-18**). Patients are usually symptomatic if adenoma is large enough to be seen on US.

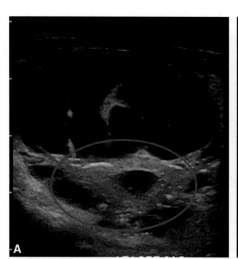
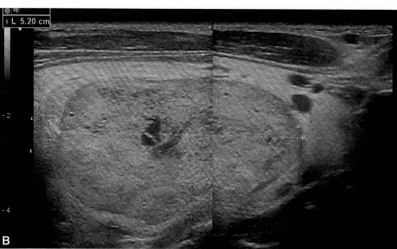

FIGURE 5-14. The solid area of this predominately cystic nodule circled in blue represents the desired region to sample on fine needle aspiration (A). Large nodule that required dual imaging to encompass the entire lesion on screen for accurate measurement (B).

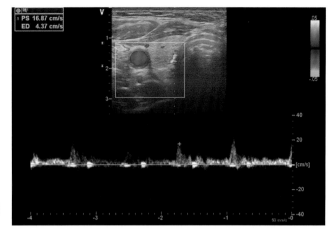

FIGURE 5-15. Blood vessel located using combination of color and pulse wave Doppler.

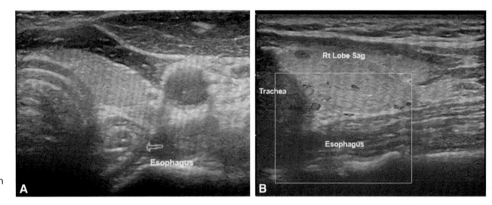

FIGURE 5-16. Image of the esophagus in the transverse (A) and sagittal (B) view.

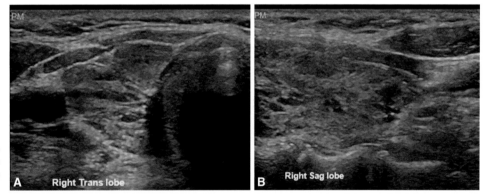

FIGURE 5-17. A patient with Hashimoto thyroiditis; gland visualized in the transverse (A) and sagittal view (B). Note the echogenic septa throughout.

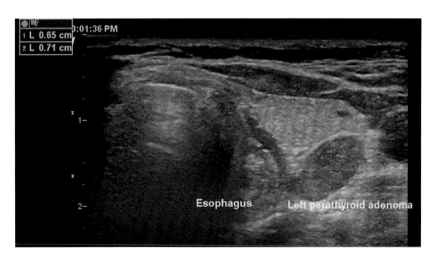

FIGURE 5-18. Transverse view of parathyroid adenoma confirmed on resection. Patient was noted to have recurrent kidney stones.

BILLING

CPT Code	Description	Global Payment	Professional Component	Technical Component
76536	Diagnostic ultrasound examination of the neck soft tissues, including the use of Doppler	$118.79	$28.71	$90.08

CPT codes and average national reimbursement for Medicare in 2016. Payment data are from https://www.cms.gov/apps/physician-fee-schedule/search/search-criteria.aspx. See Chapter 2 for details on ultrasound billing.

References

1. Vander JB. The significance of nontoxic thyroid nodules. *Ann Intern Med.* 1968;69(3):537-540.
2. Tunbridge WM, Evered DC, Hall R, et al. The spectrum of thyroid disease in a community: the Whickham survey. *Clin Endocrinol.* 1977;7(6):481-493.
3. Reiners C, Wegscheider K. Prevalence of thyroid disorders in the working population of Germany: ultrasonography screening in 96,278 unselected employees. *Thyroid.* 2004;14(11):926-932.
4. Guth S, Theune U. Very high prevalence of thyroid nodules detected by high frequency (13 MHz) ultrasound examination. *Eur J Clin Invest.* 2009;39(8):699-706.
5. Leenhardt L, Grosclaude P. Increased incidence of thyroid carcinoma in France: a true epidemic or thyroid nodule management effects? Report from the French Thyroid Cancer Committee. *Thyroid.* 2004;14(12):1056-1060.
6. Morris LG, Sikora AG, Davies L. The increasing incidence of thyroid cancer: the influence of access to care. *Thyroid.* 2013;23(7):885-891.
7. Mortensen J, Woolner LB, Bennett WA. Gross and microscopic findings in clinically normal thyroid glands. *J Clin Endocrinol Metab.* 1955;15(10):1270-1280.
8. Brito JP, Nofal AA, Montori VM. The impact of subclinical disease and mechanism of detection on the rise in thyroid cancer incidence: a population-based study in Olmsted County, Minnesota during 1935 through 2012. *Thyroid.* 2015;25(9):999-1007.
9. Aschebrook-Kilfoy B, Schechter RB, Shih Y-CT. The clinical and economic burden of a sustained increase in thyroid cancer incidence. *Cancer Epidemiol Biomarkers Prev.* 2013;22(7):1252-1259.
10. Ito Y, Uruno T. An observation trial without surgical treatment in patients with papillary microcarcinoma of the thyroid. *Thyroid.* 2003;13(4):381-387.
11. Howlett DC, Speirs A. The thyroid incidentaloma-ignore or investigate? *J Ultrasound Med.* 2007;26(10):1367-1371.
12. Rosenbaum MA, McHenry CR. Contemporary management of papillary carcinoma of the thyroid gland. *Expert Rev Anticancer Ther.* 2009;9(3):317-329.
13. Werk EE. Cancer in thyroid nodules. A community hospital survey. *Arch Intern Med.* 1984;144(3):474-476.
14. Lin JD, Chao TC. Thyroid cancer in the thyroid nodules evaluated by ultrasonography and fine-needle aspiration cytology. *Thyroid.* 2005;7:708-717.
15. Haugen BR, Alexander EK, Bible KC, et al. 2015 American Thyroid Association Management Guidelines for Adult Patients with Thyroid Nodules and Differentiated Thyroid Cancer: The American Thyroid Association Guidelines Task Force on Thyroid Nodules and Differentiated Thyroid Cancer. *Thyroid.* 2016;26(1):1-133.
16. Cappelli C, Pirola I. Is the anteroposterior and transverse diameter ratio of nonpalpable thyroid nodules a sonographic criteria for recommending fine-needle aspiration cytology? *Clin Endocrinol.* 2005;63(6):689-693.
17. Yoon DY, Lee JW. Peripheral calcification in thyroid nodules. *J Ultrasound Med.* 2007;26(10):1349-1355.
18. Campanella P, Ianni F, Rota CA, Corsello SM, Pontecorvi A. Quantification of cancer risk of each clinical and ultrasonographic suspicious feature of thyroid nodules: a systematic review and meta-analysis. *Eur J Endocrinol.* 2014;170(5):203-211.
19. Gharib H, Papini E. Thyroid nodules: clinical importance, assessment, and treatment. *Endocrinol Metab Clin North Am.* 2007;36(3):707-735.
20. Hegedüs L. The thyroid nodule. *N Engl J Med.* 2004;351(17):1764-1771.
21. Boelaert K, Horacek J. Serum thyrotropin concentration as a novel predictor of malignancy in thyroid nodules investigated by fine-needle aspiration. *J Clin Endocrinol Metab.* 2006;91(11):4295-4301.
22. AACE/AME Task Force On Thyroid Nodules; Gharib H, Papini E. American Association of Clinical Endocrinologists and Association Medical Endocrinologist Medical Guidelines for Clinical Practice for the Diagnosis and Management of Thyroid Nodules—2016 Update. *Endocr Pract.* 2016;22(1):1-60.
23. Brito JP, Gionfriddo MR, Nofal AA. The accuracy of thyroid nodule ultrasound to predict thyroid cancer: systematic review and meta-analysis. *J Clin Endocrinol Metab.* 2014;99(4):1253-1263.
24. Smith-Bindman R, Lebda P. Risk of thyroid cancer based on thyroid ultrasound imaging characteristics. *JAMA Intern Med.* 2013;173(19):1788-1796.
25. Papini E. Risk of malignancy in nonpalpable thyroid nodules: predictive value of ultrasound and color-doppler features. *J Clin Endocrinol Metab.* 2002;87(5):1941-1946.

SECTION 3
LYMPH NODE

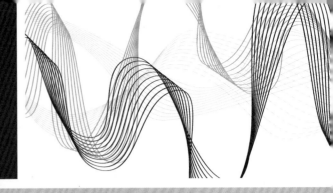

CHAPTER 6

Is This Enlarged Lymph Node Benign Appearing?

Elana Thau, MD and Charisse W. Kwan, MD, FRCPC

● Clinical Vignette

An otherwise healthy, fully immunized 7-year-old boy presented to the outpatient clinic with a 5-day history of progressive swelling on the left side of his neck. He denied fever, neck pain, or infectious symptoms. On physical examination, a mobile, nontender 2 cm × 2 cm mass was palpable in the upper anterior neck triangle. There was no overlying skin discoloration, and he had full neck range of motion. The physical examination was otherwise normal. Is this enlarged lymph node benign appearing?

LITERATURE REVIEW

Neck lumps are a common pediatric concern. It is estimated that between 17% and 62% of children have palpable cervical lymph nodes.[1] Although the majority of these represent benign reactive processes, the clinician must consider a differential diagnosis, which includes infectious, congenital, immunologic, metabolic, and neoplastic processes.[2] Obtaining a history and physical examination is necessary but may not be sufficient.[2] The structures in the neck are reliably viewed by ultrasound, and their features can be used to help make management decisions, including the need for more advanced testing.[3] Furthermore, ultrasound is relatively fast, painless, and without radiation.[3,4] In comparison to CT and MRI, ultrasound is relatively inexpensive, has good sensitivity,[5,6] and is becoming more accessible in pediatric emergency departments[7] and primary care settings.

Although no single sonographic characteristic should be used alone in deciding whether a lymph node is normal, the combination of history, physical examination findings, and ultrasound characteristics can help point toward a normal, inflamed, or malignant lymph node. It is important to be mindful that point-of-care ultrasound (POCUS) is meant to be a clinical adjunct interpreted in the context of the patient.

Most normal lymph nodes are less than 1 cm in the longest diameter. Those larger than 1 cm are considered abnormal, and this condition may also be referred to as lymphadenopathy. Size, however, has variable sensitivity for pathology, depending on what cutoff is used. Larger sizes are more specific but less sensitive.[1,5] Shape can also be a predictor of pathology. Healthy cervical lymph nodes are oval with a short- to long-axis ratio (S:L) <0.5, although this can vary depending on lymph node location.[8,9]

Infection is the most common benign cause of lymphadenopathy. This can result from a lymph node reacting to nearby infection or from infection of the lymph node itself. Ultrasound can aid in distinguishing between reactive changes, infected lymph nodes, and lymph node abscesses. Normal and reactive lymph nodes have an echogenic hilum and hypoechoic cortex.[4-6] They have vasculature confined to the hilum or are avascular[4] (**Figures 6-1 and 6-2**). Infected lymph nodes appear rounder, are often surrounded by soft tissue edema (cobblestoning of surrounding tissue), and have increased vascularity to the lymph node and surrounding tissue (**Figure 6-3**). On physical examination, the overlying skin may appear red and tender to palpation. Lymph node abscesses are round hypoechoic fluid collections, which may contain hyperechoic material[10] (**Figure 6-4**). On physical examination, the overlying skin is often red and tender to palpation. It is important to note that reactive, infected, and abscessed lymph nodes exist on a spectrum.

Malignant lymph nodes may display a thinned or absent hilum, and the cortex can become markedly hypoechoic or hyperechoic[8,11] (**Figure 6-5**). They tend to have an S:L ≥ 0.5 and thus appear abnormally round. Both malignant and severely inflamed lymph nodes can undergo necrosis, characterized by hyperechoic regions or cystic changes.[8] Malignant features can also include intranodal necrosis, calcification, ill-defined borders, matting, and adjacent soft tissue edema.[4,12] Malignant lymph nodes characteristically have peripheral or mixed vascularity.[13]

When occurring in the cervical regions, it is important to consider the differential diagnosis for cervical masses beyond lymphadenopathy. This includes congenital lesions and thyroid masses. The common congenital lesions are reviewed here. Thyroid masses and nodules are reviewed in Chapter 5.

Thyroglossal duct cysts are typically located in the midline surrounding the hyoid bone. On ultrasound, these appear as cystic structures, which are well defined, thin walled, and anechoic or

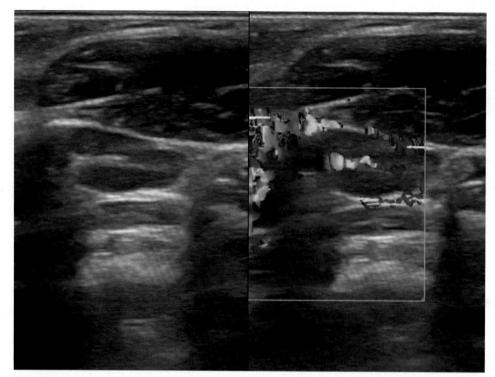

FIGURE 6-1. The normal oval lymph node has normal architecture (hilum and cortex). Color Doppler reveals central hilar flow.

hypoechoic.[14] Infected cysts may become thick walled with internal septations with vascularity to the cyst wall. Branchial cleft cysts are well-defined masses located between the thyroid gland and the sternocleidomastoid muscles (**Figure 6-6**). On ultrasound, they are well defined and round or oval in shape with a thin wall around hypoechoic fluid. Infected cysts may have thickened walls and contain echogenic fluid.[14] Cystic hygromas are lymphatic malformations (**Figure 6-7**) most commonly found in the posterior triangle of

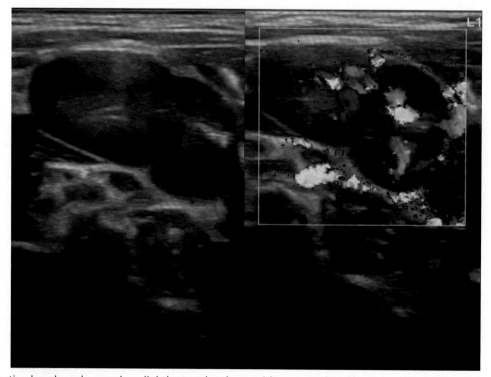

FIGURE 6-2. The reactive lymph node reveals a slightly rounder shape with preserved architecture, including the hilum and cortex. Color Doppler reveals central hilar flow.

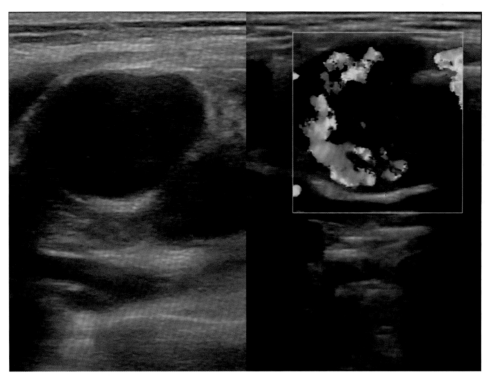

FIGURE 6-3. The infected lymph node (lymphadenitis) is round in shape with loss of normal architecture as well as surrounding loss of tissue definition, suggestive of early surrounding tissue edema. Color Doppler demonstrates increased and decentralized flow throughout.

the neck. On ultrasound, they are well-defined cystic masses that are typically avascular and multilocular with thick septa and thin walls. The internal fluid is hypoechoic or anechoic.[14] Fibromatosis colli is a hard mass palpated in the lower part of the sternocleidomastoid muscle. Ultrasound shows an elliptical hyperechoic, variably heterogeneous mass within the sternocleidomastoid.[14] Hemangiomas are soft masses, which are fluctuant on palpation. On ultrasound, they are well circumscribed with hyperechoic lobules, which are commonly homogeneous. They are hypervascular on color Doppler flow.[14]

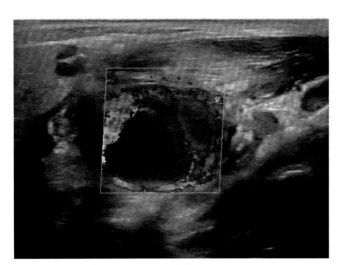

FIGURE 6-4. The abscessed or necrotic lymph node reveals a rounded structure with a hypoechoic collection. Color Doppler demonstrates increased flow of the surrounding tissue and no internal flow to the hypoechoic collection. This is highly suggestive of an abscess. Note also the thickened and ill-defined soft tissue surrounding the lymph node.

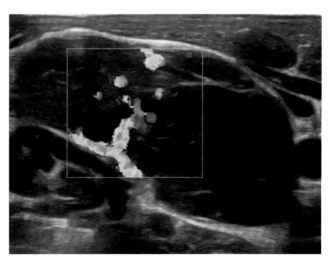

FIGURE 6-5. The malignant lymph nodes are enlarged, rounded, and lack normal lymph node architecture, with no defined hilum or cortex. Color Doppler reveals mixed vascularity rather than the typical central hilar flow on normal lymph nodes. This patient was diagnosed with lymphoma.

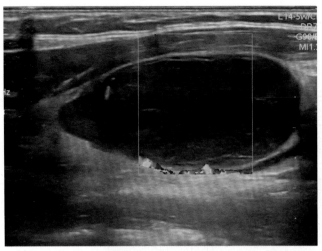

FIGURE 6-6. The branchial cleft cyst lacks the typical lymph node architecture and is well defined with mixed echotexture. Color Doppler reveals no internal flow, as would be expected of any cystic structure.

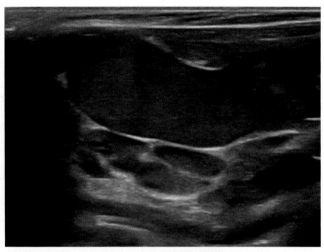

FIGURE 6-7. The lymphatic malformation has no central hilum or cortex. There are well-defined borders that surround a homogeneous echotexture. With slight pressure, the internal substance moves and appears liquid.

TABLE 6-1	Recommendations for Use of Point-of-Care Ultrasound in Clinical Practice		
Recommendation		**Rating**	**References**
When assessing a neck mass in children, POCUS can be used to help decide on medical management or referral for further imaging or surgical management.		C	1, 6, 7
When medically managing a neck mass in a child, POCUS can be used to assess response to treatment and help inform further management.		C	1, 6, 7

A = consistent, good-quality patient-oriented evidence; B = inconsistent or limited-quality patient-oriented evidence; C = consensus, disease-oriented evidence, usual practice, expert opinion, or case series. For information about the SORT evidence rating system, go to http://www.aafp.org/afpsort.

PERFORMING THE SCAN

1. **Preparation**. The patient should be positioned with neck hyperextended. A POCUS examination of a lymph node is ideally performed using a 7.5 to 15 MHz, high-frequency transducer to maximize image resolution.[1] Ample gel is applied over the area of interest to minimize patient discomfort[2] and optimize visualization of superficial lymph nodes.

2. **Examination of affected lymph node**. With the linear transducer, the cervical lymph nodes are examined in two perpendicular planes for their location, size, shape, and internal characteristics. This includes echotexture, calcifications, surrounding soft tissues (**Figures 6-8 and 6-9**), and vascular pattern by Doppler.[1,3] Power Doppler is a more sensitive modality compared with color Doppler in small lymph nodes with small blood vessels[4] but can be difficult to perform in the presence of motion artifact when examining children. Ensure that the structure of interest is examined in two planes.

PATIENT MANAGEMENT

The history and physical examination should always be considered when incorporating ultrasound findings into clinical decision making. When there are infectious symptoms such as fever, rhinorrhea, cough, pharyngitis, or local skin infection, ultrasound findings may help differentiate normal, reactive, infected, or abscessed lymph nodes. A longer duration of symptoms is more likely to accompany the presentation of an abscess or malignancy.

Normal or reactive lymph nodes are suggested by ultrasound findings of an oval or rounded well-circumscribed structure with preserved lymph node architecture (hilum and cortex) and normal vasculature. In both cases, this requires observation for progression in size, skin changes, and tenderness.

Redness and tenderness of the skin over mass accompanied by a rounded lymph node with preserved architecture but increased vascularity with or without soft tissue edema suggests an infected lymph node. This may warrant oral antibiotics. Admission and intravenous antibiotics may be required if the patient appears systemically unwell. If ultrasound findings reveal a hypoechoic fluid collection and surrounding soft tissue edema, then there is likely necrosis of the lymph node or an abscess present. Depending on local practice, this may require intravenous antibiotics with surgical consultation with or without drainage of the abscess.

Some ultrasound findings may warrant further investigation. Findings suggestive of malignancy include calcification, abnormal lymph node architecture, cystic changes, and mixed peripheral or mixed vascularity. Congenital malformations may appear as simple or complex cystic structures. In these instances, further investigations such as comprehensive ultrasound, chest radiography, CT scan, blood work, or specialist consultation should be considered. If the lymph node appears to be a primary malignancy or metastasis, consider obtaining a fine needle aspiration or core needle biopsy (**Figure 6-10**). This is discussed further in Chapter 58.

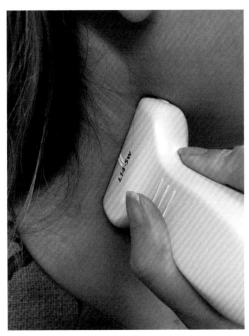

FIGURE 6-8. Scan in the long-axis orientation of the neck mass.

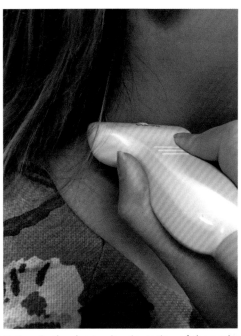

FIGURE 6-9. Scan in the short-axis orientation of the neck mass.

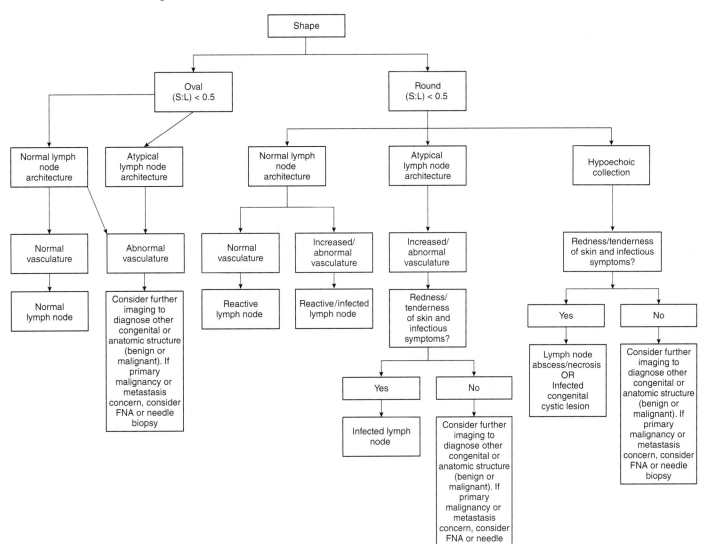

FIGURE 6-10. Management algorithm for lymph nodes larger than 1 cm in longest dimension. FNA, fine needle aspiration.

PEARLS AND PITFALLS

Pearls

- Clinical history and physical examination are important.
- Color Doppler should be used to assess vascularity and can help narrow the differential diagnosis.
- Ultrasound can be used to monitor response to antibiotics or progression of disease.

Pitfall

- Suspected malignancy, congenital abnormalities, and unrecognized structures warrant comprehensive imaging performed using radiology and further investigations.

BILLING

CPT Code	Description	Global Payment	Professional Component	Technical Component
76536	Ultrasound of soft tissues of head and neck	$116.71	$28.66	$88.05

CPT codes and average national reimbursement for Medicare in 2016. Payment data are from https://www.cms.gov/apps/physician-fee-schedule/search/search-criteria.aspx. See Chapter 2 for details on ultrasound billing.

References

1. Locke R, Comfort R, Kubba H. When does an enlarged cervical lymph node in a child need excision? A systematic review. *Int J Pediatr Otorhinolaryngol.* 2014;78:393-401.
2. Lang S, Kansy B. Cervical lymph node diseases in children. *GMS Curr Top Otorhinolaryngol Head Neck Surg.* 2014;13:1-27.
3. Wunsch R, von Rohden L, Cleaveland R, et al. Small part ultrasound in childhood and adolescence. *Eur J Radiol.* 2014;83:1549-1559.
4. Ahuja A, Ying M. Sonographic evaluation of cervical lymph nodes. *AJR Am J Roentgenol.* 2005;184:1691-1699.
5. Esen G. Ultrasound of superficial lymph nodes. *Eur J Radiol.* 2006;58:345-359.
6. Ahuja A, Ying M. Sonography of neck lymph nodes. Part II: abnormal lymph nodes. *Clin Radiol.* 2003;58:359-366.
7. Levy JA, Noble VE. Bedside ultrasound in pediatric emergency medicine. *Pediatrics.* 2008;121:e1404-e1412.
8. Chan JM, Shin LK, Jeffrey RB. Ultrasonography of abnormal neck lymph nodes. *Ultrasound Q.* 2007;23:47-54.
9. Ying M, Ahuja A, Brook F, et al. Nodal shape (s/l) and its combination with size for assessment of cervical lymphadenopathy: which cut-off should be used? *Ultrasound Med Biol.* 1999;25(8):1169-1175.
10. Zaia B. Skin. In: Shah S, Price D, Bukhman G, Shah S, Wroe E, eds. *Manual for Ultrasound for Resource-Limited Settings.* Boston, MA: Partners in Health; 2011:296.
11. Weskott HP, Yin S. Ultrasonography in the assessment of lymph node disease. *Ultrasound Clin.* 2014;9:351-371.
12. Fu X, Guo L, Lv K, et al. Sonographic appearance of cervical lymphadenopathy due to infectious mononucleosis in children and young adults. *Clin Radiol.* 2014;69:239-245.
13. Misra D, Panjwani S, Rai S, et al. Diagnostic efficacy of color Doppler ultrasound in evaluation of cervical lymphadenopathy. *Dent Res J.* 2016;13(3):217-224.
14. Rosenberg HK. Sonography of pediatric neck masses. *Ultrasound Q.* 2009;25(3):111-127.

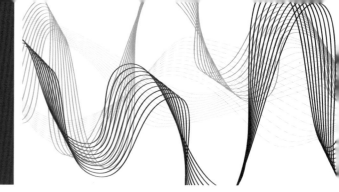

CHAPTER

7

Does This Patient Have Hydrocephalus?

Duncan Norton, MD, Sofia Markee, DO, MS, and Paul Bornemann, MD, RMSK, RPVI

● Clinical Vignette

A full-term male infant comes into the office for a routine 4-month well-baby visit. He was born by normal vaginalw delivery after an uneventful prenatal course. He has been growing well and meeting all his developmental milestones. He appears normal on examination other than a somewhat enlarged appearing head. He has no dysmorphic features. At his 2-month well-baby visit his head circumference plotted on the 95th percentile. Today it plots at the 98th percentile after repeat measurement was done and accuracy was assured. The patient has no family history of medical or genetic problems; however, his father does seem to have a somewhat unusually large head. You suspect this is a case of familial macrocephaly but you want to rule out hydrocephalus. Does this patient have hydrocephalus?

TABLE 7-1	Differential Diagnosis for Infants With Macrocephaly

- Increased brain parenchyma
  - Benign familial macrocephaly
  - Hemimegalencephaly/megalencephaly (familial or nonfamilial)
  - Overgrowth syndromes, such as Sotos syndrome or Weaver syndrome
  - Fragile X syndrome
  - Lysosomal storage diseases
  - Leukodystrophies
  - Organic acid disorders
- Increased cerebrospinal fluid
  - Hydrocephalus
  - Benign extra-axial fluid collections of infancy
- Subdural hematoma or hygroma
- Craniosynostosis
- Chiari malformations
- Dandy-Walker cysts
- Neoplastic and non-neoplastic mass lesions

LITERATURE REVIEW

Macrocephaly is a common incidental finding during well-child examinations in the primary care office. Although it is often related to benign causes, underlying pathology such as hydrocephalus must be ruled out (Table 7-1). Hydrocephalus is defined as a pathologic accumulation of cerebrospinal fluid (CSF) and dilation of the cerebral ventricles in the brain. CSF is primarily produced by the choroid plexus, which is attached to the ependyma of all four ventricles. CSF travels unidirectionally through the ventricular system. It passes from the lateral ventricles through the foramen of Monro, to the third ventricle through the cerebral aqueduct, and exits the fourth ventricle via the foramina of Luschka and Magendie. CSF then enters the subarachnoid space and is absorbed into the venous sinuses and the systemic circulation (see **Figure 7-1**). Hydrocephalus occurs when the CSF cannot be absorbed adequately because of physical or functional obstruction.[1,2]

The prevalence of hydrocephalus in infants is estimated to be between 1 and 32 per 10,000 live births, with a mortality rate of approximately 13% prior to initial hospital discharge.[2,3] Some studies suggest a morbidity of up to 78% in infants with hydrocephalus that develop residual neurologic deficits.[4,5]

The underlying pathophysiology is complex, and both genetic and environmental factors play a role. One study found hydrocephalus to be familial in up to 12% of cases, suggesting that genetics are a strong risk factor.[6] Another study revealed that male gender was an intendent risk factor, and that Asian ethnicity was inversely related to the development of hydrocephalus.[7] Other risk factors include lack of prenatal care, prematurity of less than or equal to 30 weeks gestation, multiparous gestation, maternal preexisting diabetes, pre-eclampsia, maternal chronic hypertension, maternal antidepressant use during the first trimester, and alcohol use during pregnancy.[2,6-9]

Hydrocephalus can present in many ways and may vary depending on the age of the child or underlying cause. In neonates, one of the first presenting signs of hydrocephalus is increasing head circumference. A bulging fontanelle or abnormally splayed sutures may also be apparent. Some neonates will have episodes of apnea and bradycardia; however, these symptoms are nonspecific to hydrocephalus alone and warrant further workup for other potential etiologies.[10] It is also important to consider Cushing's triad when evaluating for signs of increased intracranial pressure: hypertension, bradycardia, and irregular respirations.[10] In infants, changes in behavior and level of consciousness, such as increased irritability or lethargy, are more prominent signs associated with hydrocephalus,

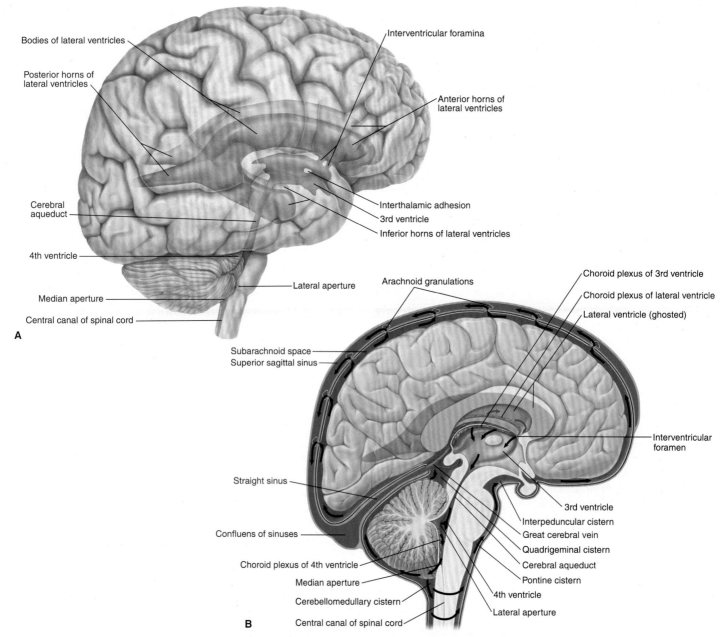

FIGURE 7-1. The location of the ventricles (A) in the brain and flow patterns of cerebrospinal fluid (B). Reprinted with permission from Gest TR. The head and the neck. In: Gest TR, ed. *Lippincott Atlas of Anatomy.* 2nd ed. Philadelphia, PA: Wolters Kluwer; 2020:384. Plate 7-58.

although these too can be seen in the neonatal period. Head size and macrocephaly remain key features for this age group.[10] In children, after the closure of sutures and fontanelles, signs and symptoms of hydrocephalus may present more acutely as there is less cranial compliance. Headaches, visual complaints, papilledema, and decreasing level of consciousness may become more prominent signs and symptoms in this age group. Some children may develop focal neurologic deficits, such as bilateral sixth cranial nerve palsies. Late-stage presentations of hydrocephalus include Parinaud syndrome, a dorsal midbrain syndrome characterized by upgaze palsy or sunset sign, and new-onset seizures. Both of these late-stage presentations warrant urgent medical attention and intervention.[11,12]

Hydrocephalus is diagnosed by imaging done via ultrasonography, computed tomography (CT), or magnetic resonance imaging (MRI). Ultrasonographic images of the brain can be obtained through the open fontanelles in the first 12 to 18 months of life.[13] Advances in

portable ultrasound have given physicians the ability to acquire rapid, radiation-free, bedside assessments of the anatomy of the newborn brain. Cranial sonography appears to be one of the most useful and highly accurate modalities for the detection of hydrocephalus in newborns and infants.[14] There are no contraindications for performing neonatal head ultrasonography.[15] However, when the fontanelles are closed, ultrasound is no longer an effective modality. In these instances, studies have shown that both CT and MRI share similar sensitivity and specificity in diagnosing hydrocephalus. MRI, along with ultrasound, has the advantage of being free of ionizing radiation. MRI can also be used to give a more detailed evaluation of the anatomy, help diagnose the underlying cause of hydrocephalus, and is useful for surgical planning when necessary.[13,16] MRI is the most expensive modality and requires sedation in infants. Fast-sequence MRI, which does not involve sedation, is an emerging modality being used more often in the diagnosis of neurologic conditions. See **Table 7-2.**

TABLE 7-2	Recommendations for Use of Point-of-Care Ultrasound in Clinical Practice		
Recommendation		Rating	Reference
Cranial sonography is one of the most useful and highly accurate modalities for detection of hydrocephalus in newborns and infants		C	14

A = consistent, good-quality patient-oriented evidence; B = inconsistent or limited-quality patient-oriented evidence; C = consensus, disease-oriented evidence, usual practice, expert opinion, or case series. For information about the SORT evidence rating system, go to http://www.aafp.org/afpsort.

PERFORMING THE SCAN

Step 1: Select the equipment and setup for the examination. Proper equipment and appropriate environment are essential to obtain adequate images. Primarily a small footprint probe, such as a phased array probe, that is between 5 and 8 MHz is needed for evaluation of the neonatal brain. A high-frequency linear array may be used if assessing superficial structures. If a high-frequency phased array probe is not available, then a typical cardiac phased array operating from 2 to 5 MHz can suffice. Warm gel should be used in a warm room when evaluating young or premature infants. See **Figure 7-2**.

Step 2: Obtain a coronal view of the brain. Begin by using a large amount of gel and placing the sector probe on the anterior fontanelle to start with a coronal view. While in the coronal plane, identify the frontal lobes and then slowly sweep posteriorly until the occipital region is identified. This will allow you to identify the frontal lobes, corpus callosum, cavum septum pellucidum (if present), lateral ventricles, third ventricle, thalami, choroid plexus in both the lateral and third ventricles, temporal lobes, parietal lobes, and occipital lobes. See **Figures 7-3 to 7-6**.

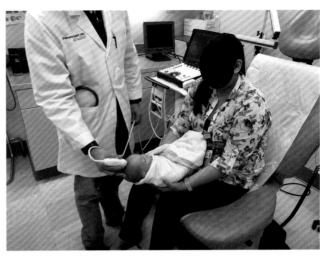

FIGURE 7-3. Probe placement, anterior fontanelle, coronal plane.

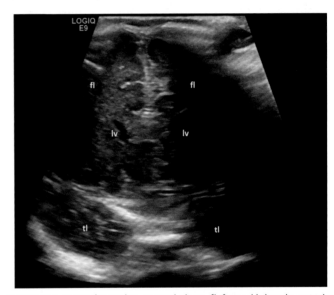

FIGURE 7-4. Normal anterior, coronal plane. fl, frontal lobes; lv, anterior horn of lateral ventricles; tl, temporal lobes.

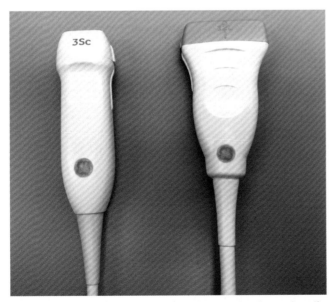

FIGURE 7-2. Picture of probes used in the examination. Primarily a small footprint probe, such as a phased array probe, that is between 5 and 8 MHz is recommended but these are not usually available in primary care. In these cases a typical cardiac phased array operating from 2 to 5 MHz can suffice (left). A high-frequency linear array 5 to 12 MHz (right) may be used if assessing superficial structures.

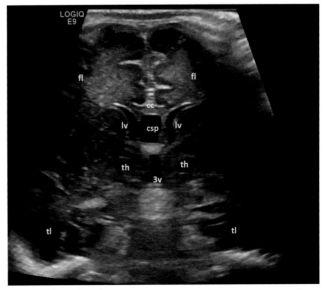

FIGURE 7-5. Normal midline, coronal plane. 3v, third ventricle; cc, corpus callosum; csp, cavum septum pellucidum; fl, frontal lobes; lv, lateral ventricles; th, thalami; tl, temporal lobes.

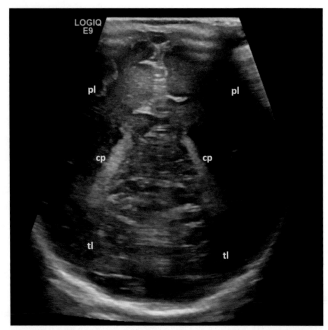

FIGURE 7-6. Normal posterior, coronal plane. cp, choroid plexus in both the lateral ventricles; pl, parietal lobes; tl, temporal lobes.

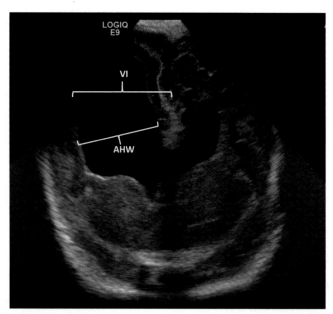

FIGURE 7-8. Midline, coronal plane in a patient with hydrocephalus. Correct caliper placements for ventricular index (VI) and anterior horn width (AHW).

Step 3: Measure the ventricular index and anterior horn width. Obtain the coronal view where the lateral ventricles are the widest, which should be at the level of the thalamus and third ventricle.

Measure the ventricular index by placing calipers across the distance between the falx cerebri and the lateral wall of the anterior horn in the coronal plane. The upper limit of normal is 14 mm in term infants. Anterior horn width should be obtained next. It is measured as the diagonal width of the anterior horn at its widest point in the coronal plane. The upper limit of normal is 4 mm.[17] See **Figures 7-7 and 7-8.**

Step 4: Obtain a sagittal view of the brain. Next, rotate the probe 90° to obtain longitudinal images in the sagittal plane. Angling to either side allows for visualization of the lateral ventricle as it courses anterior to posterior. This view is especially important to visualize the caudothalamic groove, which is the junction between

the caudate and thalamus. This is the most common site for germinal matrix hemorrhage and can appear as increased echogenicity. See **Figures 7-9 and 7-10.**

Step 5: Measure the thalamo-occipital distance. The thalamo-occipital distance should be measured from the occipital horn and should not exceed more than 21 mm.[17] See **Figures 7-11 and 7-12** and Table 7-3.

Step 6: Assess for extra-axial fluid. If available, switch to a high-frequency linear array probe. Assess for enlargement of the space overlying the frontal lobes and a prominent interhemispheric fissure. If present, use color Doppler to assess for vessels coursing through the fluid. If present, they are suggestive of fluid in the

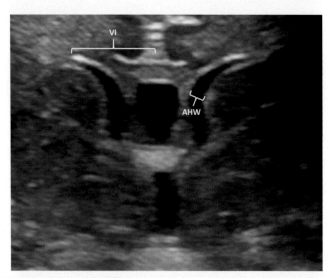

FIGURE 7-7. Normal midline, coronal plane, zoomed in. Correct caliper placements for ventricular index (VI) and anterior horn width (AHW).

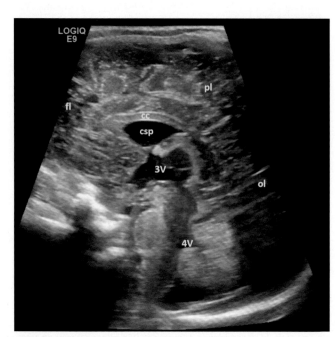

FIGURE 7-9. Normal midline, sagittal plane. 3V, third ventricle; 4V, fourth ventricle; cc, corpus callosum; csp, cavum septum pellucidum; fl, frontal lobes; ol, occipital lobes; Pl, parietal lobes.

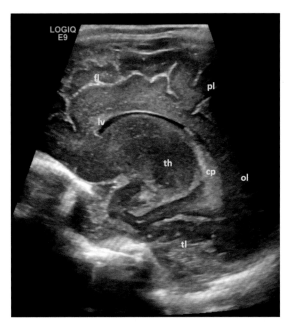

FIGURE 7-10. Normal lateral, parasagittal plane. cp, choroid plexus in both the lateral ventricles; fl, frontal lobes; lv, lateral ventricles; ol, occipital lobes; Pl, parietal lobes; th, thalami; tl, temporal lobes.

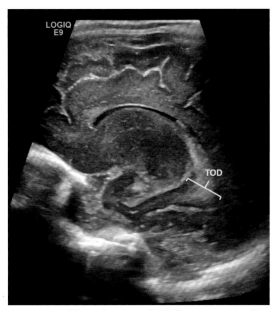

FIGURE 7-11. Normal lateral, parasagittal plane. Correct caliper placements for thalamo-occipital distance (TOD).

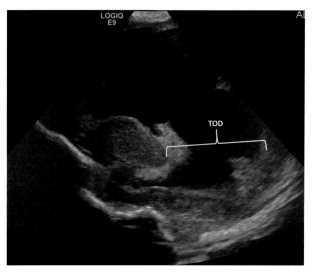

FIGURE 7-12. Lateral, parasagittal plane in a patient with hydrocephalus. Correct caliper placements for thalamo-occipital distance (TOD). Note that the hyperechoic choroid plexus located in the lateral ventricles should be included in the TOD measurement and not mistaken for extraventricular tissue.

TABLE 7-3	Normal Measurements of Lateral Ventricles in Term Infants	
Parameter	Definition	Upper Limit of Normal (mm)
Ventricular index	The distance between the falx cerebri and the lateral wall of the anterior horn in the coronal plane	14
Anterior horn width	The diagonal width of the anterior horn measured at its widest point in the coronal plane	4
Thalamo-occipital distance	The distance between the outermost point of the thalamus at its junction with the choroid plexus and the outermost part of the occipital horn in the parasagittal plane	21

subarachnoid space that is consistent with benign extra-axial fluid, if the ventricles appear normal. If there is no Doppler flow, then fluid in the subdural space such as hematoma should be considered. See **Figures 7-13 and 7-14.**

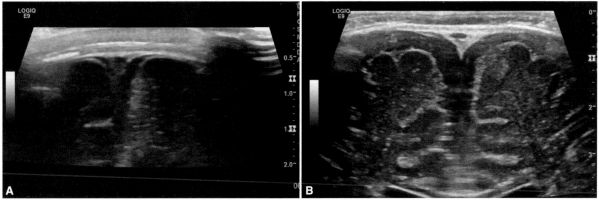

FIGURE 7-13. High-frequency coronal view of a patient with a normal amount of extra-axial fluid (A) and with increased extra-axial fluid (B).

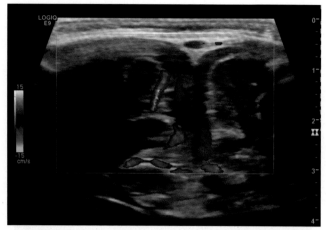

FIGURE 7-14. High-frequency coronal view of the patient with increased extra-axial fluid from Figure 7-13, with color Doppler window showing vessels in the extra-axial fluid that is consistent with benign increased extra-axial fluid.

TABLE 7-4	Red Flags for Urgent Conditions in Infants With Macrocephaly

- Concerning for increased intracranial pressure
  - Seizures
  - Bulging fontanelle
  - Papilledema
  - Lethargy
- Other red flags
  - Developmental delays
  - History of prematurity
  - History of trauma or central nervous system infection
  - Ataxia
  - Syndromic features
  - Concerning family history

PATIENT MANAGEMENT

Macrocephaly is defined as an occipitofrontal circumference (OFC) greater than 97th percentile for age, progressive enlargement that crosses two percentile lines, or a rate of growth greater than 2 cm per month in infants less than 6 months of age. When first diagnosed, measurements should be repeated by an experienced provider as errors are common. After confirming measurements, it should be immediately determined whether red flags for urgent conditions are present (Table 7-4). Especially important to recognize are signs or symptoms of increased intracranial pressure such as bulging fontanelle, papilledema, or lethargy. These patients will need urgent evaluation and this would likely be best suited for the hospital or emergency department. Other concerning findings such as developmental delays or a concerning family history will likely need early referral for specialty consultation and formal intracranial imaging.

If there are no red flags and the infant has an open anterior fontanelle that is adequate for sonography, then point-of-care ultrasound of the brain should be performed. If abnormal measurements of the ventricles are found, then the patient should be referred for specialty evaluation. Infants with hydrocephalus that is acute and rapidly progressing require emergent neurosurgical evaluation. Children without severe ventriculomegaly and are asymptomatic require a timely neurosurgical referral and can usually be managed with very close follow-up and repeat imaging.

If the ventricles are of normal size, then hydrocephalus is ruled out. If benign increased extra-axial fluid is found, then this is likely the cause of the macrocephaly. This requires no further imaging unless there is a change neurologically or head growth further deviates from the normal curve. Although considered benign, extra-axial fluid has been associated with autism spectrum disorders. Infants with this condition should be monitored for development delays, which should prompt further evaluation.

If normal ventricles and normal extra-axial fluid are found, then the infant's first-degree relatives should be examined, and their OFC measured. The patient's OFC and the average familial OFC should be plotted on a standard curve such as the Weaver curve.[18] If the patient's OFC falls within the expected range, based on the familial OFC, then familial macrocephaly is confirmed, and no further evaluation is needed.

If the entire evaluation is normal in a patient with confirmed macrocephaly, then they should be followed closely and repeat ultrasound in 1 to 2 months can be considered. See **Figure 7-15**.

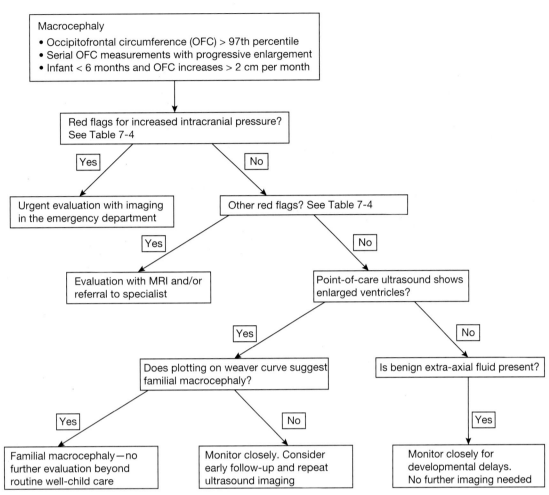

FIGURE 7-15. Algorithm for management of macrocephaly.

PEARLS AND PITFALLS

Pearls

- Infants can be scanned while they are sitting on their parent's lap. This usually helps them remain calm and makes for an easier examination.
- Using warm gel and avoiding excessive pressure on the fontanelle can help prevent vagal response and bradycardia, especially in newborns.
- Although the anterior fontanelle may remain open until 2 years of age, it becomes smaller with age and is best suited as a sonographic window in infants less than 1 year of age.

Pitfalls

- The cavum septum pellucidum is a normal variant that can be visible in some infants. It can be differentiated from the third ventricle because it is located between the lateral ventricles and the third ventricle will be located more inferiorly between the thalami.
- Frontal horn and choroid plexus cysts in the newborn likely represent clinically irrelevant normal variants.[19] Frontal horn cysts are anechoic structures located directly lateral to the frontal horn of the lateral ventricle. See **Figure 7-16**. Choroid plexus cysts appear as well-defined anechoic, circular structures within the choroid plexus. See **Figure 7-17**.
- Be careful not to mistake choroid plexus as extraventricular tissue. It will appear as hyperechoic areas of the lateral ventricles. It should not extend past the caudothalamic groove or the occipital horns as this would suggest intraventricular hemorrhage.

Pearls and Pitfalls, Continued

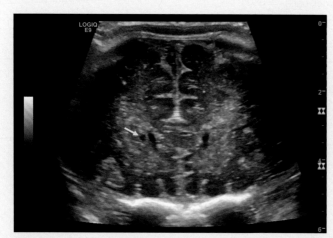

FIGURE 7-16. Normal midline, coronal plane. The arrow indicates a lateral horn cyst, which is a normal variant.

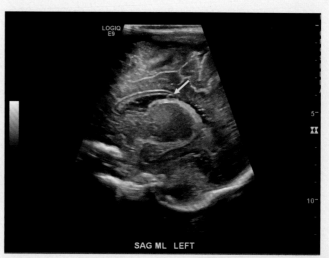

FIGURE 7-17. Normal lateral, parasagittal plane. The arrow indicates a choroid plexus cyst, which is a normal variant.

BILLING

CPT Code	Description	Global Payment	Professional Component	Technical Component
76506	Encephalogram (cranial)	$110.88	$31.23	$79.65

CPT codes and average national reimbursement for Medicare in 2016. Payment data are from https://www.cms.gov/apps/physician-fee-schedule/search/search-criteria.aspx. See Chapter 2 for details on ultrasound billing.

References

1. Damkier HH, Brown PD, Praetorius J. Cerebrospinal fluid secretion by the choroid plexus. *Physiol Rev.* 2013;93(4):1847-1892.

2. Tully HM, Dobyns WB. Infantile hydrocephalus: a review of epidemiology, classification and causes. *Eur J Med Genet.* 2014;57(8):359-368. doi:10.1016/j.ejmg.2014.06.002.

3. Jeng S, Gupta N, Wrensch M, Zhao S, Wu YW. Prevalence of congenital hydrocephalus in California, 1991-2000. *Pediatr Neurol.* 2011;45(2):67-71. doi:10.1016/j.pediatrneurol.2011.03.009.

4. Fernell E, Hagberg G, Hagberg B. Infantile hydrocephalus in preterm, low-birth weight infants—a nationwide Swedish cohort study 1979-1988. *Acta Paediatr.* 1993;82:45-48.

5. Moritake K, Nagai H, Miyazaki T, et al. Analysis of a nationwide survey on treatment and outcomes of congenital hydrocephalus in Japan. *Neurol Med Chir (Tokyo).* 2007;47:453-460.

6. Van Landingham M, Nguyen TV, Roberts A, Parent AD, Zhang J. Risk factors of congenital hydrocephalus: a 10 year retrospective study. *J Neurol Neurosurg Psychiatry.* 2009;80(2):213-217. doi: 10.1136/jnnp.2008.148932.

7. Tully HM, Capote RT, Saltzman BS. Maternal and infant factors associated with infancy-onset hydrocephalus in Washington State. *Pediatr Neurol.* 2015;52(3):320-325. doi:10.1016/j.pediatrneurol.2014.10.030.

8. Millichap JG. Congenital hydrocephalus risk factors. *Pediatr Neurol Briefs.* 2009;23(2):14–14. doi:10.15844/pedneurbriefs-23-2-8.

9. Munch TN, Rasmussen M-LH, Wohlfahrt J, Juhler M, Melbye M. Risk factors for congenital hydrocephalus: a nationwide, register-based, cohort study. *J Neurol Neurosurg Psychiatry.* 2014;85(11):1253-1259. doi:10.1136/jnnp-2013-306941.

10. Riva-Cambrin J, Shannon CN, Holubkov R, et al.; Hydrocephalus Clinical Research Network. Center effect and other factors influencing temporization and shunting of cerebrospinal fluid in preterm infants with intraventricular hemorrhage. *J Neurosurg Pediatr.* 2012;9(5):473-481. doi:10.3171/2012.1.PEDS11292.

11. Chou SY, Digre KB. Neuro-ophthalmic complications of raised intracranial pressure, hydrocephalus, and shunt malfunction. *Neurosurg Clin N Am.* 1999;10(4):587-608.

12. Cultrera F, D'Andrea M, Battaglia R, Chieregato. Unilateral oculomotor nerve palsy: unusual sign of hydrocephalus. *J Neurosurg Sci.* 2009;53(2):67-70.

13. Dinçer A, Özek MM. Radiologic evaluation of pediatric hydrocephalus. *Childs Nerv Syst.* 2011;27(10):1543-1562. doi:10.1007/s00381-011-1559-x.

14. Gupta P, Sodhi KS, Saxena AK, Khandelwal N, Singhi P. Neonatal cranial sonography: a concise review for clinicians. *J Pediatr Neurosci.* 2016;11(1):7-13. doi:10.4103/1817-1745.181261.

15. AIUM Practice parameter for the performance of neurosonography in neonates and infants. *J Ultrasound Med.* 2014. doi:10.1002/jum.15264.

16. Yue EL, Meckler GD, Fleischman RJ, et al. Test characteristics of quick brain MRI for shunt evaluation in children: an alternative modality to avoid radiation. *J Neurosurg Pediatr.* 2015;15(4):420-426. doi:10.3171/2014.9.PEDS14207.

17. Brouwer MJ, de Vries LS, Pistorius L, Rademaker KJ, Groenendaal F, Benders MJ. Ultrasound measurements of the lateral ventricles in neonates: why, how and when? A systematic review. *Acta Paediatr.* 2010;99:1298-1306.

18. Weaver DD, Christian JC. Familial variation of head size and adjustment for parental head circumference. *J Pediatr.* 1980;96(6):990-994.

19. Behnke M, Eyler FD, Garvan CW, et al. Cranial ultrasound abnormalities identified at birth: their relationship to perinatal risk and neurobehavioral outcome. *Pediatrics.* 1999;103(4). doi:10.1542/peds.103.4.e41.

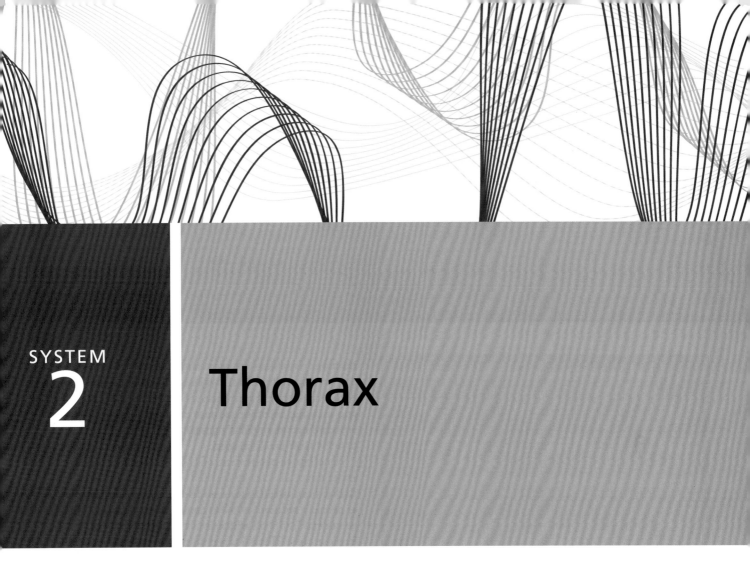

SYSTEM

2

Thorax

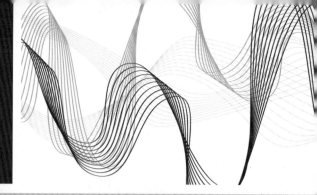

CHAPTER

8

What Is the Patient's Left Ventricular Systolic Function?

Mark E. Shaffer, MD and Andrew D. Vaughan, MD

● Clinical Vignette

A 57-year-old man with a medical history of hypertension presents to your clinic complaining of several months of progressively worsening shortness of breath with exertion. He states that he can no longer walk to his mailbox without becoming short of breath. Furthermore, he describes a worsening history of three-pillow orthopnea for the past several years. He states he occasionally has intermittent swelling of his feet. He denies chest pain and shortness of breath at rest. He has no prior history of cardiac disease. You suspect the patient has acute heart failure. What is the patient's left ventricular systolic function?

LITERATURE REVIEW

In the United States, the incidence of heart failure approaches 10 per 1 000 in those over the age of 65. In addition, mortality is as high as 50% at 5 years after diagnosis.[1] Left ventricular ejection fraction (LVEF) has been consistently demonstrated to be clinically relevant to the prognosis and treatment of heart failure. Specifically, the LVEF can identify patients who would have mortality benefit from certain therapies, inform the need for more invasive cardiac testing, and monitor patients with either acute or chronic symptoms.[2-7]

Although the left ventricle (LV) contrast angiogram was traditionally considered the gold standard for the measurement of LVEF, echocardiogram has become much more widely used for first-line assessment. LVEF measurements with echocardiogram have consistently shown a strong correlation with measurements by angiography, but with the benefits of decreased radiation exposure, lack of contrast dye complications, and decreased cost.[3,8,9]

With some degree of variability from facility to facility, echocardiograms have an estimated cost of approximately $800 per examination in the United States and can take an average of 46 minutes to complete.[10] Recently, through advancements in ultrasound technology as well as physician access to ultrasound

training, physicians are increasingly using point-of-care (POC) echocardiography. This allows instant feedback to the clinician for decision making. Rather than using the complex measurements and formulas incorporated into a formal echocardiogram, POC echocardiography typically grades LVEF by qualitative assessment or a few basic measurements.

Qualitative assessment of LVEF is dependent on provider experience but can be learned after relatively brief training. Rather than assessing for a precise percentage, function is graded as severely reduced (<30%), moderately reduced (30%-55%), or normal (>55%), which is as clinically useful as a precise EF in most cases. This is judged on the basis of the gross motion of the ventricular wall and septum viewed in several different planes. Cardiologists are routinely trained in echocardiography during their education and have been the subject of many POC echocardiogram studies.[11] When performed by cardiologists, studies suggest that a POC echocardiogram reduces need for formal studies and qualitative ventricular function assessment correlates with formal LVEF measurements with a specificity of 92%.[10,12] Noncardiologists with proper training can achieve similar results. One study showed medical residents with 3 months of training and at least 80 completed examinations were able to detect left ventricular dysfunction with a 92% sensitivity and 94% specificity.[13] Even short trainings can yield impressive results. One evaluation of noncardiology physicians with 3 hours of didactic training and five proctored scans showed a 92% agreement with normal function and 70.4% with poor function.[14]

Apart from using visual estimation of the left ventricular function to assess its ejection fraction, specific measurements have been studied that can be used to aid in the estimation of the LVEF. One of the most studied of such measurements is the E-point septal separation (EPSS).

During the rapid filling phase in early diastole, the anterior mitral-valve leaflet normally nearly touches the interventricular septum. The smallest distance of separation between the anterior leaflet of the mitral valve and the interventricular septum is the EPSS. This measurement has been shown to be a marker for LV function and is inversely correlated with the LVEF.[15] Most studies use a cutoff value of greater than 7 mm as abnormal.[15-18] Sensitivity and specificity for systolic dysfunction have been found to be roughly 83% to 100% and 50% to 75%, respectively.

Although EPSS can be very useful, it is important to also be aware of the limitations of the examination. Although it does give some quantifiable evidence to determine reduced ejection fraction, it does not allow for specific gradation of the severity of dysfunction.[19] Like all other forms of ultrasound, POC echocardiogram can be affected by artifact. Specifically, poor cardiac windows and endocardial dropout can affect measurements of the EPSS. Thus, even on a rapid bedside assessment, a qualitative assessment of LV function on the parasternal long-axis (PLAX) and parasternal short-axis (PSAX) views should still be obtained along with the EPSS measurement. Even if the study is perfectly performed, the LVEF must be interpreted in the clinical context and in the context of the entire echocardiogram, which may show signs of poor cardiac output despite a preserved LVEF. Such pathologies could include valvular stenosis or regurgitation, diastolic dysfunction, or hypertrophic obstructive cardiomyopathy.[20,21]

TABLE 8-1	Recommendations for Use of Point-of-Care Ultrasound in Clinical Practice		
Recommendation		**Rating**	**References**
Bedside echocardiogram can effectively detect the presence of left ventricle systolic dysfunction		A	10,12-14
The E-point of septal separation can be used to screen for a reduced left ventricle ejection fraction		A	15-18

A = consistent, good-quality patient-oriented evidence; B = inconsistent or limited-quality patient-oriented evidence; C = consensus, disease-oriented evidence, usual practice, expert opinion, or case series. For information about the SORT evidence rating system, go to http://www.aafp.org/afpsort.

PERFORMING THE SCAN

1. **Obtain PLAX view.** If possible, position the patient in the left lateral decubitus position to bring the heart closer to the chest wall and minimize left lung volume. If the patient is immobile, the examination may be performed in the dorsal recumbent position. Place a low-frequency cardiac probe on the left sternal border between the 4th and 5th intercostal space, with the probe marker pointed to the right shoulder. Manipulate as needed, moving up or down one interspace until the PLAX view is obtained. It should include the right ventricle, left ventricle, left atria, and aortic outflow track. Observe left ventricle squeeze, dilatation, symmetry, and thickness (**Figures 8-1 through 8-4** and ▶ **Videos 8-1 through 8-3**).

2. **Measure the EPSS.** To measure the EPSS in B-mode, capture a loop of the cardiac cycle and slowly scroll back in time to find the moment of end diastole. Identify the frame with the mitral valve at its maximum point of opening, and measure the distance between the valve and the intraventricular septum. This is the E-point of septal separation. The EPSS can also be measured in

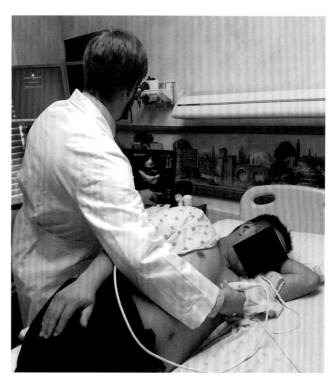

FIGURE 8-1. Proper patient positioning in the left lateral decubitus.

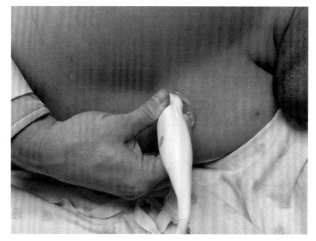

FIGURE 8-2. Probe placement for the parasternal long-axis view.

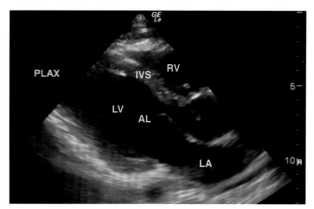

FIGURE 8-3. Parasternal long-axis (PLAX) view of normal heart at end diastole. AL, anterior leaflet of the mitral valve; IVS, interventricular septum; LA, left atrium; LV, left ventricle; RV, right ventricle.

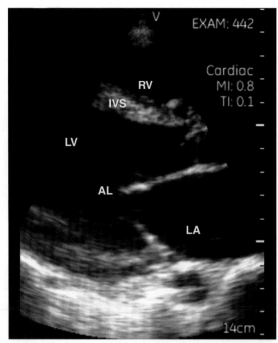

FIGURE 8-4. Parasternal long-axis view of heart with reduced left ventricular ejection fraction at end diastole. Note ventricular dilatation and poor mitral-valve excursion. AL, anterior leaflet of the mitral valve; IVS, interventricular septum; LA, left atrium; LV, left ventricle; RV, right ventricle.

M-mode, if available, by placing the M-mode spike over the tip of the mitral valve and measuring the minimal point of separation from the septum (**Figures 8-5 and 8-6**).

3. **Obtain PSAX view.** After the long-axis view has been obtained, center the probe just apical of the mitral valve and rotate 90 degrees, with the probe marker pointed to the left shoulder. The right ventricle should appear as a crescent wrapped around a circular-appearing left ventricle. Watch for even and strong contractions of this circle at three points along the ventricle, from the base (mitral-valve level) to the apex (**Figures 8-7 through 8-9** and ▶ **Videos 8-4 through 8-6**).

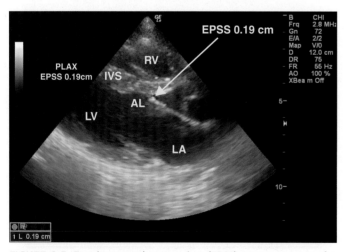

FIGURE 8-5. E-point septal separation (EPSS) measurement of a normal heart using B-mode. AL, anterior leaflet of the mitral valve; IVS, interventricular septum; LA, left atrium; LV, left ventricle; PLAX, parasternal long axis; RV, right ventricle.

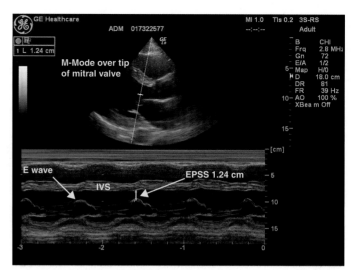

FIGURE 8-6. E-point septal separation (EPSS) measurement of a heart with reduced left ventricular ejection fraction using M-mode. IVS, interventricular septum.

PATIENT MANAGEMENT

Studies have shown that a POC echocardiogram assessment can be performed in as little as 6 minutes. Thus, the utility of the cardiac ultrasound in the POC setting is demonstrated by its ability to confirm or rule out a suspected diagnosis rapidly, and thereby decrease time to accurate diagnosis and treatment initiation.

When interpreting a POC echocardiogram that was done to evaluate left ventricular function, the examiner must consider the indication for performing the examination. The patient may have signs and symptoms that suggest a new diagnosis of left ventricular dysfunction, such as acute dyspnea with peripheral edema. Perhaps the patient has known left ventricular dysfunction, and there is a concern for new or worsening symptoms. Regardless, having a clear understanding of the indication will help the physician to understand how the evaluation of LV function will inform patient management. One example algorithm is provided (**Figure 8-10**).

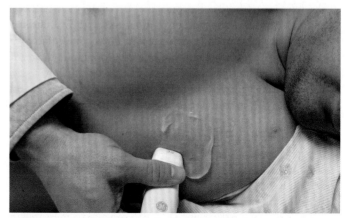

FIGURE 8-7. Probe placement for the parasternal short-axis view.

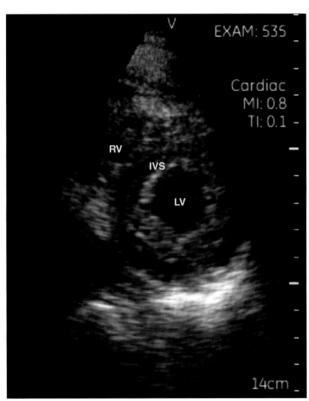

FIGURE 8-8. Parasternal short-axis view of a normal heart in systole. Left ventricle wall thickens and cavity contracts. IVS, interventricular septum; LV, left ventricle; RV, right ventricle.

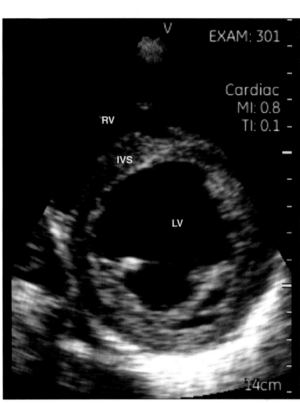

FIGURE 8-9. Parasternal short-axis view of heart with reduced ejection fraction in systole. Left ventricle wall thickens minimally and cavity minimally contracts. IVS, interventricular septum; LV, left ventricle; RV, right ventricle.

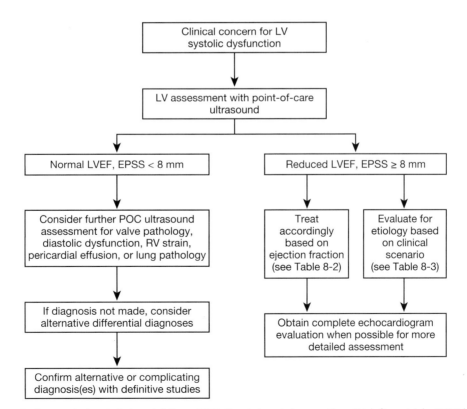

FIGURE 8-10. Management of suspected systolic heart failure. EPSS, E-point septal separation; LV, left ventricle; LVEF, left ventricular ejection fraction; POC, point-of-care; RV, right ventricle.

TABLE 8-2 **Recommended Treatment for Patients With Heart Failure With Reduced Ejection Fraction**[23-26]

Patient Characteristics	Treatment or Intervention	Mortality Reduction
Fluid retention	Diuretics	None, but can improve symptoms
All	ACEI	23%
ACEI intolerant	ARB	13%
On ACEI or ARB. NYHA class II-III symptoms. Adequate blood pressure	Angiotensin receptor-neprilysin inhibitor (must discontinue ACEI or ARB before starting)	20%
All	Beta blockers (only carvedilol, bisoprolol, and extended release metoprolol succinate have evidence for mortality benefit in heart failure)	34%
NYHA class II-IV symptoms. Creatinine clearance >30 mL/min. K$^+$ < 5.0 mEq/L.	Aldosterone antagonist	30%
On above treatments. African Americans with NYHA class III-IV symptoms	Hydralazine and isosorbide dinitrate	43%
NYHA class II-III symptoms. Sinus rhythm >70 beats/min and on maximally tolerated dose of a β-blocker	Ivabradine	None, but can decrease hospitalizations
Left ventricular ejection fraction <35%. On above treatments. NYHA class III-IV and left bundle branch block with QRS duration >150 ms and in sinus rhythm	CRT[a]	22%
Left ventricular ejection fraction <35%. On above treatments. NYHA class III-IV symptoms and life expectancy of >1 y	ICD	28%

This table is a guideline only. All interventions require consideration of full clinical context, including chronicity of the condition and comorbidities.

[a]CRT achieved through an atrial-synchronized biventricular pacemaker.

Abbreviations: ACEI, angiotensin converting enzyme inhibitor; ARB, angiotensin receptor blocker; CRT, cardiac resynchronization therapy; ICD, implantable cardioverter defibrillator; NYHA, New York Heart Association.

Should LV systolic dysfunction be confirmed, the physician may then initiate appropriate management immediately. While focusing on diuresis, afterload reduction and mortality reduction are important (**Table 8-2**). The clinician must not fail to address determining the etiology of the heart failure (**Table 8-3**). For a new onset heart failure case, this often merits a complete echocardiogram, cardiac catheterization either in the inpatient or in the ambulatory setting depending on acuity, and additional workup guided by the clinical context.

If reduced LVEF is ruled out or the diagnosis remains uncertain, the examiner should then consider alternative diagnoses. Many of these conditions can also be evaluated by POC ultrasound by inspecting the heart for pericardial effusion, right heart strain, valve dysfunction, or LV diastolic dysfunction. Further bedside evaluation by ultrasound may include examinations of the lungs for edema, consolidation, or effusion, or the vena cava for signs of distention.[22] This may lead to confirmation of an alternative diagnosis or continue to reduce the options remaining in the differential diagnosis. Additional diagnostic studies, including blood work and formal imaging, may be obtained on the basis of this narrowed differential.

TABLE 8-3 **Etiologies of New Onset or Worsening LV Heart Failure (Listed by Frequency per NHANES Database, Then Alphabetically)**[27,28]

	% Attributable Based on NHANES[27]
Coronary (ischemic) heart disease	61.6
Tobacco use	17.1
Hypertension	10.1
Obesity/overweight	8.0
Diabetes mellitus	3.1
Valvular or structural heart disease	2.2
Other endocrinopathy (hypothyroidism)	3.1
Connective tissue disease	
Electrolyte disturbance	
Idiopathic cause	
Infectious cardiomyopathy (HIV, Chagas)	
Infiltrative disease (multiple myeloma)	
Medication toxicity (doxorubicin)	
Acute myocarditis	
Peripartum cardiomyopathy	
Substance abuse (alcohol, cocaine)	

Abbreviations: LV, left ventricle; NHANES, National Health and Nutrition Examination Survey.

PEARLS AND PITFALLS

Pearls

- Apply plenty of gel for contact between rib spaces.
- The best cardiac window tends to be high on the chest in youth and lower on the chest in the elderly.
- Double check the orientation—in a cardiac mode the probe marker will be on the right side of the screen, unlike other ultrasound modes where it is on the left.

Pitfalls

- Never judge LVEF qualitatively from one view alone, which may be misleading; confirm in multiple views.
- Don't forget to ask the question "why" when a patient with reduced LVEF is identified.
- Don't assume a normal LVEF means normal cardiac output or even normal LV function; consider alternative diagnoses.

BILLING

CPT Code	Description	Global Payment	Professional Component	Technical Component
93308	Limited Transthoracic Echocardiogram	$126.03	$26.14	$99.89

CPT codes and average national reimbursement for Medicare in 2016. Payment data are from https://www.cms.gov/apps/physician-fee-schedule/search/search-criteria.aspx. See Chapter 2 for details on ultrasound billing.

References

1. Go AS, Mozaffarian D, Roger VL, et al. American Heart Association Statistics Committee and Stroke Statistics Subcommittee. Heart disease and stroke statistics—2013 update: a report from the American Heart Association. *Circulation*. 2013;127(1):e6-e245.
2. Curtis JP, Sokol SI, Wang Y, et al. The association of left ventricular ejection fraction, mortality, and cause of death in stable outpatients with heart failure. *J Am Coll Cardiol*. 2003;42(4):736-742.
3. Habash-Bseiso DE, Rokey R, Berger CJ, Weier AW, Chyou PH. Accuracy of noninvasive ejection fraction measurement in a large community-based clinic. *Clin Med Res*. 2005;3(2):75-82.
4. Grimm W, Glaveris C, Hoffmann J, et al. Noninvasive arrhythmia risk stratification in idiopathic dilated cardiomyopathy: design and first results of the Marburg Cardiomyopathy Study. *Pacing Clin Electrophysiol*. 1998;21:2551-2556.
5. Grimm W, Christ M, Bach J, Muller HH, Maisch B. Noninvasive arrhythmia risk stratification in idiopathic dilated cardiomyopathy: results of the Marburg Cardiomyopathy Study. *Circulation*. 2003;108:2883-2891.
6. Theal M, Demers C, Mckelvie RS. The role of angiotensin II receptor blockers in the treatment of heart failure patients. *Congest Heart Fail*. 2003;9:29-34.
7. Clarke CL, Grunwald GK, Allen LA, et al. Natural history of left ventricular ejection fraction in patients with heart failure. *Circ Cardiovasc Qual Outcomes*. 2013;6(6):680-686.
8. Witteles RM, Knowles JW, Perez M, et al. Use and overuse of left ventriculography. *Am Heart J*. 2012;163(4):617-623.
9. Garg N, Dresser T, Aggarwal K, et al. Comparison of left ventricular ejection fraction values obtained using invasive contrast left ventriculography, two-dimensional echocardiography, and gated single-photon emission computed tomography. *SAGE Open Med*. 2016;4:2050312116655940.
10. Khan HA, Wineinger NE, Uddin PQ, Mehta HS, Rubenson DS, Topol EJ. Can hospital rounds with pocket ultrasound by cardiologists reduce standard echocardiography? *Am J Med*. 2014;127(7):669.e1-669.e7.
11. Ryan T, Berlacher K, Lindner JR, Mankad SV, Rose GA, Wang A. COCATS 4 task force 5: training in echocardiography. *J Am Coll Cardiol*. 2015;65(17):1786-1799.
12. Kobal SL, Liel-Cohen N, Shimony S, et al. Impact of point-of-care ultrasound examination on triage of patients with suspected cardiac disease. *Am J Cardiol*. 2016;118(10):1583-1587.
13. Mjølstad OC, Andersen GN, Dalen H, et al. Feasibility and reliability of point-of-care pocket-size echocardiography performed by medical residents. *Eur Heart J Cardiovasc Imaging*. 2013;14(12):1195-1202.
14. Randazzo MR, Snoey ER, Levitt MA, Binder K. Accuracy of emergency physician assessment of left ventricular ejection fraction and central venous pressure using echocardiography. *Acad Emerg Med*. 2003;10(9):973-977.
15. McKaigney CJ, Krantz MJ, La Rocque CL, Hurst ND, Buchanan MS, Kendall JL. E-point septal separation: a bedside tool for emergency physician assessment of left ventricular ejection fraction. *Am J Emerg Med*. 2014;32(6):493-497.
16. Massie BM, Schiller NB, Ratshin RA, Parmley WW. Mitral-septal separation: new echocardiographic index of left ventricular function. *Am J Cardiol*. 1977;39(7):1008-1016.
17. Ahmadpour H, Shah AA, Allen JW, Edmiston WA, Kim SJ, Haywood LJ. Mitral E point septal separation: a reliable index of left ventricular performance in coronary artery disease. *Am Heart J*. 1983;106(1 Pt 1):21-28.
18. Elagha A, Fuisz A. Mitral valve E-point to septal separation (EPSS) measurement by cardiac magnetic resonance imaging as a quantitative surrogate of left ventricular ejection fraction (LVEF). *J Cardiovasc Magn Reson*. 2012;14(suppl 1):P154.
19. Silverstein JR, Laffely NH, Rifkin RD. Quantitative estimation of left ventricular ejection fraction from mitral valve E-point to septal separation and comparison to magnetic resonance imaging. *Am J Cardiol*. 2006;97(1):137-140.
20. Pislaru SV, Pellikka PA. The spectrum of low-output low-gradient aortic stenosis with normal ejection fraction. *Heart*. 2016;102(9):665-671.
21. Yıldırımtürk Ö, Helvacıoğlu FF, Tayyareci Y, Yurdakul S, Aytekin S. Subclinical left ventricular systolic dysfunction in patients with mild-to-moderate rheumatic mitral stenosis and normal left ventricular ejection fraction: an observational study. *Anadolu Kardiyol Derg*. 2013;13(4):328-336.
22. Anderson KL, Jenq KY, Fields JM, Panebianco NL, Dean AJ. Diagnosing heart failure among acutely dyspneic patients with cardiac, inferior vena cava, and lung ultrasonography. *Am J Emerg Med*. 2013;31(8):1208-1214.
23. Aronow WS. Update of treatment of heart failure with reduction of left ventricular ejection fraction. *Arch Med Sci Atheroscler Dis*. 2016;1(1):e106-e116.
24. Woods B, Hawkins N, Mealing S, et al. Individual patient data network meta-analysis of mortality effects of implantable cardiac devices. *Heart*. 2015;101(22):1800-1806. doi:10.1136/heartjnl-2015-307634.
25. McAlister FA, Ezekowitz J, Hooton N, et al. Cardiac resynchronization therapy for patients with left ventricular systolic dysfunction: a systematic review. *JAMA*. 2007;297(22):2502-2514.
26. Yancy CW, Jessup M, Bozkurt B, et al. 2017 ACC/AHA/HFSA focused update of the 2013 ACCF/AHA guideline for the management of heart failure: a report of the American College of Cardiology/American Heart Association Task Force on clinical practice guidelines and the Heart Failure Society of America. *J Am Coll Cardiol*. 2017;70(6):776-803.
27. He J, Ogden LG, Bazzano LA, Vupputuri S, Loria C, Whelton PK. Risk factors for congestive heart failure in US men and women: NHANES I epidemiologic follow-up study. *Arch Intern Med*. 2001;161(7):996-1002.
28. Felker GM, Thompson RE, Hare JM, et al. Underlying causes and long-term survival in patients with initially unexplained cardiomyopathy. *N Engl J Med*. 2000;342(15):1077-1084.

PART 2

Does the Patient Have Left Ventricular Hypertrophy?

Julian Reese, DO and Paul Bornemann, MD, RMSK, RPVI

● Clinical Vignette

A 60-year-old man presents to clinic for initial evaluation of high blood pressure, which was detected by his orthopedist. He has never been treated for hypertension. His only medical problem is osteoarthritis. His medications include ibuprofen as needed for pain and a daily multivitamin. In your office, seated blood pressure is 165/90 mm Hg. Additional blood pressure measured 5 minutes later is 140/90 mm Hg. His complete metabolic panel and electrocardiogram are normal. Out-of-office blood pressure measurements are unavailable. You want to know if the patient has any end organ damage that could help confirm an underlying diagnosis of hypertension. Does the patient have left ventricular hypertrophy?

LITERATURE REVIEW

In-office blood pressure measurements are easily obtained and commonly used for the diagnosis and management of hypertension. However, errors frequently occur, resulting in inaccurate measurements.[1] This can lead to overtreatment or undertreatment of hypertension. Studies estimate that 20% of patients with elevated in-office blood pressure readings have normal out-of-office blood pressure readings and that up to 20% of patients with normal in-office blood pressure readings have elevated out-of-office blood pressure readings.[2] Furthermore, another 30% of patients treated for persistently elevated in-office blood pressure readings have adequate out-of-office blood pressure readings.[3] Ultimately, three out of every four patients are treated inappropriately when in-office blood pressure readings are used exclusively to guide therapy.[2]

Out-of-office blood pressure measurements overcome many of these pitfalls. They are gaining favor owing to their improved accuracy over in-office blood pressure readings and have improved ability to predict long-term cardiovascular disease (CVD) outcomes. Several guidelines, including those from the U.S. Preventive Services Task Force (USPSTF); The Eighth Report of The Joint National Committee on Prevention, Detection, Evaluation, and Treatment of High Blood Pressure (JNC-8); and the 2017 American College of Cardiology/American Heart Association (ACC/AHA) guide for the Prevention, Detection, Evaluation, and Management of High Blood Pressure In Adults, recommend out-of-office blood pressure measurements for confirmation and titration of medication in hypertension.[1,4-7] Options for out-of-office measurements include ambulatory blood pressure measurement (ABPM) and home blood pressure measurement (HBPM). ABPM is the preferred out-of-office measurement and is considered the reference standard. Its use, however, is limited by the fact that results are not immediately available, it is expensive, and there is minimal reimbursement by third-party payers.[8-10] HBPM is often the clinical approach used when ABPM is unavailable. However, the effectiveness of this strategy is less well proven. Indeed, several studies have demonstrated lack of correlation between ambulatory readings to those obtained in the home.[11,12] Furthermore, home blood pressure readings are a poor predictor of future cardiovascular events when compared to ambulatory readings.[13] Despite the differences, both HBPM and ABPM have been shown to predict hypertensive target organ damage.[14] Their predictability, however, differs for different target organs, with ambulatory blood pressure being more closely associated with left ventricular mass (LVM) and development of left ventricular hypertrophy (LVH).[15]

In normal individuals, mass of the left ventricle (LV) is directly related to body size, with components attributable to lean body mass and obesity. Further increases or, at times, decreases in LVM may occur in response to a variety of stimuli such as exercise, valvular disease, and high blood pressure.[16] The process of increasing myocardial mass through cellular enlargement (hypertrophy) is a compensatory response to the increased volume or pressure load on the heart.[17] Depending on the underlying stimulus, different geometric patterns of hypertrophy result. The patterns are based on relative wall thickness (RWT), a ratio derived from left ventricular posterior wall thickness (PWT) and left ventricular internal diameter at end diastole (LVID$_d$)[18,19] (**Figure 9 -1**). For example, athletes who perform aerobic (isotonic) exercises such as running and swimming show a pattern of eccentric hypertrophy.[20,21] Those who perform anaerobic (isometric) exercises such as weightlifting and cross-training show a pattern of concentric hypertrophy.[20,21] In the athlete, the hypertrophy is physiologic and represents advantageous use of the Frank–Starling mechanism.

In contrast, LVH secondary to hypertension is pathologic and the result of chronic elevation in systemic blood pressure that disproportionately thickens left ventricular walls and reduces its chamber size.[22] Despite its initial adaptive nature, LVH, which is induced by hypertension, is associated with increased risk of risk sudden cardiac death, stroke, heart failure, and death after myocardial infarction.[23]

In patients with hypertension there is an incremental increase in LVM in response to increases in blood pressure.[23,24] Each increase in systolic blood pressure of 5 mm Hg is associated with an increase of 20 g in LVM.[24] The notion that LVM increases in a stepwise fashion was first demonstrated in a pioneering study by Mancia et al. In this study, LVH occurred with increasing frequency among subjects with normotension, recently discovered hypertension, and long-standing uncontrolled hypertension.[25] Several additional studies have also confirmed a clear and strong linear association between LVM and ABPM.[22,26,27] Notably, Devereux et al. demonstrated that LV mass is strongly related to ABPM and poorly correlated with in-office or HBPM.[17,23,28] Strikingly, the correlation between LVM and ambulatory blood pressure occurs across a wide range of blood pressures.[29,30] Indexing LVM for body surface area further strengthens the correlation. Additional methods of LV indexation

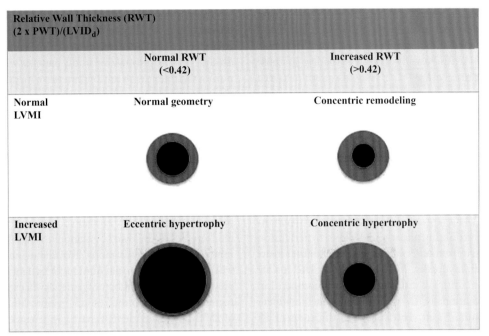

FIGURE 9 -1. Patterns of left ventricular remodeling. $LVID_d$, left ventricular internal diameter at end diastole; LVMI, left ventricular mass index; PWT, posterior wall thickness.

have also been described.[31] The methods of indexation are designed to normalize LVM for confounding variables and are also used to establish echocardiography criteria for LVH. Left ventricular mass index (LVMI) values above 95 g/m^2 for women and 115 g/m^2 for men define LVH[31] (**Table 9 -1**). Although increases in ambulatory blood pressure are associated with a higher LVMI and LVH, occasionally the increased LVMI does not reach hypertrophic values. However, parallel increases in blood pressure and LVMI place one at a higher risk for later developing LVH. As much as a 43% increase in relative risk has been reported.[32] Conversely, increases in LVMI in the absence of elevated blood pressure raises one's risk for developing high blood pressure later. In the Framingham Heart Study, adults with normotension or borderline high blood pressure and increased LVM later developed hypertension at follow-up.[32] Risk was directly related to LVM, with higher values indicating greater risk. Subsequent studies have confirmed the ability of high baseline values of LVM to predict increases in blood pressure independent of standard risk factors for hypertension.[33,34] Thus, increases in LVM and subsequent LVH are both a consequence

of and a precursor to hypertension, suggesting LVM is the ideal biomarker for evaluating and managing hypertension. Furthermore, it aids in the identification of various hypertensive phenotypes such as white coat hypertension (WCH), masked hypertension (MH), and uncontrolled hypertension.[35]

LVMI and the prevalence of LVH vary among groups with MH, WCH, normotension, and hypertension (**Figure 9 -2**). Isolated office hypertension, commonly referred to as WCH, is characterized as elevated in-office blood pressure but with normal blood pressure in the ambulatory setting. It involves up to 30% of patients with

TABLE 9 -1	Indexed Left Ventricular Mass Values with Reference Ranges for Left Ventricular Hypertrophy	
	Normal Range (g/m^2)	Left Ventricular Hypertrophy (g/m^2)
Left Ventricular Mass Assessment		
Left ventricular mass/ body surface area (BSA), women	43-95	>95
Left ventricular mass/ BSA, men	49-115	>115

Adopted from European Association of Cardiovascular Imaging (EACVI) and the American Society of Echocardiography (ASE).

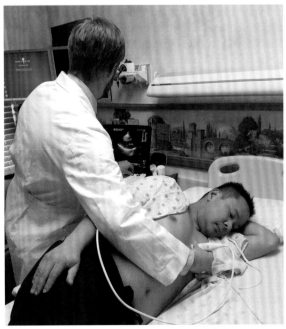

FIGURE 9 -2. Proper patient positioning in the left lateral decubitus. Provided courtesy of Mark Shaffer, MD, and Andrew Vaughan, MD.

hypertension in the office. Conversely, 37% to 50% of patients have MH, characterized as normal or prehypertensive in-office blood pressures but with elevated ambulatory blood pressure. Sega et al. demonstrated in the PAMELA study that LVMI is less in those with WCH than in those with MH.[25] They also demonstrated that LVH is less common in those with in-office hypertension and normal ambulatory blood pressures and more common in those with elevated ambulatory blood pressures.[20] Data from this study also agreed with previous correlations of LVMI and ABPM and also suggested that in the presence of elevated blood pressure (in or out of the office), cardiac structure stands a greater chance of being altered and therefore a higher likelihood of developing LVH. Thus, it is reasonable to conclude that in the absence of other stimuli, increased LVMI and LVH is representative of underlying hypertension. The challenge of attributing underlying LVH to hypertension requires differentiating it from other causes, namely, athlete's heart and hypertrophic cardiomyopathy (HCM). In the athlete, a slow resting heart rate and a history of training and sports competition are potential clues. Additionally, LV wall thickness in the athlete will rarely exceed 12 mm.[36] Left ventricular wall thickness of 15 mm or greater should raise suspicion for HCM.[37] Hypertensive LVH rarely approaches this value.

From a diagnostic point of view, LVH can be detected by electrocardiography (ECG) or echocardiography. ECG is inexpensive and perhaps the most readily available to clinicians. Although its specificity is high, its sensitivity is low, and thus ECG cannot be used to rule out LVH.[38] Echocardiography is much more sensitive than ECG and, if available, is the test of choice to assess for LVH.[39,40] Despite its superiority, guidelines including those from the 2017 AHA/ACC do not support the routine use of screening echocardiography for detection of LVH in the initial evaluation of hypertension. The cost associated with the inappropriate use of echocardiography appears to be the major factor driving current recommendations.[31,41]

Measurement of LV mass with point-of-care ultrasound (POCUS) devices bypasses many of the costs associated with formal echocardiography. Previously believed to be a measurement limited to those with specialized echocardiographic training, LVM can be measured using POCUS and limited echocardiography. Even those inexperienced primary care providers who are unfamiliar with POCUS can calculate LVM quickly and accurately with a few hours of training.[19,42] Use of POCUS ultrasound may be especially helpful in patients where the diagnosis of hypertension is not completely clear. The ACC/AHA guidelines recommend "Assessment of LVH in a patient with borderline hypertension without LVH on ECG to guide decision making regarding initiation of therapy. A limited goal-directed echocardiogram may be indicated for this purpose."[43]

Measurement of LVM requires measurement of the interventricular septum (IVS), posterior wall (PW), and internal diameter of LV cavity. LV mass is then calculated using the American Society of Echocardiography (ASE)-recommended Devereux's formula.[19] The formula subtracts LV cavity volume from the volume enclosed by the LV epicardial surface, then multiples this value by density to determine mass.[19] LVM is then indexed to body surface area (see above) to determine LVMI and presence of LVH (Table 9 -1). Calculation of RWT characterizes the pattern of LVH as concentric or eccentric (Figure 9 -1).

Therapy for established LVH improves survival, reduces cardiovascular morbidity, and improves myocardial performance.[44,45] Evidence benefiting the treatment of LVH was examined in The LIFE Study.[44] In this prospective study, patients who had a lower LVMI during treatment with antihypertensive medication had lower rates of cardiovascular morbidity and all-cause mortality. The results from this trial suggested a potential role not only for treating LVH but also for monitoring for a reduction LVMI, similar to the way hemoglobin A1C is used in diabetic patients. The ability to promote LVH regression differs among antihypertensive medications. The Treatment of Mild Hypertension Study (TOMHS) has shown that the long-acting diuretic chlorthalidone is slightly more effective than other agents.[27] A 2003 meta-analysis of antihypertensive medication in the treatment of LVH also showed that angiotensin receptor blockers (ARBs) followed by angiotensin-converting enzyme (ACE) inhibitors are also efficacious. Treatment-induced LVH regression will occur in a substantial number of patients with adequate blood pressure control.[46] A subset of patients will experience a lack of LVH regression despite optimal blood pressure control. The maintenance of LVH in these patients is partly independent of blood pressure, and modification of lifestyle and additional CVD risk factors may be of benefit.[46] Current guidelines do not make specific recommendations regarding the treatment of LV regression.[33,41]

TABLE 9 -2	**Recommendations for Use of Point-of-Care Ultrasound in Clinical Practice**	
Recommendation	**Rating**	**Reference**
Use limited goal-directed echocardiogram to guide treatment in patients with borderline hypertension without left ventricular hypertrophy on electrocardiography.	C	43

A = consistent, good-quality patient-oriented evidence; B = inconsistent or limited-quality patient-oriented evidence; C = consensus, disease-oriented evidence, usual practice, expert opinion, or case series. For information about the SORT evidence rating system, go to http://www.aafp.org/afpsort.

PERFORMING THE SCAN

1. **Preparation**. The patient should be in the supine position. It may be necessary to place him or her in the left lateral decubitus position with the left arm above the head to proximate the heart to the chest wall and to open the rib interspaces (Figure 9 -2).

2. **Parasternal long-axis view**. Once the patient is positioned in the proper orientation, a phased-array transducer is placed on the chest wall just left of the sternum in the 3rd or 4th intercostal space. The transducer marker should be pointed toward the patient's right shoulder. Tilt and slide the transducer to obtain the parasternal long-axis (PLAX) view (**Figure 9 -3**). In the optimal view, the aortic and mitral valves are just right of center, and the left ventricular walls are parallel to one another. The right ventricular outflow tract is seen in the near field (**Figure 9 -4**).

3. **Measurement of LVID_d**. The LV internal diameter is measured in the PLAX view in end diastole. Once this view is properly obtained, freeze the image and scroll to the frame immediately after mitral

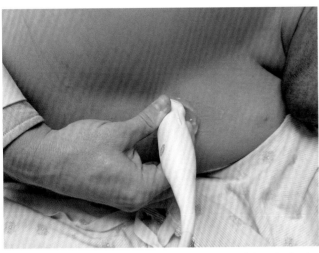

FIGURE 9-3. Probe placement for the parasternal long-axis view. Provided courtesy of Mark Shaffer, MD, and Andrew Vaughan, MD.

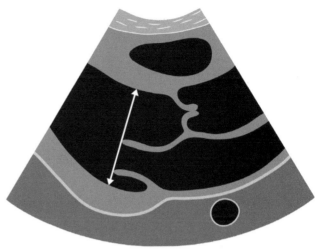

FIGURE 9-5. Left ventricular internal diameter at end diastole.

valve closure. This frame corresponds to end diastole and represents the largest cardiac diameter. Next, using the measurement function, position electronic calipers longitudinally at the tip of the mitral valve leaflets, between the interfaces of the myocardial walls and internal cavity perpendicular to the long axis of the LV (**Figure 9 -5**).

4. **Measurement of IVS and PWT**. Measure the thickness of the left ventricular walls at the same time that you measure $LVID_d$. To measure PWT, place electronic calipers at the interface between the left ventricular myocardial wall and the pericardium. IVS thickness is measured by placing electronic calipers between the septum at the internal cavity interfaces of the LV and right ventricle. The chordae tendineae and papillary muscles must be carefully excluded when measuring PWT and the moderator band from right ventricle cavity when measuring the IVS. Measurements should again be perpendicular to the long axis of the LV (**Figures 9-6 and 9-7**).

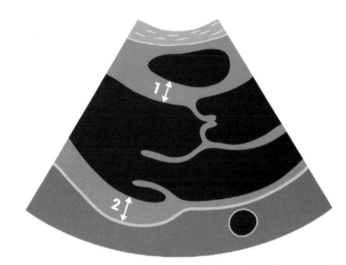

FIGURE 9-6. Interventricular septum (1) and posterior wall thickness (2).

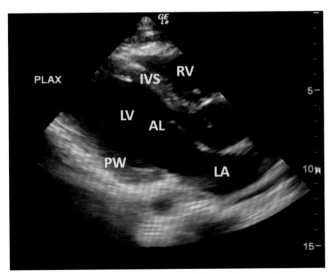

FIGURE 9-4. Parasternal long-axis (PLAX) view of normal heart at end diastole. AL, anterior leaflet of the mitral valve; IVS, interventricular septum; LA, left atrium; LV, left ventricle; PW, posterior wall of left ventricle; RV, right ventricle. Provided courtesy of Mark Shaffer, MD, and Andrew Vaughan, MD.

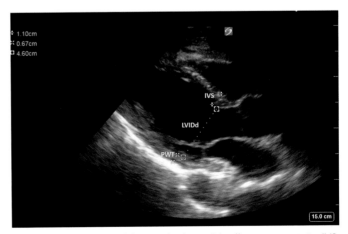

FIGURE 9-7. Parasternal long-axis view with all measurements. IVS, interventricular septum; $LVID_d$, left ventricular internal diameter at end diastole; PWT, posterior wall thickness.

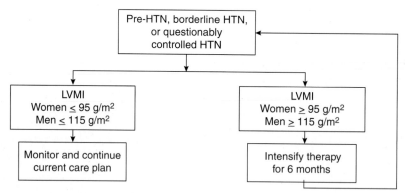

FIGURE 9-8. Left ventricular mass index (LVMI) algorithm for evaluation and management of hypertension (HTN).

5. **Determination of LVMI.** Calculate the LV mass using the preceding values for IVS, PWT, and LVID and Devereux's formula: $[(IVS_d + LVID_d + PWT_d)^3 - (LVID_d)^3] \times 1.05$. It is recommended to index the LV mass to the patient's body size by dividing the LV mass by the patient's calculated body surface area. The formula for body surface area is BSA (m^2) = $\sqrt{([Height (in) \times Weight (lb)]/3131)}$. For ease of use, an online calculator for LVMI is found at http://www.csecho.ca/wp-content/themes/twentyeleven-csecho/cardiomath/?eqnHD=echo&eqnDisp=lvmlvmi.

PATIENT MANAGEMENT

Measurement of blood pressure using proper tools is the first step in the evaluation and management of hypertension. Once an accurate measurement of the patient's blood pressure is obtained, the level of blood pressure can be categorized as normal, prehypertension, or stage 1 or stage 2 hypertension.

When in-office blood pressure measurements are elevated or in the prehypertensive range, ABPM is recommended for confirmation readings and to help further guide management. However, because it is not always available, and given that LVMI directly correlates with ABPM, we propose that bedside measurement of LVMI can serve as a surrogate. Thus, when ABPM is not available and in-office blood pressure is elevated, the next step is to measure LVMI. For those not currently receiving treatment, if LVH is demonstrated, therapy should be initiated. For patients who demonstrate LVH, it is important to document regression, and a 6-month follow-up is recommended to repeat LVMI. If a patient is already receiving treatment for hypertension and LVH is demonstrated, then adherence to therapy should be assessed, and intensification of antihypertensive therapy should be considered. Alternatively, if calculated LVMI is below the hypertrophic range, then antihypertensive therapy should be continued for those currently being treated for hypertension.

Antihypertensive therapy is usually not necessary for patients with elevated in-office blood pressures who have no history of hypertension when bedside LVMI is below the range for LVH. However, repeat LVMI in 6 months is advisable in these patients because of the greater tendency toward increases in LV mass and subsequent development of underlying hypertension and LVH.

It is important to always consider other causes of LVH such as HCM, and athlete's heart, especially when there is disagreement between blood pressure and expected LVMI. Athletes will have a PWT and IVS that are almost always less than 12 mm, an LVID$_d$ that is usually above 55 mm, a slow resting heart rate, and a history of training and sports competitions. In contrast, if the patient has a left ventricular wall thickness that exceeds 15 mm (in any segment) and/or LVID$_d$ that is less than 45 mm, then suspect pathologic LVH. A family history of sudden cardiac death and a systolic heart murmur are clues to the diagnosis of HCM. A formal echocardiogram and referral to a specialist should be considered in these cases (**Figure 9-8**).

PEARLS AND PITFALLS

Pearls

- Clearly define the endocardial border and structure you are measuring (do not measure what you cannot see!).
- Measurements do not have to be in a straight line but must be perpendicular to the structure being measured and in the basal section of the heart.
- An anechoic space separates the papillary muscle from the endocardial border of the PW. Include the papillary muscle in the measurements of LVID$_d$ to prevent underestimation.

- Be sure to scan up and down the chest between the different intercostal spaces starting near the sternum and moving laterally. Look for the best window where the PLAX view is clearly seen. Look at several different windows before choosing the best one.

If you are having difficulty finding a good window, be sure the patient is in the left lateral decubitus position, and then have him or her slowly exhale and hold their breath at end-exhalation. This will help reduce lung artifact that can shadow out the cardiac window.

Pearls and Pitfalls, Continued

Pitfalls

- Failure to identify the correct frame within the cardiac cycle. Remember, measurements are taken from the frame immediately after mitral valve closure (end diastole).
- Measuring right ventricular trabeculations (moderator band) as part of the IVS. Adjust gain and depth to clearly define the endocardial border of IVS and right ventricular trabeculations.

- Off-axis PLAX views result in an oblique section and can overestimate LVMI results. Avoid off-axis views by making sure the IVS and PW are parallel to one another.
- Some older adults will have a slightly S-shaped IVS, which is known as a "sigmoid septum." This is considered normal but can make the measurements of the left ventricular dimensions difficult. In this case, it is reasonable to take the measurements slightly more toward the apex than at the normal location at the tip of the mitral valve leaflets.

BILLING

CPT Code	Description	Global Payment	Professional Component	Technical Component
93308	Echocardiography, transthoracic, real time with image documentation (2D); follow-up or limited study	$125.75	$26.15	$99.60

CPT codes and average national reimbursement for Medicare in 2016. Payment data are from https://www.cms.gov/apps/physician-fee-schedule/search/search-criteria.aspx. See Chapter 2 for details on ultrasound billing.

References

1. Whelton PK, Carey RM, Aronow WS, et al. 2017 ACC/AHA/AAPA/ABC/ACPM/AGS/APhA/ASH/ASPC/NMA/PCNA guideline for the prevention, detection, evaluation, and management of high blood pressure in adults: executive summary: a report of the American College of Cardiology/American Heart Association Task Force on clinical practice guidelines. *Hypertension.* 2018;71(6):1269-1324.

2. Peacock J, Diaz KM, Viera AJ, Schwartz JE, Shimbo D. Unmasking masked hypertension: prevalence, clinical implications, diagnosis, correlates and future directions. *J Hum Hypertens.* 2014;28(9):521-528.

3. Vongpatanasin W. Resistant hypertension: a review of diagnosis and management. *JAMA.* 2014;311(21):2216-2224. Review. Erratum in: *JAMA.* 2014;312(11):1157.

4. Uhlig K, Balk EM, Patel K, et al. *Self-Measured Blood Pressure Monitoring: Comparative Effectiveness.* Rockville, MD: Agency for Healthcare Research and Quality (U.S.); 2012.

5. Margolis KL, Asche SE, Bergdall AR, et al. Effect of home blood pressure telemonitoring and pharmacist management on blood pressure control: a cluster randomized clinical trial. *JAMA.* 2013;310:46-56.

6. McManus RJ, Mant J, Haque MS, et al. Effect of self-monitoring and medication self-titration on systolic blood pressure in hypertensive patients at high risk of cardiovascular disease: the TASMIN-SR randomized clinical trial. *JAMA.* 2014;312:799-808.

7. Siu AL. Screening for high blood pressure in adults: U.S. Preventive Services Task Force recommendation statement. *Ann Intern Med.* 2015;163:778-786.

8. Krakoff LR. Cost-effectiveness of ambulatory blood pressure: a reanalysis. *Hypertension.* 2006;47(1):29-34.

9. Rickerby J. The role of home blood pressure measurement in managing hypertension: an evidence-based review. *J Hum Hypertens.* 2002;16(7):469-472. Review.

10. Krakoff LR, Eison H, Phillips RH, Leiman SJ, Lev S. Effect of ambulatory blood pressure monitoring on the diagnosis and cost of treatment for mild hypertension. *Am Heart J.* 1988;116(4):1152-1154.

11. Hodgkinson J, Mant J, Martin U, et al. Relative effectiveness of clinic and home blood pressure monitoring compared with ambulatory blood pressure monitoring in diagnosis of hypertension: systematic review. *BMJ.* 2011;342:d3621.

12. Stergiou GS, Salgami EV, Tzamouranis DG, Roussias LG. Masked hypertension assessed by ambulatory blood pressure versus home blood pressure monitoring: is it the same phenomenon? *Am J Hypertens.* 2005;18:772-778.

13. Mancia G, Facchett R, Bombelli M, Grassi G, Sega R. Long-term risk of mortality associated with selective and combined elevation in office, home, and ambulatory blood pressure. *Hypertension.* 2006;47:846-853.

14. Bliziotis IA, Destounis A, Stergiou GS. Home versus ambulatory and office blood pressure in predicting target organ damage in hypertension: a systematic review and meta-analysis. *J Hypertens.* 2012;30(7):1289-1299.

15. Hara A, Tanaka K, Ohkubo T, et al. Ambulatory versus home versus clinic blood pressure: the association with subclinical cerebrovascular disease: the Ohasama Study. *Hypertension.* 2012;59(1):22-28.

16. Katholi RE, Couri DM. Left ventricular hypertrophy: major risk factor in patients with hypertension: update and practical clinical applications. *Int J Hypertens.* 2011;2011:495349.

17. Devereux RB, Roman MJ. Left ventricular hypertrophy in hypertension: stimuli, patterns, and consequences. *Hypertens Res.* 1999;22(1):1-9.

18. Verma A, Meris A, Skali H, et al. Prognostic implications of left ventricular mass and geometry following myocardial infarction: the VALIANT (VALsartan In Acute myocardial iNfarcTion) Echocardiographic Study. *JACC Cardiovasc Imaging.* 2008;1(5):582-591.

19. Marwick TH, Gillebert TC, Aurigemma G, et al. Recommendations on the use of echocardiography in adult hypertension: a report from the European Association of Cardiovascular Imaging (EACVI) and the American Society of Echocardiography (ASE)†. *Eur Heart J Cardiovasc Imaging.* 2015;16(6):577-605.

20. Morganroth J, Maron BJ, Henry WL, Epstein SE. Comparative left ventricular dimensions in trained athletes. *Ann Intern Med.* 1975;82(4):521-524.

21. Sugishita Y, Koseki S, Matsuda M, Yamaguchi T, Ito I. Myocardial mechanics of athletic hearts in comparison with diseased hearts. *Am Heart J.* 1982;105(2):273-280.

22. Verdecchia P, Carini G, Circo A, et al. Left ventricular mass and cardiovascular morbidity in essential hypertension: the MAVI study. *J Am Coll Cardiol.* 2001;38(7):1829-1835.

23. Devereux RB, Pickering TG, Harshfield GA, et al. Left ventricular hypertrophy in patients with hypertension: importance of blood pressure response to regularly recurring stress. *Circulation.* 1983;68:470-476.

24. Iso H, Kiyama M, Doi M, et al. Left ventricular mass and subsequent blood pressure changes among middle-aged men in rural and urban Japanese populations. *Circulation.* 1994;89(4):1717-1724.

25. Mancia G, Carugo S, Grassi G, et al; Pressioni Arteriose Monitorate E Loro Associazioni (PAMELA) Study. Prevalence of left ventricular hypertrophy in hypertensive patients without and with blood pressure control: data from the PAMELA population. Pressioni Arteriose Monitorate E Loro Associazioni. *Hypertension.* 2002;39(3):744-749.

26. Sokolow M, Werdegar S, Kain H, Hinman AT. Relationship between level of blood pressure measured casually and by portable recorders and severity of complications in essential hypertension. *Circulation.* 1966;34:279-298.

PART 2

27. Giaconi S, Levanti C, Fommei E, et al. Microalbuminuria and casual and ambulatory blood pressure monitoring in normotensives and in patients with borderline and mild essential hypertension. *Am J Hypertens*. 1989;2:259.

28. Omboni S, Ravogli A, Parati G, et al. Prognostic value of ambulatory blood pressure monitoring. *J Hypertens*. 1991;9(suppl 3):S25-S28.

29. Stanton A, Mullaney PB, Mee F, O'Malley K, O'Brien ET. Fundal blood vessel alterations are associated with mild-to-moderate hypertension. *J Hypertens*. 1991;9(suppl 6):S488.

30. American College of Cardiology Foundation Appropriate Use Criteria Task Force; American Society of Echocardiography; American Heart Association; Douglas PS, Garcia MJ, Haines DE, et al. ACCF/ASE/AHA/ANSC/HFSA/HRS/SCAI/SCCM/SCCT/SCMR 2011 appropriate use criteria for echocardiography. A report of the American college of cardiology foundation appropriate use criteria task force, American society of echocardiography, American heart association, American society of nuclear cardiology, heart failure society of America, heart rhythm society, society for cardiovascular angiography and interventions, society of critical care medicine, society of cardiovascular computed tomography, society for cardiovascular magnetic resonance American college of chest physicians. *J Am Soc Echocardiogr*. 2011;24:229-267.

31. Post WS, Larson MG, Levy D. Impact of left ventricular structure on the incidence of hypertension: the Framingham Heart Study. *Circulation*. 1994;90:179-185.

32. De Simone G, Devereux RB, Roman MJ, Schlussel Y, Alderman MH, Laragh JH. Echocardiographic left ventricular mass and electrolyte intake predict subsequent arterial hypertension in initially normotensive adults. *Ann Intern Med*. 1991;114:202.

33. Sega R, Trocino G, Lanzarotti A, et al. Alterations of cardiac structure in patients with isolated office, ambulatory, or home hypertension: data from the general population (Pressione Arteriose Monitorate E Loro Associazioni [PAMELA] Study). *Circulation*. 2001;104(12):1385-1392.

34. Cuspidi C, Sala C, Tadic M, Rescaldani M, Grassi G, Mancia G. Untreated masked hypertension and subclinical cardiac damage: a systematic review and meta-analysis. *Am J Hypertens*. 2015;28(6):806-813.

35. Pelliccia A, Maron BJ, Spataro A, Proschan MA, Spirito P. The upper limit of physiologic cardiac hypertrophy in highly trained elite athletes. *N Engl J Med*. 1991;324(5):295-301.

36. Maron BJ, Pelliccia A, Spirito P. Cardiac disease in young trained athletes. Insights into methods for distinguishing athlete's heart from structural heart disease, with particular emphasis on hypertrophic cardiomyopathy. *Circulation*. 1995;91(5):1596-1601.

37. Okin PM, Roman MJ, Devereux RB, Kligfield P. Electrocardiographic identification of left ventricular hypertrophy: test performance in relation to definition of hypertrophy and presence of obesity. *J Am Coll Cardiol*. 1996;27(1):124-131.

38. Klingbeil AU, Schneider M, Martus P, Messerli FH, Schmieder RE. A meta-analysis of the effects of treatment on left ventricular mass in essential hypertension. *Am J Med*. 2003;115(1):41-46.

39. Cuspidi C, Ambrosioni E, Mancia G, et al. Role of echocardiography and carotid ultrasonography in stratifying risk in patients with essential hypertension: the assessment of prognostic risk observational survey. *J Hypertens*. 2002;20:1307.

40. Lee JH, Park JH. Role of echocardiography in clinical hypertension. *Clin Hypertens*. 2015;21:9.

41. Bornemann P, Johnson J, Tiglao S, et al. Assessment of primary care physicians' use of a pocket ultrasound device to measure left ventricular mass in patients with hypertension. *J Am Board Fam Med*. 2015;28(6):706-712.

42. Devereux RB, Dahlöf B, Gerdts E, et al. Regression of hypertensive left ventricular hypertrophy by losartan compared with atenolol: the Losartan Intervention for Endpoint Reduction in Hypertension (LIFE) trial. *Circulation*. 2004;110(11):1456-1462.

43. Cheitlin MD, Armstrong WF, Aurigemma GP, et al. American College of Cardiology; American Heart Association; American Society of Echocardiography. ACC/AHA/ASE 2003 guideline update for the clinical application echocardiography: summary article: a report of the American College of Cardiology/American Heart Association Task Force on Practice Guidelines (ACC/AHA/ASE Committee to Update the 1997 Guidelines for the Clinical Application of Echocardiography). *Circulation*. 2003;108(9):1146-1162.

44. Liebson PR, Grandits GA, Dianzumba S, et al. Comparison of five antihypertensive monotherapies and placebo for change in left ventricular mass in patients receiving nutritional-hygienic therapy in the Treatment of Mild Hypertension Study (TOMHS). *Circulation*. 1995;91:698-706.

45. Pierdomenico SD, Lapenna D, Cuccurullo F. Regression of echocardiographic left ventricular hypertrophy after 2 years of therapy reduces cardiovascular risk in patients with essential hypertension. *Am J Hypertens*. 2008;21(4):464-470.

46. Lønnebakken MT, Izzo R, Mancusi C, et al. Left ventricular hypertrophy regression during antihypertensive treatment in an outpatient clinic (the Campania Salute Network). *J Am Heart Assoc*. 2017;6(3). doi:10.1161/JAHA.116.004152.

Does the Patient Have a Pericardial Effusion?

Mark E. Shaffer, MD

• Clinical Vignette

A 35-year-old woman from East Africa comes to your office with chest tightness, shortness of breath, and dizziness. Symptoms have been worsening for weeks to months and are now affecting her daily activities. An examination reveals mild tachycardia and hypotension (HR 109 BP 80/60). She has clear lung sounds throughout, distant heart sounds, and elevated jugular venous pressure. From her history, you know she has had many exposures to tuberculosis. Does the patient have a pericardial effusion?

LITERATURE REVIEW

Pericardial effusion refers to a pathologic level of fluid in the pericardial cavity surrounding the heart. The causes of pericardial effusions are numerous. Worldwide, tuberculosis is a dominant cause of both massive slow-growing effusions and constrictive pericarditis. Other common causes in developed nations include neoplasm, trauma, congestive heart failure, myocardial infarction, and aortic dissection.[1,2] A physician may consider evaluating for pericardial effusion on the basis of patient symptoms or when assessing for asymptomatic complications of a known disease process, such as tuberculosis in a patient with acquired immunodeficiency syndrome. Bedside point-of-care ultrasound by the physician can easily demonstrate the presence of an effusion, characterize the effusion, and provide evidence for the presence or absence of pericardial tamponade.

Identifying and Characterizing the Effusion

Early in embryonic development, membranes form which divide our body into discrete chambers. Even before our dominant blood vessels twist into heart shape, they are bound within a primitive pericardial cavity bordered by what will be the fibrous pericardium.[1] This cavity is usually filled by a small quantity (<50 mL) of lubricating material, which may be seen as a small anechoic retrocardiac streak on echocardiogram. Any fluid beyond this amount is considered pathologic and must be addressed.[2] The detection of pericardial effusion is easily performed by bedside ultrasound with sensitivities of over 95% by noncardiologist physician sonographers.[3,4] The size of the effusion can be described by measuring in one dimension the greatest depth of the effusion. Fluid accumulation that is more than trace but less than 1 cm and located predominantly in the posterior atrioventricular groove is considered small and is likely under 300 mL. Effusions measuring 1 to 2 cm in size are possibly seen around the entire heart and are considered moderate, roughly 300 to 700 mL. Large effusions are greater than 2 cm in size and may contain more than 700 mL[1] (Table 10-1).

TABLE 10-1 Sensitivity and Specificity of Echocardiography Findings for Pericardial Tamponade

Finding	Sensitivity	Specificity	Comments
Inferior vena cava distention	97%	40%	Seen with many conditions
Right atrium collapse	50%-100%	33%-100%	100% specificity if defined as 1/3 cycle length
Right ventricle diastolic collapse	48%-100%	72%-100%	Less sensitive in setting of right ventricular hypertrophy

Adapted by permission from Springer: Guntheroth WG. Sensitivity and specificity of echocardiographic evidence of tamponade: implications for ventricular interdependence and pulsus paradoxus. *Pediatr Cardiol.* 2007;28(5):358-362. Copyright © 2007 Springer Nature.

In addition to size, the examiner must also pay attention to the quality of the effusion to aid in the differential diagnosis. Purely anechoic lesions are most likely serous, whereas particulate or echogenic material suggests infectious, inflammatory, or hemorrhagic material (Table 10-2).

Pericardial Tamponade

Pericardial tamponade is an emergent, potentially life-threatening condition in which the pressure in the pericardial sac has increased to be equal or greater than that of the right ventricle (RV). This prevents filling of the RV during diastole and leads to pulses paradoxus and findings of right heart failure such as increased jugular venous distention. As pressures increase, the patient develops tachycardia and hypotension and eventually cardiovascular collapse. Pericardial tamponade can occur at low volumes of effusion (150-200 mL) if rapidly accumulating as in trauma or pericarditis.[5] Although subacute presentations do occur, many cases of pericardial tamponade are truly life-threatening emergencies, and a rapid diagnosing of the condition by bedside ultrasound may be essential in performing life-saving pericardiocentesis in a timely manner.

TABLE 10-2 Causes of Pericardial Effusion

Etiology	Examples
Neoplastic	Cardiac, leukemia/lymphoma or metastatic from lung, breast, or melanoma
Infectious	Viral, bacterial, mycobacterial, parasitic
Traumatic	Trauma, iatrogenic, aortic dissection
Cardiac	Postmyocardial infarction, congestive heart failure
Other	Uremia, collagen vascular disease, radiation therapy, idiopathic

Echocardiographic evidence for tamponade mirrors clinical findings. The single most sensitive finding is a dilated, nonresponsive inferior vena cava (IVC), suggesting elevated right-sided filling pressures. This is not a very specific finding but is concerning for emerging tamponade, given the presence of a pericardial effusion. Right atrial collapse is more specific, especially if it lasts over one-third of the cardiac cycle.[6] Even more specific but less sensitive is right ventricular collapse.[7] The ventricle is seen to constrict with systole and then not open immediately with diastole. As the pericardium becomes constricted, the intraventricular septum may be visualized bouncing back and forth between right and left heart to pump blood, rather than the chambers dilating and contracting as usual. This is also known as a "dancing" or "bouncing" septum. In more advanced cases, the left heart chambers may also show collapse. Overall sensitivity and specificity estimates are given in Table 10-1.[8] More and more data suggest that pericardial tamponade is just one end of a spectrum of pericardial disease and that even small effusions may have hemodynamic effects on cardiac output.

Pericardiocentesis

Pericardial fluid may need to be drained for emergent relief of tamponade or for diagnostic purposes. Options include bedside pericardiocentesis, pericardial drain placement, and pericardectomy performed by video-assisted thoracoscopic surgery or thoracotomy. Bedside ultrasound greatly aids the performance of pericardiocentesis, but the procedure should be performed only by appropriately trained medical professionals with careful cardiac monitoring. Complications can include arrhythmia and ventricular rupture, which may be life threatening.[9]

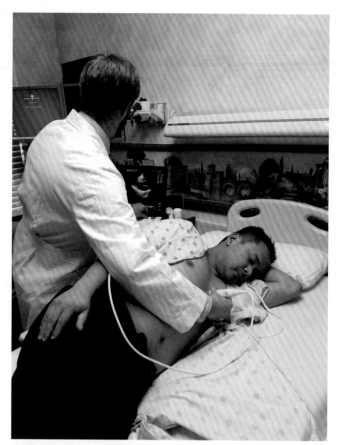

FIGURE 10-1. Proper patient positioning in the left lateral decubitus position.

TABLE 10-3	Recommendations for Use of Point-of-Care Ultrasound in Clinical Practice	
Recommendation	Rating	References
Bedside ultrasound can effectively detect the presence of pericardial effusion.	A	5, 6
Bedside ultrasound can effectively detect a pericardial tamponade.	A	8, 9

A = consistent, good-quality patient-oriented evidence; B = inconsistent or limited-quality patient-oriented evidence; C = consensus, disease-oriented evidence, usual practice, expert opinion, or case series. For information about the SORT evidence rating system, go to http://www.aafp.org/afpsort.

PERFORMING THE SCAN

1. **Prepare the patient for bedside echocardiogram.** Explain to the patient what to expect from your exam as well as possible findings and limitations. The patient should be draped to expose the anterior chest and upper abdomen and positioned in left lateral decubitus position initially. A cardiac probe with acardiac preset is ideal for the exam. An abdominal probe will work as well, but note that the probe marker will be reversed if an abdominal preset is used. Apply a sufficient quantity of gel to assure good contact with the chest wall (**Figure 10-1**).

2. **Obtain a parasternal long-axis view.** Position the probe on the patient's chest along the left sternal border between the third and fourth ribs. Aim the probe marker to the patient's right

shoulder. If the heart cannot be visualized, shift up or down one intercostal space. Once the heart is visualized, manipulate the probe slightly to obtain the parasternal long-axis view including the RV, left ventricle (LV), and left atrium. Adjust depth to ensure that the posterior border of the heart is well seen. Assess for the presence of an effusion, measure its size if present, and note the echogenicity. Next, assess for signs of tamponade by observing the RV and left atrial filling and intraventricular septal motion (**Figures 10-2 through 10-4**).

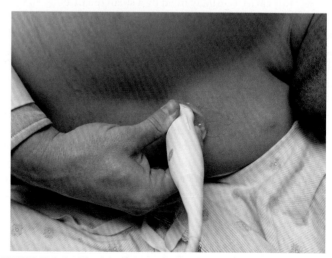

FIGURE 10-2. Positioning of the probe for the parasternal long-axis view.

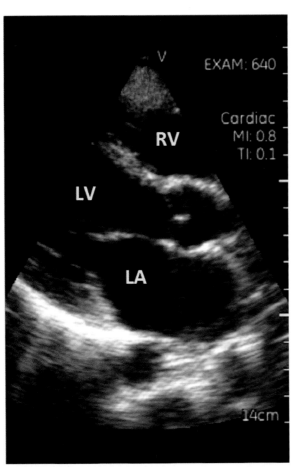

FIGURE 10-3. A normal parasternal long-axis view in mid-diastole. LA, left atrium; LV, left ventricle; RV, right ventricle.

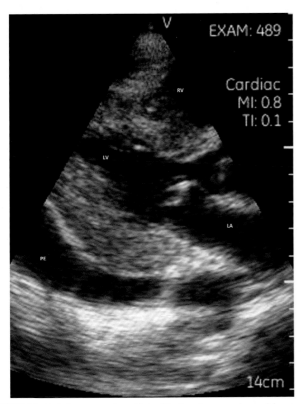

FIGURE 10-4. A large pericardial effusion in parasternal long-axis view—note anterior and posterior anechoic regions. LA, left atrium; LV, left ventricle; PE, pericardial effusion; RV, right ventricle.

3. **Obtain a four-chamber subcostal view.** Have the patient lie supine with knees bent. Place cardiac probe 3 to 4 cm below the xiphoid process in a vertical position with a probe marker to the patient's left. Flatten the angle of the probe until all four chambers of the heart are visible, which may require slight pressure into the abdomen and an anterior angulation. This view uses the liver as a window to reveal the RVs and LVs, and atria and is one of the most sensitive views for a pericardial effusion and the most likely to be used in ultrasound-guided pericardiocentesis (**Figures 10-5 through 10-7**).

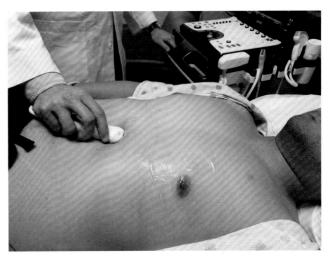

FIGURE 10-5. Proper probe placement for the four-chamber subcostal view.

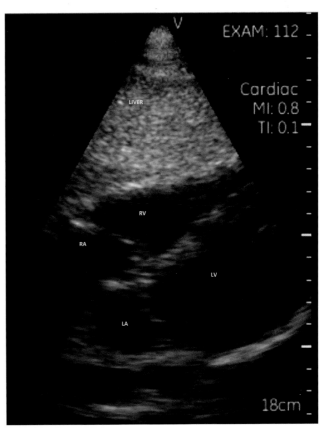

FIGURE 10-6. A normal four-chamber subcostal view of the heart through the liver. LA, left atrium; LV, left ventricle; RA, right atrium; RV, right ventricle.

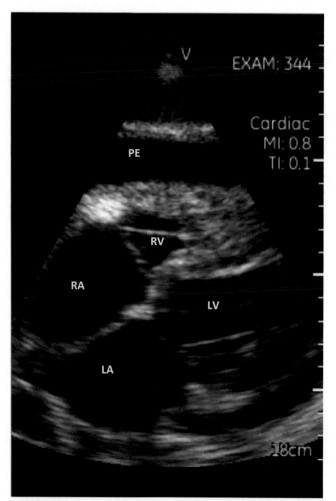

FIGURE 10-7. A large pericardial effusion in a four-chamber subcostal view. LA, left atrium; LV, left ventricle; PE, pericardial effusion; RA, right atrium; RV, right ventricle.

4. **Obtain an IVC subcostal view.** With the patient in supine position, place probe 3 to 4 cm below the xyphoid just right of the midline, with the probe marker pointed to the patient's head. Use gentle downward pressure and slight upward angulation to view the IVC passing through the liver and its entry into the right atrium. Measure the diameter of the IVC at rest, which should be less than 20 mm. Observe the diameter as the patient takes a rapid breath in—the sniff test—which should cause the IVC diameter to decrease by over 50% (**Figures 10-8 through 10-10**).

PATIENT MANAGEMENT

Beside ultrasound for pericardial effusion will yield three possible results: no pathologic effusion, pathologic effusion without tamponade, or pathologic effusion with signs of tamponade (▶ **Videos 10-1 and 10-2**). The findings of the tamponade can also be seen in the setting of constrictive pericarditis, but this is outside the scope of this chapter.

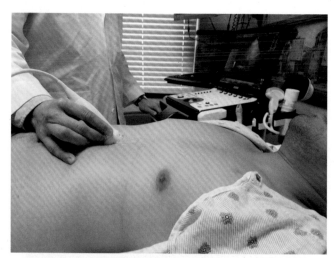

FIGURE 10-8. Proper probe placement for the inferior vena cava subcostal view.

Most echocardiograms will reveal no effusion or a trace physiologic effusion not contributing to the patient's presentation, and therefore, other causes for the symptoms must be found.

If a pathologic effusion is noted without signs of tamponade, it may not be the direct cause of symptoms, and other options must be explored, as stated earlier. If the effusion is significant,

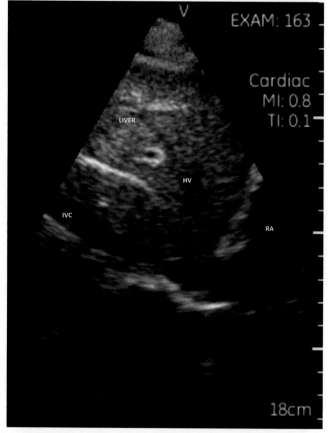

FIGURE 10-9. A normal inferior vena cava (IVC) with a positive "sniff" test—near collapse with inhalation. HV, hepatic vein; RA, right atrium.

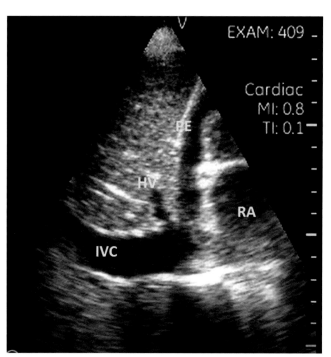

FIGURE 10-10. An abnormal, dilated inferior vena cava (IVC) with negative sniff. Pericardial effusion noted as the IVC approaches the right atrium. HV, hepatic vein; PE, pericardial effusion; RA, right atrium.

periodic reassessment for tamponade is recommended as the patient's condition may change rapidly, especially if there is a decrease in preload. Keep in mind that the amount of fluid present does not correlate directly with the risk of tamponade. The rapidity in whichever fluid collects is a much more important factor. After the patient is otherwise stabilized, the risks and benefits of nonemergent pericardiocentesis must be considered. Pericardiocentesis may be performed for diagnostic or therapeutic indications. Furthermore, information like bacterial culture results can be helpful to guide treatment. In a controlled prepared environment, the risk for major complications is low at 1.2%.[9]

Emergent pericardiocentesis is warranted for any echocardiographic findings of tamponade when concordant with the patient's clinical presentation. Under these circumstances it is a life-saving procedure but also carries a risk of arrhythmia, ventricular puncture, and death. Therefore, it should be performed by the most skilled provider in the most controlled environment possible. Ultrasound may be used during the procedure, guiding the physician to the largest pocket of fluid and optimal approach. Many cases will require drain placement or pericardectomy. Note that emergent pericardiocentesis is not indicated for ultrasound findings of tamponade in the patient who is clinically asymptomatic (**Figure 10-11**).

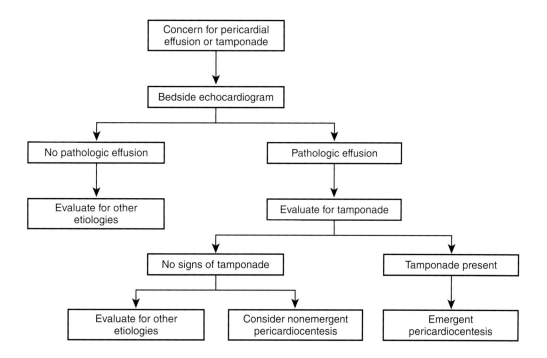

FIGURE 10-11. Basic algorithm for management of pericardial effusion. IVC, inferior vena cava.

Grading of Effusions

Size	Volume	Measurement
Trace	Trace	Trace, nonpathologic
Small	<300 cc	<1 cm posterior only
Moderate	300–700 cc	1–2 cm, circumferential
Large	>700 cc	<2 cm, circumferential

Findings of Tamponade

Ultrasound	Clinical
Distended IVC	Tachycardia
Right atrium collapse	Hypotension
Right ventricle diastolic collapse	Pulsus paradoxus

PART 2

PEARLS AND PITFALLS

Pearls

- Pericardial effusions stay anterior to the descending thoracic aorta, pleural effusions stay posterior. Obtain multiple views to clarify if needed.
- Pericardial effusion patients are preload dependent—avoid diuresis if there is any concern about tamponade.

Pitfalls

- PE may be present but not the cause of the patient's symptoms; look for other causes as well.
- Many patients have a pericardial fat pad, which may be confused for an effusion. This is typically only anterior and is partially echoic thus distinguishable from a mild effusion (**Figure 10-12**).
- Right heart chambers will not collapse if right heart pressures are high enough due to another cause (cor pulmonale), even in a true tamponade.

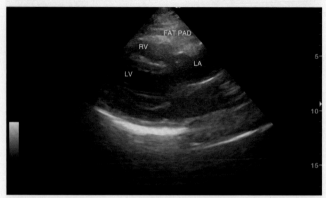

FIGURE 10-12. Parasternal long-axis view of a normal heart with a pericardial fat pad. LA, left atrium; LV, left ventricle; RV, right ventricle.

BILLING

CPT Code	Description	Global Payment	Professional Component	Technical Component
93308	Limited transthoracic echocardiogram	$126.03	$26.14	$99.89

CPT codes and average national reimbursement for Medicare in 2016. Payment data are from https://www.cms.gov/apps/physician-fee-schedule/search/search-criteria.aspx. See Chapter 2 for details on ultrasound billing.

References

1. Sadler TW. *Langman's Medical Embryology*. 9th ed. Philadelphia, PA: Lippincott Williams and Wilkins; 2004.
2. Dudzinski DM, Mak GS, Hung JW. Pericardial diseases. *Curr Probl Cardiol.* 2012;37(3):75-118. doi:10.1016/j.cpcardiol.2011.10.002.
3. Mandavia DP, Hoffner RJ, Mahaney K, Henderson SO. Bedside echocardiography by emergency physicians. *Ann Emerg Med.* 2001;38(4):377-382.
4. Labovitz AJ, Noble VE, Bierig M. Focused cardiac ultrasound in the emergent setting: a consensus statement of the American Society of Echocardiography and American College of Emergency Physicians. *J Am Soc Echocardiogr.* 2010;23(12):1225-1230. doi:10.1016/j.echo.2010.10.005.
5. Cummings K, Green D, Johnson W, Javidan-Nejad, C, Bhalla S. Imaging of pericardial diseases. *Semin Ultrasound CT MR.* 2016;37(3):238-254. doi:10.1053/j.sult.2015.09.001.
6. Gillam LD, Guyer DE, Gibson TC, King ME, Marshall JE, Weyman AE. Hydrodynamic compression of the right atrium: a new echocardiographic sign of cardiac tamponade. *Circulation.* 1983;68(2):294-301.
7. Argulian E, Messerli F. Misconceptions and facts about pericardial effusion and tamponade. *Am J Med.* 2013;126(10):858-861. doi:10.1016/j.amjmed.2013.03.022.
8. Guntheroth WG. Sensitivity and specificity of echocardiographic evidence of tamponade: implications for ventricular interdependence and pulsus paradoxus [review]. *Pediatr Cardiol.* 2007;28(5):358-362.
9. Tsang TS, Enriquez-Sarano M, Freeman WK, et al. Consecutive 1127 therapeutic echocardiographically guided pericardiocenteses: clinical profile, practice patterns and outcomes spanning 21 years. *Mayo Clin Proc.* 2002;77(5):429-436.

Does the Patient Have Right Heart Strain?

Mark E. Shaffer, MD and Joseph C. Lai, DO

● Clinical Vignette

A 55-year-old man with a past history significant for hypertension and hyperlipidemia presents to the emergency department for shortness of breath, chest pain, and right lower extremity swelling after a trans-Atlantic flight. Patient's vitals currently read HR: 115, BP: 85/49, R: 26, T: 99.7, Sao_2: 85% on RA (improves to 95% on high flow oxygen). An electrocardiogram shows no ST segment elevation but does have nonspecific T-wave abnormalities. You are clinically concerned about a pulmonary embolism (PE). Does the patient have right heart strain?

LITERATURE REVIEW

By strict definition, right heart strain is a measurement referring to the percent change in myocardial deformation in the right ventricle (RV) during systole.[1] More commonly among clinicians the term is used to refer to the presence of RV systolic dysfunction or RV chamber hypertrophy. The role of ultrasound in patients with RV strain is to better define the condition, prioritize further testing, and assist with treatment decisions. Although this chapter focuses on right heart strain related to PE, it is important to review the echocardiographic findings of chronic right heart strain that are frequently encountered in primary care. Most causes of right heart strain are related to chronic pulmonary hypertension, which has been described as five separate categories of disease (Table 11-1).

Assessing Right Heart Function in Chronic Pulmonary Hypertension

The role of diagnostic testing in chronic pulmonary hypertension is to confirm its existence, quantify its severity, and identify its cause. Any clinical suspicion of pulmonary hypertension warrants an evaluation by echocardiography.[2] Pulmonary artery hypertension is typically diagnosed at late stages of disease simply because of the nature of its nonspecific symptoms. Echocardiogram is used to estimate pulmonary pressures at rest and during exercise and may help exclude any secondary causes of pulmonary hypertension, predict the prognosis, and monitor the efficacy of specific therapeutic interventions.[3]

On echocardiogram, common stigmata from right heart strain from chronic pulmonary hypertension may include RV wall thickening greater than 5 mm, chamber dilatation, and D-Shaping of the left ventricle (LV). It may be associated with peripheral edema and a dilated inferior vena cava (IVC). These findings will be accompanied by the hallmark sonographic finding of pulmonary hypertension—increased tricuspid valve regurgitant velocities. Although a relatively common abnormality, the severity of tricuspid regurgitation (TR) may be an independent predictor of mortality.[4]

Although a simple bedside echocardiogram with Color Flow Doppler will show TR, this mode is not sufficient to estimate pulmonary artery systolic pressures (PASP). In a complete echocardiogram, peak tricuspid velocities may be measured using pulse wave or continuous wave Doppler and then used to estimate right ventricle systolic pressures (RVSP) using a simplified Bernoulli equation:

$$\text{RVSP (mm Hg)} = 4(V_{max}\ [m/s])^2 + \text{RA pressure (mm Hg)},$$

where RA pressure is estimated on the basis of IVC diameter and response to respiration.

Assuming there is no flow limited lesion such as pulmonary artery stenosis, RVSP will equal PASP.

It is important to remember that even on formal echocardiogram, PASP are estimates based on TR velocities and IVC dynamics and that the definitive diagnosis of pulmonary hypertension can be made only by pulmonary artery catheterization. In practice, this is usually reserved for diagnostically challenging cases because of the risks and costs of the procedure.

TABLE 11-1	Classification of Chronic Pulmonary Hypertension by Etiology				
Group	1: Pulmonary artery Hypertension	2: Left heart disease	3: Chronic lung disease/hypoxia	4: Chronic thromboembolism	5: Multifactorial
Example diseases	Congenital, connective tissue disease, toxin	LV dysfunction, valve disease	COPD, sleep apnea, interstitial lung disease	Thromboembolism	Sarcoidosis, Gaucher Disease
Diagnostic testing	Right heart catheterization, echocardiogram, disease specific	Echocardiogram	PFTs, sleep study, chest x-ray or CT	Chest CT angiogram	Disease specific

Abbreviations: COPD, chronic obstructive pulmonary disease; CT, computed tomography; LV, left ventricular; PFTs, pulmonary function tests.

TABLE 11-2   Prevalence of Echocardiographic Signs for Stable and Unstable Pulmonary Embolism

	All PE (%)	Unstable PE (%)
RVD > 90% LVD in four-chamber view	20	81
McConnell sign (dilated RV with preserved apical contractility)	19.8	75
Flattened intraventricular septum	18.4	69
Distended inferior vena cava	13	19
Free thrombus in RV	1.8	31

Abbreviations: LVD, left ventricle diameter; PE, pulmonary embolism; RV, right ventricle; RVD, right ventricle diameter.

Adapted from Kurnicka K, Lichodziejewska B, Goliszek S, et al. Echocardiographic pattern of acute pulmonary embolism: analysis of 511 consecutive patients. *J Am Soc Echocardiogr*. 2016;29(9):907-913. Copyright © 2016 by the American Society of Echocardiography. With permission.

Assessing Right Ventricle Strain in Acute Pulmonary Embolism

PE is a common and life-threatening cause of acute right heart strain. Although small embolisms may produce subtle symptoms, such as chest pain and hypoxia, a large embolism can cause an acute increase of pulmonary pressure, which if severe, can precipitate acute right heart failure.[5] In contrast to chronic pulmonary hypertension, the ventricle does not have time to hypertrophy and may over dilate to the point of poor contractility. RV dilatation and dysfunction are important factors that are associated with a 2-fold higher in-hospital mortality rates and other poor early outcomes for patients with PE.[6] Ultrasound can be used to identify hemodynamically significant PEs by observing the RV dilated to a size greater than the LV, reduced RV systolic function, or rarely, by visualizing free-floating thrombus.[7] The visualization of severe right heart strain, combined with clinical suspicion, can lead to faster identification, diagnosis, and treatment in hemodynamically unstable patients, which will usually include thrombolysis. Echocardiographic signs of acute PE are shown in Table 11-2. Note that a dilated IVC, while frequently present in chronic pulmonary hypertension, is less frequently seen in PE, even where severe.[8] Furthermore, RV wall thickening (>5 mm) will almost always be secondary to a chronic process.

Standard Measurements of the Right Ventricle

Although a global gestalt of dilatation, function, and wall thickening are clinically useful, uniform guidelines are necessary for cardiac chamber quantification to provide objective information. These will always be referenced in a formal echocardiogram and

TABLE 11-3   Normal Measurements of Right Heart in Adults

Site of Measurement	Normal Range for Adults (mm)
RV base diameter	25-41
RV mid diameter	19-35
RV longitudinal diameter	59-83
RV wall thickness	1-5

Abbreviation: RV, right ventricle.

TABLE 11-4   Recommendations for Use of Point-of-Care Ultrasound in Clinical Practice

Recommendation	Rating	References
Bedside ultrasound can effectively detect right heart dysfunction.	A	3, 5, 8, 9
Unstable patients with suspected pulmonary embolism and right heart dysfunction should be considered for thrombolytic therapy.	A	13, 14

A = consistent, good-quality patient-oriented evidence; B = inconsistent or limited-quality patient-oriented evidence; C = consensus, disease-oriented evidence, usual practice, expert opinion, or case series. For information about the SORT evidence rating system, go to http://www.aafp.org/afpsort.

may be useful in the point-of-care setting as well. Recommended standard measurements and their ranges per the American Society of Echocardiography are summarized in Table 11-3.[9]

PERFORMING THE SCAN

1. **Prepare the patient for bedside echocardiogram.** Explain to the patient what to expect from your examination, as well as possible findings and limitations. As with other echocardiogram exams, the patient should be ideally draped to expose the anterior chest and upper abdomen and initially positioned in left lateral decubitus position. A cardiac probe in the cardiac setting is ideal for the exam but an abdominal probe will work, but note that the probe marker will be reversed if abdominal settings are used. Apply a sufficient quantity of gel for good contact on the chest wall (**Figure 11-1**).

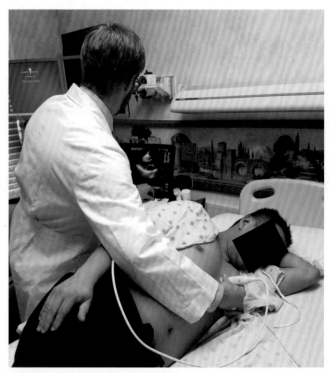

FIGURE 11-1. Proper patient positioning in left lateral decubitus.

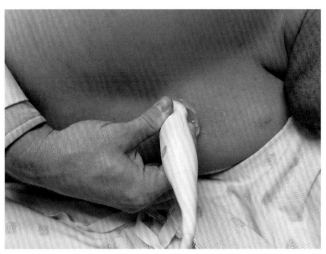

FIGURE 11-2. Probe positioning for the parasternal long-axis view.

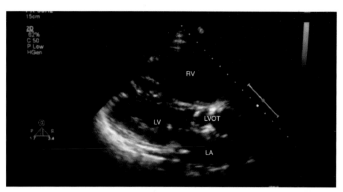

FIGURE 11-4. Parasternal long-axis view showing right heart strain. Note the dominance of the right ventricle and in-bowing of the intraventricular septum. LA, left atrium; LV, left ventricle; LVOT, left ventricular outflow tract; RV, right ventricle.

2. **Obtain a parasternal long-axis view.** Place a low-frequency cardiac probe on the left of the sternum in between the fourth and fifth interspace with the probe marker pointed toward the right shoulder. Manipulate the probe, down or up an interspace, as needed to obtain the best view. It should include the RV, LV, left atria, and aortic outflow tract. Observe global motion and RV size and contractility. Capture a loop of the cardiac cycle and advance to end diastole, the closure of the mitral valve, when the maximum dilatation of the ventricles can be identified. The RV should appear visibly smaller than the LV and the anterior wall of the RV should be thinner than the intraventricular septum. A bulging right ventricle or thickened ventricle wall suggests elevated pulmonary pressures (**Figures 11-2 through 11-4** and ▶ **Video 11-1**).

3. **Obtain a parasternal short-axis view.** From a PLAX view, focus the probe on the mitral valve and rotate 90°, with the probe marker now aimed at the left shoulder. Fan the probe apically for a cross-section view of the ventricles as they contract. The RV should appear as a crescent shape wrapped around a "doughnut shaped" LV. A bulging RV or "D-shaped" LV suggests high right heart pressures pushing on the cardiac septum[10] (**Figures 11-5 through 11-7** and ▶ **Videos 11-2 and 11-3**).

4. **Obtain an apical four-chamber view.** Move the probe to the point of maximal impulse on the patient's chest, usually under the left nipple. Point the probe marker to the patient's left and then rotate slightly toward the left shoulder while aiming the probe toward the cardiac base (sternum). Use fine manipulation to obtain a view of all four cardiac chambers, with ventricles appearing closest to the probe and atria on the far side of the screen. The ventricles should appear almost symmetric, with the LV being the larger of the two ventricles—a wider chamber with thicker walls. Observe global motion and RV contractility. Capture a loop of the cardiac cycle and advance to end diastole, the closure of the mitral valve, when the maximum dilatation of the ventricles can be identified. This is the best view for estimating RV volume and performing measurements if desired. Back in real-time scanning, apply Color Doppler, if available, over the RV and the tricuspid valve to evaluate for the presence and severity of regurgitation. Some regurgitation may be normal. This is also an appropriate view to apply pulse wave or continuous wave Doppler to measure velocities if performing a more advanced scan (**Figures 11-8 through 11-10**).

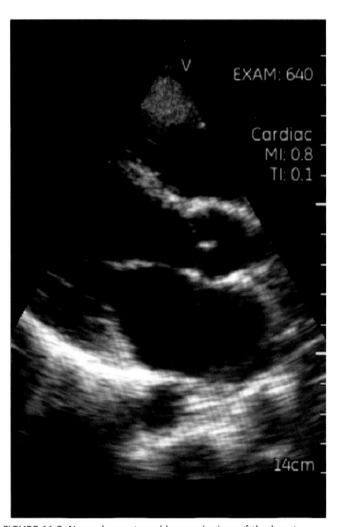

FIGURE 11-3. Normal parasternal long-axis view of the heart.

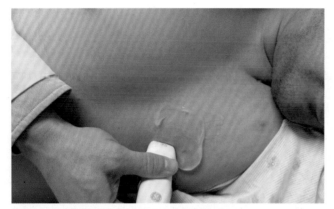

FIGURE 11-5. Probe positioning for the parasternal short-axis view.

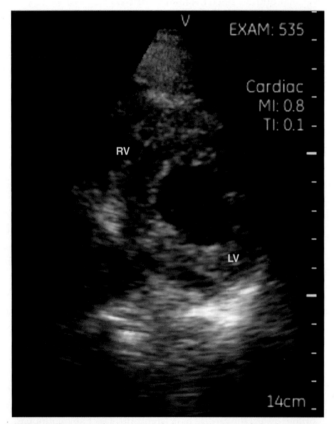

FIGURE 11-6. Normal parasternal short-axis view of the heart. Note the circular left ventricle and the crescent-shaped right ventricle. LV, left ventricle; RV, right ventricle.

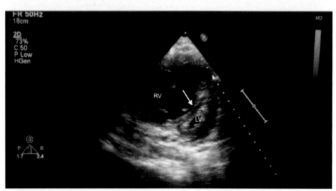

FIGURE 11-7. Parasternal short-axis view showing right heart strain with D-shaping of the left ventricle. LV, left ventricle; RV, right ventricle.

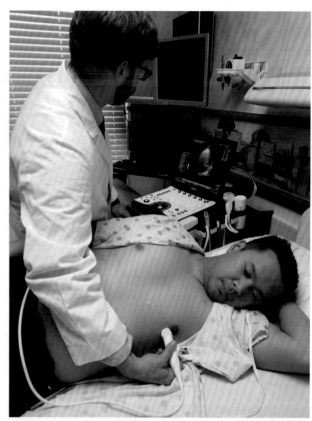

FIGURE 11-8. Probe positioning for the apical four-chamber view.

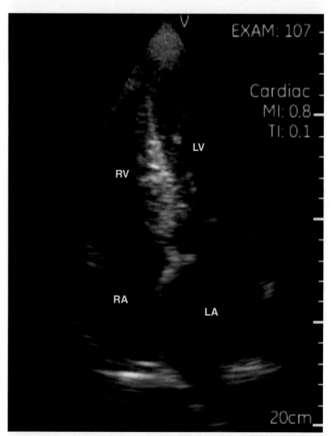

FIGURE 11-9. B mode apical four-chamber view of a normal heart. Note the dominance of the left ventricle (right side of the image). LA, left atrium; LV, left ventricle; RA, right atrium; RV, right ventricle.

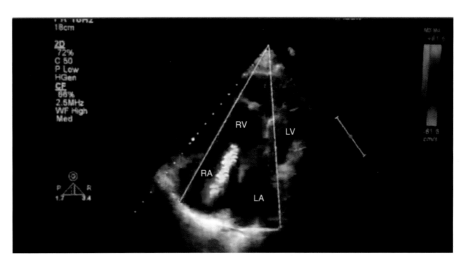

FIGURE 11-10. Apical four-chamber view with Color Doppler over the tricuspid valve in a patient with right heart strain. Note the dominance of the right ventricle and the high-velocity regurgitation jet. LA, left atrium; LV, left ventricle; RA, right atrium; RV, right ventricle.

PATIENT MANAGEMENT

Bedside ultrasound for right heart strain is useful in both acute and chronic settings. For the patient with chronic dyspnea, an abnormal bedside exam leads the physician to pursue a more aggressive workup for pulmonary hypertension. This may include formal echocardiogram, right heart catheterization, and workup for likely etiologies based on the clinical scenario. The etiologies of chronic pulmonary hypertension are divided by the WHO into five standard categories, as described in Table 11-1.[11]

In acute illness, evaluating for right heart strain may aid in the management of any acute cardiac or respiratory condition, but has a particular role in the management of acute PE. Being able to perform the scan at bedside upon first contact with the patient reduces time to definitive and possibly lifesaving intervention.

When a patient presents with clinical concerns for PE, he or she should be immediately assessed for hemodynamic stability. Unstable patients are frequently treated with intravenous saline to increase preload and raise blood pressure. However, in a severe PE, this may actually worsen symptoms by further dilating a hyperexpanded RV.[12] Current CHEST guidelines recommend systemic thrombolytics in patients with acute PE with hypotension in order to restore perfusion, but many of these patients are too unstable for a confirmatory CTA.[13] Bedside cardiac ultrasound bridges the gap by confirming RV dysfunction which, in the high-risk patient, can be interpreted as a confirmation of embolism. Thrombolytics are a lifesaving, yet risky, intervention, with 1 in 18 patients suffering a major bleed and 1 in 78 an intracranial hemorrhage.[14] The algorithm presented in **Figure 11-11** reflects current guidelines but must be tailored to individual patient risks and goals of care as well as the clinical setting. Catheter-directed interventions may be preferable to systemic thrombolysis in some centers depending on resources.

Some data suggest that hemodynamically stable patients with RV dysfunction seen on echocardiogram may also have a net benefit from thrombolytics.[14] Even if thrombolytics are not given, RV strain in the stable patient with PE is helpful in prognosis and may influence the decision of their initial disposition and duration of anticoagulation therapy upon hospital discharge. Recent studies suggest that many patients will benefit from lifelong anticoagulation therapy after just a single unprovoked PE, also reflected in current CHEST guidelines.[15]

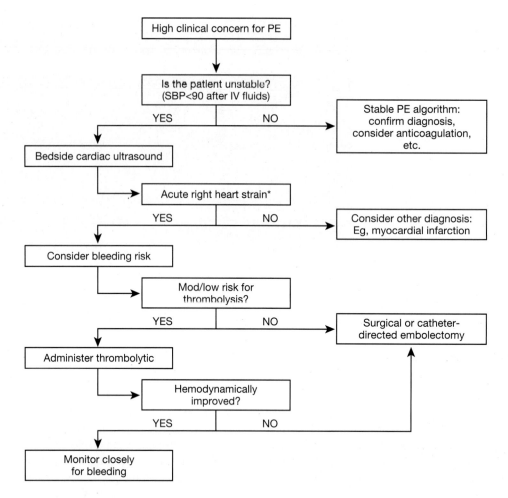

*Note: Right heart strain findings of acute PE include a dilated or dysfunctional RV and flattening of the intraventricular septum. If signs of chronic right heart strain are present, such as wall thickening and IVC dilatation, workup for chronic pulmonary hypertension is indicated starting with formal echocardiogram after acute condition has been stabilized.

FIGURE 11-11. Simplified algorithm for management of acute pulmonary embolism. IV, intravenous fluids; IVC, inferior vena cava; PE, pulmonary embolism; RV, right ventricle; SBP, systolic blood pressure.

PEARLS AND PITFALLS

Pearls

- RV dimensions are best estimated in the apical four-chamber view at end diastole.
- Assess tricuspid regurgitation (TR) during inspiration where the degree of TR will be at its greatest.
- RV can be distinguished from LV by the presence of the moderator band and the location of the tricuspid valve just slightly apical to the mitral valve.
- The IVC is infrequently dilated in acute PE, even if severe.
- RV wall thickening (>5 mm) will almost always be secondary to a chronic process.

Pitfalls

- Double-check probe settings: Typical orientation in the cardiac mode will have the probe marker on the right side of the screen, reversed from other ultrasound settings.
- Avoid making a diagnosis of RV strain on one set of measurements that is dependent on probe positioning and angle—especially the PLAX. Obtain multiple views to confirm when possible.
- LV dilatation will make RV dilatation less obvious on exam.
- A normal echocardiogram does not exclude a PE.

BILLING

CPT Code	Description	Global Payment	Professional Component	Technical Component
93308	Limited transthoracic echocardiogram	$126.03	$26.14	$99.89
93321	Doppler echo limited	$27.63	$7.54	$20.10

CPT codes and average national reimbursement for Medicare in 2016. Payment data are from https://www.cms.gov/apps/physician-fee-schedule/search/search-criteria.aspx. See Chapter 2 for details on ultrasound billing.

References

1. Rudski LG, Lai WW, Afilalo J, et al. Guidelines for the echocardiographic assessment of the right heart in adults: a report from the American Society of Echocardiography. *J Am Soc Echocardiogr.* 2010;23:685-713.
2. McLaughlin VV, Archer SL, Badesch DB, et al. ACCF/AHA 2009 Expert Consensus Document on pulmonary hypertension. *Circulation.* 2009;119(16):2252-2292.
3. Bossone E, Bodini BD, Mazza A, Allegra L. Pulmonary arterial hypertension: the key role of echocardiography. *Chest.* 2005;127(5):1836-1843.
4. Nath J, Foster E, Heidenreich PA. Impact of tricuspid regurgitation on long-term survival. *J Am Coll Cardiol.* 2004;43(4):405-409.
5. Matthews JC, McLaughlin V. Acute right ventricular failure in the setting of acute pulmonary embolism or chronic pulmonary hypertension: a detailed review of the pathophysiology, diagnosis, and management. *Curr Cardiol Rev.* 2008;4(1):49-59.
6. ten Wolde M, Söhne M, Quak E, Mac Gillavry MR, Büller HR. Prognostic value of echocardiographically assessed right ventricular dysfunction in patients with pulmonary embolism. *Arch Intern Med.* 2004;164(15):9-23.
7. Patel AN, Nickels LC, Flach FE, De Portu G, Ganti L. The use of bedside ultrasound in the evaluation of patients presenting with signs and symptoms of pulmonary embolism. *Case Rep Emerg Med.* 2013;2013:312632.
8. Kurnicka K, Lichodziejewska B, Goliszek S, et al. Echocardiographic pattern of acute pulmonary embolism: analysis of 511 consecutive patients. *J Am Soc Echocardiogr.* 2016;29(9):907-913.
9. Lang RM, Badano LP, Mor-Avi V, et al. Recommendations for cardiac chamber quantification by echocardiography in adults: an update from the American Society of Echocardiography and the European Association of Cardiovascular Imaging. *J Am Soc Echocardiogr.* 2015;14(28):1-39.
10. Bleeker GB, Steendijk P, Holman ER, et al. Acquired right ventricular dysfunction. *Heart.* 2006;92(suppl 1):i14-i18.
11. Simonneau G, Gatzoulis M, Adiata I, et al. Updated clinical classification of pulmonary hypertension. *J Am Coll Cardiol.* 2013;62:S34.
12. Wood KE. Review of a pathophysiologic approach to the golden hour of hemodynamically significant pulmonary embolism. *Chest.* 2002;121(3):877-905.
13. Kearon C, Akl EA, Ornelas J, et al. Antithrombotic therapy for VTE disease: CHEST guideline and expert panel report. *Chest.* 2016;149(2):315-352.
14. Chatterjee S, Chakraborty A, Weinberg I, et al. Thrombolysis for pulmonary embolism and risk of all-cause mortality, major bleeding, and intracranial hemorrhage: a meta-analysis. *JAMA.* 2014;311(23):2414-2421.
15. Couturard F, Sanchez O, Pernod G, et al. Six months vs extended oral anticoagulation after a first episode of pulmonary embolism: the PADIS-PE randomized clinical trial. *JAMA.* 2015;314(1):31-40.

PART 2

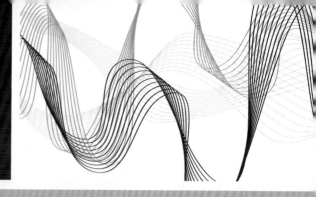

CHAPTER

12

Does the Patient Have Pulmonary Edema?

Michael Wagner, MD, FACP, RDMS and Keith R. Barron, MD, FACP

● Clinical Vignette

A 66-year-old man with a history of chronic obstructive pulmonary disease (COPD), obstructive sleep apnea, and heart failure with preserved ejection fraction presents to the clinic with chest tightness, dyspnea, and cough, which have increased over the past week. Review of systems is remarkable for orthopnea and increased sputum production. Physical examination reveals distant heart sounds without murmurs, mild wheezing bilaterally, and lower extremity edema. An electrocardiogram shows sinus tachycardia and nonspecific T-wave flattening in the lateral leads.

At this point in the outpatient evaluation, there is insufficient evidence to conclusively determine the etiology of the patient's symptoms. The two most likely causes, COPD exacerbation and heart failure exacerbation, can be distinguished by answering the question: Does the patient have pulmonary edema?

LITERATURE REVIEW

The detection of pulmonary edema or congestion on physical examination is often challenging, as patients with significant symptoms may have few objective signs. Further, even when present, many traditional physical examination findings, including crackles on auscultation, have likelihood ratios that result in minimal or small changes in diagnostic probability.[1,2] Crackles can occur in COPD, whereas interstitial fluid from heart failure can result in bronchospasm and wheezing. Chest radiography has been traditionally used for the detection of pulmonary edema, and whereas the typical findings of vascular congestion and interstitial edema have high specificity, they have poor sensitivity and are absent in as many as 20% of patients with acute decompensated heart failure (ADHF).[3] In patients who have both COPD and heart failure, syndromes that commonly overlap and are underrecognized, the accuracy of chest x-ray may be even worse[4] and the optimal cutoff for natriuretic peptides in this population is unclear.[2]

Artifacts generated by lung ultrasound called sonographic "B-lines" are emerging as an excellent marker for pulmonary edema and have been shown to correlate with Kerley B-lines and lung water scores on chest radiography[5] as well as water-thickened interlobular septa and ground glass opacities seen on computed tomography.[6] Although B-lines are related to measures of hemodynamic compromise in patients with heart failure, with increasing numbers corresponding with higher pulmonary capillary wedge pressures,[7] natriuretic peptides,[8,9] and measurements of diastolic dysfunction on echocardiography,[10] they may provide additional information about the integrity of the alveolar-capillary membrane. B-lines are a real-time, noninvasive tool to detect and quantify extravascular lung water (EVLW), corresponding to measurements by invasive techniques in humans[7] and dissection in animal models.[11,12] Because they appear rapidly and are detectable even prior to symptoms or hypoxemia,[11-13] and clear after adequate treatment of ADHF or volume overload,[14,15] B-lines represent an ideal tool for the early detection of pulmonary congestion as well as monitoring the response to therapy, both in the inpatient and outpatient setting.

The clinical utility of lung ultrasound for the detection of pulmonary edema was first recognized in critically ill patients and found to be helpful in distinguishing ADHF from COPD exacerbation in patients with respiratory failure.[16] Subsequently, the majority of studies have been done in intensive care units and emergency departments,[17] with the largest multicenter study demonstrating a sensitivity and specificity >97% in differentiating ADHF from noncardiac causes of acute dyspnea.[18] There is a linear correlation between the number of B-lines present and the extent of pulmonary edema, and the number of B-lines decreases in real time as volume is removed in dialysis patients.[14] Although studies on the diagnostic accuracy of lung ultrasound for pulmonary edema in the outpatient setting have yet to be performed, the detection of B-lines on lung ultrasound has been shown to provide useful prognostic information in clinic patients. A high degree of congestion as assessed by lung ultrasound, even with handheld devices, markedly increases the risk of death or hospitalization, whereas the absence or a low number of B-lines identifies patients at a very low risk for adverse events, better than natriuretic peptides.[19-21] This information can lead to better adjustment and titration of therapies, arrangement of timely follow-up, while achieving better allocation of resources.

Understanding and identifying the structures and artifacts that arise around the pleural surface is essential for successful identification of pulmonary edema. Unlike most other uses of B-mode ultrasound, where organs or tissues appear similar to visual representations or cross-sections of actual anatomy, the presence of air and ribs creates many artifacts at the pleural surface. Thus, normally aerated lung parenchyma does not resemble lung tissue, and is obscured by artifacts. Artifact interpretation is, therefore, a critical component of lung ultrasonography. In pulmonary edema, fluid initially fills and thickens the interstitial space before spilling into the alveoli. This change in density of the lung alters the normal artifacts found at the pleural surface. Recognition of the change in artifacts allows for detection of changes in lung density as the lung becomes "wet," allowing for the diagnosis of pulmonary edema with ultrasound. The identification of a pathologic number of "B-lines" in a diffuse and bilateral pattern significantly increases the likelihood of pulmonary edema, whereas the absence of "B-lines" excludes pulmonary edema with high sensitivity.

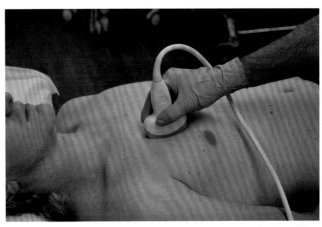

FIGURE 12-1. In each zone, place a low-frequency probe (curvilinear shown) so that the center is between two ribs with the probe marker pointed cephalad. Adjust the probe to ensure the probe face is perpendicular to the lung surface.

TABLE 12-1	Recommendations for Use of Point-of-Care Ultrasound in Clinical Practice		
Recommendation		Rating	References
In resource-limited settings, lung ultrasound should be considered as a particularly useful diagnostic modality in the evaluation of interstitial syndrome.		A	21
The presence of multiple diffuse bilateral B-lines indicates interstitial syndrome. Causes of interstitial syndrome include the following conditions: • Pulmonary edema of various causes • Interstitial pneumonia or pneumonitis • Diffuse parenchymal lung disease (pulmonary fibrosis)		A	21
Lung ultrasound is superior to conventional chest radiography for ruling in significant interstitial syndrome.		A	21
In patients with suspected interstitial syndrome, a negative lung ultrasound examination is superior to conventional chest radiography in ruling out significant interstitial syndrome.		A	21

A = consistent, good-quality patient-oriented evidence; B = inconsistent or limited-quality patient-oriented evidence; C = consensus, disease-oriented evidence, usual practice, expert opinion, or case series. For information about the SORT evidence rating system, go to http://www.aafp.org/afpsort.

PERFORMING THE SCAN

1. **Patient position and equipment.** Place the patient in the supine position. The assessment for pulmonary edema or B-lines may be more accurate if the patient is lying completely flat. Alternatively, the patient may remain upright if this is not feasible. Although the exam can be performed around loose-fitting clothing if required, it is best if the patient is undressed from the waist up, using a sheet or gown if needed to maintain comfort/modesty.

   Select a low-frequency probe: either a sector probe or curvilinear probe is acceptable. Although some studies have utilized a high-frequency linear probe, most have used low-frequency probes.

Choose a depth setting of 16 to 18 cm using the lung or pleural preset. If this is not available, an abdominal or cardiac preset is acceptable. Note that if a cardiac preset is used, the probe marker orientation will be the opposite of the other presets.

2. **Identify the lung "home screen" and normal artifacts.** Although scanning technique and anatomy can be variable, when first learning lung ultrasound, avoid disorientation or confusion by framing the image in the same way every time using certain key landmarks. This starting point or "home screen" should be easily acquired and rapidly allows the user to recognize issues with depth, gain, and orientation. For either the right or left side, begin the examination by placing the transducer on the anterior chest in the second intercostal space just lateral to the sternum with the probe marker toward the patient's feet for cardiac settings and toward the head for all noncardiac settings (**Figure 12-1**). Position the probe over the two ribs, which will appear as rounded, partially echogenic structures with posterior shadowing. Next, identify the echogenic horizontal pleural line (PL), which appears posterior to and between the ribs. When framed correctly, the PL should be in the center of the screen and the superior and inferior ribs should be on the left and right (**Figure 12-2A and B**). The PL is the junction of static parietal pleura of the chest wall and dynamic visceral pleura of the lung. The visceral pleura of the lung moves along the chest wall during normal respiration, which causes a subtle shimmering or glimmering appearance of the PL. This sliding, often described as "ants marching on a log" or "beads on a string," is a normal finding indicating that the parietal and visceral pleura are opposed at the site of probe placement (▶ **Video 12-1**). In normally aerated lung, an A-line pattern will be present. A-lines are horizontal, echogenic reverberation artifacts that appear in an equidistant repeating fashion below, and parallel to, the PL (**Figure 12-2C**). The PL and subsequent artifacts are most visible when the transducer is perpendicular to the PL, so subtly fanning or angulating the probe may be necessary to maximally interpret the artifacts.

3. **Use a systematic approach.** An eight-zone approach is typically utilized, with each hemithorax divided into four zones: two anterior and two lateral. The anterior chest wall is defined as the

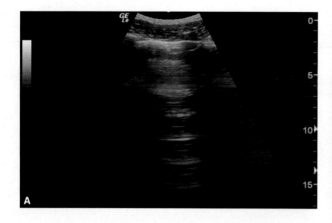

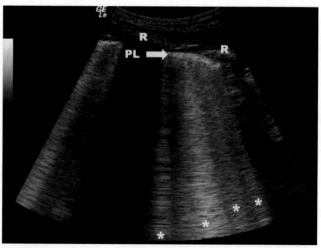

FIGURE 12-2. A, Unlabeled view of the lung ultrasound "home-screen." B, Labeled view of the lung ultrasound "homescreen." Two ribs (R), can be seen just anterior to the pleural line (PL) which appears to shimmer or slide with respirations when viewed in real time. The region above the PL appears like tissue and is similar to the ultrasound of other solid organs. The region below the PL is all artifacts and not truly representative of the lung parenchyma. C, Equidistant from the probe to the PL are repeating horizontal hyperechoic artifacts called "A-lines" (<), suggesting the absence of pulmonary edema at the examined site. Two ribs (R) help frame the image.

region from the sternum to the anterior axillary line, whereas the lateral zone is defined as the region from the anterior to the posterior axillary line (**Figure 12-3**). Each zone is scanned, and the artifact pattern interpreted, with the overall pattern being concluded only after all zones have been examined.

4. **Look for "B-lines."** After becoming oriented at the home screen, evaluate for pulmonary edema by identifying the

presence of an A-line or B-line pattern in each zone. As the lung begins to develop early pulmonary edema and thickening of the interstitium, B-lines begin to replace A-lines. According to the international consensus conference on lung ultrasound, B-lines are defined as "discrete laser-like vertical hyperechoic artifacts that arise from the PL, extend to the bottom of the screen without fading, and move synchronously with lung

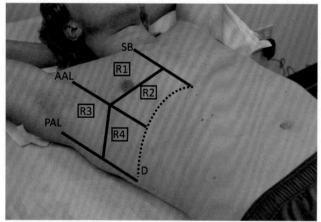

FIGURE 12-3. The zones and approximate probe positions in thoracic ultrasonography as described by Volpicelli et al. Each area is the same on the opposing left side (L1-4), with a complete scan for pulmonary edema consisting of eight examined zones. AAL, anterior axillary line; D, diaphragm (dotted line represents approximate location); PAL, posterior axillary line; R1, right upper anterior zone; R2, right lower anterior zone; R3, right upper lateral zone; R4, right lower lateral zone; SB, sternal border.

FIGURE 12-4. Here, four vertical hyperechoic artifacts (*) can be seen streaming down from the pleural line (PL), which constitutes a positive zone. At least two positive zones in both left and right hemithoraces would be considered a diffuse B-pattern, consistent with pulmonary edema. Two ribs (R) appropriately frame the image.

sliding"[22] (**Figure 12-4**). One to two B-lines may be seen in a single intercostal space in normal subjects without pulmonary edema, particularly in the posterior-lateral zones. B-lines serve as a densitometer of the lungs,[22] with fewer and thinner B-lines in mild edema and thicker, more confluent B-lines in more severe disease. A zone is considered "positive" or abnormal by the presence of three or more B-lines in a longitudinal plane between two ribs. If confluent B-lines are present, the zone should be considered positive if >30% of the rib space is occupied by B-lines. In severe disease, the B-lines may coalesce to occupy the entire rib space and a "white lung" pattern is present (**Figure 12-5**). A "white lung" pattern is also considered a positive zone (**Tables 12-2 and 12-3**).

5. **Interpret the distribution/pattern of B-lines in the clinical context.** The presence of at least two positive zones bilaterally (four zones total) is referred to as a "B-pattern" and defines the sonographic diffuse interstitial syndrome. Patients who have positive zones that do not meet this criteria are felt to have a "focal B-line pattern." A focal (localized) sonographic pattern of interstitial syndrome may be seen in the presence of any of the following: pneumonia and pneumonitis, atelectasis, pulmonary contusion, pulmonary infarction, pleural disease, and neoplasia.[23]

In the proper clinical context, "diffuse B-pattern" is most often EVLW due to increased hydrostatic pressure. It is important to note that this pattern can also be seen with infections causing interstitial inflammation and vessel permeability (noncardiogenic pulmonary edema). Examining the heart and inferior vena cava are helpful exam adjuncts if the etiology of the lung water is in question. Finally, just as crackles can be heard in both pulmonary fibrosis and pulmonary edema, pulmonary fibrosis or other infiltrative processes of the interstitium may also result in a "B-pattern." Additional clues of pulmonary fibrosis can include a thickened and irregular pleural surface with or without small subpleural consolidations (**Figure 12-6**).

TABLE 12-2	Normal Artifacts
Understanding artifacts is essential to understanding pleural ultrasound	
Pleural line	An echogenic, or bright white, linear artifact that arises deep to the ribs that "slides" with respiration.
Ribs and rib shadows	Ribs are highly reflective of ultrasound waves and appear as echogenic, curved structures with posterior shadowing. Cartilaginous portions close to the sternum appear less echogenic and create less shadow than more ossified portions laterally.
Lung sliding	A dynamic artifact occurring in a normal, aerated lung that is generated by the translational movement of the visceral along the parietal pleura during respiration. It appears as shimmering of the PL like "ants marching on a log," or moving "beads on a string."
A-line	Horizontal, echogenic artifact that appears in an equidistant repeating fashion below, and parallel to, the PL. A-lines should be the same distance apart as the distance from the probe to the pleural surface. A normal finding in aerated lung, but also present in pneumothorax.

Abbreviation: PL, pleural line.

TABLE 12-3	Abnormal Artifacts
Interpretation of both normal and abnormal artifacts is key to diagnosis of pulmonary edema	
B-line	An echogenic vertical artifact that arises at the pleural line, moves with respiration and extends to the edge of the screen, usually at depth settings >16 cm. A sign of interstitial edema or fibrosis. Greater than three B-lines in a single intercostal space is considered abnormal.

Although these findings may be helpful in the patient without an established diagnosis of fibrotic lung disease, they likely preclude sonographic assessment for EVLW by all but the most advanced users.

PATIENT MANAGEMENT

The presence of a B-line pattern in at least two zones on both left and right sides is suggestive of pulmonary edema, particularly in a patient with a history of heart failure. This pattern is associated with adverse outcomes and warrants strong consideration for adjustments to therapy. Conversely, a diffuse A-line pattern (with normal lung sliding) suggests "dry" lungs and is associated with a low risk of admission for heart failure and adverse events in patients with a history of heart failure. If the patient is having symptoms, it argues strongly against ADHF with higher sensitivity than chest x-ray, and alternative etiologies should be considered.

Patients with some pathologic B-lines but do not meet the criteria for a diffuse interstitial pattern, for example those with a focal B-line pattern, may have an infectious process like pneumonia,

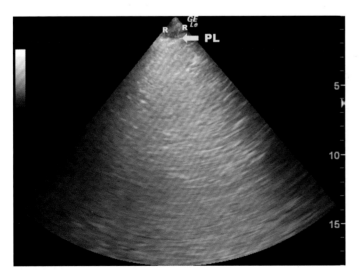

FIGURE 12-5. Here, in a case of severe pulmonary edema, the B-lines are confluent, and the lung appears diffusely echogenic. This is the so called "white lung" pattern. PL, pleural line; R, ribs.

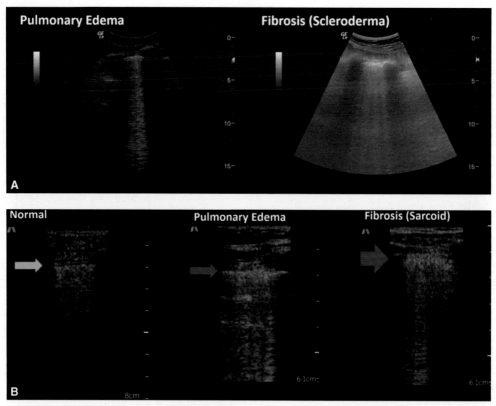

FIGURE 12-6. A, B-lines from pulmonary edema (left) compared with B-lines from pulmonary fibrosis (right) with a low-frequency probe. B, Using a high-frequency probe, the pleural line (arrows) can be more clearly seen. In pulmonary edema, it is usually smooth, whereas in pulmonary fibrosis it is often thickened and irregular appearing.

particularly if unilateral. If bilateral, in addition to infectious causes, the possibility of mild or early pulmonary congestion should be considered. Additional lung findings on ultrasound are helpful diagnostically. The presence of bilateral pleural effusions suggests chronic heart failure, whereas B-lines associated with visible consolidations strongly suggest pneumonia (**Figure 12-7**).

Ultrasound examination of the heart and inferior vena cava may also be helpful when interpreting a focal B-line pattern. A suggested algorithm for incorporation of lung ultrasound in the evaluation of a patient with suspected pulmonary edema can be found in **Figure 12-8**. See **Table 12-4** for a list of common differential diagnoses to consider.

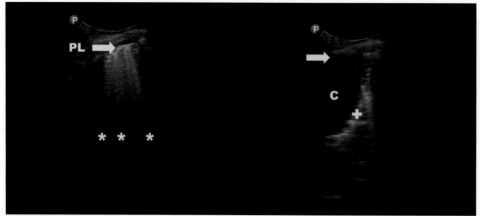

FIGURE 12-7. Consolidations are often surrounded by a region of focal B-lines. A focal B-line pattern (*) was seen in zones R3 and R4 in a patient with fever, cough, and pleuritic chest pain. By sliding the probe just laterally and posteriorly, using the B-lines as a signal to examine further, a consolidation (C) reaching the surface of the lung (arrow) was discovered just next to the focal B-line pattern. The hyperechoic irregular border between consolidation and the rest of the aerated lung is often referred to as the "shred sign" and is also supportive of a diagnosis of pneumonia.

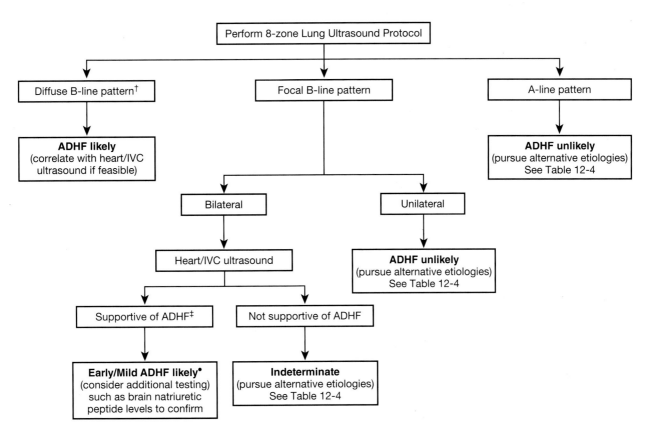

Suggested algorithm for diagnosis of pulmonary edema
†Requires ≥2 positive zones on right and left hemithorax.
‡IVC plethoric (>2.2 cm), Left atrium enlarged, +/– Left ventricular function reduced.
•B-lines should generally be confined to basolateral zones in mild cases of ADHF

FIGURE 12-8. Suggested clinical algorithm incorporating lung ultrasound into the evaluation of the patient with signs or symptoms of pulmonary edema in the primary care setting. ADHF, acute decompensated heart failure; IVC, inferior vena cava.

TABLE 12-4	Differential Diagnosis of Dyspnea Based on Lung Ultrasound Findings
Primary Lung Ultrasound Findings	**Common Differential Diagnoses and Supportive Ultrasound Findings**
Diffuse bilateral B-lines	Pulmonary edema • Supported by bilateral pleural effusions, and findings consistent with ADHF on evaluation of the IVC and heart Pulmonary fibrosis • Supported by thickened and irregular pleural surface with or without small subpleural consolidations
Unilateral focal B-lines	Pneumonia or atelectasis • Supported by the presence of consolidation (see Chapter 15) Pulmonary contusion
Bilateral focal (patchy) B-lines	Pneumonia or atelectasis • Supported by the presence of consolidation (see Chapter 15) Early ADHF • Supported by bilateral pleural effusions, and findings consistent with ADHF on evaluation of the IVC and heart Pulmonary fibrosis • Supported by thickened and irregular pleural surface with or without small subpleural consolidations Acute respiratory distress syndrome • Supported by anterior subpleural consolidations. Absence or reduction of lung sliding. Irregular, thickened, or fragmented pleural line. Pulmonary hemorrhage
Diffuse A-lines	Asthma or COPD Pneumothorax • Supported by the absence of lung sliding (see Chapter 14) Pulmonary infarction • Supported by the presence of deep vein thrombosis on lower extremity venous ultrasound (see Chapter 45). May also see focal B-lines or wedge-shaped subpleural consolidation.

Abbreviations: ADHF; acute decompensated heart failure, COPD, chronic obstructive pulmonary disease; IVC, inferior vena cava.

PEARLS AND PITFALLS

Pearls

- The artifact pattern (A-lines or B-lines) is best detected when the maximum amount of ultrasound waves return to the probe face. To ensure the beam is perpendicular to the lung pleural surface, the probe may require slight fanning (tilting), even though the face may be perpendicular to the skin and chest wall. This is evidenced by a brighter PL and more pronounced lung ultrasound artifact pattern (more echogenic A-lines or B-lines).
- Although we are traditionally taught that B-lines must erase A-lines, in our experience, this may not always be true with modern ultrasounds and pocket-sized devices. This is especially true in mild disease. The presence of three or more B-lines in a single intercostal space should be considered a positive zone, regardless of the presence or absence of A-lines (**Figure 12-9**).
- The distribution pattern should be carefully considered when interpreting a B-line pattern. Cardiogenic pulmonary edema begins in dependent positions and progresses superiorly and then anteriorly. It is almost always bilateral. Significant B-lines in the superior and anterior zones with absent B-lines in the lateral and dependent regions is more likely to be noncardiogenic pulmonary edema.

Pitfalls

- Failure to visualize the pleural surface clearly at a perpendicular angle may result in missed B-lines.
- B-lines are gain-dependent artifacts. This is most relevant in mild cases of pulmonary edema or when examining otherwise normal lungs. If the gain settings are too low, B-lines can be presumed absent when they are actually present. If gain settings are too high, one can potentially overcall otherwise normal artifact patterns.
- Recognition of appropriate anatomic landmarks is essential to this technique. Inadvertently scanning caudal to the diaphragm in the abdomen may result in misinterpretation of air–fluid interfaces in stomach/bowel as B-lines.
- Not seeking additional diagnostic information in borderline cases or ignoring clinical data that do not support the lung ultrasound findings. Lung ultrasound is a powerful diagnostic tool, but is just one part of the clinical assessment when evaluating a patient. It should supplement, not replace, a clinician's judgment.

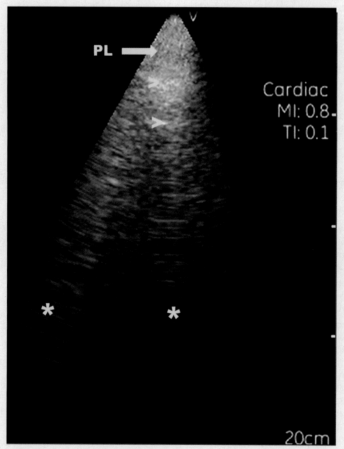

FIGURE 12-9. A modern pocket-sized ultrasound image in a patient with radiographic pulmonary edema. In real time, the pleural line (PL) can be seen sliding, and B-lines (*) stream down off it. However, a few A-lines are visible (>) despite the presence of B-lines.

BILLING

CPT Code	Description	Global Payment	Professional Component	Technical Component
76604	Ultrasound, chest, real time with image documentation	$89.56	$27.58	$61.97

CPT codes and average national reimbursement for Medicare in 2016. Payment data are from https://www.cms.gov/apps/physician-fee-schedule/search/search-criteria.aspx. See Chapter 2 for details on ultrasound billing.

References

1. McGee S. *Evidence-Based Physical Diagnosis*. Philadelphia, PA: WB Saunders; 2001.
2. Wang CS, FitzGerald JM, Schulzer M, Mak E, Ayas NT. Does this dyspneic patient in the emergency department have congestive heart failure? *JAMA*. 2005;294:1944-1956.
3. Collins SP, Lindsell CJ, Storrow AB, Abraham WT; ADHERE Scientific Advisory Committee Investigators and Study Group. Prevalence of negative chest radiography results in the emergency department patient with decompensated heart failure. *Ann Emerg Med*. 2006;47:13-18.
4. Hawkins NM, Petrie MC, Jhund PS, Chalmers GW, Dunn FG, McMurray JJ. Heart failure and chronic obstructive pulmonary disease: diagnostic pitfalls and epidemiology. *Eur J Heart Fail*. 2009;11(2):130-139.
5. Jambrik Z, Monti S, Coppola V, et al. Usefulness of ultrasound lung comets as a nonradiologic sign of extravascular lung water. *Am J Cardiol*. 2004;93:1265-1270.
6. Lichtenstein DA, Meziere G, Biderman P, Gepner A, Barre O. The comet-tail artifact. An ultrasound sign of alveolar-interstitial syndrome. *Am J Respir Crit Care Med*. 1997;156:1640-1646.
7. Agricola E, Bove T, Oppizzi M, et al. Ultrasound comet-tail images: a marker of pulmonary edema: a comparative study with wedge pressure and extravascular lung water. *Chest*. 2005;127:1690-1695.
8. Gargani L, Frassi F, Soldati G, Tesorio P, Gheorghiade M, Picano E. Ultrasound lung comets for the differential diagnosis of acute cardiogenic dyspnoea: a comparison with natriuretic peptides. *Eur J Heart Fail*. 2008;10:70.
9. Liteplo AS, Marill KA, Villen T, et al. Emergency thoracic ultrasound in the differentiation of the etiology of shortness of breath (ETUDES): sonographic B-lines and N-terminal pro-brain-type natriuretic peptide in diagnosing congestive heart failure. *Acad Emerg Med*. 2009;16:201-210.
10. Frassi F, Gargani L, Gligorova S, Ciampi Q, Mottola G, Picano E. Clinical and echocardiographic determinants of ultrasound lung comets. *Eur J Echocardiogr*. 2007;8:474.
11. Gargani L, Lionetti V, Di Cristofano C, Bevilacqua G, Recchia FA, Picano E. Early detection of acute lung injury uncoupled to hypoxemia in pigs using ultrasound lung comets. *Crit Care Med*. 2007;35:2769-2774.
12. Jambrik Z, Gargani L, Adamicza Á, et al. B-lines quantify the lung water content: a lung ultrasound versus lung gravimetry study in acute lung injury. *Ultrasound Med Biol*. 2010;36:2004-2010.
13. Agricola E, Picano E, Oppizzi M, et al. Assessment of stress-induced pulmonary interstitial edema by chest ultrasound during exercise echocardiography and its correlation with left ventricular function. *J Am Soc Echocardiogr*. 2006;19:457-463.
14. Noble VE, Murray AF, Capp R, Sylvia-Reardon MH, Steele DJR, Liteplo A. Ultrasound assessment for extravascular lung water in patients undergoing hemodialysis. Time course for resolution. *Chest*. 2009;135:1433-1439.
15. Volpicelli G, Caramello V, Cardinale L, Mussa A, Bar F, Francisco MF. Bedside ultrasound of the lung for the monitoring of acute decompensated heart failure. *Am J Emerg Med*. 2008;26:585-591.
16. Lichtenstein D, Mezière G. A lung ultrasound sign allowing bedside distinction between pulmonary edema and COPD: the comet-tail artifact. *Intensive Care Med*. 1998;24:1331-1334.
17. Al Deeb M, Barbic S, Featherstone R, Dankoff J, Barbic D. Point-of-care ultrasonography for the diagnosis of acute cardiogenic pulmonary edema in patients presenting with acute dyspnea: a systematic review and meta-analysis. *Acad Emerg Med*. 2014;21:843-852.
18. Pivetta E, Goffi A, Lupia E, et al. Lung ultrasound-implemented diagnosis of acute decompensated heart failure in the ED: a SIMEU multicenter study. *Chest*. 2015;148:202-210.
19. Gustafsson M, Alehagen U, Johansson P. Imaging congestion with a pocket ultrasound device: prognostic implications in patients with chronic heart failure. *J Card Fail*. 2015;21(7):548-554.
20. Platz E, Lewis EF, Uno H, et al. Detection and prognostic value of pulmonary congestion by lung ultrasound in ambulatory heart failure patients. *Eur Heart J*. 2016;37:1244-1251.
21. Miglioranza MH, Gargani L, Sant'Anna RT, et al. Lung ultrasound for the evaluation of pulmonary congestion in outpatients: a comparison with clinical assessment, natriuretic peptides, and echocardiography. *JACC Cardiovasc Imaging*. 2013;6:1141-1151.
22. Volpicelli G, Elbarbary M, Blaivas M, et al; International Liaison Committee on Lung Ultrasound (ILC-LUS) for International Consensus Conference on Lung Ultrasound (ICC-LUS). International evidence-based recommendations for point-of-care lung ultrasound. *Intensive Care Med*. 2012;38(4):577-591.
23. Volpicelli G. Lung sonography. *J Ultrasound Med*. 2013;32:165-171.

Does the Patient Have a Pleural Effusion?

Kevin Bergman, MD and Jennifer Madeline Owen, MD

● Clinical Vignette

A 54-year-old immigrant farmer with no known prior medical history presents with 3 weeks of progressive shortness of breath, cough, and fatigue. He has dyspnea on exertion and intermittent pleuritic chest pain. On examination, the patient has decreased breath sounds and decreased tactile fremitus at the left base without other adventitial lung sounds. The remainder of his physical examination is unremarkable. Does the patient have a pleural effusion?

LITERATURE REVIEW

A pleural effusion is an abnormal collection of fluid in the space between the parietal and visceral pleura. A total of 1.5 million cases of pleural effusion are diagnosed in the United States every year.[1] They are most commonly seen because of underlying congestive heart failure (CHF), pneumonia, and malignancy, but are also present in many other conditions. They are often manifestations of a complicated presentation of the underlying disease process (see Table 13-1), and timely recognition and treatment has been shown to improve patient outcomes. For example, the presence of a parapneumonic effusion in a patient with pneumonia is associated with higher morbidity and mortality, but if identified and treated, it typically resolves without complication.[1] In the setting of cancer, a malignant effusion qualifies as a stage 4 diagnosis and portends a very poor prognosis.[1]

Patients usually present with nonspecific complaints of shortness of breath, cough, and pleuritic chest pain.[1] Physical examination findings include asymmetric chest expansion, decreased or absent breath sounds, crackles, pleural rub, decreased tactile fremitus, dullness to percussion, and diminished resonance with auscultatory percussion. Based on a systematic review in *JAMA*, the most accurate physical examination findings to rule in a pleural effusion are dullness to percussion (+LR 8.7) and asymmetric chest expansion (+LR 8.1), and the most accurate finding to

rule out an effusion was normal tactile fremitus (−LR 0.21).[2] However, physical examination findings alone are not sensitive or specific enough and further imaging is required for the definitive diagnosis.

Chest radiography is the traditional imaging method for evaluating for a pleural effusion but has several limitations. First, chest x-ray is dependent on the amount of fluid present and different views need to be obtained. At least 200 mL of pleural fluid is needed to see blunting of the costophrenic recesses on a posteroanterior x-ray, and the literature shows that even an effusion of 500 mL can be missed on a chest x-ray.[3] A lateral x-ray is more sensitive because the fluid accumulates in the posterior costophrenic recess first and it has been shown to detect 50 mL of fluid.[3] A lateral decubitus x-ray can potentially detect an effusion starting at 5 to 20 mL and is the most sensitive view for detecting fluid.[4] Second, pleural effusions can be mistaken for parenchymal opacities on portable anteroposterior radiography. In fact, in 2010 Kitazono et al. showed that radiologists either misdiagnose small or medium-sized effusions as parenchymal opacities 45% of the time or fail to see these effusions 55% of the time.[5] Lastly, there is no way to further characterize the type of effusion such as transudative or exudative when seen on radiography alone.

Computed tomography (CT) overcomes many of the limitations of chest radiography and is often considered the gold standard for the detection of pleural effusions. However, even CT is limited in its ability to distinguish small effusions from atelectasis, tumor, or thickened pleura.[6] Additionally, CT is expensive and requires a patient to be transported to the machine, which may not be possible emergently. It also may not always be readily available depending on the location of the patient care facility. Finally, CT is associated with high doses of radiation. One CT scan of the chest exposes the patient to 7 mSv of radiation, the radiation dose of which is equivalent to 350 chest x-rays.[7] The seventh National Academy of Science report on Biological Effects of Ionizing Radiation estimated that a single dose of 10 mSv produces a lifetime risk of developing a solid cancer or leukemia of 1 in 1 000.[8]

TABLE 13-1 Physical Examination and Ultrasound Findings by Etiology of Pleural Effusion

Disease Associated with Pleural Effusion	Physical Examination Findings	Ultrasound Findings
Congestive heart failure	Jugular venous distention, S3, rales, peripheral edema	Bilateral B-lines, diminished ejection fraction, plethoric IVC, mitral regurgitation
Pneumonia	Fever, decreased breath sounds, rhonchi	Focal B-lines, adjacent alveolar consolidation, dynamic air bronchograms, lung hepatization
Malignancy	Weight loss, lymphadenopathy, focal decreased breast sounds	Pleural thickness >7 mm, diaphragmatic thickness >10 mm, nodules on pleura
Pulmonary embolism	Dyspnea, pleuritic chest pain, leg pain, cough, new arrhythmia	Subpleural lesion, right heart strain, +DVT in leg

Abbreviations: DVT, deep vein thrombosis; IVC, inferior vena cava.

TABLE 13-2	Recommendations for Use of Point-of-Care Ultrasound in Clinical Practice		
Recommendation		Rating	Reference
In opacities identified by chest radiography, lung ultrasound should be used because it is more accurate than chest radiography in distinguishing between effusion and consolidation.		A	25
For the detection of effusion, lung ultrasound is more accurate than supine radiography and is as accurate as CT.		A	25
In the evaluation of pleural effusion in adults, the microconvex transducer is preferable. If not available, a phased array or a convex transducer can be used.		B	25
The optimal site to detect a nonloculated pleural effusion is at the posterior axillary line above the diaphragm.		B	25
Both of the following signs are present in almost all free effusions: – A space (usually anechoic) between the parietal and visceral pleura – Respiratory movement of the lung within the effusion ("sinusoid sign")		A	25
A pleural effusion with internal echoes suggests that it is an exudate or hemorrhage. Although most transudates are anechoic, some exudates are also anechoic. Thoracentesis may be needed for further characterization.		A	25

A = consistent, good-quality patient-oriented evidence; B = inconsistent or limited-quality patient-oriented evidence; C = consensus, disease-oriented evidence, usual practice, expert opinion, or case series. For information about the SORT evidence rating system, go to http://www.aafp.org/afpsort.

Point-of-care ultrasound (POCUS) improves greatly upon the diagnostic accuracy of chest radiography and avoids many of the negative aspects of CT. Ultrasound has been used by radiologists to evaluate for pleural effusions for decades. Even with older technology, a 1976 study demonstrated the ultrasound's ability to identify pleural effusions of as little as 3 to 5 mL of fluid.[9] A 2016 meta-analysis found a pooled sensitivity and specificity of 94% and 98%, respectively, for ultrasound to accurately detect pleural effusion, compared with a sensitivity and specificity of only 51% and 91%, respectively, for chest x-ray.[10] In fact, pleural ultrasound can reliably detect 20 mL of fluid in the thorax and has been found to be 100% sensitive for effusions over 100 mL.[11] Ultrasound also has the added benefits of being able to visualize septations better than CT, discern certain pleural fluid characteristics, as well as accurately assess lung parenchyma for pleural, alveolar, or interstitial pathology. Additionally, ultrasound is portable, nonradiating, and repeatable. This allows for it to be performed and interpreted by the treating clinician, giving actionable information in real time. Studies have also shown that after just 3 hours of training, novice sonographers can diagnose pleural effusions with good agreement with experts.[12]

PERFORMING THE SCAN

A phased array or curvilinear probe should be used for this examination. A high-frequency (linear) probe is excellent for assessing for a pneumothorax or the pleural line, but does not penetrate deep enough to adequately assess for pleural effusion in an adult.

1. **Have the patient be in the sitting or semi-recumbent position.** Supine position is also possible for critically ill or bedbound patients. Gravity dictates that free-flowing effusions collect in the dependent portions of the thorax, best seen in the costophrenic recess just above the diaphragm. Place the probe at the **mid-axillary line** (**Figure 13-1**) at the level of the diaphragm with probe indicator pointing cephalad and scan toward the **posterior axillary line** (**Figure 13-2**).
2. **Identify the liver or spleen, then the diaphragm, then the lung and chest wall.** Optimize your gain and depth appropriately.

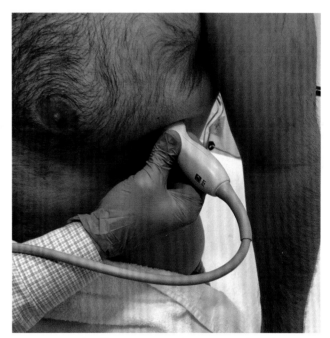

FIGURE 13-1. Mid-axillary position. Begin your scan here for a pleural effusion with the probe in coronal orientation and the probe marker cephalad.

The **diaphragm** (**Figure 13-3**) appears as a convex, curved, bright white line overlying the abdominal contents. A **pleural effusion** (**Figure 13-4**) appears as an anechoic space above the diaphragm between the visceral and parietal pleura of the lung. Of note, the diaphragm is lower in patients with chronic obstructive pulmonary disease (COPD) and higher in patients with abdominal obesity.

3. **Assess for visualization of the thoracic spine above the diaphragm.** Air-filled lung parenchyma typically obscures the view of the thoracic spine above the diaphragm (Figure 13-3); however, the presence of a pleural effusion or dense consolidation makes the spine visible. This is known as the **"spine sign"** (Figure 13-4) and is reliably seen with a pleural effusion.

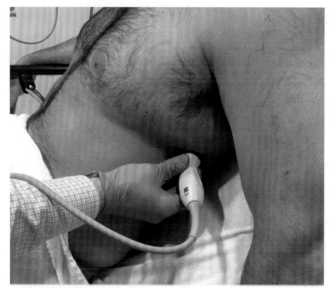

FIGURE 13-2. Posterior axillary position. Scan from the mid-axillary position toward the posterior axillary position with the probe in coronal orientation and the probe marker cephalad, visualizing the diaphragm.

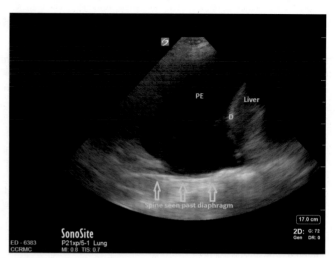

FIGURE 13-4. Appearance of pleural effusion with positive spine sign. D, diaphragm; PE, pleural effusion. Note the anechoic pleural effusion above the diaphragm, with visualization of the thoracic spine deep to the effusion. This is the spine sign and is reliably seen with pleural effusions.

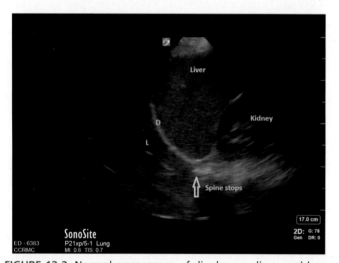

FIGURE 13-3. Normal appearance of diaphragm, liver, and lung. Negative spine sign. D, diaphragm; L, lung. Normal apposition of lung, liver, and diaphragm. The spine sign (not seen here) indicates visualization of the thoracic spine above diaphragm.

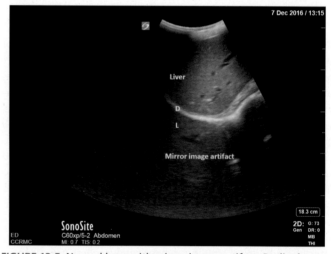

FIGURE 13-5. Normal lung with mirror image artifact. D, diaphragm; L, lung. The mirror image artifact is seen in normal lung without a pleural effusion, where the mirror image of certain details of the liver is seen on the thoracic side of the diaphragm. The mirror image artifact is a normal finding, indicating the presence of aerated lung above the diaphragm and effectively ruling out a pleural effusion.

4. **Look for the loss of *mirror image artifact*** (Figures 13-5 and 13-6). The mirror image artifact is a normal artifact indicating the presence of aerated lung above the diaphragm and effectively ruling out a pleural effusion. However, the lack of this sign indicates that there is fluid above the diaphragm. Also look for the loss of the **"curtain sign,"** which is the lung parenchyma obscuring the diaphragm and costovertebral angle by respirophasic excursion with each breath.

5. **Assess for respirophasic movement of lung within the effusion to verify that it is not a solid mass or consolidation.** When this respirophasic movement is seen on M-mode, it is called **"the sinusoid sign"** (Figure 13-7). Color Doppler may also be used to help determine if the anechoic contents are free-flowing (Figure 13-8).

6. **Assessing volume.** It is useful to know the relative size of an effusion. Once an effusion is >1 cm as measured on lateral decubitus chest x-ray on ultrasound, a thoracentesis can be performed safely.[13]

7. **Assessing characteristics.** Once a pleural effusion has been identified, the next step is to determine the cause. This is often done by distinguishing between an exudative or transudative process based on analysis of the pleural fluid obtained with thoracentesis. POCUS examination can also give clues to the type of fluid present. Effusions can be characterized by several specifications: simple versus complex, homogenous versus heterogeneous, and the amount of echogenicity. In general, a simple anechoic effusion is usually a transudate. Complex effusions are usually exudative and can be further divided into

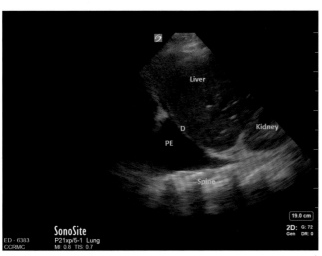

FIGURE 13-6. Pleural effusion with loss of mirror image artifact. D, diaphragm; PE, pleural effusion. Note the loss of the mirror image of the liver above the diaphragm and, instead, the presence of an anechoic pleural effusion.

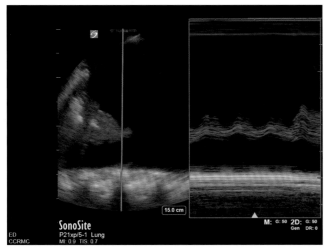

FIGURE 13-7. Sinusoidal sign. The sinusoid sign describes the appearance on M-mode of respirophasic movement of lung within the effusion, indicating that it is indeed fluid and not a solid mass or consolidation above the diaphragm.

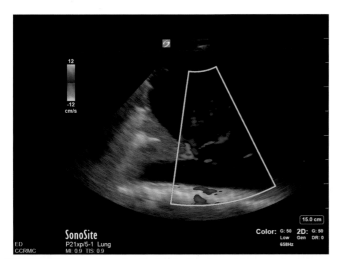

FIGURE 13-8. Color Doppler. Similar to the sinusoid sign, color Doppler may also be used to help verify that the anechoic contents are indeed free-flowing and not solid.

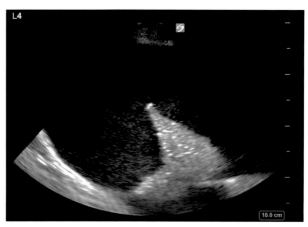

FIGURE 13-9. A homogenous echogenic effusion. This example is from a patient with an acute hemothorax secondary to left ventricular rupture. Image courtesy of David Schrift, MD.

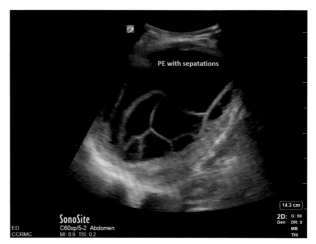

FIGURE 13-10. Septated effusion. PE, pleural effusion. Note the multiple lattice-like septations in this complex pleural effusion. Because of this, the patient went for VATS (video-assisted thoracoscopic surgery) instead of having a bedside thoracentesis.

septate and nonseptate. A homogenous echogenic effusion is likely an empyema or hemorrhagic effusion. See **Figure 13-9** and **Video 13-1**. See Table 13-3 for more examples. **Figure 13-10** shows septations.

PATIENT MANAGEMENT

Because the signs and symptoms of a pleural effusion are nonspecific, such as dyspnea, cough, pleuritic chest pain, and adventitial or decreased lung sounds, we recommend that assessing for a pleural effusion be a part of a general lung ultrasound examination. Once you have identified a pleural effusion via the focused assessment described earlier, the next step is to place the effusion in the context of the patient's clinical condition. Pleural effusions are signs of an underlying disease process rather than a diagnosis in and of themselves, and it is the clinical context itself that can help guide workup and management.

First, any unstable patients should be evaluated and treated in an acute care or hospital environment, especially those who appear acutely dyspneic, in respiratory distress, or septic. Next, it is extremely useful to categorize the patient's clinical context as fluid

TABLE 13-3	Specific Ultrasound Findings That Are Predictive of or Most Consistent with Certain Conditions[14,15]	
Ultrasound Findings	**Condition**	
Simple anechoic	Usually transudative	
Complex echogenic, homogenous or heterogeneous, with or without septations	Usually exudative	
Heterogeneous echogenicity with swirling	High cellular content, associated with malignancy	
Fibrinous stranding, septations, loculations	Exudative, associated with tuberculosis and pneumonia	
Homogenous echogenicity with layering effect in costophrenic recesses (hematocrit sign)	Hemothorax	
Homogenous echogenicity with speckling, does not change with patient's position	Empyema	
Pleural thickness >10 mm, pleural nodularity and diaphragmatic thickness >7 mm	Underlying malignancy	

overload, pneumonia, malignancy, or other. (See **Figures 13-11 and 13-12** and Table 13-1.)

1. **Fluid overload**. If the patient has known CHF with dyspnea, orthopnea, pulmonary edema, and bilateral, small, symmetric effusions, then decompensated CHF is the most likely etiology of the effusions, especially if the patient is also found to have bilateral B-lines, depressed ejection fraction, and a plethoric inferior vena cava (IVC). Similarly, if the patient has a history of cirrhosis with hypoalbuminemia and ascites in addition to bilateral pleural effusions, fluid overload from decompensated cirrhosis is the most likely etiology. Diagnostic thoracentesis is usually unnecessary in these cases, and treatment should focus on judicious diuresis and therapeutic optimization of the underlying disease process. Clinic follow-up within 3 days is appropriate. If the effusions are atypical or refractory to medical management, then diagnostic or therapeutic thoracentesis is indicated.

2. **Pneumonia**. If the patient's effusion is associated clinically with cough or fever, or other signs and symptoms of pneumonia, especially with adjacent alveolar consolidation, a timely diagnosis of a parapneumonic effusion or empyema is essential. Although most parapneumonic effusions are small and resolve without drainage, patients with complicated parapneumonic effusions or empyema—defined by the presence of pleural pus, loculations, fluid pH <7.0, or positive Gram stain or cultures—usually have longer hospitalizations, are subject to complications such as fibrosing

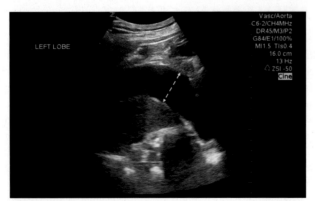

FIGURE 13-11. Here a pleural effusion is being measured in the transverse plane at the base of the lung. The calipers (yellow hashed line) are placed in the longest distance from the visceral to parietal pleura. The effusion volume (in mL) can be estimated by multiplying this measurement (in cm) by 20.

pleuritis, and have an overall increased morbidity and mortality. In these cases, prompt diagnosis and drainage is essential. Not only can bedside ultrasound aid in a timely initial diagnosis of the effusion, the characteristics and size of the effusion can help risk-stratify these patients. Thoracentesis and pleural fluid analysis should be performed on all parapneumonic effusions >1 cm to further classify them, because complicated effusions or empyema will need tube thoracostomy.[16] If loculations or septations are visualized on ultrasound, tube drainage is indicated and may be done in place of a diagnostic thoracentesis.[17]

3. **Malignancy**. If the patient has signs and symptoms of a malignancy without known pleural or pulmonary involvement, then prompt thoracentesis is indicated to assess for evidence of malignant cells in the pleural fluid or another explanation for the effusion. Although a full workup is indicated, additional ultrasound findings such as a pleural thickness >10 mm, nodular pleura, and a diaphragmatic thickness >7 mm (see ▶ Video 13-2) are strongly suggestive of a lung malignancy in a recent study and were shown to have positive and negative predictive values of 82.8% and 81.2%, respectively.[18] For those who meet criteria for a malignant pleural effusion, lung cancer accounted for 40%, breast cancer 25%, lymphoma 10%, and gastric and ovarian each with 5% of malignancies.[19] A malignant pleural effusion is a significant diagnosis for those with lung cancer because it changes staging to a stage 4 and heralds an extremely poor prognosis. Mean survival after diagnosis is only 4 to 8 months, so expeditiously establishing this diagnosis helps appropriately counsel patients and usually alters diagnostic and treatment decisions to a more palliative strategy.

4. **Other**. At least 50 different lung and/or systemic disorders can cause a pleural effusion. If the patient with an effusion has no signs or symptoms of fluid overload, pneumonia, or malignancy, then they will need thoracentesis for pleural fluid analysis to help ascertain the etiology. Given this extensive possibilities, it is essential to do a thorough morphologic, chemical, and cytologic workup of the fluid including applying Light's criteria rule for characterization as an exudate or transudate.[20] A few of the most common causes of exudative effusions include: viral pleurisy, pulmonary embolism (PE), tuberculosis, coronary artery bypass grafting, systemic lupus erythematosus, and rheumatoid arthritis.[21] (See Table 13-4.) Of note, tuberculous pleural effusions are the second most common extrapulmonary manifestation

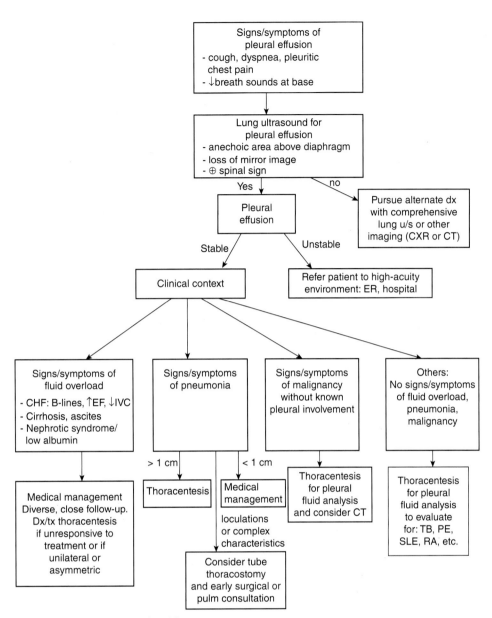

FIGURE 13-12. Management algorithm.

of mycobacterium tuberculosis, and early drainage may reduce residual symptomatic pleural thickening. Additionally, between 21% and 47% of patients with PE have pleural effusions, most of which are unilateral and small and can be missed on chest x-rays, thereby missing a clue to this important diagnosis.[22]

Once the effusion patient has been placed in these clinical categories, systematic and focused ultrasound can substantiate or corroborate the presumed bedside diagnosis. For example, just as we assess for rales, jugular venous distention (JVD), peripheral edema, and an S3 in our physical examination for CHF, so can we look for B-lines, depressed ejection fraction, plethoric IVC, and mitral regurgitation in a presumed CHF-related effusion. Similarly, it is highly recommended to also assess for signs of a deep vein thrombosis (DVT) and right heart strain in a suspected PE, adjacent alveolar consolidation and focal B-lines in a suspected pneumonia, pleural/diaphragmatic thickening and nodules in a possible malignancy, and signs of a positive Focused Assessment by Sonography for HIV-associated Tuberculosis (FASH) examination for a human immunodeficiency virus (HIV) patient with presumed extrapulmonary tuberculosis.[23] This systematic, focused, and integrated approach to the patient will greatly improve sensitivity and specificity and help you efficiently arrive at your patient's correct diagnosis.

TABLE 13-4	Common Conditions in Primary Care Associated With Pleural Effusions

Viral infection

Ascites

Nephrotic syndrome or other cause of hypoalbuminemia

Tuberculosis

Postcardiac surgery

Empyema

Pancreatitis

Medications such as nitrofurantoin, amiodarone, phenytoin, methotrexate

Rheumatoid arthritis

Systemic lupus erythematosus

Pericarditis

PEARLS AND PITFALLS

Pearl

- The volume in milliliters of pleural fluid can be estimated by measuring the maximal distance in centimeters between parietal and visceral pleura at the lung base and then multiplying by 20.[24]

Pitfalls

- Be sure to identify the diaphragm. Ascites with an elevated hemidiaphragm can mimic a pleural effusion. A hepatized lung or a complicated effusion can appear to be liver or spleen.
- Be sure to adjust your gain appropriately. Undergained images could impair visualization of the lung or even overestimate the size of an effusion. Overgained images could mischaracterize the pleural fluid as being more complex than it actually is.

- Up to 20% of anechoic effusions are actually solid per one study. Lymphomas and neurogenic neoplasms mimic effusions but are actually solid. Look for respirophasic movement of lung parenchyma into the effusion ("sinusoid sign") and/or color Doppler to help distinguish.
- Subcutaneous emphysema, pneumothorax, pleural calcifications all impair visualization of pleural effusions and can give a false-negative result.
- Wounds or bandages covering the lower thorax may impede comprehensive ultrasound scanning for a pleural effusion.
- Avoid an overreliance on pleural fluid characteristics to guide decision-making because simple-appearing effusions can be exudative and complex-appearing effusions can be transudative.

BILLING

CPT Code	Description	Medicare Global Payment	Professional Component	Technical Component	APC Code	APC Payment
76604	Ultrasound chest (includes mediastinum)	$89.56	$27.58	$61.97	0265	$90.05

CPT codes and average national reimbursement for Medicare in 2016. Payment data are from https://www.cms.gov/apps/physician-fee-schedule/search/search-criteria.aspx. See Chapter 2 for details on ultrasound billing.

References

1. Bhatnagar R, Maskell N. The modern diagnosis and management of pleural effusions. *BMJ.* 2015;351:h4520.
2. Wong CL, Holroyd-Leduc J, Straus SE. Does this patient have a pleural effusion? *JAMA.* 2009;301(3):309-317.
3. Blackmore CC, Black WC, Dallas RV, Crow HC. Pleural fluid volume estimation: a chest radiograph prediction rule. *Acad Radiol.* 1996;3(2):103-109.
4. Moskowitz H, Platt RT, Schachar R, Mellins H. Roentgen visualization of minute pleural effusion. An experimental study to determine the minimum amount of pleural fluid visible on a radiograph. *Radiology.* 1973;109(1):33-35.
5. Kitazono MT, Lau CT, Parada AN, Renjen P, Miller WT Jr. Differentiation of pleural effusions from parenchymal opacities: accuracy of bedside chest radiography. *AJR Am J Roentgenol.* 2010;194(2):407-412.
6. Esmadi M, Lone N, Ahmad DS, Onofrio J, Brush RG. Multiloculated pleural effusion detected by ultrasound only in a critically-ill patient. *Am J Case Rep.* 2013;14:63-66.
7. Fazel R, Krumholz HM, Wang Y, et al. Exposure to low-dose ionizing radiation from medical imaging procedures. *N Engl J Med.* 2009;361(9):849-857.
8. Committee to Assess the Health Risks from Exposure to Low Levels of Ionizing Radiation, BEIR VII, National Research Council. *Health Risks from Exposure to Low Levels of Ionizing Radiation.* Washington, DC: National Academies Press; 2006.
9. Gryminski J, Kradowki P, Lypacewicz G. The diagnosis of pleural effusion by ultrasonic and radiologic techniques. *Chest.* 1976;70(1):33-37.
10. Yousefifard M, Baikpour M, Ghelichkhani P, et al. Screening performance characteristic of ultrasonography and radiography in detection of pleural effusion; a meta-analysis. *Emerg (Tehran).* 2016;4(1):1-10.
11. Kalokairinou-Motogna M, Maratou K, Paianid I, et al. Application of color Doppler ultrasound in the study of small pleural effusion. *Med Ultrason.* 2010;12(1):12-16.
12. Begot E, Grumann A, Duvoid T, et al. Ultrasonographic identification and semiquantitative assessment of unloculated pleural effusions in critically ill patients by residents after a focused training. *Intensive Care Med.* 2014;40(10):1475-1480. doi:10.1007/s00134-014-3449-7.

13. Saguil A, Wyrick K, Hallgren J. Diagnostic approach to pleural effusion. *Am Fam Physician.* 2014;90(2):99-104.
14. Soni NJ, Franco R, Velez MI, et al. Ultrasound in the diagnosis and management of pleural effusions. *J Hosp Med.* 2015;10(12):811-816.
15. Yang PC, Luh KT, Chang DB, et al. Value of sonography in determining the nature of pleural effusion: analysis of 320 cases. *AJR Am J Roentgenol.* 1992;159(1):29-33.
16. Mandell LA, Wunderink RG, Anzueto A, et al. Infectious Diseases Society of America/American Thoracic Society consensus guidelines on the management of community-acquired pneumonia in adults. *Clin Infect Dis.* 2007;44(suppl 2):S27-S72.
17. Colice GL, Curtis A, Deslauriers J, et al. Medical and surgical treatment of parapneumonic effusions: an evidence-based guideline. *Chest.* 2000;118(4):1158-1171.
18. Bugalho A, Ferreira D, Dias SS, et al. The diagnostic value of transthoracic ultrasonographic features in predicting malignancy in undiagnosed pleural effusions: a prospective observational study. *Respiration.* 2014;87:270-278.
19. Sahn SA. Malignant pleural effusions. In Fishman AP, Elias JA, Fishman JA, et al, eds. *Pulmonary Disease and Disorders.* 3rd ed. New York, NY: McGraw-Hill; 1998:1429-1438.
20. Light RW. *Pleural Diseases.* 5th ed. Baltimore, MD: Lippincott, Williams and Wilkins; 2007.
21. Porcel JM, Light RW. Diagnostic approach to pleural effusion in adults. *Am Fam Physician.* 2006;73(7):1211-1220.
22. Worsley DF, Alavi A, Aronchick JM, Chen JT, Greenspan RH, Ravin CE. Chest radiographic findings in patients with acute pulmonary embolism: observations from the PIOPED Study. *Radiology.* 1993;189:133-136.
23. Heller T, Wallrauch C, Goblirsch S, Brunetti E. Focused assessment with sonography for HIV-associated tuberculosis (FASH): a short protocol and a pictorial review. *Crit Ultrasound J.* 2012;4(1):21.
24. Balik M, Plasil P, Waldauf P, et al. Ultrasound estimation of volume of pleural fluid in mechanically ventilated patients. *Intensive Care Med.* 2006;32(2):318.
25. Volpicelli G, Elbarbary M, Blaivas M, et al. International evidence-based recommendations for point-of-care lung ultrasound. *Intensive Care Med.* 2012;38(4):577-591.

Does the Patient Have a Pneumothorax?

Keith R. Barron, MD, FACP and Michael Wagner, MD, FACP, RDMS

Clinical Vignette

A 77-year-old man presents to your clinic with sudden onset of dyspnea and pleuritic, right-sided chest pain that began earlier in the day after a vigorous coughing episode. He uses inhalers daily for chronic obstructive pulmonary disease and has a 50 pack-year smoking history. Breath sounds are asymmetrically diminished over the right chest. Does the patient have a pneumothorax?

LITERATURE REVIEW

Pneumothorax (PTX) is a potentially life-threatening condition that refers to the presence of air in the pleural space that may occur either spontaneously or as a result of thoracic trauma or procedures, among other causes.[1] The annual rate of general practitioner consultations for PTX may be as high as 24 per 100 000 and 9.8 per 100 000 every year for men and women, respectively.[2]

Although history and physical examination may be suggestive of PTX, imaging is essential for establishing the diagnosis and guiding treatment. Historically, chest radiography has been used; however, timely access may be limited in the primary care setting. When compared with computed tomography (CT) scan, the sensitivity of chest radiography is limited, especially if performed with the patient supine or semirecumbent.[3,4] CT remains the reference standard, but its use is limited due to cost, portability, and availability, as well as radiation concerns.

Although first described in horses as early as 1986, the use of ultrasound for the diagnosis of PTX received increased attention after a series of articles by Daniel Lichtenstein described its clinical utility in critical care settings.[5-7] The addition of lung ultrasound to the focused assessment with sonography in trauma exam in the early 2000s resulted in the technique becoming widespread in emergency departments.[8] Since then, multiple studies and meta-analyses have found that ultrasound is more sensitive than supine chest x-ray (CXR) and equally specific.[9-11] This use of point-of-care ultrasound (POCUS) for the diagnosis of PTX is now widespread as a convenient, accurate, and safe alternative to ionizing radiation in emergency and critical care medicine. Although further research will need to establish its test characteristics outside of these settings, its use appears particularly well-suited for primary care as well.

Understanding and identifying the structures and artifacts that arise around the pleural surface is essential for the successful identification of PTX. Unlike most other uses of B-mode ultrasound, where organs or tissues appear similar to visual representations or cross-sections of actual anatomy, the presence of air and ribs creates many artifacts at the pleural surface. As a result, normally aerated lung parenchyma does not resemble lung tissue and is obscured by

artifacts. In PTX, free air dissects through the potential space that exists between the parietal and visceral pleura, which, in turn, alters the normal artifacts found at the pleural surface. Interpretation of the change in artifacts allows the diagnosis of PTX.

Each step of the examination will be explained in detail, but the overall goal is to first identify that the normal artifact of "lung sliding" is absent at the pleural surface, suggesting the presence of PTX, followed by imaging the exact transition point on the thorax called a "lung point" that occurs between the aerated lung and the free intrathoracic air of the PTX. Identification of this lung point should be considered pathognomonic for PTX. M-mode ultrasound is an optional modality that may assist in diagnosis as well.

TABLE 14-1	Recommendations for Use of Point-of-Care Ultrasound in Clinical Practice		
Recommendation		Rating	References
Lung ultrasound performed by expert operators compares favorably with chest computed tomography for the diagnosis of PTX.		A	8, 9
Lung ultrasound more accurately rules in and rules out the diagnosis of PTX than supine anterior chest radiography.		A	8-10
Lung ultrasound should be used in clinical settings when PTX is in the differential diagnosis.		A	10

A = consistent, good-quality patient-oriented evidence; B = inconsistent or limited-quality patient-oriented evidence; C = consensus, disease-oriented evidence, usual practice, expert opinion, or case series. For information about the SORT evidence rating system, go to http://www.aafp.org/afpsort.

PERFORMING THE SCAN

1. **Preparation.** Patient positioning is key to the diagnosis of PTX. Free intrapleural air will rise to the least-dependent portion of the thorax; therefore, position the patient supine, with the head of the bed at zero degrees (**Figure 14-1**). Intrapleural air should rise to the anterior chest wall, allowing examination of an area that is easily accessible. Further, this allows for standardization of examination techniques that were developed in critical or acute care settings, where the patient is already recumbent. Performing a PTX examination in any other position may reduce the sensitivity of the study, as air in small PTXs may rise apically into the supraclavicular area, which is difficult to image with ultrasound (**Figure 14-2**).

   Many probe types may be used, according to physician preference, location, and patient body habitus. In thin individuals and children, a high-frequency transducer allows for easy identification of the pleural surface, which is a superficial

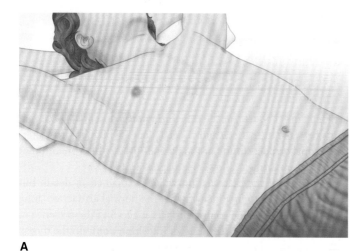

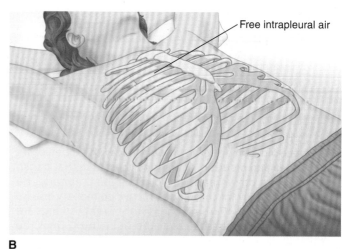

Free intrapleural air

A

B

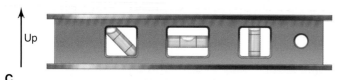

Up

C

FIGURE 14-1. Position the patient supine, at zero degrees (A), as intrapleural air will rise to the anterior chest wall, facilitating examination (B). It may be helpful to think of a simple level, where the position of the air bubble varies with positioning (C).

structure. Some authorities advocate for microconvex probes, but other low-frequency probes, such as curvilinear/convex, or even a multiphased array or sector-scanning probe, may be used, especially in scenarios where multiorgan examination in a rapid sequence is desired. Many machines have a "pleural" or "lung" preset now and should be used when available. However, other settings that minimize image processing (and therefore obscure artifact interpretation) have not been shown to adversely affect diagnostic accuracy, so they may be used if needed.

2. **Identify the lung "home screen" and normal artifacts.** For either the right or left side, begin the examination by placing the transducer on the anterior chest in the second intercostal space just lateral to the sternum, with the probe marker directed toward the patient's head. Position the probe over the two ribs, which will appear as rounded, partially echogenic structures with posterior shadowing. Next, identify the echogenic horizontal pleural line, which appears posterior to and between the ribs. When framed correctly, the pleural line should be in the center of the screen and the superior and inferior ribs should be on the left and right; this view constitutes the lung "home screen," which allows for the identification of normal architecture and artifacts (**Figure 14-3**).

Free intrapleural air

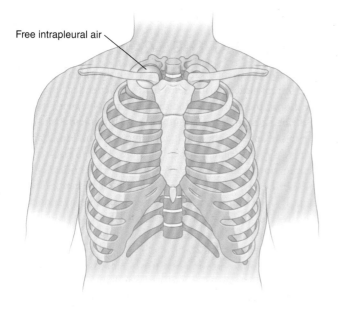

FIGURE 14-2. In an upright position, air may rise apically, below the clavicles, limiting the ability to diagnose pneumothorax.

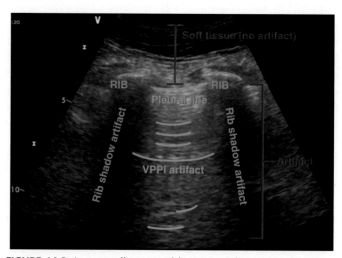

FIGURE 14-3. In normally aerated lung, an A-line pattern appears below the pleural line that is a repeating pattern of the visceral parietal pleural interface (VPPI) artifact. Note that when properly framed within the intercostal space, two ribs can be seen with posterior shadowing artifact.

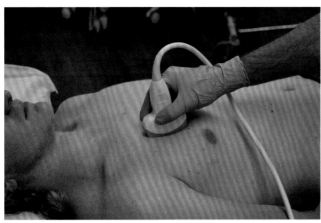

FIGURE 14-4. With the probe marker pointed toward the patient's head, place the transducer over an intercostal space adjacent to the sternum.

The pleural line is the junction of static parietal pleura of the chest wall and dynamic visceral pleura of the lung. The visceral pleura of the lung moves along the chest wall during normal respiration, which causes a subtle shimmering or glimmering appearance of the pleural line. This sliding, often described as "ants marching on a log" or "beads on a string," is a normal finding indicating that the parietal and visceral pleura are opposed at the site of probe placement (▶ **Videos 14-1 and 14-2**). In normally aerated lung, an A-line pattern will be present. A-lines are horizontal, echogenic reverberation artifacts that appear in an equidistant repeating fashion below,

and parallel to, the pleural line (Figure 14-3). The pleural line and subsequent artifacts are most visible when the transducer is perpendicular to the pleural line, so subtly fanning or angulating the probe may be necessary to maximally interpret the artifacts.

3. **Look for lung "sliding" to *rule out* PTX.** After becoming oriented at the home screen, evaluate for PTX by looking for intrapleural air. Free pleural air generally migrates to the least-gravitationally dependent portion of the thorax which, in a supine patient at 0°, occurs along the anterior chest, often in rib spaces 3-6 (**Figure 14-4**). The presence of lung sliding in these locations excludes PTX with high sensitivity.

In patients with PTX, pleural air dissects between the parietal and visceral pleura. Ultrasound beams are reflected by the intrapleural air just beyond the chest wall, and the moving visceral pleura of the collapsed lung is no longer detected by the ultrasound probe, causing a loss of lung sliding (▶ **Video 14-3**, **Figure 14-5**, and Table 14-2). Note that in PTX an A-line pattern will still be present, without lung sliding, as this artifact occurs when ultrasound waves encounter both normally aerated lung and free pleural air. B-lines, laser-like vertical artifacts that arise at the pleural line and move with respiration, are a sign of interstitial edema or fibrosis (▶ **Video 14-4**, **Figure 14-6**, and Table 14-2). Like lung sliding, they are seen only where the lung touches the chest wall, so their presences also rules out PTX at that probe position.

Absent lung sliding is the first sign of PTX, but may be present in other conditions where minimal visceral pleural movement occurs, such as pleural adhesions or contralateral

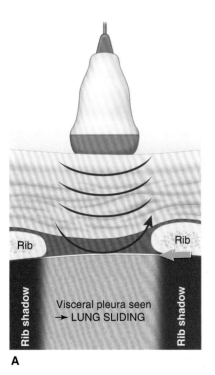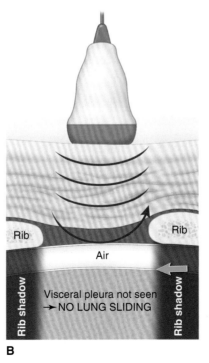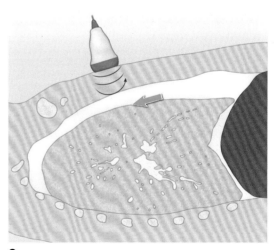

A   B   C

FIGURE 14-5. The normal lung "home screen" may show an A-line pattern both in normally aerated lung and in pneumothorax. When present, free pleural air dissects between the parietal and visceral pleura (A). Because air is highly reflective of ultrasound waves, the free air that is present in the potential space between the pleural layers obscures visualization of the deeper visceral pleura (B and C). In dynamic ultrasound scanning, this inability to image the visceral pleura is indicated by a loss of lung sliding.

TABLE 14-2	Normal Artifacts
Understanding artifacts is essential to understanding pleural ultrasound.	
Pleural line	An echogenic, or bright white, linear artifact that arises deep to the ribs that "slides" with respiration.
Ribs and rib shadows	Ribs are highly reflective of ultrasound waves and appear as echogenic, curved structures with posterior shadowing. Cartilaginous portions close to the sternum appear less echogenic and create less shadow than more ossified portions laterally.
Sliding	A dynamic artifact occurring in a normal, aerated lung that is generated by the translational movement of the visceral pleura along the parietal pleura during respiration. It appears as shimmering of the pleural line like "ants marching on a log," or moving "beads on a string."
A-line	Horizontal, echogenic artifact that appears in an equidistant repeating fashion below, and parallel to, the pleural line. A-lines should be the same distance apart as the distance from the probe to the pleural surface. A normal finding in aerated lung, but also present in pneumothorax.
Lung pulse	Subtle, horizontal, pulsations of the pleural surface that occur simultaneously with the cardiac cycle.
"Seashore" sign	A normal finding in M-mode. Lung sliding below the pleural line in M-mode generates a characteristic granular "sandy beach" pattern below the more stationary subcutaneous tissue and muscles that generate a linear "waves" pattern.

mainstem bronchus intubation. Usually in these situations a subtle, rhythmic, horizontal pulsation of the pleural line occurs synchronized with the cardiac cycle and is called the "lung pulse." This finding should be considered equivalent to lung sliding and does not occur at the site of PTX (Table 14-2).

4. **If lung sliding is absent, find the "lung point" to *rule in* PTX.** In the absence of lung sliding, angle the transducer in an oblique plane in an intercostal space and track laterally along the chest wall until a lung point is found (**Figure 14-7** and Table 14-2). A lung point is the artifact pattern generated along the pleural line by the dynamic transition point between partially collapsed lung, causing lung sliding, and the free pleural air, causing the A-line pattern without sliding. This point, with both patterns seen in a single view, varies with respiration as the air meniscus and partially aerated lung migrate along the chest wall (⏵ **Video 14-5**). A lung point should be considered pathognomonic for PTX, with a specificity of nearly 100% when performed by experienced operators.

In general, the further lateral and posterior the lung point is, the larger is the PTX. In a small number of cases, when the lung is completely and circumferentially collapsed away from the chest wall, the return of lung sliding or a lung point will not be visible no matter how far laterally or posteriorly the probe is positioned. A pattern where lung sliding is absent along the anterior chest but present over the lateral chest, without direct visualization of a lung point, is suggestive of, but not diagnostic for, a PTX.

5. **M-mode may be used to support the diagnosis.** In situations when the presence of lung sliding artifact is unclear, such as with low-resolution probes or with novice practitioners, M-mode is often advocated to support the diagnosis of PTX. With the transducer placed in the least-dependent portion

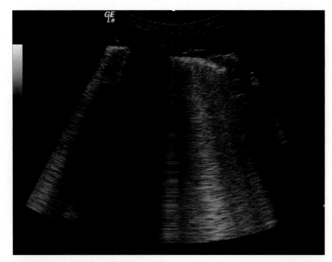

FIGURE 14-6. In this still image of an intercostal space, B-lines appear as laser-like vertical artifacts that arise at the pleural line. They are a sign of interstitial edema or fibrosis and rule out pneumothorax at that site.

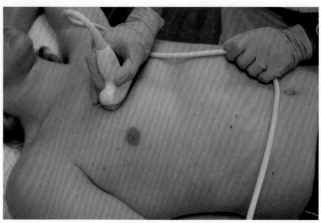

FIGURE 14-7. If lung sliding is absent, rotate the probe to an oblique position within the intercostal space and track laterally until a lung point is found.

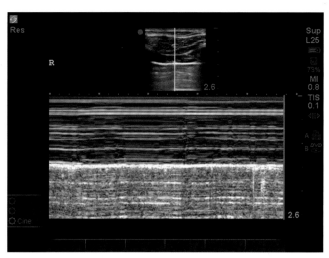

FIGURE 14-8. In normally aerated lung, M-mode within an intercostal space will generate a characteristic "seashore" pattern, as if waves (upper portion of screen) are lapping against a sandy beach (lower portion of screen).

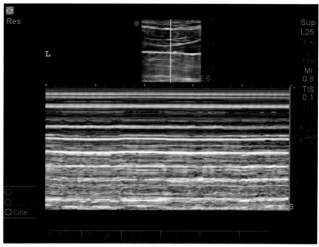

FIGURE 14-9. M-mode within an intercostal space when pneumothorax is present will generate the "barcode" sign, with static lines (or waves, see Figure 14-7), present across the screen throughout the respiratory cycle.

TABLE 14-3	Abnormal Artifacts
Interpretation of both normal and abnormal artifacts is key to the diagnosis of PTX.	
Loss of sliding	Absence of the normal shimmering of the pleural line that occurs when air is interposed between the parietal and visceral pleura. An A-line pattern with a loss of sliding is necessary for the diagnosis of PTX; however, the loss of sliding alone is not a sufficient condition for diagnosis, as other conditions may also rarely abolish sliding.
Lung point	An artifact that is pathognomonic for PTX. Usually best visualized with the ultrasound transducer oriented in the oblique plane, it signals the "air meniscus" or dynamic transition point between aerated lung and pleural air/PTX.
B-line	An echogenic vertical artifact that arises at the pleural line, moves with respiration, and extends to the edge of the screen. A sign of interstitial edema or fibrosis. The presence of this artifact rules out PTX at that point.
"Barcode" sign	Indicates PTX on M-mode. The loss of lung sliding generates similar patterns above and below the pleural line of M-mode, as if like a barcode.

Abbreviation: PTX, pneumothorax.

of the anterior chest in a supine patient, image the pleural line and home screen artifacts in B-mode, then switch to M-mode, placing the line down the center of the screen. A normally aerated lung will generate a characteristic "seashore sign": the inferior portion of the screen that corresponds to the portion of aerated lung that is sliding with respiration will appear like sand on a beach, with the more stationary subcutaneous tissue anterior to the pleural surface appearing like waves (**Figure 14-8** and Table 14-2). In the absence of lung sliding, the linear wave-like pattern will extend across the entire portion of the screen, generating the "barcode" sign (**Figure 14-9** and Table 14-3).

PATIENT MANAGEMENT

The presence of lung sliding at the least-dependent regions on the chest of a supine patient makes PTX unlikely. An A-line pattern without sliding or lung pulse is an indirect sign of PTX, which should prompt a search for the lung point. When found, a lung point confirms the diagnosis of PTX.

The next steps of management of PTX detected by POCUS depend on the stability of the patient. Although ultrasound findings can be specific for the diagnosis of PTX, emergent, bedside pleural drainage may not be the best initial step, as oxygen administration and observation may be appropriate for patients who are stable and have small-volume PTXs.

In emergency situations with a critically ill, unstable patient when tension PTX is suspected, some experienced practitioners will perform pleural drainage when encountering a unilateral A-line pattern without lung sliding. Indeed, the procedure itself may be guided by ultrasound at the bedside without need for further imaging. Conversely, in stable patients, especially in an outpatient or noncritical setting, the demonstration of a "lung point" should be required for a definitive diagnosis of PTX in the absence of further imaging (**Figure 14-10**).

There is some disagreement about the role of POCUS in quantifying the size of PTX, but the lung point may move laterally and past the midaxillary line in larger PTXs. In stable patients, further imaging may be required to definitively quantify the size of PTX. Ultrasound is more sensitive than CXR in supine patients, so CT may be required if quantification of PTX is needed in this population, especially in patients with emphysema.

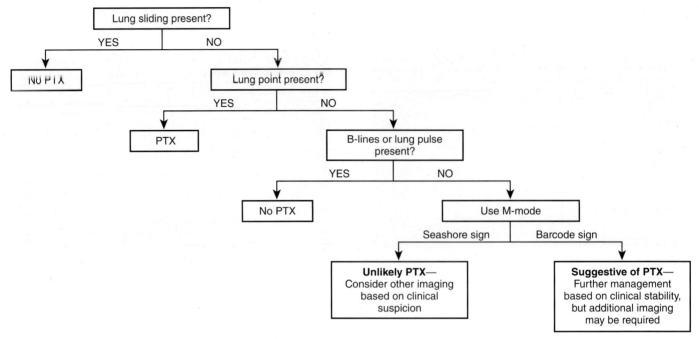

FIGURE 14-10. Suggested algorithm for the diagnosis of pneumothorax (PTX).

PEARLS AND PITFALLS

Pearl

- Over the left anterior chest wall, the heart may obscure lung sliding. Although often frustrating to learners, the visualization of a beating heart muscle, and not a static A-line pattern, excludes pleural air at that location as well.

Pitfall

- The absence of lung sliding is suggestive of PTX, but other conditions such as bullous emphysema, highly inflammatory pneumonias, or contralateral mainstem bronchus intubation may abolish or diminish lung sliding.
- Do not mistake the junction of lung and nonlung (rib, pericardium, diaphragm) as a lung point.

- Do not mistake a rib cortex for the pleural line. To an untrained eye, the linear, hyperechoic line of the rib cortex may appear similar to the pleural line when imaged in a plane parallel to its long axis. M-mode performed through a rib cortex will generate a barcode sign.
- The presence of the barcode sign in M-mode is not diagnostic of PTX by itself. Novice practitioners often assign too much importance to this sign.
- Intercostal muscle retractions will still be visible in PTX and novice practitioners may mistake this vertical translational movement that occurs with chest wall contraction to indicate lung pulse or even sliding.

BILLING

CPT Code	Description	Global Payment	Professional Component	Technical Component
76604	Ultrasound, chest, real time with image documentation	$89.56	$27.58	$61.97

CPT codes and average national reimbursement for Medicare in 2016. Payment data are from https://www.cms.gov/apps/physician-fee-schedule/search/search-criteria.aspx. See Chapter 2 for details on ultrasound billing.

References

1. Light R, Lee YGL. Pneumothorax, chylothorax, hemothorax, and fibrothorax. In: Broaddus VC, ed. *Murray and Nadel's Textbook of Respiratory Medicine*. 6th ed. Philadelphia, PA: Saunders; 2016:1439.e1410-1460.e1410.
2. Gupta D, Hansell A, Nichols T, Duong T, Ayres JG, Strachan D. Epidemiology of pneumothorax in England. *Thorax*. 2000;55(8):666-671.
3. Tocino IM, Miller MH, Fairfax WR. Distribution of pneumothorax in the supine and semirecumbent critically ill adult. *AJR Am J Roentgenol*. 1985;144(5):901-905.
4. Ball CG, Kirkpatrick AW, Laupland KB, et al. Factors related to the failure of radiographic recognition of occult posttraumatic pneumothoraces. *Am J Surg*. 2005;189(5):541-546; discussion 546.
5. Rantanen NW. Diseases of the thorax. *Vet Clin North Am Equine Pract*. 1986;2(1):49-66.
6. Lichtenstein DA, Menu Y. A bedside ultrasound sign ruling out pneumothorax in the critically ill. Lung sliding. *Chest*. 1995;108(5):1345-1348.
7. Lichtenstein D, Mezière G, Biderman P, Gepner A. The "lung point": an ultrasound sign specific to pneumothorax. *Intensive Care Med*. 2000;26(10):1434-1440.
8. Kirkpatrick AW, Sirois M, Laupland KB, et al. Hand-held thoracic sonography for detecting post-traumatic pneumothoraces: the Extended Focused Assessment with Sonography for Trauma (EFAST). *J Trauma*. 2004;57:288-295.
9. Alrajhi K, Woo MY, Vaillancourt C. Test characteristics of ultrasonography for the detection of pneumothorax: a systematic review and meta-analysis. *Chest*. 2012;141(3):703-708.
10. Alrajab S, Youssef AM, Akkus NI, Caldito G. Pleural ultrasonography versus chest radiography for the diagnosis of pneumothorax: review of the literature and meta-analysis. *Crit Care*. 2013;17(5):R208.
11. Volpicelli G, Elbarbary M, Blaivas M, et al. International evidence-based recommendations for point-of-care lung ultrasound. *Intensive Care Med*. 2012;38(4):577-591.

PART 2

Does the Patient Have Pneumonia?

Andrew W. Shannon, MD, MPH and William Chotas, MD

● Clinical Vignette

An 8-year-old female presents with a 3-day history of worsening cough. According to her mother, her breathing has progressively been more labored and she developed a fever of 39°C the morning prior to presentation. She has no significant past medical history and is up-to-date with her vaccinations.

Her vital signs show a temperature of 39.3°C, a heart rate of 130 beats per minute, a respiratory rate of 40 breaths per minute, and a blood pressure of 102/75 mm Hg. She has a room air oxygen saturation of 95%. Her examination shows a well-appearing girl with a moderately increased work of breathing evidenced by abdominal breathing and subcostal retractions. Her lung exam reveals bilateral coarse breath sounds that appear decreased over the bases. She has a benign abdomen and her head, eyes, ear, nose, and throat (HEENT) exam is unremarkable. Does the patient have pneumonia?

LITERATURE REVIEW

Community-acquired pneumonia (CAP) is the leading cause of death in pediatric patients worldwide,[1] and along with influenza is the eighth leading cause of death in the adult population.[2] For the purposes of this chapter, CAP will refer to pneumonia of both bacterial and viral etiologies.

CAP develops outside of the health care setting and is the most frequent form of pneumonia encountered in the emergency department and outpatient clinic. In the past, health care–associated pneumonia (HCAP) was a term that referred to pneumonia that developed in the outpatient setting in patients with exposure to health care settings with a high risk for exposure to drug-resistant organisms.[3] However, HCAP was removed from the 2016 Infectious Disease Society of America (IDSA) Guidelines as it was found that the pathogens encountered were similar to those found in CAP, and that there was less risk for the multidrug-resistant organisms than previously thought.[4] Hospital-acquired pneumonia (HAP) is pneumonia that develops 48 hours or more after admission.[3] The primary care physician will be concerned mostly with CAP, and therefore, the diagnosis and management of HAP will not be covered in this chapter.

Pneumonia has classically been diagnosed clinically through a combination of symptoms, vital signs, and findings on chest auscultation. However, clinical findings have been found to lack the sensitivity and specificity of chest imaging, and new guidelines from the IDSA require that an infiltrate be visualized for diagnosis.[5,6] The type of imaging is not specified in the guidelines but has traditionally been x-ray or computed tomography (CT).

Chest imaging is not always needed in children who are deemed well enough to be treated in the outpatient setting; however, it is recommended for children with hypoxemia, respiratory distress, or who otherwise require care in the inpatient setting.[7] It should also be considered in children without respiratory symptoms but with a temperature of 39.0°C or greater and a white blood cell count that is

greater than 20 000 cells/μL because they are at a high risk for occult pneumonia.[8,9] It is additionally recommended in cases of failed antibiotic therapy or clinical worsening to exclude complications such as parapneumonic effusions, necrotizing pneumonia, or pneumothorax.[7]

However, chest x-ray (CXR) and CT have considerable limitations. They both require exposure to ionizing radiation, which is especially problematic in children and pregnant adults. Furthermore, they are expensive, time-consuming, and require specialized equipment and interpretation. Thus, in both high- and low-resource environments, other diagnostic modalities have been sought.

The use of lung ultrasound (LUS) for the diagnosis of pneumonia has been studied in the medical literature for more than 30 years, with the first description in children as early as 1986.[10] Recently, several meta-analyses on the use of LUS for the diagnosis of pneumonia have been published for both pediatric and adult populations. Results showed a high accuracy of LUS for the diagnosis of pneumonia, with sensitivity ranging between 88% and 97% and specificity between 86% and 96% when compared with CXR or CT.[11-14] An international consensus document published in 2011 supported the use of LUS for the diagnosis of pneumonia citing comparable accuracy to CXR in adults and children. LUS was also noted to be faster than x-ray, reduce exposure to ionizing radiation, and to be able to distinguish pneumonia from atelectasis and other causes of consolidation.[15]

As the evidence continues to accumulate on the benefits of lung ultrasonography, some questions remain.[16] Studies have not directly examined the differences in accuracy of the scanning protocols used. Although the majority of studies in the pediatric literature employ a protocol established by Copetti and Cattarossi,[17] there has been a lack of consensus in the adult literature, with 2, 8, and 28 rib interspace protocols described.[15] What has been employed most frequently is some variant of Lichtenstein's bedside lung ultrasound in emergency (BLUE) protocol, an algorithmic approach to LUS used to diagnose multiple etiologies of lung pathology.[18]

Summary recommendations and strength of evidence for LUS for pneumonia are listed in (Table 15-1).[19]

TABLE 15-1	**Recommendations for Use of Point-of-Care Ultrasound in Clinical Practice**	
	Rating	References
LUS is a useful tool for ruling-in consolidation and can be applied in the point-of-care setting	A	11-13,15,17
LUS can effectively rule in and rule out pneumonia in both adult and pediatric patients	B	11-13,15
Lung ultrasonography is faster than CT and CXR, taking on average only 7 min	C	15,28

A = consistent, good-quality patient-oriented evidence; B = inconsistent or limited-quality patient-oriented evidence; C = consensus, disease-oriented evidence, usual practice, expert opinion, or case series. For information about the SORT evidence rating system, go to http://www.aafp.org/afpsort.
Abbreviations: CT, computed tomography; CXR, chest x-ray; LUS, lung ultrasound.

PERFORMING THE SCAN

1. **Position the patient.** The patient's anterior chest may be examined in either supine or upright positions. The lateral and posterior chest may be examined with patient upright, semirecumbent, or supine, especially when the patient cannot be moved. Because of the variation in body size between pediatric and adult patients, two probe placement protocols will be described. The findings and diagnostic criteria are the same in the diagnosis of pneumonia for both pediatric and adult patients.

2. **Select the probe.** For the pediatric patient, a higher-frequency 7.5 to 10 MHz linear probe offering better resolution may be selected, as the pleural line will be relatively superficial due to the lack of intervening soft tissues. A 5 to 7.5 MHz microconvex probe can also be used, and may provide better visualization of the supraclavicular thoracic regions. Adult patients are better examined using the lower-frequency microconvex or curvilinear array probes to provide for deeper tissue penetration.

3. **Visualize the pleura.** Place the probe in the long axis of the body with the marker pointing cephalad. Visualize the hyperechoic pleural line deep to the soft tissue of the chest wall in between the adjacent ribs. The hyperechoic cortices of the ribs will be seen superficial to the pleural line and produce shadows that obscure deeper structures. The normal pleural line demonstrates lung sliding, which is caused by the interface of the parietal and visceral pleura as they move along each other with respiration. This lung sliding may be obvious or it may be only a "shimmering,"

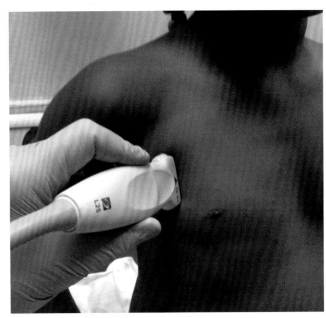

FIGURE 15-2. Pediatric chest scanning technique.

often described as "marching ants." The absence of normal lung sliding is concerning for possible pneumothorax but can also be seen in pneumonia.

4. **Scan the chest.** Begin scanning with the probe in a parasagittal orientation at the level of the second intercostal space in the anterior axillary line. Scan caudally until the diaphragm is visualized. It will appear as an echogenic line that moves inferiorly with respiration. It should be less echogenic than the pleural line. When using a high-frequency transducer, the diaphragm may, in fact, appear as two distinct echogenic lines with the muscle layer apparent in between them (**Figure 15-1**). Next, move the transducer medially toward the sternum and continue to scan cephalad to the clavicle. The pleural–pericardial interface will be apparent higher in the thorax on the left anterior chest, and is effectively the caudal limit of the pleural line until scanning more laterally. Repeat this "up and down" motion of the transducer along the pleural–chest wall interface until all areas of the thorax are imaged (**Figure 15-2**).

Because of the surface area of the adult thorax, an exhaustive "up and down" tracing of the pleural interface is not as practical as in the pediatric patient. Instead, begin by scanning the anterior chest wall in the midclavicular line at the 2nd or 3rd intercostal space with the transducer in the longitudinal or parasagittal orientation (**Figure 15-3**). Then, scan the anterolateral chest wall in the 4th or 5th intercostal space at the anterior axillary line. It may be necessary to orient the transducer somewhat obliquely to the long axis at this position due to the curvature of the ribs (**Figure 15-4**). Next, move the probe to the lower aspect of the ribs in the mid-axillary line with the transducer in a coronal orientation to the body to view the costophrenic angle. This view is equivalent to a supradiaphragmatic extended-focused assessment with sonography in trauma (E-FAST) view for pleural fluid (**Figure 15-5**). The pleural line–diaphragm interface should be visible as described earlier. The final view will be the posterior-lateral alveolar and/or pulmonary syndrome

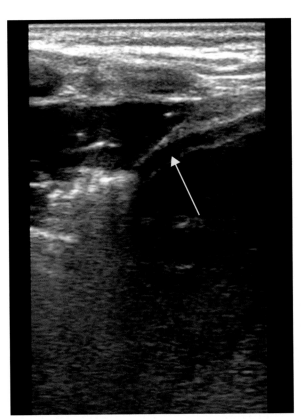

FIGURE 15-1. Visualization of the diaphragm with a high-frequency transducer. Note that the diaphragm appears as two distinct echogenic lines with the muscle layer apparent in between them. Arrow, diaphragm.

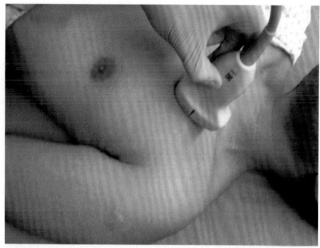

FIGURE 15-3. Anterior mid-clavicular positioning.

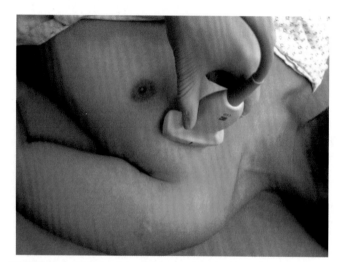

FIGURE 15-4. Anterior lateral lung positioning.

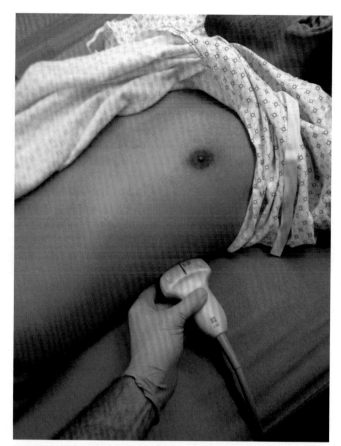

FIGURE 15-5. Lateral pleural space positioning.

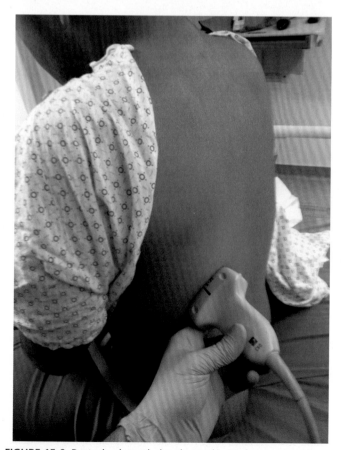

FIGURE 15-6. Posterior-lateral alveolar and/or pulmonary syndrome probe positioning, seated.

view, which will be at approximately the 4th or 5th intercostal space in the posterior axillary line[18] (**Figure 15-6**).

5. **Assess the pleural artifact pattern.** A-lines are artifacts seen on real-time 2D scanning that are also indicative of normal anatomy. They are visualized as horizontal, echogenic lines deep to the pleural line that lose signal strength the deeper they are seen (**Figure 15-7**). They are caused by reverberation of ultrasound pulses between the pleural line in the normal air-filled lung and the transducer surface.

B-lines are bright vertical artifacts that extend from the pleural line down to the bottom of the screen. They erase A-lines and move with lung sliding[20] (**Figure 15-8**). Although several B-lines can be normal, especially in dependent lung zones, when there are three or more visualized in one intercostal space they are thought to represent abnormal thickening of the interstitial septa of the lung (**Figure 15-9**). When three or more are present in a longitudinal intercostal space in more than two regions, it has been termed "alveolar-interstitial syndrome," the most common cause of which is interstitial edema.[21]

When a pattern of multiple B-lines is seen in a localized region, it suggests focal interstitial thickening that can be caused by

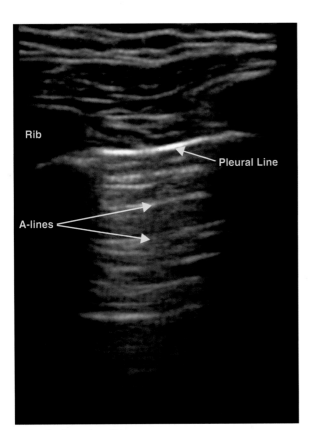

FIGURE 15-7. Thoracic A-lines.

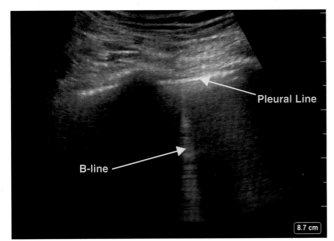

FIGURE 15-8. Thoracic B-line.

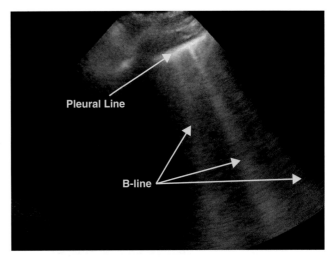

FIGURE 15-9. Multiple thoracic B-lines.

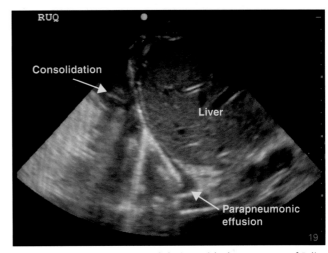

FIGURE 15-10. Pulmonary consolidation with the presence of B-lines and a parapneumonic effusion.

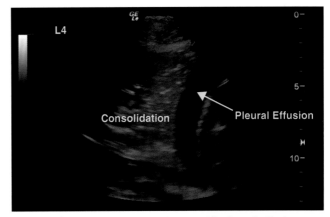

FIGURE 15-11. Pulmonary consolidation with pleural effusion.

pneumonia as well as atelectasis, pulmonary infarction, pulmonary contusion, and pleural disease. Multiple B-lines presenting diffusely throughout the chest would be more suggestive of an atypical or viral interstitial pneumonia, but the differential also includes bronchiolitis, pulmonary edema, and pulmonary fibrosis. B-lines may also be seen at the periphery of a consolidated pneumonia.

Lung sliding in pneumonia is typically reduced or absent, and the pleural line may lose its distinct echogenicity.[17] An adjacent parapneumonic effusion may also be seen (**Figure 15-10**).

6. **Assess for consolidation.** Consolidation in the lung appears as a spectrum from a hypoechoic area below the pleura to a "tissue-like" appearance similar to the echotexture of the liver (**Figure 15-11**). A common finding observed in consolidations is the air bronchogram.[22] Air bronchograms are bright hyperechoic densities visualized within the homogenous appearance of

a consolidation (**Figure 15-12**). They are intense reflections of the bronchial tree seen within the consolidated lung parenchyma. In dynamic air bronchograms, there is movement of air through the bronchial tree with respiration, causing these artifacts to move within and throughout the consolidation. This movement of the bronchogram artifacts with respiration is not seen in the consolidated appearance of the lung tissue in atelectasis.[23]

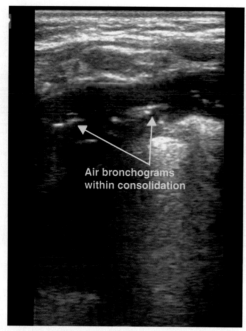

FIGURE 15-12. Consolidation with air bronchograms.

PATIENT MANAGEMENT

In pediatric patients, the degree of hypoxemia and respiratory distress can determine if they are well enough to be treated in the outpatient setting or if they require inpatient management (**Figure 15-13**). Children with a sustained oxygen saturation that is lesser than 90%

on room air (at sea level) and respiratory distress, aged less than 3 to 6 months, or children with suspected methicillin-resistant *Staphylococcus aureus* (or other organisms with increased virulence) should all be managed in a hospital setting, whereas those requiring invasive ventilation should be taken care of in the intensive care unit (ICU).[7]

In well-appearing children with no respiratory distress and oxygen saturation greater than 90% suspected to have pneumonia, there is no need for routine imaging. Although these patients can be treated empirically in the outpatient setting according to guidelines, because of the accuracy of LUS and the lack of ionizing radiation, we recommend the use of LUS to confirm the diagnosis so as to promote the judicious use of antibiotics. Children requiring hospitalization should have chest imaging performed to document the infiltrate and identify potential complications necessitating further therapy such as parapneumonic effusion, necrotizing pneumonia, or pneumothorax.[7] Substituting LUS for CXR resulted in fewer radiographs without an increase in adverse events in at least one recent prospective pediatric trial.[24]

In adult patients, clinical decision tools such as CURB-65 or the pneumonia severity index can help identify patients who could safely be treated in the outpatient setting.[25] ICU-level care is needed for patients with septic shock requiring vasopressors, those requiring mechanical ventilation, and patients with other markers of organ dysfunction.[5] All adults in whom pneumonia is suspected should receive imaging to confirm the presence of pneumonia.[5]

Antibiotic therapy should be given empirically to patients with pneumonia, and therapy should be tailored when specific pathogens are suspected or identified. Suggested empiric antibiotic regimens are detailed in **Tables 15-2**[7] and **15-3**.[5]

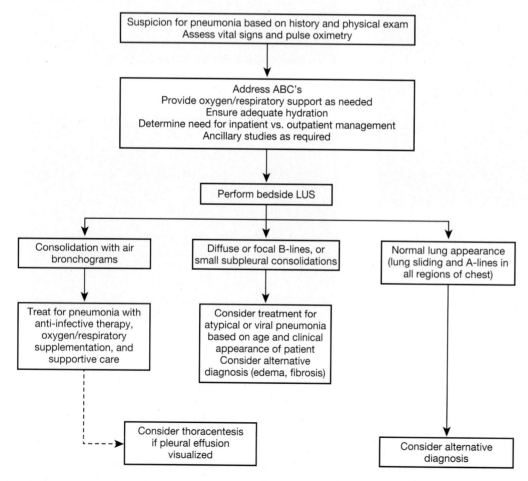

FIGURE 15-13. Lung ultrasound (LUS) pneumonia management algorithm.

TABLE 15-2 **Empiric Antibiotic Regimen for Community-Acquired Pneumonia (Pediatrics)**

Patient Characteristics	Presumed Bacterial Pneumonia	Presumed Atypical Pneumonia
Outpatient		
<5 y old	Amoxicillin, oral Alternative: amoxicillin clavulanate	Azithromycin, oral Alternative: oral clarithromycin or erythromycin
>5 y old	Amoxicillin, oral Alternative: amoxicillin clavulanate ± macrolide	Azithromycin, oral Alternative: oral clarithromycin, erythromycin, doxycycline (>7 y old)
Inpatient		
Fully immunized (vs. *Haemophilus influenzae* type b and *Streptococcus pneumoniae*); local PCN resistance in invasive pneumococcus significant	Ampicillin or PCN G; ceftriaxone or cefotaxime; addition of vancomycin or clindamycin if suspected CA-MRSA	Azithromycin ± β-lactam Alternative: clarithromycin, erythromycin; doxycycline or levofloxacin for older children
Not fully immunized (vs. *H. influenzae* type b and *S. pneumoniae*); local PCN resistance in invasive pneumococcus significant	Ceftriaxone or cefotaxime; alternatively levofloxacin; addition of vancomycin or clindamycin if suspected CA-MRSA	Azithromycin ± β-lactam Alternative: clarithromycin, erythromycin; doxycycline or levofloxacin for mature children

Abbreviations: CA-MRSA, community-associated methicillin-resistant *Staphylococcus aureus*; PCN, penicillin.

From Bradley JS, Byington CL, Shah SS, et al. The management of community-acquired pneumonia in infants and children older than 3 months of age: clinical practice guidelines by the Pediatric Infectious Diseases Society and the Infectious Diseases Society of America. *Clin Infect Dis.* 2011;53(7):e25-e76. Reproduced with permission from Infectious Diseases Society of America.

TABLE 15-3 **Empiric Antibiotic Regimen for Community-Acquired Pneumonia (Adults)**

Patient Characteristics	Antibiotic Choice	Strength of Recommendation
Previously healthy; No use of antimicrobials in previous 3 mo	Macrolide	Strong recommendation; level I evidence
	Doxycycline	Weak recommendation; level III evidence
Presence of comorbidities (chronic heart, lung, liver or renal disease; diabetes mellitus; alcoholism; malignancies; asplenia; immunosuppressing conditions or use of immunosuppressing drugs)	Respiratory fluoroquinolone (moxifloxacin, gemifloxacin, levofloxacin [750 mg])	Strong recommendation; level I evidence
Use of antimicrobials within previous 3 mo (in which case an alternative from a different class should be selected)	β-lactam plus a macrolide	Strong recommendation; level I evidence
Inpatient, not ICU		
	Respiratory fluoroquinolone	Strong recommendation; level I evidence
	β-lactam plus a macrolide	Strong recommendation; level I evidence

From Mandell LA, Wunderink RG, Anzueto A, et al. Infectious Diseases Society of America/American Thoracic Society consensus guidelines on the management of community-acquired pneumonia in adults. *Clin Infect Dis.* 2007;44(suppl 2):S27-S72. Reproduced with permission from Infectious Diseases Society of America.

PEARLS AND PITFALLS

Pearls

- Dynamic air bronchograms, when present, can help differentiate pneumonia from atelectasis in a consolidated lung.
- Focal, pathologic B-lines and subpleural consolidations smaller than 1 cm, when found together, are highly suggestive of viral pneumonia (**Figure 15-14**).[26]

Pitfalls

- When LUS is negative for pneumonia, pneumothorax or other interstitial syndrome, do not forget to consider alternative diagnoses including pulmonary embolism and myocardial infarction.
- Be aware of short vertical artifacts such as I-lines or Z-lines that may be confused with B-lines. They also arise from the pleura, or just below it, but are short path reverberations and will not continue to the bottom of the screen. They are not related to lung pathology.[15,27]
- Consolidations that do not reach the pleura, although rare, can be missed by LUS but diagnosed by CXR.
- A small area of consolidation can be missed or confused with the spleen when in the left lower lobe.

Pearls and Pitfalls, Continued

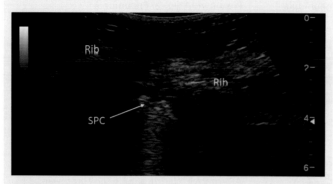

FIGURE 15-14. A small subpleural consolidation (SPC) that is specific for viral pneumonia in children.

BILLING[29,30]

CPT Code	Description	Global Payment	Professional Component	Technical Component
76604	US Exam Chest	$90.08	$27.63	$62.45

CPT codes and average national reimbursement for Medicare in 2016. Payment data are from https://www.cms.gov/apps/physician-fee-schedule/search/search-criteria.aspx. See Chapter 2 for details on ultrasound billing.

References

1. Liu L, Hill K, Oza S, et al. Levels and causes of mortality under age five years. In: Black RE, Laxminarayan R, Temmerman M, Walker N, eds. *Reproductive, Maternal, Newborn, and Child Health: Disease Control Priorities.* Vol 2, 3rd ed. Washington, DC: The International Bank for Reconstruction and Development/The World Bank; 2016.

2. National Center for Health Statistics (US). *Health, United States, 2015: With Special Feature on Racial and Ethnic Health Disparities.* Hyattsville, MD: National Center for Health Statistics (US); 2016. https://www.ncbi.nlm.nih.gov/books/NBK367640.

3. American Thoracic Society; Infectious Diseases Society of America. Guidelines for the management of adults with hospital-acquired, ventilator-associated, and healthcare-associated pneumonia. *Am J Respir Crit Care Med.* 2005;171(4):388-416. doi:10.1164/rccm.200405-644ST.

4. Kalil AC, Metersky ML, Klompas M, et al. Management of adults with hospital-acquired and ventilator-associated pneumonia: 2016 Clinical Practice Guidelines by the Infectious Diseases Society of America and the American Thoracic Society. *Clin Infect Dis.* 2016;63(5):e61-e111. doi:10.1093/cid/ciw353.

5. Mandell LA, Wunderink RG, Anzueto A, et al. Infectious Diseases Society of America/American Thoracic Society consensus guidelines on the management of community-acquired pneumonia in adults. *Clin Infect Dis.* 2007;44(suppl 2):S27-S72. doi:10.1086/511159.

6. Wipf JE, Lipsky BA, Hirschmann JV, et al. Diagnosing pneumonia by physical examination: relevant or relic? *Arch Intern Med.* 1999;159(10):1082-1087.

7. Bradley JS, Byington CL, Shah SS, et al. The management of community-acquired pneumonia in infants and children older than 3 months of age: clinical practice guidelines by the Pediatric Infectious Diseases Society and the Infectious Diseases Society of America. *Clin Infect Dis.* 2011;53(7):e25-e76. doi:10.1093/cid/cir531.

8. Murphy CG, van de Pol AC, Harper MB, Bachur RG. Clinical predictors of occult pneumonia in the febrile child. *Acad Emerg Med.* 2007;14(3):243-249. doi:10.1197/j.aem.2006.08.022.

9. Bachur R, Perry H, Harper MB. Occult pneumonias: empiric chest radiographs in febrile children with leukocytosis. *Ann Emerg Med.* 1999;33(2):166-173.

10. Weinberg B, Diakoumakis EE, Kass EG, Seife B, Zvi ZB. The air bronchogram: sonographic demonstration. *Am J Roentgenol.* 1986;147(3):593-595. doi:10.2214/ajr.147.3.593.

11. Pereda MA, Chavez MA, Hooper-Miele CC, et al. Lung ultrasound for the diagnosis of pneumonia in children: a meta-analysis. *Pediatrics.* 2015;135(4):714-722. doi:10.1542/peds.2014-2833.

12. Chavez MA, Shams N, Ellington LE, et al. Lung ultrasound for the diagnosis of pneumonia in adults: a systematic review and meta-analysis. *Respir Res.* 2014;15:50. doi:10.1186/1465-9921-15-50.

13. Hu QJ, Shen YC, Jia LQ, et al. Diagnostic performance of lung ultrasound in the diagnosis of pneumonia: a bivariate meta-analysis. *Int J Clin Exp Med.* 2014;7(1):115-121.

14. Long L, Zhao HT, Zhang ZY, Wang GY, Zhao HL. Lung ultrasound for the diagnosis of pneumonia in adults: A meta-analysis. *Medicine (Baltimore).* 2017;96(3):e5713. doi:10.1097/md.0000000000005713.

15. Volpicelli G, Elbarbary M, Blaivas M, et al. International evidence-based recommendations for point-of-care lung ultrasound. *Intensive Care Med.* 2012;38(4):577-591. doi:10.1007/s00134-012-2513-4.

16. Zar HJ, Andronikou S, Nicol MP. Advances in the diagnosis of pneumonia in children. *BMJ.* 2017;358:j2739.

17. Copetti R, Cattarossi L. Ultrasound diagnosis of pneumonia in children. *Radiol Med.* 2008;113(2):190-198. doi:10.1007/s11547-008-0247-8.

18. Lichtenstein DA, Mezière GA. Relevance of lung ultrasound in the diagnosis of acute respiratory failure: the BLUE protocol. *Chest.* 2008;134(1):117-125. doi:10.1378/chest.07-2800.

19. Ebell MH, Siwek J, Weiss BD, et al. Strength of recommendation taxonomy (SORT): a patient-centered approach to grading evidence in the medical literature. *Am Fam Physician.* 2004;69(3):548-556.

20. Lichtenstein DA. Ultrasound in the management of thoracic disease. *Crit Care Med.* 2007;35(5 suppl):S250-S261. doi:10.1097/01.ccm.0000260674.60761.85.

21. Lichtenstein DA, Mezière GA, Lagoueyte JF, Biderman P, Goldstein I, Gepner A. A-lines and B-lines: lung ultrasound as a bedside tool for predicting pulmonary artery occlusion pressure in the critically ill. *Chest.* 2009;136(4):1014-1020. doi:10.1378/chest.09-0001.

22. Copetti R, Cattarossi L. Lung ultrasound in newborns, infants, and children. In: Mathis G, ed. *Chest Sonography.* Berlin, Heidelberg: Springer Berlin Heidelberg; 2011:241-245.

23. Lichtenstein D, Mezière G, Seitz J. The dynamic air bronchogram. A lung ultrasound sign of alveolar consolidation ruling out atelectasis. *Chest.* 2009;135(6):1421-1425. doi:10.1378/chest.08-2281.

24. Jones BP, Tay ET, Elikashvili I, et al. Feasibility and safety of substituting lung ultrasonography for chest radiography when diagnosing pneumonia in children: a randomized controlled trial. *Chest.* 2016;150(1):131-138. doi:10.1016/j.chest.2016.02.643.

25. Lim W, van der Eerden MM, Laing R, et al. Defining community acquired pneumonia severity on presentation to hospital: an international derivation and validation study. *Thorax.* 2003;58(5):377-382. doi:10.1136/thorax.58.5.377.

26. Tsung JW, Kessler DO, Shah VP. Prospective application of clinician-performed lung ultrasonography during the 2009 H1N1 influenza A pandemic: distinguishing viral from bacterial pneumonia. *Crit Ultrasound J.* 2012;4(1):16. doi:10.1186/2036-7902-4-16.

27. Lee FC. Lung ultrasound: a primary survey of the acutely dyspneic patient. *J Intensive Care.* 2016;4(1):57. doi:10.1186/s40560-016-0180-1.

28. Shah VP, Tunik MG, Tsung JW. Prospective evaluation of point-of-care ultrasonography for the diagnosis of pneumonia in children and young adults. *JAMA Pediatr.* 2013;167(2):119-125. doi:10.1001/2013.jamapediatrics.107.

29. Physician Fee Schedule Search [database online]. Baltimore MD: U.S. Centers for Medicare and Medicaid Services; 2013. https://www.cms.gov/apps/physician-fee-schedule/search/search-criteria.aspx. Accessed April 14, 2017.

30. CPT Assistant; May, 2009;19(5).

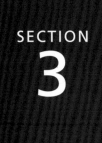
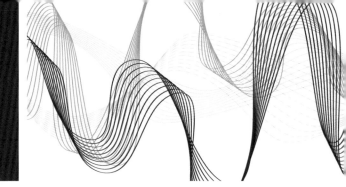

SECTION 3 BREAST

CHAPTER 16

Does the Patient's Breast Mass Need to Be Biopsied?

Esther Kim, MD, Andrew Kim, MD, John Rocco MacMillan Rodney, MD, FAAFP, RDMS, and William MacMillan Rodney, MD, FAAFP, FACEP

● Clinical Vignette

A 42-year-old female presents to your clinic complaining of a palpable left breast lump. She had received free screening at a local community event and was told that she would need to follow-up with a physician. On examination, the left breast lump is retroareolar and approximately 3 cm × 3 cm on palpation with some breast asymmetry, although there is no nipple retraction or overlying skin changes. Does the patient's breast mass need to be biopsied?

LITERATURE REVIEW

Imaging of the breast is performed with a variety of different techniques, the most prominent of which are mammography, magnetic resonance imaging (MRI), and ultrasound. The American College of Radiology (ACR) BI-RADS 5th edition acknowledges these three modalities in assessing the risk of breast cancer in patients.[1] Of these three, mammography is the most commonly recommended imaging modality in the assessment of breast lesions. Mammographic findings often dictate the necessity of ultrasound, but ultrasound can also be used without mammography on the basis of the patient's age and risk.

Ultrasound technology has improved significantly in the last 20 years, and so has the utility of ultrasound in diagnosing breast lesions. Although its initial use was primarily in diagnosing simple cysts, breast ultrasound is now used to characterize all types of breast lesions and to estimate their risk of malignancy. The seminal work by Stavros et al. showed that ultrasound could be used to distinguish breast lesions as benign or malignant with an negative predictive value (NPV) of 99.5%.[2] Subsequently, the use of the BI-RADS lexicon and categories for ultrasound has proven consistent with mammography in several studies.[3-6] Therefore, the BI-RADS categories are a natural framework for determining whether a patient needs a breast biopsy.

Breast ultrasound has three primary uses today. The first is as an adjunct to mammography, further characterizing mammographic abnormalities. The second is in the workup and diagnosis of breast masses. The final use for breast ultrasound is ultrasound-guided percutaneous breast biopsies, and Table 16-2 provides a list of general indications for this procedure. If percutaneous biopsy is not available, ultrasound can also be used for mapping prior to excisional biopsy.

In terms of primary screening for breast cancer, ultrasonography is in general not recommended except when mammography is not feasible.[7] Breast ultrasound as secondary screening following mammography has also been extensively studied. Although adding breast ultrasound to mammographic breast cancer screening improves its sensitivity, especially with dense breast tissue, it also increases the rate of false positives, leading to a larger number of breast biopsies with benign results. Therefore, ultrasound is not currently recommended for screening but rather as an adjunct to mammography to better characterize mammographic findings.[8]

TABLE 16-1 Recommendations for Use of Point-of-Care Ultrasound in Clinical Practice		
Recommendation	Rating	References
Breast ultrasound can be used to accurately characterize a lesion as benign.	A	1,2,4,6,11
Women under 30 years with a palpable breast mass should obtain an ultrasound for initial evaluation instead of mammography.	C	12-15

A = consistent, good-quality patient-oriented evidence; B = inconsistent or limited-quality patient-oriented evidence; C = consensus, disease-oriented evidence, usual practice, expert opinion, or case series. For information about the SORT evidence rating system, go to http://www.aafp.org/afpsort.

TABLE 16-2	Indications for Ultrasound-Guided Breast Interventional Procedures	
Type of Lesions	**When to Biopsy**	
Simple and complicated cysts	1. Symptomatic 2. Unclear if the lesion is a complicated cyst or solid lesion	
Complex cyst and solid masses	1. Masses assessed as BI-RADS Category 4 or 5 2. >1 suspicious mass in a multicentric distribution 3. Masses assessed as BI-RADS 3 but with clinical concerns or when short term interval imaging follow-up would be difficult 4. Masses seen on ultrasound exam correlate with suspicious areas of enhancement seen on contrast-enhanced breast MRI.	
Microcalcifications	1. If seen on directed ultrasound exam and correlate with suspicious calcifications seen on mammography	
Lymph nodes in axilla or axillary tails	1. In cases of known or suspected malignancy	

Abbreviation: MRI, magnetic resonance imaging.
Adapted from Newell MS, Barke LD, Argus AD, et al. *ACR Practice Parameter for the Performance of Ultrasound-guided Percutaneous Breast Interventional Procedures.* American College of Radiology. https://www.acr.org/-/media/ACR/Files/Practice-Parameters/US-GuidedBreast.pdf. Accessed November 26, 2016.

PERFORMING THE SCAN

1. **Preparation.** Have the patient undress and put on a gown. Have a chaperone in the room during the exam. Perform ultrasound exam with the patient in supine position. Other positions may be utilized to obtain the best image. These include the upright position and the contralateral decubitus position for the lateral half of the breast to minimize the breast density. If the patient had previous imaging results (mammography, MRI, etc.), have the results available to help guide your scan. Ask the patient in what position he or she best feels the mass. If the patient feels the mass best when he or she is supine, standing, or sitting, the ultrasound can be performed in that position.

2. **Equipment.** We recommend using the linear-array transducer probe with a frequency of 10 to 15 MHz. The focal zone should be adjusted to center the lesion. For superficial masses, place a large amount of gel on the patient to place the mass of interest in the focal zone of the transducer and to avoid volume averaging (**Figure 16-1**).

3. **Scan the breast tissue.** The skin is hyperechoic and typically less than 2 mm thick. The subcutaneous fat, anterior to the anterior mammary fascia, contains the hyperechoic bands of the suspensory ligaments (also known as Cooper's ligaments) running through it. The mammary layer, which is the breast parenchyma, is posterior to the subcutaneous fat and is where the majority of breast cancers are detected. The parenchyma is typically hyperechoic but may be heterogeneous. It contains approximately 15 to 20 lobes of the glandular tissue, which drain into ducts that appear as thin echogenic lines, although they can appear as hypoechoic tubes when filled with fluid. Next is the retromammary layer that is composed mostly of fat and contains the deep pectoral fascia. The ribs, the pectoralis and intercostal muscles, and the lung pleura can be visualized posterior to this layer (**Figures 16-2 through 16-4**).

4. **Documentation.** Images should be clearly labeled, such as right or left breast, location of the lesion using clock-face notation, distance from the nipple, and orientation of the transducer. Do not measure the distance from the areola, because areolar sizes

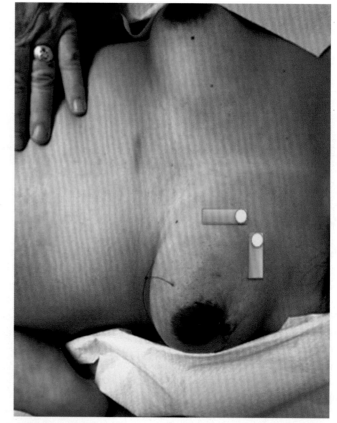

FIGURE 16-1. The patient is placed in the left lateral decubitus position. Ultrasound probe marker is pointed caudal or toward the patient's right.

may be different (**Figure 16-5**). The size of the lesion should be measured in at least two planes; in general, orthogonal planes are recommended but not necessary. Color Doppler may be used to assess the vascularity of the lesion. Be careful to use as little pressure as possible because the breast vasculature is easily compressed. Like the BI-RADS characterization used in mammography, use the BI-RADS ultrasound lexicon to describe the sonographic features of the mass.

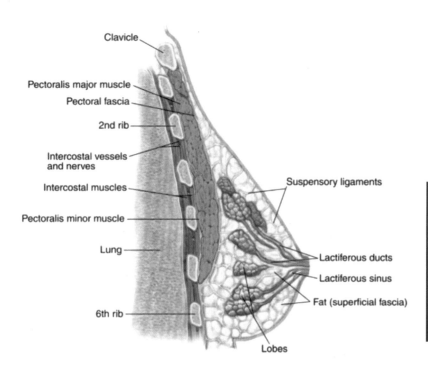

FIGURE 16-2. Graphical depiction of normal breast anatomy. Reprinted with permission from Tank PW. *Lippincott Williams & Wilkins Atlas of Anatomy*. Philadelphia, PA: Wolters Kluwer Health/Lippincott Williams & Wilkins; 2009. Plate 2-10.

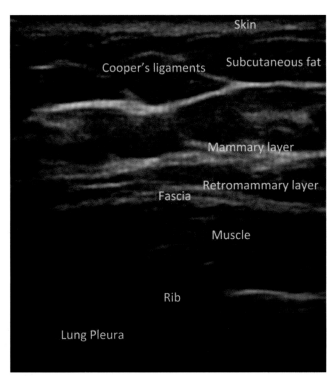

FIGURE 16-3. Sample sonographic image of normal breast tissue from the midclavicular sagittal view.

PATIENT MANAGEMENT

Palpable masses should always receive an ultrasound, although it is unclear how significant palpability is in determining the risk for malignancy.[9] The patient's age is crucial in estimating the patient's risk of malignancy and in assessing the value of obtaining mammography, given that dense breast tissue may make interpretation difficult. For example, the ACR specifically recommends using ultrasound for

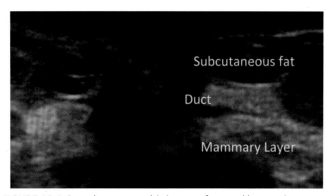

FIGURE 16-4. Sample sonographic image of normal breast tissue over the nipple in sagittal view.

initial imaging when the patient is less than 30 years of age and not at a high risk for developing breast cancer.[10]

The decision to biopsy a breast mass is primarily dependent on the suspected diagnosis and the risk of malignancy. The BI-RADS

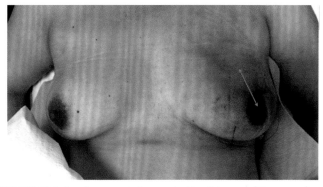

FIGURE 16-5. For documentation, note the distance of the mass from the nipple, not the areola.

TABLE 16-3 Ultrasound BI-RADS Assessment Categories and Management

	Management
Category 0: Incomplete—need additional imaging evaluation	Additional imaging
Category 1: Negative	Routine screening
Category 2: Benign	Routine screening
Category 3: Probably Benign	Short-Interval (6-mo) follow-up
Category 4: Suspicious • 4A: Low suspicion for malignancy • 4B: Moderate suspicion for malignancy • 4C: High suspicion for malignancy	Tissue diagnosis
Category 5: Highly Suggestive of Malignancy	Tissue diagnosis
Category 6: Known Biopsy-Proven Malignancy	Surgical excision when clinically appropriate

Adapted with permission from Mendelson EB, Böhm-Vélez M, Berg WA, et al. ACR BI-RADS® Ultrasound. In: D'Orsi CJ, Sickles EA, Mendelson EB, Morris EA, eds. *ACR BI-RADS® Atlas, Breast Imaging Reporting and Data System.* 5th ed. Reston, VA: American College of Radiology; 2013.

classification allows for a reasonable approach on the basis of the probability of malignancy (**Table 16-3**). Lesions with BI-RADS categories 1 and 2, which represents ~0% chance of malignancy, do not require biopsy; lesions with BI-RADS category 3, which represents a 0% to 2% chance of malignancy, need short-term follow-up at 6 months; and lesions with BI-RADS categories 4 or 5, which represents a >2% chance of malignancy, require biopsy.[1] **Figure 16-6** provides an algorithm for working up palpable breast masses with ultrasonography that utilizes these BI-RADS categories. A synopsis of the various ultrasound findings for benign, probably benign, and suspicious lesions are listed with their associated BI-RADS categories in **Tables 16-4 to 16-6** along with some common diagnoses seen on breast ultrasound in **Table 16-7** (**Figures 16-6 through 16-9**).

TABLE 16-4 Benign Findings

Benign Ultrasound Findings (Compatible With BI-RADS 2)

• Lack of any suspicious findings
• Marked hyperechogenicity (relative to fat)
• May be isoechoic or mildly hypoechoic
• Circumscribed margins
• Parallel orientation to the skin ("wider than tall")
• Ellipsoid shape (may include two or three undulations)
• Thin echogenic pseudocapsule
• Homogeneous low-level internal echoes
• No acoustic shadowing
• No microcalcification
• No ill-defined cystic changes

TABLE 16-5 Probably Benign Findings

Probably Benign Ultrasound Findings (Compatible With BI-RADS 3)

• A solid hypoechoic oval or gently lobulated mass with circumscribed margins
• An oval- or round-shaped mass
• A mass with slight or no lobulation
• Lesions with an abrupt interface and a parallel orientation
• Complicated cysts
• Clustered microcysts

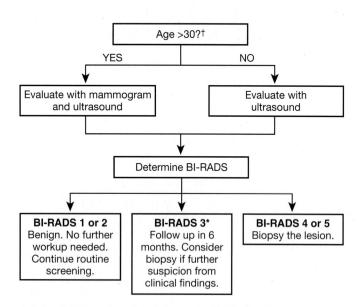

† Age cutoff may differ depending on institutional policy.
∘ If BI-RADS 0, patient will need further imaging before determining biopsy status. If BI-RADS 6, biopsy depends on previous malignancy workup.
* If findings are stable at 6, 12, and 24 months, the mass becomes BI-RADS 2.

FIGURE 16-6. Algorithm for working up a palpable breast lesion.

TABLE 16-6 Suspicious Findings

Suspicious Ultrasound Findings (Compatible With BI-RADS 4 or 5)

• Spiculated margins
• Nonparallel ("taller than wide") orientation to the skin
• Indistinct, angular, or microlobulated margins
• Posterior shadowing
• Markedly hypoechoic echotexture
• Associated calcifications (visible as echogenic foci)
• Heterogeneous texture
• Hypervascularity on Doppler
• Ductal extension

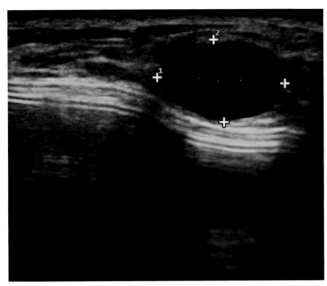

FIGURE 16-7. Anechoic, well-circumscribed, thin echogenic capsule, with posterior acoustic enhancement. Simple cyst compatible with BI-RADS category 2.

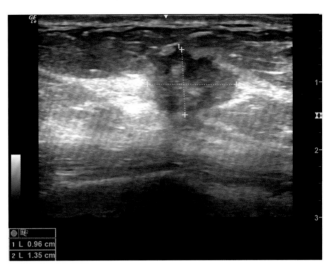

FIGURE 16-9. Indistinct, angular margins, posterior shadowing, and heterogeneous texture. Suspicious mass consistent with BI-RADS category 5. Biopsy showed infiltrating ductal carcinoma.

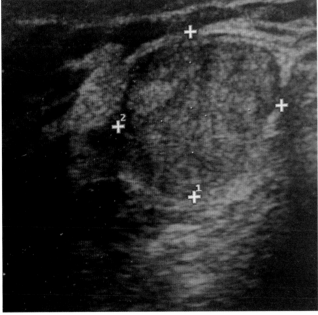

FIGURE 16-8. Solid, oval-shaped, well-circumscribed, uniformly hypoechoic mass with parallel orientation. Fibroadenoma compatible with BI-RADS category 3.

TABLE 16-7	Common Diagnoses
Common Findings	
Simple cyst	• Anechoic, well-circumscribed, thin echogenic capsule, posterior acoustic enhancement • Can aspirate if symptomatic or if preventing adequate mammography • Consistent with BI-RADS 2
Complicated cyst	• Similar to simple cyst, except that it contains internal echoes or fluid-fluid levels • Differential dx: galactocele, hematoma, oil cyst, abscess • Consistent with BI-RADS 3
Complex cyst	• Similar to complicated cyst, except that it has a discrete solid component • Differential dx: hematoma, fat necrosis, abscess, malignancy • Consistent with BI-RADS 4
Fibroadenoma	• Most common benign breast tumor • Firm, mobile mass clinically • Oval, circumscribed, uniformly hypoechoic • Parallel orientation • May have gentle lobulation • May be isoechoic

PEARLS AND PITFALLS

Pearls

- Ultrasound all palpable breast masses
- Fibroadenoma is the most common diagnosis of a palpable breast mass
- Always obtain images in at least two planes for abnormal findings

Pitfalls

- Do not forget to consider the clinical context and physical exam in your final judgment on the need for a biopsy. The BI-RADS classification is solely based off the imaging findings.
- Avoid using breast ultrasonography for primary breast cancer screening unless mammography is not an option.

BILLING

CPT Code	Description	Global Payment	Professional Component	Technical Component
76641	Complete ultrasound, breast, unilateral, real time with image documentation	$108.85	$37.24	$71.61
76642	Limited ultrasound, breast, unilateral, real time with image documentation	$89.51	$34.73	$54.78

CPT codes and average national reimbursement for Medicare in 2016. Payment data are from https://www.cms.gov/apps/physician-fee-schedule/search/search-criteria.aspx. See Chapter 2 for details on ultrasound billing.

References

1. Mendelson EB, Böhm-Vélez M, Berg WA, et al. ACR BI-RADS® Ultrasound. In: D'Orsi CJ, Sickles EA, Mendelson EB, Morris EA, eds. *ACR BI-RADS® Atlas, Breast Imaging Reporting and Data System.* Reston, VA: American College of Radiology; 2013.
2. Stavros AT, Thickman D, Rapp CL, Dennis MA, Parker SH, Sisney GA. Solid breast nodules: use of sonography to distinguish between benign and malignant lesions. *Radiology.* 1995;196:123-134.
3. Lee S, Jung Y, Bae Y. Synchronous BI-RADS Category 3 lesions on preoperative ultrasonography in patients with breast cancer: is short-term follow-up appropriate? *J Breast Cancer.* 2015;18(2):181-186.
4. Hong AS, Rosen EL, Soo MS, Baker JA. BI-RADS for sonography: positive and negative predictive values of sonographic features. *AJR Am J Roentgenol.* 2005;184:1260-1265.
5. Graf O, Helbich TH, Hopf G, Sickles EA. Probably benign breast masses at US: is follow-up an acceptable alternative to biopsy? *Radiology.* 2007;244(1):87-93.
6. Heinig J, Witterler R, Schmitz R, Kiesel L, Steinhard J. Accuracy of classification of breast ultrasound findings based on criteria used for BI-RADS. *Ultrasound Obstet Gynecol.* 2008;32(4):573.
7. Nelson HD, Tyne K, Naik A, et al. Screening for breast cancer: an update of the U.S. Preventive Services Task Force. *Ann Intern Med.* 2009; 151(10):727.
8. Berg WA, Blume JD, Cormack JV, et al. Combined screening with ultrasound and mammography vs mammography alone in women at elevated risk of breast cancer. *JAMA.* 2008;299(18):2151-2163.
9. Shin JH, Han BK, Ko EY, Choe YH, Nam SJ. Probably benign breast masses diagnosed by sonography: is there a difference in the cancer rate according to palpability? *AJR Am J Roentgenol.* 2009;192(4):W187-W191.
10. Newell MS, Barke LD, Argus AD, et al. *ACR Practice Parameter for the Performance of a Breast Ultrasound Examination.* American College of Radiology. https://www.acr.org/-/media/ACR/Files/Practice-Parameters/US-Breast.pdf. Accessed November 26, 2016.
11. Soo MS, Rosen EL, Baker JA, Vo TT, Boyd BA. Negative predictive value of sonography with mammography in patients with palpable breast lesions. *AJR Am J Roentgenol.* 2001;177:1167-1170.
12. Miyake KK, Ikeda DM. *Breast Imaging: The Requisites.* St. Louis, MO: Elsevier Inc; 2017:chap 4.
13. Loving VA, DeMartini WB, Eby PR, Gutierrez RL, Peacock S, Lehman CD. Targeted ultrasound in women younger than 30 years with focal breast signs or symptoms: outcomes analyses and management implications. *AJR Am J Roentgenol.* 2010;195(6):1472.
14. Morrow M, Wong S, Venta L. The evaluation of breast masses in women younger than 40 years of age. *Surgery.* 1998;124:634.
15. Lehman CD, Lee AY, Lee CI. Imaging management of palpable breast abnormalities. *AJR Am J Roentgenol.* 2014;203:1142-1153.

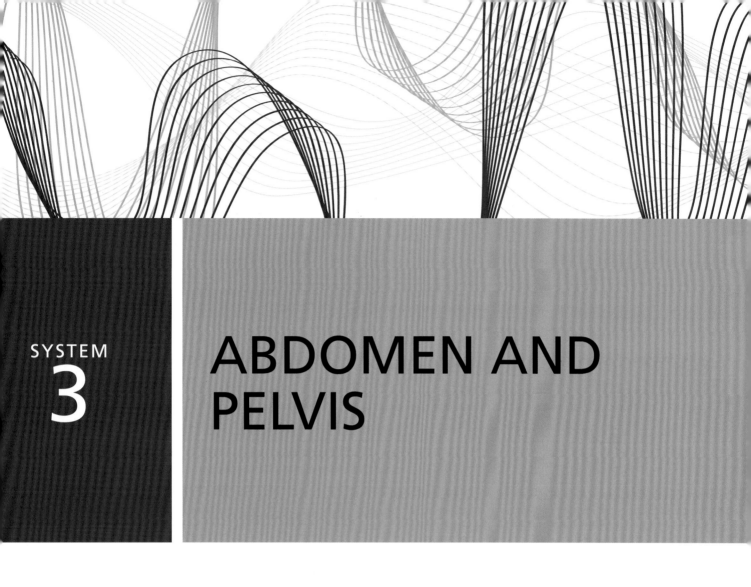

ABDOMEN AND PELVIS

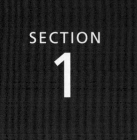

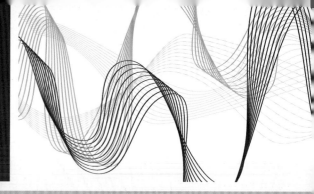

CHAPTER
17

Does the Patient Have Nephrolithiasis?

David Flick, MD, Holly Beth Crellin, MD, and Nicholas Adam Kohles, MD

● Clinical Vignette

A 38-year-old male presents with waxing and waning right-sided flank pain over the past 6 hours. He reports that at times the pain is severe enough to cause nausea and even emesis. He denies fever, chills, dysuria, or testicular symptoms. Prior to this, he was well and spent the entire prior day hiking in the summer heat. His past medical history is notable for a similar episode that was diagnosed as an uncomplicated nephrolithiasis. Family history is notable for hypertension and diabetes mellitus. Vital signs are normal and physical examination is benign. Urine dipstick is positive for blood only. Does the patient have nephrolithiasis?

LITERATURE REVIEW

Nephrolithiasis is a common reason for presentation for medical care, leading to as many as 2.7 million outpatient visits annually.[1,2] An estimated 13% of men and 7% of women will experience nephrolithiasis over their lifetime.[1,2] The condition is seen more often in middle age, low socioeconomic groups, and non-Hispanic whites. Additional risk factors include higher body mass index, obesity, gout, diabetes, and a positive family history.[3] Recurrence rates are high, with up to 50% of patients having a second episode.[1,2] Among industrialized countries, the rate of nephrolithiasis has been increasing, paralleling increasing rates of metabolic syndrome.[1-3]

The vast majority of nephroliths contain calcium, with about 75% consisting of either calcium oxalate or calcium phosphate.[1,2] Uric acid stones are less commonly encountered, accounting for approximately 10% of nephroliths. These are often found in patients with gout and are notably radiolucent on standard films. Struvite stones encompass roughly 10% of nephroliths but should be considered a special case as these are more often found in the presence of urease-producing bacteria and have more potential for complication. Cysteine stones are much rarer and encompass only 1% of all nephroliths.[1,2] Nephroliths typically form either on the renal papillae or in the collecting duct, causing no symptoms until they break loose and become lodged in the ureter. Although nephroliths can become lodged anywhere in the urinary tract, the most common sites are the narrow ureterovesicular junction, ureteropelvic junction, and pelvic brim.[4] Approximately 90% of the time, nephroliths measuring 5 mm or less will spontaneously pass, whereas this number decreases to only 5% when nephroliths reach 8 mm.[4,5] As a nephrolith lodges along the ureter, it causes irritation and edema to the surrounding tissues. Obstruction of urine flow can cause pressure to build proximally, resulting in ureteral and renal pelvic dilatation.[5]

Patients commonly describe sharp, spasmodic pain correlating with increased peristaltic activity from ureteral irritation. Others may note constant aching pain with radiation to the groin or flank pain due to renal capsular distension. Additional signs and symptoms such as nausea, vomiting, costovertebral angle pain, and hematuria may be apparent, but the presence of fever, chills, hypotension, testicular tenderness, or abdominal masses should clue the provider to rule out other additional diagnoses.[1,4]

The diagnosis of nephrolithiasis has changed dramatically over the past two decades with the emergence of computed tomographic (CT) scanners as standard equipment. Prior to the availability of CT, intravenous pyelography (IVP) was the gold standard for diagnosis, with abdominal x-rays commonly used to monitor therapy.[6] In 1995, Smith et al showed that non-contrast-enhanced CT (NCCT) was superior to IVP for the diagnosis of nephrolithiasis in patients with flank pain.[7] Additional advantages to CT include the ability to identify a wide variety of differential diagnoses. Current guidelines including the American College of Radiology list NCCT as the standard for diagnosing nephroliths in most patients.[8] However, recent concerns have begun to grow regarding the cumulative impact of ionizing radiation exposure, especially in young stone formers who may receive additional radiation over the years.

The use of ultrasound to detect renal calculi was first documented in 1961 when Schlegel described the use of A mode ultrasound intraoperatively to detect a nephrolith.[9] Since then, the evidence in favor for the use of ultrasound has continued to mount. In 2014, a large multisystem study showed no difference in major complications, return ER visits, serious adverse events, hospitalizations or even overall pain when comparing ultrasound, both formal and point of care, to NCCT.[10] All this with lower radiation exposure and shorter ER care times. Although ultrasound is not as sensitive in detecting nephroliths themselves compared with CT, it is very sensitive in detecting and quantifying the degree of hydronephrosis.[11] The degree of hydronephrosis correlates with the size of the nephrolith. Small stones will cause none or very mild hydronephrosis, which are most likely to pass spontaneously. Larger stones will cause an increasing degree of hydronephrosis and are much less likely to pass spontaneously.[12,13] With this in mind, the true utility of point-of-care ultrasound for nephrolithiasis is the ability to triage patients into those that are likely to pass the stone spontaneously, or those that are not and warrant further imaging with CT.[10] Ultrasound is considered a first-line method for the detection of renal calculi in pregnant patients, pediatric patients, and other special groups such as those with contrast allergy or renal insufficiency.[8,10,14] Ultrasound remains an acceptable method for detection, although NCCT is preferred by most groups.[10] In conclusion, although ultrasound cannot match the sensitivity of NCCT, its advantage lies in the absence of ionizing radiation, its ability to provide real-time imaging at the bedside, and the ability to triage stones that are likely to pass versus those that are not by way of evaluating the presence, absence, or degree of hydronephrosis.

TABLE 17-1	Recommendations for Use of Point-of-Care Ultrasound in Clinical Practice		
Recommendation		**Rating**	**References**
Limited renal ultrasonography can effectively aid in the diagnosis of nephrolithiasis and associated hydronephrosis at the bedside.		A	6,8,10,15,16
Point-of-care ultrasound for the evaluation of nephrolithiasis and hydronephrosis can be performed at the bedside effectively by nonradiologists with brief training.		A	5,8-10,16

A = consistent, good-quality patient-oriented evidence; B = inconsistent or limited-quality patient-oriented evidence; C = consensus, disease-oriented evidence, usual practice, expert opinion, or case series. For information about the SORT evidence rating system, go to http://www.aafp.org/afpsort.

PERFORMING THE SCAN

1. **Preparation.** The patient should be positioned in the supine position. A lateral decubitus position can be used for particularly posterior lying kidneys by allowing more access to the patient's flank (**Figure 17-1**). Position the ultrasound equipment next to the patient's bed and select a probe. The curvilinear probe provides a large field of view but with multiple rib shadows. A phased array probe will give a smaller view but can be placed in between the ribs to avoid shadow artifact (**Figure 17-2**). Both probes offer a lower frequency that allows for a greater depth of scanning.

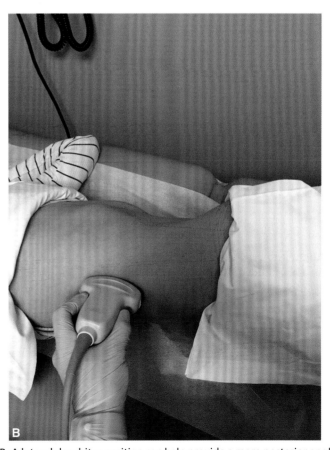

FIGURE 17-1. A, Standard supine position for scanning the right kidney. B, A lateral decubitus position can help provide a more posterior angle for imaging the kidneys.

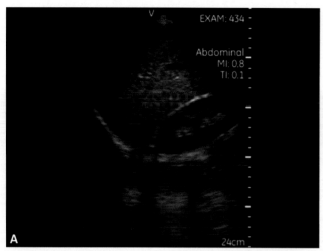

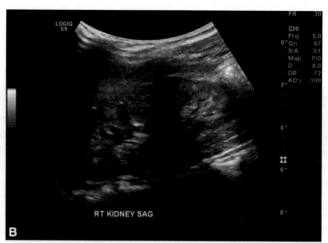

FIGURE 17-2. A, Image of the kidney with a phased array probe. Note the relative smaller field of view but the lack of rib shadows. B, Image of the kidney with a curvilinear probe. Note the greater field of view but obstructing rib shadows.

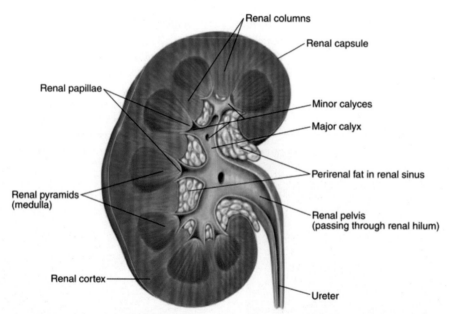

FIGURE 17-3. Cross-sectional anatomy of the kidney for reference. Reprinted with permission from Gest TR. The abdomen. In: Gest TR, ed. *Lippincott Atlas of Anatomy*. 2nd ed. Philadelphia, PA: Wolters Kluwer; 2020:266. Plate 5-34.

2. **Right kidney**

a. **Longitudinal view.** Place the probe in the anterior axillary line of the right lower intercostal spaces (around ribs 10-11) with the indicator pointing toward the patient's head (Figure 17-1A). The probe should be fanned slightly posteriorly, as the kidneys are retroperitoneal structures. Using the liver as an acoustic window, locate the kidney by fanning posteriorly or sliding the probe inferiorly. Adjust the probe as necessary to align the view with the axis of the kidney. Examine the entire length of the kidney, including the upper and lower poles, by rocking the probe up and down. Fan the probe back and forth to examine the kidney from posterior to anterior. In this view,

the kidney is stretched out in a classic "kidney bean" type shape (**Figure 17-3**). The normal kidney has a sharp, clear interface between itself and the liver known as the hepatorenal space or Morrison's pouch. The normal kidney has a cortex that is very similar in echogenicity to the liver with a medulla slightly hyperechoic. At the junction of the cortex and the medulla, the renal pyramids may be visible as hypoechoic or anechoic areas. In the setting of obstruction, hydronephrosis will be seen, which will appear as dilated, balloon-like, calyces (**Figure 17-4**). Severe hydronephrosis is characterized by calyceal dilation to a degree that the renal cortex becomes thinned. A normal renal cortex is usually greater than 1 cm

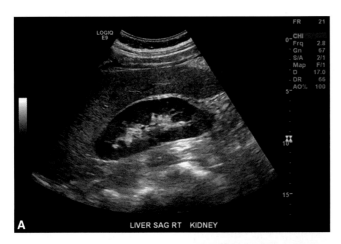

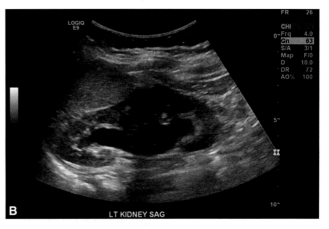

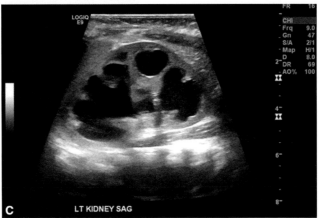

FIGURE 17-4. A, The normal right kidney in its long axis. Note the use of the liver as an acoustic window that provides excellent contrast (from LWW Anatomy Atlas). B, Moderate hydronephrosis of the left kidney. Note the dilated, anechoic draining system. C, Severe hydronephrosis. The draining system is dilated to the point of obscuring the normal appearance of the kidney parenchyma and the renal cortex becomes thin (<1 cm) because of compression. Note the "bear-claw"-like appearance of the dilated calyces.

in thickness. If nephroliths are present within the kidney, they will appear as bright, echogenic foci with accompanying posterior acoustic shadowing (**Figure 17-5**). Note that intrarenal nephroliths are asymptomatic and are usually incidental findings. The presence of a nephrolith within the

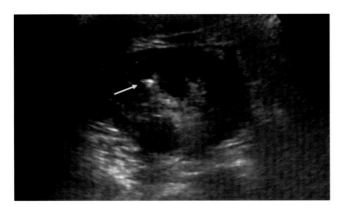

FIGURE 17-5. Intrarenal nephrolith. Note the echogenic nephrolith identified by the yellow arrow.

kidney does not necessarily correlate with nephroliths further along the urothelial tract.

   b. **Transverse view.** The transverse view can be used to help clarify something seen in the longitudinal view by adding an element of dimension, but is not strictly necessary in this application. After completing the longitudinal view, rotate the probe 90 degrees counterclockwise. The indicator should be facing toward the patient's right/back. Adjust the probe to bring the transverse view of the kidney into the image window. Here, the kidney takes on a horseshoe shape with the hypoechoic cortex wrapping around the more echogenic medulla (**Figure 17-6**). Scan the kidney from the upper to the lower pole by fanning the probe superior and posteriorly.

3. **Left kidney**

   a. **Longitudinal view.** The left kidney should be examined using a slightly modified technique. Start slightly higher in the anterior axillary line of the left lower intercostal spaces (around ribs 9-10). The probe should be angled slightly posteriorly with the probe marker in the cephalic position (**Figure 17-7**). At times, the spleen may be used as an acoustic

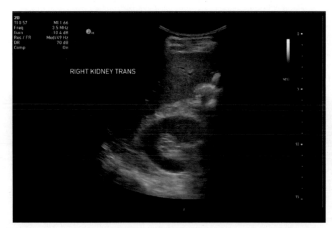

FIGURE 17-6. Transverse view of the kidney.

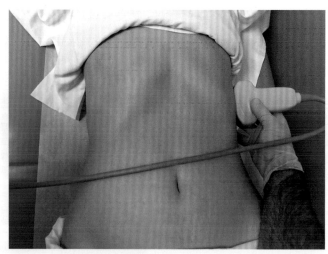

FIGURE 17-7. Standard supine position for scanning the left kidney. Note the more posterior position of the probe. When scanning across the bed, it is often a useful reference point to start by placing the pinky on the exam table.

window. Perform the same series of movements as described for the right kidney.

4. **Ureters.** The ureters may be seen exiting the renal pelvis if dilated, but otherwise are generally not appreciable as they dive down toward the bladder among the abdominal organs. If seen, they will appear as an anechoic, tube-like structure when stretched out in a longitudinal plane (**Figure 17-8**).

5. **Bladder.** In the setting of nephrolithiasis, the bladder should be examined to evaluate for the signs of obstruction. This can be performed directly by looking for obstructing stones in

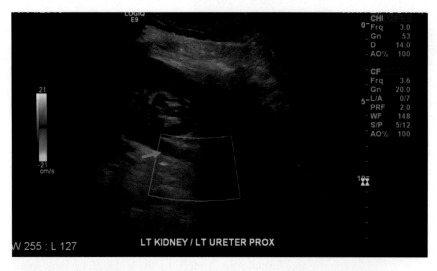

FIGURE 17-8. Dilated proximal ureter (blue arrow). Note the tube-like, anechoic structure. The lack of color flow helps differentiate hydroureter from renal vasculature.

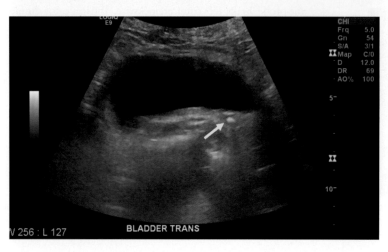

FIGURE 17-9. A nephrolith is seen obstructing the left ureterovesicular junction (yellow arrow). This image actually shows the actual offending stone causing hydroureter shown in Figure 17-8.

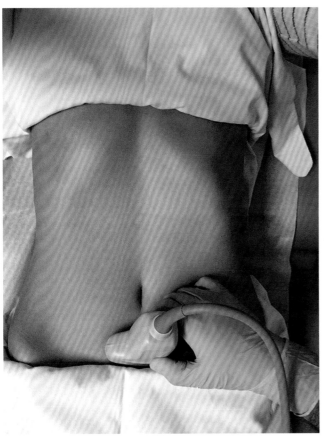

FIGURE 17-10. Supine position for evaluating the bladder.

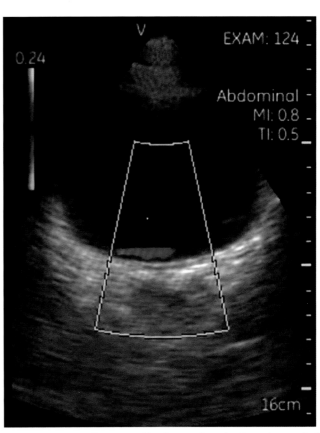

FIGURE 17-11. A right ureteral jet is seen in color Doppler mode in this image captured by a portable ultrasound device. [Video 17-1 included for e-book version]

the ureterovesicular junction itself or indirectly by looking for ureteral emptying into the bladder (**Figure 17-9**). wwwwwwwIf the ureter is obstructed by a stone, there will be no flow. Any probe can be used for this part of the examination, but the curvilinear probe offers the largest footprint. Start by examining the bladder in the axial plane with the indicator pointed toward the patient's right (**Figure 17-10**). Fan the probe superior to inferior looking for a "saddle" appearance of the posterior portion of the bladder. This is the location of the trigone where the ureters empty into the bladder. The normal bladder appears as a large, box-shaped anechoic, fluid-filled structure. Just deep to the bladder will lie either the prostate in a man or the uterus in a woman. Switch from B mode to power or color Doppler mode and center the box at the posterior portion of the bladder. Ensure the patient is well hydrated and simply wait. In the absence of pathology, "bladder jets" can be seen as the ureters peristalse and drain into the bladder. With the Doppler box in position, pulses of color will be seen representing this movement of fluid into the bladder (**Figure 17-11** and ▶ **Video 17-1**). In the setting of obstruction, these jets will be absent on the affected side. Strictly speaking, there does not appear to be any literature to show any increased diagnostic or prognostic value with this step, and thus may be skipped in the interest of time.

PATIENT MANAGEMENT

Traditional management of nephrolithiasis with the aid of NCCT is largely based on the size of the nephrolith. Nephroliths 5 mm or smaller are likely to pass spontaneously and are usually managed initially with conservative measures. Management with ultrasound uses the degree of hydronephrosis to make inferences about the size of the nephrolith, as discussed earlier. If there is only mild or moderate hydronephrosis, then the nephrolith has the highest likelihood to pass spontaneously. The mainstay of acute management is pain control. As nephroliths cause significant pain, this is usually achieved with opioid analgesics with or without nonsteroidal anti-inflammatory drugs. If there are no signs of infection, pain is controlled, and only mild or moderate hydronephrosis is seen, the patient can be managed conservatively. The patient should be started on expulsive therapy (see **Table 17-2**) and instructed to drink at least 2 L of water per day. He or she should also be instructed to strain the urine and, if collected, any nephrolith should be sent for analysis. Most stones will pass in 1 to 4 weeks. Periodic evaluation should be arranged in the interim. Imaging with NCCT and referral to urology are indicated at any point if the patient develops signs of infection or severe hydronephrosis or if the nephrolith is not passed spontaneously after initial observation.[14-21] **Figure 17-12** demonstrates a step-by-step approach in evaluating and managing suspected nephrolithiasis with the aid of bedside ultrasound.

TABLE 17-2	Acute Management of Nephrolithiasis[16-24]	
Management Type	**Treatment**	**Dosage**
Medical expulsive therapy (Antispasmodics)[c]	**Alpha Blockers**[a]	
	Tamsulosin[b]	0.4 mg PO daily (adults and children age >2)
	Doxazosin	4 mg PO daily
	Terazosin	5 mg PO daily for up to 2 wk
	Calcium Channel Blockers	
	Nifedipine	30 mg PO daily
Fluids	PO water or IV NS if PO intolerant	At least 3 L daily
		0.9% normal saline solution if blood pressure is low; consider decreasing sodium chloride in patients with calciuria (5% dextrose in water and 0.45% normal saline)
Pain management[d]	**Opioid Narcotics**	
	Codeine/acetaminophen	One or two tablets (5-10 mg codeine/325-500 mg acetaminophen) orally every 4-6 h as needed
	Hydrocodone/ acetaminophen (Vicodin)	5-10 mg orally every 4-6 h as needed Peds: <50 kg Hydrocodone 0.1-0.2 mg/kg/dose every 4-6 h as needed

[a]Preferred agents for medical expulsive therapy.
[b]Preferred agent in pediatric populations.
[c]Often administered for up to 4 wk before performing follow-up imaging studies to determine whether the stone has passed.
[d]Caution using nonsteroidal anti-inflammatory drugs as they may decrease glomerular filtration.

Abbreviations: IV, intravenous; NS, normal saline; PO, per os (by mouth).

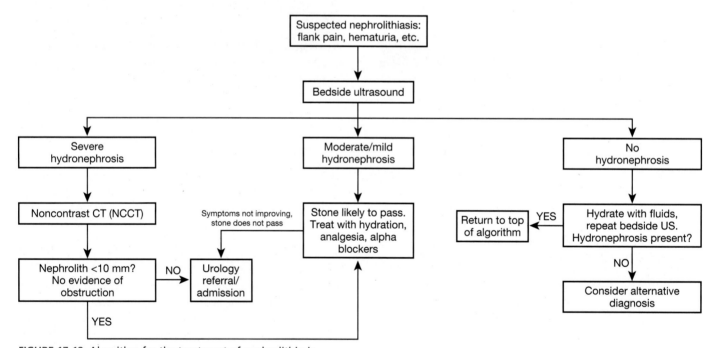

FIGURE 17-12. Algorithm for the treatment of nephrolithiasis.

PEARLS AND PITFALLS

Pearls

- The phased array transducer is useful to look through small acoustic windows such as between ribs. The curvilinear probe offers a large footprint to visualize the kidney at the expense of rib shadow. Aligning the curvilinear probe in an oblique plane more parallel with the ribs can help eliminate rib shadow.
- If the intercostal window is not satisfactory, place the probe below the 12th rib and have the patient take a large breath and hold to bring the kidney inferiorly toward the probe.
- For instances of mild hydronephrosis, scan the unaffected kidney for reference of normal.
- To differentiate between hydroureter and the renal vasculature, apply color flow. Hydroureter should show no color flow.

Pitfalls

- Mild hydronephrosis may be a normal finding. If this is the case, hydronephrosis will be seen bilaterally without evidence of obstruction. Overhydration and pregnancy are two potential causes.
- Simple renal cysts may be confused with hydronephrosis. Scanning completely through the structure and identifying if it connects with the rest of the collecting system will help differentiate the two.
- Chronic kidney disease may alter the kidney's appearance and echogenicity causing the identification of normal structures to be difficult (**Figure 17-13**).
- Hydronephrosis will not be present initially following obstruction. It can take several days to accumulate, especially in the setting of poor hydration. IV fluid boluses can help aid in the sensitivity of the scan.[25]

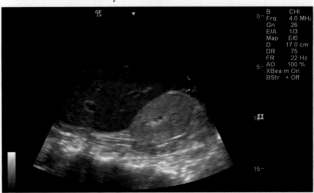

FIGURE 17-13. Chronic kidney disease. Note the hyperechoic and small kidney as well as the distorted contour. Incidentally, there is also a small pocket of perirenal fluid measured at the inferior pole of the kidney.

BILLING

CPT Code	Description	Global Payment	Professional Component	Technical Component
76770	Ultrasound, Retroperitoneal, Complete	$114.93	$37.59	$77.34
76775	Ultrasound, Retroperitoneal, Limited	$58.72	$29.36	$29.36

CPT codes and average national reimbursement for Medicare in 2016. Payment data are from https://www.cms.gov/apps/physician-fee-schedule/search/search-criteria.aspx. See Chapter 2 for details on ultrasound billing.

References

1. Pearle MS, Calhoun EA, Curhan GC. Urologic diseases of America Project: urolithiasis. *J Urol.* 2005;173(3):848-857.
2. Ziemba JB, Matlaga BR. Epidemiology and economics of nephrolithiasis. *Investig Clin Urol.* 2017;58(5):299-306.
3. Scales CD, Smith AC, Hanley JM, Saigal CS, and Urologic Diseases in America Project. Prevalence of kidney stones in the United States. *Eur Urol.* 2012;62(1):160-165.
4. Menckhoff C. Nephrolithiasis. In: Adams JG, Barton ED, Colling JL, DeBlieux P, Gisondi MA, Nadel ES, eds. *Emergency Medicine Clinical Essentials.* Philadelphia, PA: Elsevier/Saunders; 2013:P976-P983.
5. Dalziel PJ, Noble VE. Bedside ultrasound and the assessment of renal colic: a review. *Emerg Med J.* 2013;30(1):3-8.
6. Nobel VE, Brown DFM. Renal ultrasound. *Emerg Med Clin N Am.* 2004;22:641-659.
7. Smith RC, Rosenfield AT, Kyuran AC. Acute Flank pain: comparison of non-contrast enhanced CT and Intravenous urography. *Radiology.* 1995;194:789-794.
8. Moreno Coursey C, Beland MD, Goldfarb S, et al. *Expert Panel on Urologic Imaging. ACR Appropriateness Criteria Acute Onset Flank Pain—Suspicion of Stone Disease (urolithiasis).* Reston, VA: American College of Radiology; 2015:11.
9. Schlegel JU, Diggdon P, Cuellar J. The use of ultrasound for localizing renal calculi. *J Urol.* 1961;86:367-369.
10. Smith-Bindman R, Aubin C, Bailitz J, et al. Ultrasonography versus computed tomography for suspected nephrolithiasis. *N Engl J Med.* 2014;371(12):1100-1110.
11. Fowler KA, Locken JA, Duchesne JH, Williamson MR. US for detecting renal calculi with nonenhanced CT as a reference standard. *Radiology.* 2002;222(1):109-113.
12. Goertz JK, Lotterman S. Can the degree of hydronephrosis on ultrasound predict kidney stone size? *Am J Emerg Med.* 2010;28(7):813-816.
13. Moak JH, Lyons MS, Lindsell CJ. Bedside renal ultrasound in the evaluation of suspected ureterolithiasis. *Am J Emerg Med.* 2012;30(1):218-221. doi:10.1016/j.ajem.2010.11.024.
14. Masselli G, Weston M, Spencer J. The role of imaging in the diagnosis and management of renal stone disease in pregnancy. *Clin Radiol.* 2015;70(12):1462-1471.
15. Daniels B, Gross CP, Molinaro A, et al. STONE PLUS: evaluation of emergency department patients with suspected renal colic, using a clinical prediction tool combined with point-of-care limited ultrasonography. *Ann Emerg Med.* 2016;67(4):439-448.
16. Chu DI, Tasian, GE, Copelovitch L. Pediatric kidney stones—avoidance and treatment. *Curr Treat Options Peds.* 2016;2:104.
17. Frassetto L, Kohlstadt I. Treatment and prevention of kidney stones: an update. *Am Fam Physician.* 2011;84(11):1234-1242.
18. Gurbuz MC, Polat H, Canat L, et al. Efficacy of three different alpha 1-adrenergic blockers and hyoscine N-butylbromide for distal ureteral stones. *Int Braz J Urol.* 2011;37(2):195-200.
19. Mokhless I, Zahran AR, Youssif M, Fahmy A. Tamsulosin for the management of distal ureteral stones in children: a prospective randomized study. *J Pediatr Urol.* 2012;8(5):544-548.

PART 2

20. Preminger GM, Tiselius HG, Assimos DG, et al; EAU/AUA Nephrolithiasis Guideline Panel. 2007 guideline for the management of ureteral calculi. *J Urol.* 2007;178(6):2418-2434.

21. Tasian GE, Copelovitch L. Evaluation and medical management of kidney stones in children. *J Urol.* 2014;192(5):1329-1336.

22. Tasian GE, Cost NG, Granberg CF, et al. Tamsulosin and spontaneous passage of ureteral stones in children: a multi-institutional cohort study. *J Urol.* 2014;192(2):506-511.

23. Veláquez N, Zapata D, Wang HH, et al. Medical expulsive therapy for pediatric urolitiasis: systemic review and meta-analysis. *J Pediatr Urol.* 2015;11(6):321-327.

24. Xu H, Zisman AL, Coe FL, Worcester EM. Kidney stones: an update on current pharmacological management and future directions. *Expert Opin Pharmacother.* 2013;14(4):435-447.

25. Henderson SO, Hoffner RJ, Aragona JL, Groth DE, Esekogwu VI, Chan D. Bedside emergency department ultrasonography plus radiography of the kidneys, ureters, and bladder vs intravenous pyelography in the evaluation of suspected ureteral colic. *Acad Emerg Med.* 1998;5(7):666-671.

Does the Patient Have Chronic Kidney Disease?

Melissa Ferguson, MD and Jason Reinking, MD

Clinical Vignette

A 62-year-old man with a history of essential hypertension presents for follow-up after routine screening labs that demonstrated a creatinine of 2.0 mg/dL. He denies any symptoms, and his physical examination is normal. No prior lab values are available. You feel it is unlikely to be an acute issue, but the etiology and chronicity of his kidney disease are unclear. Does the patient have chronic kidney disease?

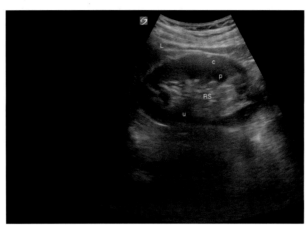

FIGURE 18-1. Normal renal ultrasound anatomy. c, cortex; L, liver; p, pyramid; RS, renal sinus; u, ureter.

LITERATURE REVIEW

Chronic kidney disease (CKD) is defined as abnormalities of kidney structure or function present for greater than 3 months. CKD (stages 1-5) affects approximately 15% of the American population, a prevalence that has been roughly stable over the last several decades.[1] Risk factors include hypertension, diabetes, increasing age, and low socioeconomic status. It is a worldwide public health problem whose patients experience significant mortality and morbidity. Early recognition and intervention can prove valuable in treating this disease process.

Traditionally, CKD is classified using three main categories: prerenal (decreased renal perfusion), intrinsic renal (pathology of the vessels or interstitium), and postrenal (obstruction). In developed countries, the most common etiologies of CKD are overwhelmingly related to diabetic nephropathy and hypertensive nephrosclerosis.[2]

CKD often presents incidentally on laboratory screening or with nonspecific symptoms later attributed to CKD. A thorough workup of CKD to determine the exact etiology includes multiple lab tests, imaging, and possible biopsy. Here, we will discuss how ultrasonography can be used to supplement the clinical diagnosis at the point of care.

Ultrasound is the ideal imaging modality for CKD because of its safety profile, low cost, easy visualization, and interpretation simplicity. It should be performed on all patients presenting with renal failure of unclear etiology (see **Figure 18-1** for normal renal anatomy). It is important to understand that although obtaining an ultrasound is usually helpful in the CKD workup, it is not always definitively diagnostic. Although certain etiologies of undiagnosed renal failure can be clearly seen with ultrasound such as chronic hydronephrosis (obstruction), multiple cysts (polycystic kidney disease), masses (renal carcinoma), or asymmetry (renovascular disease), statistically such diagnoses comprise a relatively small proportion of overall CKD.[3] More commonly, it is the constellation of small, hyperechoic kidneys with a thinning cortex that are associated with progression and irreversibility regardless of the etiology in CKD.

The most useful ultrasound findings associated with CKD are renal size, cortical echogenicity, and parenchymal thickness (Table 18-1). Normal renal size is 9 to 13 cm when measured

TABLE 18-1	Ultrasound Findings Associated With Chronic Kidney Disease (CKD)		
	Normal Parameters	**Nondiabetic CKD**	**Diabetic Nephropathy**
Kidney size: Length measured in longitudinal plane	~9–13 cm	<9 cm (ie, small kidneys)	>13 cm (nephromegaly in early disease) OR <9 cm (small in later disease)
Cortical echogenicity	Hypo- or isoechoic compared to liver	Hyperechoic compared to liver	Variable, similar to nondiabetic in later stages
Parenchymal thickness	Approx. 15–20 mm	<15 mm	Variable, similar to nondiabetic in later stages
Other findings: • Cysts • Hydronephrosis • Undifferentiated mass • Asymmetry	Benign cysts can be present	Multiple cysts, masses, asymmetry (>2 cm difference), hydronephrosis indicate pathology and should have further workup	Similar to nondiabetic

Dietrich C. EFSUMB—European Course Book. EFSUMB. 2011; Sanusi A, Arogundade FA, Famurewa OC, et al. Relationship of ultrasonographically determined kidney volume with measured GFR, calculated creatinine clearance and other parameters in chronic kidney disease (CKD). *Nephrol Dial Transplant.* 2009;24:1690-1694; Fiorini F, Barozzi L. The role of ultrasonography in the study of medical nephropathy. *J Ultrasound.* 2007;10(4):161-167; Lucisano G, Comi N, Pelagi E, Cianfrone P, Fuiano L, Fuiano G. Can renal sonography be a reliable diagnostic tool in the assessment of chronic kidney disease? *J Ultrasound Med.* 2015;34:299-306; O'Neil W. Renal relevant radiology: use of ultrasound in kidney disease and nephrology procedures. *Clin J Am Soc Nephrol.* 2014;9:373-381.

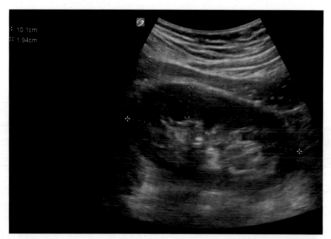

FIGURE 18-2. A 33-year-old man with normal renal function and size (10.1 cm), hypoechoic parenchyma compared to liver, and normal renal parenchymal thickness (19 mm).

TABLE 18-2 **Classification of Renal Parenchymal Echogenicity**

Echogenicity	Definition	General Association
HYPOechoic	Darker when compared to liver parenchyma	Normal
ISOechoic	Similar when compared to liver	Normal
HYPERechoic	Brighter when compared to liver	Pathologic—associated with chronic kidney disease

Reprinted from Fiorini F, Barozzi L. The role of ultrasonography in the study of medical nephropathy. *J Ultrasound.* 2007;10(4):161-167. Copyright © 2007 Elsevier Masson Srl. With permission.

longitudinally (**Figure 18-2**).[4] Studies have demonstrated a positive correlation between renal size and renal function,[5,6] with longitudinal length <9 cm generally agreed upon by experts as abnormal (**Figure 18-3**).[7] Renal cortical echogenicity is generally comparable or hypoechoic to the adjacent liver, whereas a hyperechoic cortex is more commonly associated with chronic disease (Figure 18-3 and Table 18-2).[8,9] Lastly, normal range for parenchymal thickness (measurement of pyramids plus cortex) is considered to be 15 to 20 mm.[8] Studies have correlated CKD with parenchymal thickness <15 cm (**Figure 18-4**).[10] Specifically, the findings most suggestive of irreversible CKD are the combination of small, hyperechoic kidneys with a thinning parenchyma (**Figure 18-5** and Table 18-1). Of note, there is also a strong association with decreasing cortical thickness and CKD; however, this measurement can be technically challenging in view of the often indistinct appearance of the

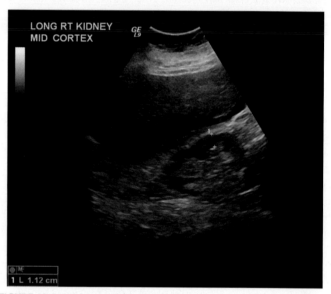

FIGURE 18-4. A 64-year-old woman with known chronic kidney disease with decreased parenchymal thickness (11 mm).

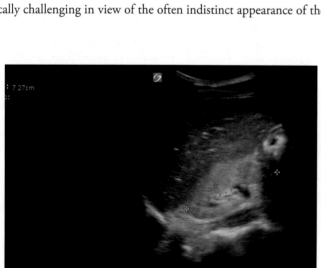

FIGURE 18-3. An 18-year-old man presenting with nausea and vomiting, with renal failure of unknown duration (BUN/Cr of 80/8.0). Small (7.27 cm) hyperechoic renal cortex causing loss of cortical–medullary boundary. BUN, blood urea nitrogen.

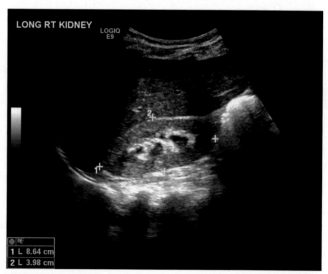

FIGURE 18-5. A 68-year-old woman with known chronic kidney disease with decreased size (8.6 cm), hyperechoic parenchyma compared to liver, and decreased parenchymal thickness.

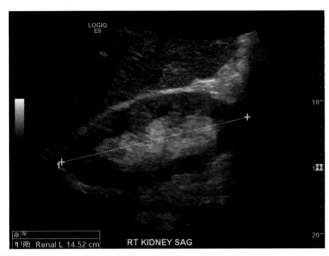

FIGURE 18-6. Nephromegaly.

medullary pyramids, resulting in high inter- and intraoperator variability.[11] Any of these findings alone can often be nonspecific and, if used in isolation, have the potential to be misleading. For instance, combining smaller kidney size and increased echogenicity can greatly increase the specificity of CKD compared to utilizing either parameter alone.[12] Additionally, it is important to utilize multiple measurements for renal size to ensure accuracy, as it is an important component of the assessment.[13]

Ultrasonographic findings of late stage kidney failure can indicate the impending need for referral and possible renal replacement therapy.[14] This may preclude the need for biopsy if the process is irreversible at this stage. Although ultrasound is frequently utilized to assess for evidence of irreversible disease, it is important to note that the presence of normal or large kidneys on ultrasound does not exclude chronic disease. This is especially true in diabetic nephropathy, where nephromegaly (>13 cm longitudinal length) is typically associated with early disease, followed by decrease in size with disease progression **(Figure 18-6)**. Therefore, it can be difficult to predict end stage renal disease with imaging alone in diabetic nephropathy. It should be noted that up to 20% of diabetics will develop nondiabetic renal disease, which can display the classic findings mentioned earlier.[15]

TABLE 18-3	Recommendations for Use of Point-of-Care Ultrasound in Clinical Practice		
Recommendation	**Rating**	**References**
Point-of-care ultrasound can be used in the evaluation of CKD using the combination of kidney size, cortical echogenicity, and parenchymal thickness.	C	10, 13
When measuring kidney size utilizing point-of-care ultrasound, practitioners should use multiple measurements to determine largest longitudinal size.	C	10, 13

A = consistent, good-quality patient-oriented evidence; B = inconsistent or limited-quality patient-oriented evidence; C = consensus, disease-oriented evidence, usual practice, expert opinion, or case series. For information about the SORT evidence rating system, go to http://www.aafp.org/afpsort.

PERFORMING THE SCAN

1. **Preparation.** The patient should be in the supine position for the entire examination. Position the ultrasound equipment appropriately and select a low-frequency (abdominal) probe. If unavailable, a phased-array probe can also be used.
2. **Evaluate the right kidney.** Place the probe in the right midaxillary line centered on the last intercostal space, probe marker toward the patient's head **(Figure 18-7)**. Direct the transducer slightly posteriorly using the liver as an acoustic window. Slightly rock and twist the transducer to obtain images of the kidney, ensuring the full length is in view for proper measurements.
3. **Evaluate the left kidney.** As the left kidney is typically superior and posterior compared to the right, place the probe in the posterior axillary line in the intercostal space, slightly superior to the right side with the probe marker to the patient's head **(Figure 18-8)**. If necessary, angle probe anteriorly from the posterior axillary line.
4. **Measurement of kidney size.** On localization of a kidney, measure the renal length using on-screen calipers in the longitudinal plane from the superior capsule to the inferior

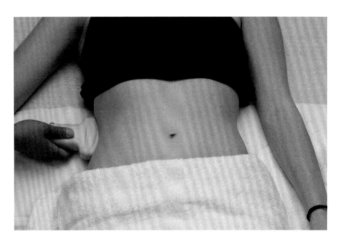

FIGURE 18-7. Approximate location of transducer when obtaining right kidney images.

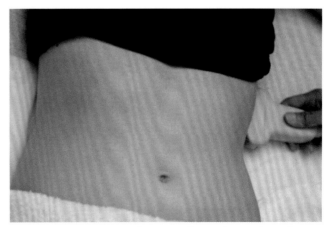

FIGURE 18-8. Approximate location of transducer when obtaining left kidney images.

capsule (Figure 18-2). Rotate the transducer on its vertical axis to find the maximal length as the kidney lies obliquely in the abdomen.

5. **Evaluate cortical echogenicity.** Start with the assessment of the echogenicity of the right kidney. Obtain several views of the renal cortex and assess subjectively when compared to the liver if it is hypoechoic, isoechoic, or hyperechoic (Figure 18-3 and Table 18-2). Do the same on the left, using the spleen as a comparison.

6. **Assess parenchymal thickness.** Measure parenchymal thickness in the longitudinal plane. Parenchymal thickness comprises both the cortex and the inner medullary pyramid to the border of the renal sinus (Figure 18-2).

7. **Evaluate for other abnormalities.** Scan completely through the transverse and longitudinal planes to completely evaluate the parenchyma to assess for cysts, hydronephrosis, and masses.

PATIENT MANAGEMENT

When a patient presents to care with an elevated creatinine on laboratory tests of unclear duration and etiology, point-of-care ultrasound can be utilized to determine the need for further diagnostic testing, which may include a renal biopsy. The initial ultrasound should assess for symmetry, presence of hydronephrosis, and presence of masses, each of which contains an appropriate workup. In their absence, the size and echogenicity can help determine etiology.

In a nondiabetic patient, small and hyperechoic kidneys with thin parenchyma are often associated with irreversible chronic sclerosis, and thus a renal biopsy should be considered. In nondiabetic patients with normal-sized kidneys (defined as 9-13 cm), further diagnostic testing may reveal variable etiologies. For those patients with suspected diabetic nephropathy, renal ultrasounds with no evidence of pathology can be found despite the subsequent diagnosis of significant chronic renal pathology. Specifically, diabetic patients often have normal appearing kidneys or nephromegaly (size > 13 cm) in the earlier stages of disease. In diabetic nephropathy, it is difficult to predict the reversibility based on imaging.[13] Additionally, diabetics can develop nondiabetic kidney disease, and therefore consideration of the clinical context and concurrent etiology is of utmost importance[16] (see **Figure 18-9** for point-of-care ultrasound CKD algorithm).

It should be noted that for a patient in the early stages of disease and without evidence of pathology, a baseline ultrasound can be useful in comparison to future images when disease has progressed. Serial ultrasounds are limited in their utility in established CKD and are generally not considered useful unless there is evidence of progression of disease or new onset of symptoms. However, repeat ultrasounds in the context of potential acute or chronic disease can be useful to determine acute reversible causes, such as hypovolemia or obstruction. Ultimately, the timing and frequency of ultrasounds in CKD should be determined on a case-by-case basis.[17]

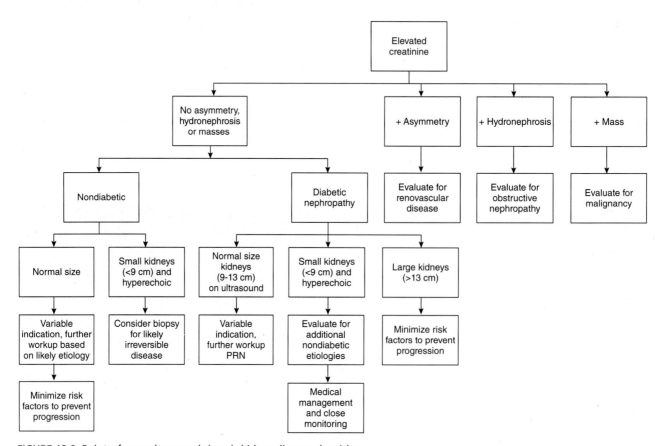

FIGURE 18-9. Point-of-care ultrasound chronic kidney disease algorithm.

PEARLS AND PITFALLS

Pearls

- The kidney can be one of the more readily imaged structures found by ultrasound novices; however, an unobstructed view can be difficult to obtain secondary to rib shadows. If this occurs, have the patient take a deep breath and hold, using the diaphragm to inferiorly displace the kidneys into better view. If still unable to see, use a "rib window" by placing the patient's ipsilateral arm over his or her head, thereby maximizing the intercostal space.
- Use the "knuckles-to-the-bed" technique to best visualize the left and more posterior of the two kidneys. Allow the knuckles of the hand holding the transducer to touch the bed, angling the transducer anteriorly to view the left kidney.
- The right kidney is generally easier to obtain than the left, and therefore it is recommended to start with the right and proceed to the left. Using the right as a baseline, the left kidney is generally more superior and posterior compared to the right.

- On obtaining an initial view of the kidney, be sure to rock the probe to obtain the plane demonstrating the greatest diameter, thereby ensuring the kidney is bisected symmetrically. Renal length measurements depend on accuracy of views with a symmetrical plane as they can infer important prognostic information.

Pitfalls

- Normal appearing kidneys do not rule out the presence of CKD.
- Mean renal size is related to multiple variables, most notably height.[18] It is important to remember that height extremes may influence size measurements when considering CKD in the context of renal size.
- Renal cysts can sometimes be mistaken for hydronephrosis. Remember that cysts occur typically within the parenchyma and are smooth walled, circular, and thin without connecting to the pelvis or collecting system.

BILLING

CPT Code	Description	Global Payment	Professional Component	Technical Component
76770	Ultrasound, retroperitoneal (renal), real time with image documentation; complete	$114.93	$37.59	$77.34
76775	Ultrasound, retroperitoneal (renal), real time with image documentation; limited	$58.72	$29.36	$29.36

CPT codes and average national reimbursement for Medicare in 2016. Payment data are from https://www.cms.gov/apps/physician-fee-schedule/search/search-criteria.aspx. See Chapter 2 for details on ultrasound billing.

References

1. Centers for Disease Control and Prevention. Chronic kidney disease surveillance system—United States. CDC Website. http://nccd.cdc.gov/CKD
2. Hernandez GT, Nasri H. World Kidney Day 2014: increasing awareness of chronic kidney disease and aging. *J Renal Inj Prev.* 2014;3(1):3-4.
3. Snyder S, Pendergraph B. Evaluation and detection of chronic kidney disease. *Am Fam Physician.* 2005;72(9):1723-1732.
4. Dietrich C. EFSUMB—European Course Book. EFSUMB. 2011.
5. Makusidi MA, Chijioke A, Braimoh KT, Aderibigbe A, Olanrewaju TO, Liman HM. Usefulness of renal length and volume by ultrasound in determining severity of chronic kidney disease. *Saudi J Kidney Dis Transpl.* 2014;25(5):1117-1121.
6. Yaprak M, Çakır Ö, Turan MN, et al. Role of ultrasonographic chronic kidney disease score in the assessment of chronic kidney disease. *Int Urol Nephrol.* 2017;49(1):123-131.
7. Sanusi A, Arogundade FA, Famurewa OC, et al. Relationship of ultrasonographically determined kidney volume with measured GFR, calculated creatinine clearance and other parameters in chronic kidney disease (CKD). *Nephrol Dial Transplant.* 2009;24:1690-1694.
8. Fiorini F, Barozzi L. The role of ultrasonography in the study of medical nephropathy. *J Ultrasound.* 2007;10(4):161-167.
9. Hricak H, Cruz C, Romanski R, et al. Renal parenchymal disease: sonographic-histologic correlation. *Radiology.* 1982;144(1):141-147.
10. Lucisano G, Comi N, Pelagi E, Cianfrone P, Fuiano L, Fuiano G. Can renal sonography be a reliable diagnostic tool in the assessment of chronic kidney disease? *J Ultrasound Med.* 2015;34:299-306.
11. Meola M, Petrucci I, Ronco C. Ultrasound imaging in acute and chronic kidney disease. *Karger.* 2016;188:I-VIII.
12. Moghazi S, Jones E, Schroepple J, et al. Correlation of renal histopathology with sonographic findings. *Kidney Int.* 2005;67(4):1515-1520.
13. O'Neil W. Renal relevant radiology: use of ultrasound in kidney disease and nephrology procedures. *Clin J Am Soc Nephrol.* 2014;9:373-381.
14. Buturovic-Ponikvar J, Visnar-Perovic A. Ultrasonography in chronic renal failure. *Eur J Radiol.* 2003;46(2):115-122.
15. Ritz E, Orth SR. Nephropathy in patients with type 2 diabetes mellitus. *N Engl J Med.* 1999;341:1127-1133.
16. Remuzzi G, Schieppati A, Ruggenenti P. Nephropathy in patients with Type 2 diabetes. *N Engl J Med.* 2002;346:1145-1151.
17. Meola M, Petrucci I. Ultrasound and color Doppler applications in chronic kidney disease. *G Ital Nefrol.* 2012;29(6):699-715.
18. Raza M, Hameed A, Khan MI. Sonographic assessment of renal size and its correlation with body mass index in adults without known renal disease. *J Ayub Med Coll Abbottabad.* 2011;23(3):64-68.

HEPATOBILIARY

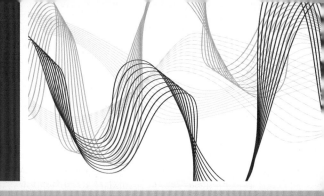

Does the Patient Have Hepatosplenomegaly?

Androuw Carrasco, MD

● Clinical Vignette

A 16-year-old female presents with sore throat for 5 days. She has a dry cough and some nausea. She denies fever, voice changes, or sick contacts. On physical examination, she is afebrile, has palpable posterior cervical adenopathy, and bilateral tonsillar exudate and swelling. Her uvula is midline and she has no splenomegaly on palpation. A rapid strep test was negative. You suspect acute viral pharyngitis, possibly mononucleosis. The patient's mother wants to know if it is safe for her to return to contact sports. Does the patient have hepatosplenomegaly?

LITERATURE REVIEW

Studies have demonstrated that the physical examination is widely variable in its ability to detect hepatosplenomegaly and is very dependent on the ability of the examiner.[1-4] Imaging techniques are, therefore, preferable when available. The spleen and liver are well evaluated by computed tomography and magnetic resonance imaging; however, sonography has certain advantages, including its availability, lack of ionizing radiation, and low cost.

Hepatosplenomegaly should not be considered a diagnosis in itself but a compensatory reaction to disease processes, and its discovery at bedside should prompt further workup. The broad differential for hepatosplenomegaly reflects the diverse physiologic processes of these organs: immunologic functions, extramedullary hematopoiesis, distinct circulatory pathways, and multiple metabolic functions. It is helpful for the primary care provider to group the etiologies of hepatosplenomegaly into categories on the basis of clinical suspicion including hepatitis, mononucleosis, hematologic abnormalities, and other systemic processes.

Hepatitis can be associated with hepatomegaly and can be caused by multiple etiologies which can include viral infection, alcoholic toxicity, nonalcoholic steatohepatitis, drug toxicity, and autoimmune causes. Ultrasonography can be useful in differentiating these etiologies, but this evaluation is beyond the scope of this chapter.[5,6] Further research is necessary to explore the impact of hepatomegaly detection on patient-oriented outcomes in patients found to have hepatitis.

The finding of splenomegaly has the highest diagnostic specificity of all examination findings in distinguishing infectious mononucleosis from other causes of sore throat.[7] In patients actively involved in contact sports, ascertaining if splenomegaly is present is crucial, as 50% to 60% of adolescents with mononucleosis have splenomegaly. Because an enlarged spleen is at risk for rupture and adolescents are often involved in formal or informal play, patients should not compete in contact or collision sports for a minimum of three to four weeks after the onset of symptoms.

Hematologic diagnoses like leukemia are often first encountered by primary care physicians. Hepatosplenomegaly is present in about 50% of adults with acute lymphoblastic leukemia.[8] In one large, retrospective review, 75% of patients with chronic myelogenous leukemia had a palpable spleen.[9] Hence, if a degree of clinical suspicion and the finding of splenomegaly are both present, further evaluation with a complete blood count (CBC) with differential and peripheral blood smear is recommended. These studies will identify leukemias as well as sickle cell disease, spherocytosis, and other hereditary hemolytic anemias. Polycythemia vera (PV), a chronic myeloproliferative disorder, is another hematologic diagnosis where ultrasound evaluation can assist. It has been reported with an incidence of 2.3 per 100 000 persons per year.[10] Therefore, a typical family physician can expect to make a diagnosis of PV at some point in his or her career. Untreated, the rates of life expectancy are 6 to 18 months. Diagnosis is made using criteria developed by the Polycythemia Vera Study Group; criteria include elevated red blood cell mass, normal oxygen saturation, and palpable splenomegaly. The known lack of sensitivity by palpation has led the organization to discuss the utility of ultrasound, although such a finding by sonography might be relegated to the status of a minor criterion, and this has not been established yet.[11]

Algorithms for an expedited diagnosis of other diseases by point-of-care ultrasound are being investigated and have found utility when paired with current diagnostic practices. One group determined that the finding of hepatosplenomegaly had high enough specificity in a subpopulation of adults in Tanzania to classify the patient as having "severe malaria" and guiding treatment decisions appropriately.[12] For the primary care provider in the United States of America, an examination for malaria should occur for refugees from endemic areas who present with recurring fever, splenomegaly, fatigue, pallor, or anemia and thrombocytopenia.[13]

TABLE 19-1	Recommendations for Use of Point-of-Care Ultrasound in Clinical Practice		
Recommendation		**Rating**	**References**
Ultrasound is more reliable than physical examination in identifying splenomegaly or hepatomegaly.		A	1-4

A = consistent, good-quality patient-oriented evidence; B = inconsistent or limited-quality patient-oriented evidence; C = consensus, disease-oriented evidence, usual practice, expert opinion, or case series. For information about the SORT evidence rating system, go to http://www.aafp.org/afpsort.

PERFORMING THE SCAN

1. **Preparation.** The presence of hepatomegaly is best examined with the patient in the supine position, using a 3 to 5 MHz curvilinear probe, with the probe placed in the longitudinal orientation on the subcostal margin of the right upper abdominal quadrant at the midclavicular line (**Figure 19-1A**). The spleen can be examined with the patient in the supine position, using a 3 to 5 MHz curvilinear probe, with the probe placed in the coronal orientation in left mid-auxiliary line at the 10th intercostal space (**Figure 19-1B**). The normal liver and spleen are homogenous, contain fine-level echoes, with the liver minimally hyperechoic compared with the renal cortex but hypoechoic compared with the spleen (**Figure 19-2**).

2. **Assess for hepatomegaly.** The liver length will be the longest superior–inferior dimension that can be obtained with this view. For image optimization, attempt to project the ultrasound as perpendicular to the superior most portion of the liver dome as possible by slowly rocking and fanning the probe to obtain the most hyperlucent image of the liver edge and diaphragm dome in view (**Figures 19-3 and 19-4**).

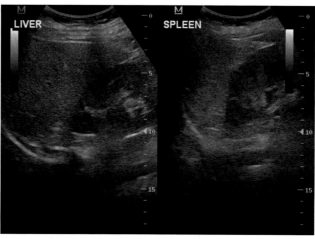

FIGURE 19-2. Liver and spleen have similar echogenicity on ultrasound.

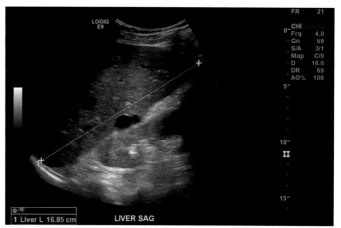

FIGURE 19-3. Borderline normal liver length.

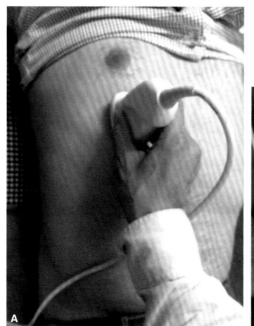
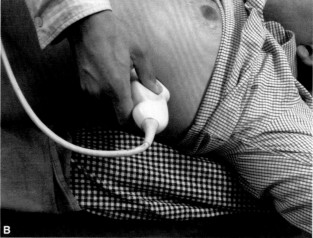

FIGURE 19-1. A, Patient position/probe position for hepatomegaly evaluation. B, Patient position/probe position for splenomegaly evaluation.

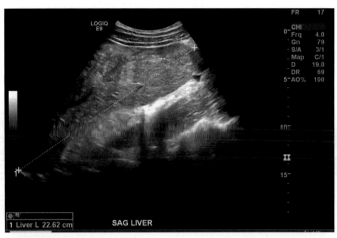

FIGURE 19-4. Hepatomegaly.

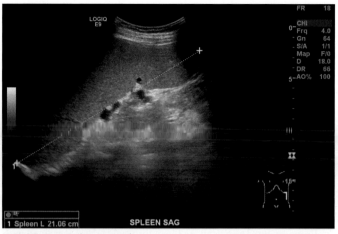

FIGURE 19-6. Splenomegaly.

Prospective studies have validated that measuring the liver length in the midclavicular line along the superior–inferior dimension suffices to assess for hepatomegaly and is defined as greater than 16 cm in length.[14]

3. **Assess for splenomegaly**. The maximum spleen length is in an oblique orientation and the probe should be oriented as such in the intercostal space to avoid rib shadowing. For image optimization, slowly fanning posteriorly and anteriorly along the coronal plane will help you find the maximum length (**Figures 19-5 and 19-6**). Occasionally, visualization can also be obscured from overlying bowel or gastric gas and overlying lung in the costophrenic angle. Holding mid inspiration and having the patient in the right lateral decubitus positions can help. Sonographic measurement of spleen length >13 cm measured from diaphragm to spleen tip is consistent with splenomegaly. This threshold accounts for patient body-height differences and inherent changes during

TABLE 19-2	Splenic Length by Sonography in Children	
Age (y)	Mean Spleen Length (cm) ± 1 SD	
5-8	8.5 ± 1.0	
9-10	8.6 ± 1.1	
11-12	9.7 ± 1.0	
13-14	10.1 ± 1.2	
15-16	10.1 ± 1.0	

Spleen sizes for younger population.[16]

digestion.[15] Importantly, when considering mononucleosis in the pediatric population, the upper limit of normal values varies slightly[16] (Table 19-2).

PATIENT MANAGEMENT

The clinical significance of hepatosplenomegaly will depend on the provider's suspicion of a particular diagnosis and its prevalence in the community. It is important to consider that the diagnostic criteria for various diseases have historically been based on a palpable spleen, as mentioned earlier. Therefore, the clinical or diagnostic significance of an enlarged spleen sonographically but not palpably ("scanomegaly") is less certain and is being researched. We present an algorithm that considers pathology where palpable hepatosplenomegaly can be verified sonographically (**Figure 19-7**). The presence of splenomegaly in a suspected case of mononucleosis should prompt the recommendation to avoid play for three to four weeks after the onset of symptoms, given the risk of splenic rupture. The presence of hepatosplenomegaly in a patient with weight loss or night sweats should prompt the practitioner to ordering a CBC, blood smear, and further workup if indicated.

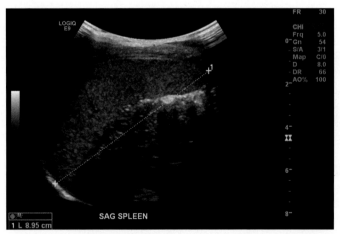

FIGURE 19-5. Normal spleen length.

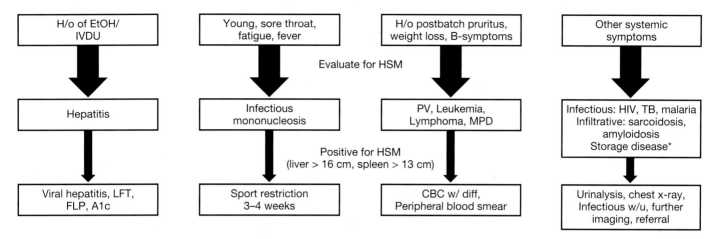

FIGURE 19-7. Hepatosplenomegaly can be assessed in the following grouped categories and worked up according to clinical suspicion. *Storage disease including lipid, glycogen, lysosomal/Goucher's, alpha-1-antitrypsin disease, hemochromatosis. A1c, hemoglobin A1c; CBC, complete blood count; EtOH, alcohol; FLP, fasting lipid profile; HIV, human immunodeficiency virus; HSM, hepatosplenomegaly; IVDU, intravenous drug user; LFT, liver function tests; MPD, myeloproliferative disease; PV, polycythemia vera; TB, tuberculosis.

PEARLS AND PITFALLS

Pearls

- When assessing for hepatomegaly, suspended inspiration enables examination of the dome of the liver the best.
- When assessing for hepatomegaly, include the entire liver span even if it has differing degrees of echogenicity. This commonly occurs in a nonuniform distribution among the lobe segments in nonalcoholic hepatosteatosis.
- The presence of splenomegaly, nodular liver edge, and ascites suggests that a patient has cirrhosis and portal hypertension.

Pitfall

- When assessing for splenomegaly, if the patient is instructed to take too deep a breath, the lung may descend enough to introduce artifact into the visual field. Ask the patient to hold at mid-inspiration for best results.

BILLING

CPT Code	Description	Global Payment	Professional Component	Technical Component
76705	Limited abdominal ultrasound	$101.31	$32.86	$68.45

CPT codes and average national reimbursement for Medicare in 2016. Payment data are from https://www.cms.gov/apps/physician-fee-schedule/search/search-criteria.aspx. See Chapter 2 for details on ultrasound billing.

References

1. Tamayo SG, Rickman LS, Mathews WC, et al. Examiner dependence on physical diagnostic tests for the detection of splenomegaly: a prospective study with multiple observers. *J Gen Intern Med*. 1993;8(2):69.
2. Joshi R, Singh A, Jajoo N, Pai M, Kalantri SP. Accuracy and reliability of palpation and percussion for detecting hepatomegaly: a rural hospital-based study. *Indian J Gastroenterol*. 2004;23(5):171-174.
3. Gupta K, Dhawan A, Abel C, Talley N, Attia J. A re-evaluation of the scratch test for locating the liver edge. *BMC Gastroenterol*. 2013;13:35.
4. Olson AP, Trappey B, Wagner M, Newman M, Nixon LJ, Schnobrich D. Point-of-care ultrasonography improves the diagnosis of splenomegaly in hospitalized patients. *Crit Ultrasound J*. 2015;7(1):13.
5. Loria P, Adinolfi LE, Bellentani S, et al; NAFLD Expert Committee of the Associazione Italiana per lo studio del Fegato. Practice guidelines for the diagnosis and management of nonalcoholic fatty liver disease. A decalogue from the Italian Association for the Study of the Liver (AISF) Expert Committee. *Dig Liver Dis*. 2010;42(4):272-282.
6. Ma X, Holalkere NS, Kambadakone RA, Mino-Kenudson M, Hahn PF, Sahani DV. Imaging-based quantification of hepatic fat: methods and clinical applications. *Radiographics*. 2009;29(5):1253-1277.
7. Aronson MD, Komaroff AL, Pass TM, Ervin CT, Branch WT. Heterophil antibody in adults with sore throat: frequency and clinical presentation. *Ann Intern Med*. 1982;96:507.
8. Cornell RF, Palmer J. Adult acute leukemia. *Dis Mon*. 2012;58(4):219-238.
9. Savage DG, Szydlo RM, Goldman JM. Clinical features at diagnosis in 430 patients with chronic myeloid leukaemia seen at a referral centre over a 16-year period. *Br J Haematol*. 1997;96(1):111-116.
10. Tefferi A. Polycythemia vera: a comprehensive review and clinical recommendations. *Mayo Clin Proc*. 2003;78:174-194.
11. Pearson TC. Evaluation of diagnostic criteria in polycythemia vera. *Semin Hematol*. 2001;38(1 suppl 2):21-24.
12. Zha Y, Zhou M, Hari A, et al. Ultrasound diagnosis of malaria: examination of the spleen, liver, and optic nerve sheath diameter. *World J Emerg Med*. 2015;6(1):10-15.
13. Barnett ED. Infectious disease screening for refugees resettled in the United States. *Clin Infect Dis*. 2004;39(6):833-841.
14. Niederau C, Sonnenberg A, Muller JE, et al. Sonographic measurements of the normal liver, spleen, pancreas, and portal vein. *Radiology*. 1983;149:537-540.
15. Spielmann AL, DeLong DM, Kliewer MA. Sonographic evaluation of spleen size in tall healthy athletes. *AJR Am J Roentgenol*. 2005;184:45-49.
16. Dittrich M, Milde S, Dinkel E, Baumann W, Weitzel D. Sonographic biometry of liver and spleen size in childhood. *Pediatr Radiol*. 1983;13(4):206-211.

Does the Patient Have Hepatic Steatosis?

Gina Bornemann, MMIS, MS and Paul Bornemann, MD, RMSK, RPVI

● Clinical Vignette

A 59-year-old man presents for hyperlipidemia follow-up and refill of his statin medication. His blood pressure is 140/90 mm Hg and body mass index (BMI) is 29. His physical examination is otherwise normal. Fasting glucose levels are 110 mg/dL; lipid profile demonstrates cholesterol levels of 213 mg/dL, triglycerides of 146 mg/dL, low-density lipoprotein (LDL) of 129 mg/dL, and high-density lipoprotein (HDL) of 55 mg/dL. Past medical history is remarkable for obesity, hyperlipidemia, and a recent ear infection treated with amoxicillin/clavulanate. He denies use of alcohol apart from the occasional social drink. Baseline liver function test before he started on the statin showed slightly elevated levels of aspartate aminotransferase (AST) and alanine aminotransferase (ALT); acute viral hepatitis panel was negative. Does the patient have hepatic steatosis?

LITERATURE REVIEW

Elevated transaminases is a common incidental laboratory finding in primary care, and nonalcoholic fatty liver disease (NAFLD) is the most common cause.[1] NAFLD is a digestive disorder characterized by the accumulation of mostly triglycerides in the liver, a clinical finding called hepatic steatosis. NAFLD is a condition in which hepatic steatosis exists but is not caused by other hepatic insults such as alcohol consumption or viral hepatitis. NAFLD exists along a continuum, ranging from relatively benign nonalcoholic fatty liver (NAFL) to the more severe nonalcoholic steatohepatitis (NASH). NAFL is associated with minimal hepatic inflammation and a very low risk of progressing to cirrhosis. On the other hand, NASH is associated with hepatocyte inflammation and has an increased risk of progression to fibrosis and cirrhosis. Cirrhosis that occurs secondary to NASH or that is otherwise associated with steatosis is referred to as NASH cirrhosis.[2] Once cirrhosis occurs, it is generally irreversible and is associated with a high rate of complications including liver failure, variceal bleeding, infection, and hepatocellular carcinoma.

Rates of NASH-associated morbidity and mortality have been increasing worldwide. It is currently estimated that up to 30% of adults in the United States have NAFLD and up to 10% of those have NASH.[1] Chronic liver disease and cirrhosis are responsible for increasing rates of mortality and morbidity worldwide and in the United States liver disease had been listed by the Centers for Disease Control and Prevention (CDC) as the 12th leading cause of death in 2015. About 4.9 million adults in the United States received a liver disease diagnosis in 2015. These figures are expected to increase.[3-6] Additionally, it has been observed that liver disease may also contribute to damage to other organs. Individuals with liver disease may be particularly vulnerable to cardiovascular disease, the top cause of death in the United States.[7]

The cause of NAFLD is not fully understood, but there is a good understanding of underlying risk factors. It is highly associated with obesity, hypertension, dyslipidemia, and insulin resistance.[8] It mostly occurs in middle-aged adults, although it can occur at any age, including in children. NAFLD is a diagnosis of exclusion and other secondary causes of hepatic steatosis must be ruled out. See Table 20-1. Alcohol consumption is another common cause of hepatic steatosis. NAFLD can only be considered in patients without a history of significant alcohol consumption. Significant alcohol consumption is defined as more than 20 g/day or >14 drinks/week for females and more than 30 g/day or >21 drinks/week for males.[3,9,10]

Liver biopsy is the gold standard for the diagnosis of NAFLD and for differentiating benign steatosis from NASH or cirrhosis. However, biopsy remains an invasive technique with the risk of complications and sampling error.[11] Less invasive methods of diagnosis have been sought. Serum transaminases are often positive in NAFLD; however, they are neither sensitive nor specific by themselves. Computed tomography, magnetic resonance imaging, and ultrasound are all sensitive and specific for detecting hepatic steatosis. Ultrasound was shown in a meta-analysis to be accurate at diagnosing steatosis with a sensitivity of 84.8% and specificity of 93.6%.[12] Additionally, point-of-care ultrasound (POCUS) using five criteria taught during a 20-minute training period has been shown to have a sensitivity of 80% and a specificity of 99% for detecting moderate to severe steatosis.[13] Imaging is not able to differentiate NAFL from NASH; however, if surface nodularity is seen, then cirrhosis can be confidently diagnosed. Ultrasound

TABLE 20-1	Differential Diagnosis for Hepatic Steatosis

- Nonalcoholic fatty liver disease
- Excessive alcohol consumption
- Hepatitis C
- Medications (amiodarone, methotrexate, tamoxifen, corticosteroids, valproate, antiretroviral medicines)
- Wilson's disease
- Lipodystrophy
- Starvation
- Parenteral nutrition
- Abetalipoproteinemia
- Reye's syndrome
- Acute fatty liver of pregnancy
- HELLP (hemolysis, elevated liver enzymes, low platelet count) syndrome
- Inborn errors of metabolism

Adapted from Chalasani N, Younossi Z, Lavine JE, et al. The diagnosis and management of nonalcoholic fatty liver disease: practice guidance from the American Association for the Study of Liver Diseases. *Hepatology*. 2018;67(1):328-357. Copyright © 2017 by the American Association for the Study of Liver Diseases. Reprinted by permission of John Wiley & Sons, Inc.

TABLE 20-2	Recommendations for Use of Point-of-Care Ultrasound in Clinical Practice		
Recommendation		Rating	References
Point-of-care ultrasound is a sensitive and specific test in the evaluation of nonalcoholic fatty liver disease (NAFLD).		B	23
NAFLD fibrosis score is an effective noninvasive method to stratify the risk of severe fibrosis or cirrhosis in patients with NAFLD.		A	15
All patients diagnosed with NAFLD should receive lifestyle modification counseling with a goal of 5% to 7% decrease in weight.		A	17

A = consistent, good-quality patient-oriented evidence; B = inconsistent or limited-quality patient-oriented evidence; C = consensus, disease-oriented evidence, usual practice, expert opinion, or case series. For information about the SORT evidence rating system, go to http://www.aafp.org/afpsort.

assessment for hepatic nodularity has a sensitivity and specificity of 54% and 95%, respectively, for diagnosing cirrhosis.[14] Thus, imaging modalities, including POCUS, can effectively diagnose steatosis, but are still limited by an inability to differentiate NAFL from NASH.

Noninvasive scoring systems that utilize serum markers have shown the ability to determine fibrosis risk in different liver diseases including NAFLD. The NAFLD Fibrosis Score (NFS) and FIB-4 index are two examples that are recommended by the American Association for the Study of Liver Diseases guidelines.[2] We prefer the NFS as it has more evidence behind its use in NAFLD.[15] The NFS considers age, AST, ALT, platelet (PLT) count, BMI, hyperglycemia, and albumin. Results are most valuable when they are at the high or low extremes. For the NFS, a score < -1.455 had 90% sensitivity to exclude advanced fibrosis, whereas a score > 0.676 had 97% specificity to rule in advanced fibrosis.[15] However, when results are in the intermediate range (-1.455 to 0.676) they are less helpful. In these instances, further noninvasive testing such as shear wave elastography (SWE) is an option, if available. SWE is a special type of ultrasound and is not currently readily available to most primary care providers. It measures hepatic stiffness, which correlates with the degree of fibrosis. It also tends to be most useful when results are very high or low. As with noninvasive serum markers, SWE can have indeterminate results as well.[16] If SWE is indeterminate or not otherwise available, liver biopsy can be considered.

PERFORMING THE SCAN

1. **Preparation.** The patient should be lying comfortably in a supine position and measures should be taken to ensure the privacy of the patient. If necessary, the patient could be rolled to the right lateral decubitus position. We recommend the use of two transducers, the curvilinear transducer and the linear transducer, that will be used for better imaging of the liver contour. Start with the curvilinear transducer (2-5 MHz). Select the "Abdomen" preset. Ultrasound gel should be warmed, if possible, for the comfort of the patient (**Figure 20-1**).

2. **Assess the liver in the sagittal plane.** Start with the transducer below the sternum and angle the transducer cephalad. The probe indicator should be pointing to the patient's head. Find the left lobe of the liver and slowly slide the transducer laterally through the entire left and right lobe for a complete visualization of the liver (**Figures 20-2 to 20-5**).

3. **Assess the liver in the transverse plane.** Place the transducer below the costal margin or in one of the lower intercostal spaces

in the right upper quadrant. Rotate the transducer into the transverse plane with the marker pointing to the patient's right. Angle as cephalad as possible to visualize the superior liver at the level of the border of the right cardiac ventricle. Slowly scan inferiorly to the level of the right kidney. Take care to visualize the entire liver in the transverse plane (**Figures 20-6 to 20-10**).

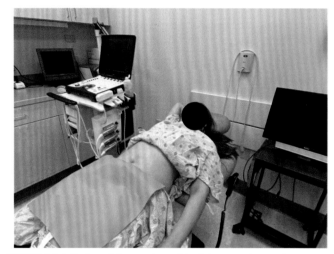

FIGURE 20-1. Patient lying supine with right arm elevated.

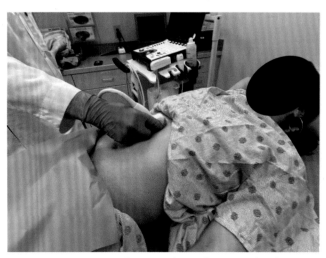

FIGURE 20-2. Correct starting transducer placement for the sagittal plane scan. The transducer is inferior to the sternum and angled cephalad. The probe maker points toward the patient's head.

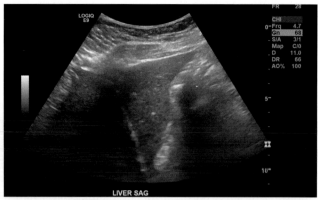

FIGURE 20-3. Sagittal, left lobe of liver. This is the starting position for the sagittal scan.

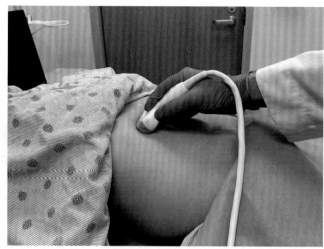

FIGURE 20-6. Correct starting transducer placement for the transverse plane scan. The transducer is inferior to the 12th rib in the mid-clavicular line and angled cephalad. The probe maker points toward the patient's right.

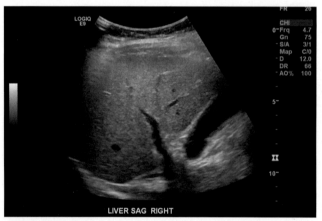

FIGURE 20-4. Sagittal, midline of liver. The gallbladder and porta hepatis will be seen between the right and left hepatic lobes.

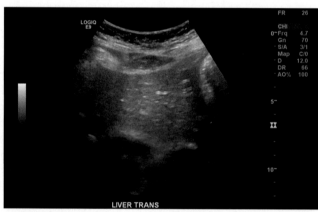

FIGURE 20-7. Transverse, superior liver. The heart will be visualized adjacent to the liver. This is the starting position for the transverse scan.

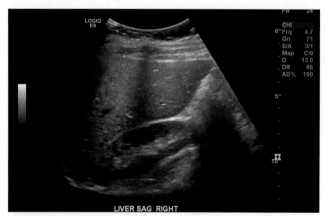

FIGURE 20-5. Sagittal, right lobe of liver. The sagittal scan is completed by continuing through the entire right lobe of the liver past the right kidney.

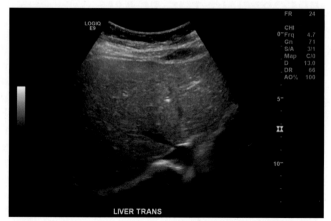

FIGURE 20-8. Transverse, mid-liver. Continuing to scan inferiorly, the hepatic veins and inferior vena cava will be visualized next.

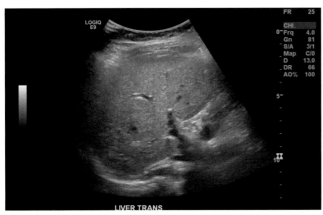

FIGURE 20-9. Transverse, mid-liver. Continuing to scan inferiorly, the porta hepatis and gallbladder will be visualized inferior to the hepatic veins and inferior vena cava.

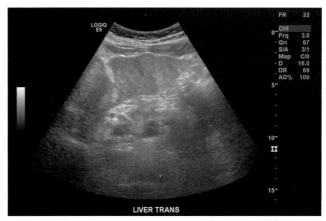

FIGURE 20-12. Low-frequency transducer image of liver with nodularity consistent with cirrhosis.

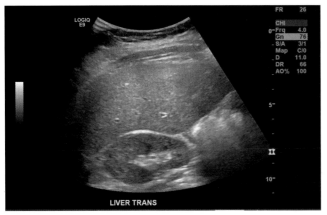

FIGURE 20-10. Transverse, inferior liver at the right kidney. The transverse scan is completed by continuing through the entire liver past the right kidney.

4. **Assess for signs of steatosis.** Place the probe in the right upper quadrant in the 10th or 11th intercostal space in a transverse plane. Assess for the five signs of steatosis that, when present, have been validated in a POCUS protocol (**Figure 20-11**).[13]

   1. Abrupt attenuation of the liver image in the first 4 to 5 cm of depth, making the deeper part of the liver very dark and difficult, if not impossible, to visualize.

   2. Diffusely hyperechoic liver parenchyma, within at least the first 2 cm of depth.

   3. A uniformly heterogeneous or coarse-appearing liver parenchyma.

   4. Subcutaneous tissue that is at least 2 cm in depth visualized in the near field.

   5. An enlarged liver that fills the entire field of view (considered a helpful finding if present but not necessary for diagnosis).

5. **Evaluate for signs of cirrhosis.** Evaluate the entire liver surface for nodularity with the curvilinear transducer. Switch to a high-frequency linear array transducer and evaluate superficial surface of the liver for nodularity (**Figures 20-12 to 20-14**).

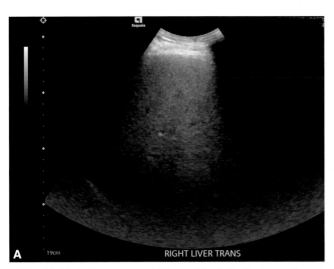

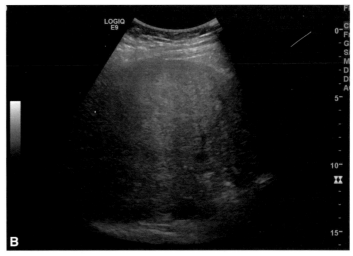

FIGURE 20-11. A, Transverse, mid-liver with all the features of steatosis. Abrupt attenuation of the liver. Diffusely hyperechoic liver parenchyma. Uniformly heterogeneous liver parenchyma. Subcutaneous tissue greater than 2 cm in depth. Enlarged liver that fills the entire field of view. Compare this to the similar view of the normal liver in **Figure 20-8**. B, A liver similar in appearance to Figure 20-11A with the same features of steatosis, but with slightly less attenuation.

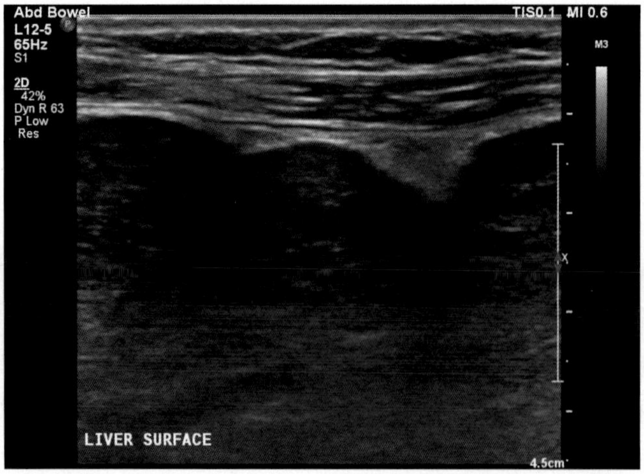

FIGURE 20-13. High-frequency transducer image of liver with nodularity consistent with cirrhosis. High-frequency images of the liver may be more sensitive for finding nodularity than low-frequency images.

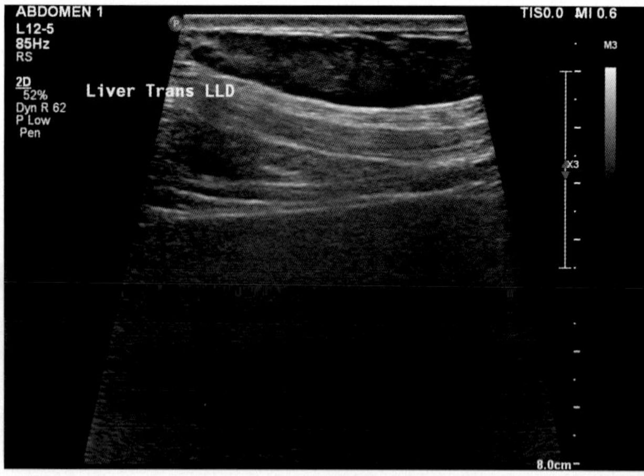

FIGURE 20-14. High-frequency transducer image of liver with normal, smooth margin.

PATIENT MANAGEMENT

The diagnostic evaluation for NAFLD frequently begins when a patient presents to primary care with nonspecific elevations in their liver transaminases. The first step is to take a thorough history of risk factors for potential causes including hepatotoxins such as medications, supplements, or alcohol consumption. If their history is positive for potential hepatotoxins or alcohol use, they should be instructed to discontinue these for several months and then repeat testing can be performed. If their status is not already known, it is recommended that all patients be assessed for hepatitis B and C. This is because of the prevalence, risk of spreading unrecognized infection, and availability of effective treatments, especially for hepatitis C.

If patients have no history of heavy alcohol use, or hepatotoxin ingestion and test negative for viral hepatitis, the next step is to perform a POCUS assessment for steatosis. If steatosis is found, then the diagnosis is likely NAFLD. If findings of cirrhosis are found on ultrasound then there is no further need for fibrosis evaluation. However, if not, there is still the possibility of significant underlying fibrosis or cirrhosis and noninvasive serum markers for fibrosis risk assessment should be obtained. The NFS is the preferred method and can be easily calculated in the primary care office. An online NFS calculator can be found at http://gihep.com/calculators/hepatology/nafld-fibrosis-score/. If the NFS is less than −1.455, then significant fibrosis is unlikely. If the score is greater than 0.676, then the patient likely has significant fibrosis or cirrhosis. In these instances, the patient may be referred for biopsy or just treated as if they had cirrhosis. Patients with indeterminate results (−1.455 to 0.676) can be referred for SWE or liver biopsy for further evaluation.

In patients where POCUS does not confirm NAFLD, the clinician should consider further laboratory evaluation for less common causes of transaminitis including Wilson's disease, hemochromatosis, autoimmune hepatitis, primary biliary cirrhosis, alpha-1 antitrypsin, and Celiac disease.

In all patients diagnosed with NAFLD, lifestyle modification counseling should be given. The most effective intervention for NAFLD by far is weight loss. A 5% to 7% decrease in weight is associated with improvement in NAFL and NASH.[17] In patients with biopsy-proven NASH, both vitamin E (800 IU/day) and pioglitazone (30 mg/day) have been shown to improve histology, although patient-oriented outcomes data are currently lacking. Vitamin E data are only available for patients without diabetes, whereas pioglitazone has data for patients with or without diabetes.[2]

In addition to the above specific treatments, any patient with presumed cirrhosis should have additional treatment considerations. Patients should be vaccinated against hepatitis A and B if not already done as they are at high risk for poor outcomes of acute hepatitis given their underlying liver impairment. Given their increased risk of morbidity from infections, routine vaccination against pneumococcus (PPSV23) and influenza is also recommended. All patients with cirrhosis should be referred for upper endoscopy to screen for esophageal varices. If found, prophylactic treatment with beta-blockers or banding can decrease the risk of major hemorrhage. Additionally, all patients with cirrhosis are at increased risk for hepatocellular carcinoma and should undergo ultrasound of liver for screening every 6 months. Findings of decompensated cirrhosis include variceal hemorrhage, ascites, spontaneous bacterial peritonitis, hepatocellular carcinoma, hepatorenal syndrome, or hepatopulmonary syndrome. When decompensation is present, a Model for End-Stage Liver Disease (MELD) score should be calculated to determine overall prognosis.[18] MELD score is derived from lab findings including the international normalized ratio (INR), bilirubin, and creatinine and predicts mortality related to liver failure. An online calculator can be found at https://www.mayoclinic.org/medical-professionals/transplant-medicine/calculators/meld-model/itt-20434705. If the MELD score is greater than or equal to 15, patients should be referred to a transplant center for evaluation for liver transplantation (**Figure 20-15**).[19]

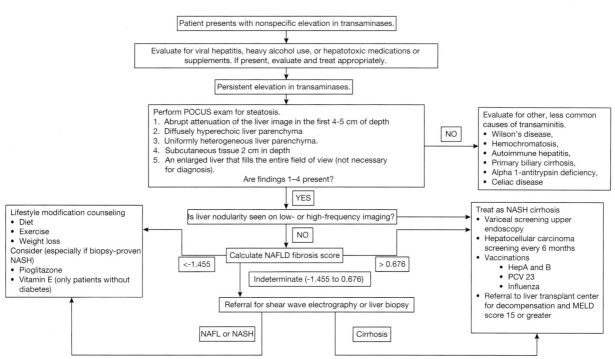

FIGURE 20-15. Algorithm for management of suspected nonalcoholic fatty liver disease (NAFLD). MELD, Model for End-Stage Liver Disease; NAFL, nonalcoholic fatty liver; NASH, nonalcoholic steatohepatitis.

PEARLS AND PITFALLS

Pearls

- It is highly recommended that the patient fast for 4 to 6 hours prior to the examination.
- When obtaining hepatic views through intercostal windows, angling the transducer slightly oblique and parallel to the ribs will decrease rib shadows in the image.
- Mild steatosis can be difficult to detect and may not show all the signs mentioned earlier. In these cases, the liver may demonstrate only mildly increased echogenicity. The liver is normally hyperechoic to the renal cortex, and this doesn't make for a good comparison. However, the liver is usually hypoechoic to the spleen. A split screen image of the liver and spleen can be obtained using the same gain settings to make the comparison (**Figure 20-16**).

Pitfalls

- When the transducer is perfectly perpendicular to the liver, the surface may appear nodular when it is in fact normal. Always be sure to confirm nodularity by tilting the transducer to a perpendicular angle with the liver surface.
- A liver with NAFLD may have areas of focal steatosis or focal sparing, which can be mistaken for a neoplasm. Focal areas tend to involve the area around the gallbladder, porta hepatis, the dorsal left lobe, or the caudate lobe.

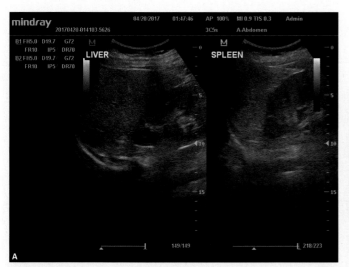

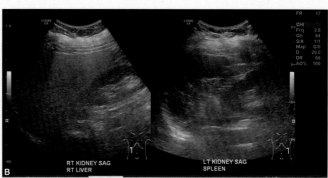

FIGURE 20-16. A, Split screen image of a normal liver and spleen. Note that the liver is hyperechoic to the renal cortex but hypoechoic compared to the spleen. B, Split screen image of a liver with mild steatosis. Note that the liver is hyperechoic to the renal cortex and to the spleen.

BILLING

CPT Code	Description	Global Payment	Professional Component	Technical Component
76705	"Ultrasound, abdominal, real time (with image documentation); limited (e.g., single organ, quadrant, follow-up)"	$92.73	$30.88	$62.66

CPT codes and average national reimbursement for Medicare in 2016. Payment data are from https://www.cms.gov/apps/physician-fee-schedule/search/search-criteria.aspx. See Chapter 2 for details on ultrasound billing.

References

1. Torres DM, Harrison SA. Diagnosis and therapy of nonalcoholic steato-hepatitis. *Gastroenterology*. 2008;134(6):1682-1698.

2. Chalasani N, Younossi Z, Lavine JE, et al. The diagnosis and management of nonalcoholic fatty liver disease: Practice guidance from the American Association for the Study of Liver Diseases. *Hepatology*. 2018;67(1):328-357.

3. Severson TJ, Besur S, Bonkovsky HL. Genetic factors that affect nonalcoholic fatty liver disease: a systematic clinical review. *World J Gastroenterol*. 2016;22(29):6742-6756. doi:10.3748/wjg.v22.i29.6742.

4. Kochanek KD, Murphy SL, Xu J, Tejada-Vera B. National vital statistics report. *Natl Vital Stat Rep*. 2016;65(4). https://www.cdc.gov/nchs/data/nvsr/nvsr65/nvsr65_04.pdf.

5. Chronic liver disease and cirrhosis. Centers for Disease Control and Prevention Website. https://www.cdc.gov/nchs/fastats/liver-disease.htm. Updated October 6, 2016.

6. Younossi ZM, Stepanova M, Afendy M, et al. Changes in the prevalence of the most common causes of chronic liver diseases in the United States from 1988 to 2008. *Clin Gastroenterol Hepatol*. 2011;9(6):524.e1-530.e1. doi:10.1016/j.cgh.2011.03.020.

7. Misra VL, Khashab M, Chalasani N. Nonalcoholic fatty liver disease and cardiovascular risk. *Curr Gastroenterol Rep*. 2009;11(1):50-55. doi:10.1007/s11894-009-0008-4.

8. Marchesini G, Bugianesi E, Forlani G, et al. Nonalcoholic fatty liver, steatohepatitis, and the metabolic syndrome. *Hepatology*. 2003;37(4):917-923. Erratum in: *Hepatology*. 2003;38(2):536.

9. Brunt EM, Janney CG, Di Bisceglie AM, Neuschwander-Tetri BA, Bacon BR. Nonalcoholic steatohepatitis: a proposal for grading and staging the histological lesions. *Am J Gastroenterol*. 1999;94(9):2467-2474. doi:10.1111/j.1572-0241.1999.01377.x.

10. Younossi ZM, Koenig AB, Abdelatif D, Fazel Y, Henry L, Wymer M. Global epidemiology of nonalcoholic fatty liver disease-Meta-analytic assessment of prevalence, incidence, and outcomes. *Hepatology*. 2016;64(1):73-84. doi:10.1002/hep.28431.

11. Regev A, Berho M, Jeffers LJ, et al. Sampling error and intraobserver variation in liver biopsy in patients with chronic HCV infection. *Am J Gastroenterol*. 2002;97(10):2614-2618. doi:10.1016/S0002-9270(02)04396-4.

12. Hernaez R, Lazo M, Bonekamp S, et al. Diagnostic accuracy and reliability of ultrasonography for the detection of fatty liver: a meta-analysis. *Hepatology*. 2011;54(3):1082-1090. doi:10.1002/hep.24452.

13. Riley TR, Mendoza A, Bruno MA. Bedside ultrasound can predict nonalcoholic fatty liver disease in the hands of clinicians using a prototype image. *Dig Dis Sci*. 2006;51(5):982-985. doi:10.1007/s10620-006-9343-6.

14. Colli A, Fraquelli M, Andreoletti M, Marino B, Zuccoli E, Conte D. Severe liver fibrosis or cirrhosis: accuracy of US for detection—analysis of 300 cases. *Radiology*. 2003;227:89-94.

15. Musso G, Gambino R, Cassader M, Pagano G. Meta-analysis: natural history of non-alcoholic fatty liver disease (NAFLD) and diagnostic accuracy of non-invasive tests for liver disease severity. *Ann Med*. 2011;43:617-649.

16. Tapper EB, Challies T, Nasser I, Afdhal NH, Lai M. The performance of vibration controlled transient elastography in a US cohort of patients with nonalcoholic fatty liver disease. *Am J Gastroenterol*. 2016;111:677-684.

17. Musso G, Cassader M, Rosina F, Gambino R. Impact of current treatments on liver disease, glucose metabolism and cardiovascular risk in non-alcoholic fatty liver disease (NAFLD): a systematic review and meta-analysis of randomised trials. *Diabetologia*. 2012;55:885-904.

18. Kamath PS, Wiesner RH, Malinchoc M, et al. A model to predict survival in patients with end-stage liver disease. *Hepatology*. 2001;33(2):464-470.

19. Selvaggi G. Patient selection in liver transplant: when is it the right time to list? *Mayo Clin Proc*. 2008;83(2):140-142.

Does the Patient Have Ascites?

Erin Stratta, MD and Kendra Johnson, MD

● Clinical Vignette

A 55-year-old male presents to clinic having just relocated from another state. He complains of progressive weight gain, especially in his belly, and, in the past week, difficulty breathing. This is his first visit to a physician in years. He admits to many years of heavy alcohol use and notes, "I feel like my belly is so swollen I'm pregnant!" On examination, you note faintly jaundiced skin and a distended, tympanic abdomen. Does the patient have ascites?

LITERATURE REVIEW

Ascites is an abnormal accumulation of fluid in the peritoneal cavity. It is most commonly associated with portal hypertension. In the United States, over 80% of ascites cases are caused by cirrhosis, specifically from alcohol use, followed by hepatitis C and nonalcoholic steatohepatitis (NASH). Other less common causes include malignancy, heart failure, tuberculosis, kidney disease, vascular obstruction, or infection[1,2] (see **Table 21-1**).

Diagnosis of ascites starts with a good history and physical examination. This allows the clinician to form an appropriate differential diagnosis, determine the likelihood that a patient may have ascites, and give clues as to the underlying cause. A history of recent trauma may lean toward blood, rather than ascites, in the abdomen. In contrast, a long history of drinking, with slowly progressive peripheral edema and abdominal distention, is classic for ascites.

On physical examination, classic findings of possible ascites include a distended abdomen with tympany on percussion and fluid wave on palpation (**Figure 21-1**). However, not all patients will exhibit obvious signs of ascites. This is why a combination of concerning patient history and clinical suspicion should prompt clinicians to utilize point-of-care ultrasound (POCUS) to evaluate for ascites.

As there is little downside to doing an ultrasound examination for ascites, clinicians should have a low threshold to perform this as part of their physical examination. For example, patients with new or progressive abdominal distention, jaundice, history of heavy alcohol use, peripheral edema, abdominal pain, shortness of breath, and/or congestive heart failure could benefit from a bedside evaluation for ascites. Because over 50% of those diagnosed with cirrhosis will develop ascites within 10 years, having a low threshold for ultrasound in these patients is also prudent.[3]

Ascites is often classified on the basis of content of different components in the fluid. This makes paracentesis, or sampling of the ascitic fluid, diagnostically important. Paracentesis also has a therapeutic role for many people, because it can alleviate the shortness of breath common with significant ascites. Ultrasound is useful to demonstrate the presence of ascites, identify the optimal location for performing a paracentesis, and provide live guidance during the procedure.

Formal ultrasound has been used to detect ascites for decades and can detect as little as 100 mL of ascitic fluid.[4] Multiple studies have demonstrated that even after a brief training, POCUS is a reliable and effective way to detect ascites. One study trained 12 medical students in basic abdominal ultrasound, including evaluation for ascites. After this brief training, the students had a sensitivity and specificity of 100% for identifying the presence or absences of ascites in five hospitalized patients.[5] In another study, 31 physicians were randomized to either a 4-hour abdominal ultrasound course, or no additional training, and the group that completed the ultrasound

TABLE 21-1 Causes of Ascites and Frequency Reported in Literature

Causes of Ascites	Frequency (%)
Cirrhosis	81
Malignancy	7-10
Tuberculosis	2-7
Heart failure	3
Nephrotic syndrome	1
Dialysis	1
Pancreatic disease	1
Other	2

Note that these frequencies will vary depending on the local prevalence of underlying causes such as tuberculosis.

From Runyon BA. Care of patients with ascites. *N Engl J Med*. 1994;330(5): 337-342. Copyright © 1994 Massachusetts Medical Society. Reprinted with permission from Massachusetts Medical Society; Shaikh MA, Khan J, Almani S, Dur-e-Yakta, Saikh D. Frequency of causes of ascites in patients at a medical unit of a tertiary medical care facility. *J Ayub Med Coll*. 2019;22(2):88-92.

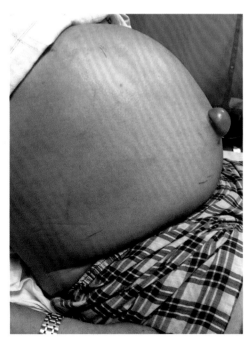

FIGURE 21-1. A patient with ascites and a significantly distended and tense abdomen.

course could accurately diagnose fluid in the abdomen of a patient with ascites 82% of the time, compared to 43% in the control group.[6] In addition to the standard ultrasound, a small pocket portable ultrasound device can also be used effectively to determine the presence or absence of ascites. A study based in the emergency room found a sensitivity of 0.96 and a specificity of 0.82 of portable ultrasound for this purpose.[7]

In addition to reliably diagnosing or excluding ascites, the use of ultrasound guidance during paracentesis has been shown in multiple studies to result in a higher chance of success and a lower complication rate. A prospective, randomized study in the emergency room setting found that of patients randomized to bedside ultrasound assistance during paracentesis, 95% had ascitic fluid successfully obtained, as compared to only 61% of patients randomized to traditional landmark-based paracentesis.[8] Another study found that ultrasound guidance reduced the risk of bleeding complications after paracentesis by 68%.[9] See Chapter 55 for details about the technique of ultrasound-guided paracentesis.

The literature supports the use of bedside ultrasound for ascites in a variety of clinical settings, including the emergency room, inpatient medicine,[10] and palliative care.[11] Its utility is equally applicable in the ambulatory care setting, where quick diagnosis of ascites by ultrasound can guide clinical decision making. This chapter will explore how and when to use POCUS to detect and manage ascites.

TABLE 21-2	Recommendations for Use of Point-of-Care Ultrasound in Clinical Practice

Recommendation	Rating	References
Point-of-care ultrasound for evaluation of ascites can be performed effectively by practitioners after a brief training.	A	6, 7
Use of ultrasound to identify an appropriate fluid pocket to perform paracentesis results in higher chance of success and lower complication rate.	A	9, 10

A = consistent, good-quality patient-oriented evidence; B = inconsistent or limited-quality patient-oriented evidence; C = consensus, disease-oriented evidence, usual practice, expert opinion, or case series. For information about the SORT evidence rating system, go to http://www.aafp.org/afpsort.

PERFORMING THE SCAN

1. **Preparation.** Place the patient in a semiupright, supine, or lateral decubitus position for this scan, depending on patient comfort. Ascites collects in the abdomen in a gravity-dependent fashion, and, therefore, most practitioners will place the patient semiupright (**Figure 21-2**). For most cases, select a low-frequency (2-5 MHz), curvilinear probe to best perform this scan, with an abdominal preset. A phased array probe may also be used.
2. **Overview.** The technique for the ascites ultrasound examination is similar to the focused assessment with sonography in trauma (FAST) or eFAST examinations and involves scanning of all four quadrants of the abdomen as well as the suprapubic

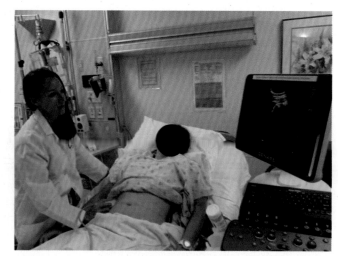

FIGURE 21-2. Patient positioning for the ascites examination.

region. Scanning each quadrant methodically will reduce the likelihood of missing an abnormal finding or a collection of free fluid. The goal is to obtain an image deep enough to see the structures typical in that region. For example, in the right upper quadrant, visualizing the diaphragm, liver, and kidney is important (**Figure 21-3**). In some patients, whether as a result of obesity or large amounts of ascitic fluid, the depth may need to be increased significantly to optimally visualize all structures. Remember to scan in both the longitudinal (sagittal) and the transverse planes. As in any ultrasound examination, experiment with different levels of pressure, and make small sweeping movements with the transducer to obtain optimal images. Ascitic fluid will appear anechoic (black) and darker than surrounding structures, and will often float or move freely as it is untethered to surrounding structures.

3. **Evaluate the right upper quadrant (Figure 21-4).** Place the transducer in the midaxillary line near the bottom of the ribs, and move toward the midclavicular line. Adjust the transducer up or down rib spaces as needed to obtain an image of structures in the right upper quadrant. Identify the diaphragm, liver, and

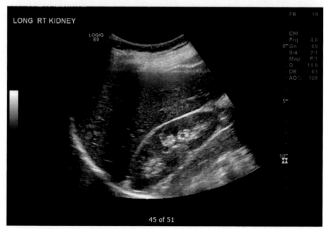

FIGURE 21-3. Normal anatomy in right upper quadrant, including view of the diaphragm, liver, and kidney.

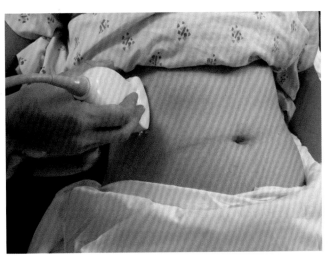

FIGURE 21-4. Probe placement for right upper quadrant evaluation.

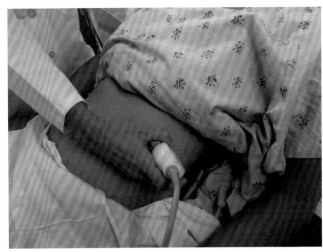

FIGURE 21-6. Probe placement for left upper quadrant evaluation.

kidney. Evaluate for anechoic fluid around the liver and kidney or below the diaphragm (**Figure 21-5**).

4. **Evaluate the left upper quadrant (Figures 21-6 and 21-7).** Move to the midaxillary line at the lower rib border on the left side. Again, adjust the rib space level as needed. Identify the diaphragm, spleen, and kidney. Ensure adequate views of the kidneys on both sides.

5. **Evaluate the right and left lower quadrants (Figures 21-8 to 21-11).** Identify bowel and any free fluid that may be in these regions. Bowel segments are typically floating or undulating

echoic shapes that connect. Ascitic fluid in these areas will typically appear to be pushing the bowel down or floating above it. Ask the patient to sit up, or roll to one side, and repeat the evaluation, as this may allow for better visualization of free fluid in the abdomen. Scan from the right lower quadrant up to the right upper quadrant, and do the same on the left, including the paracolic gutters, in a methodical manner.

6. **Evaluate the suprapubic space (Figure 21-12).** Identify the bladder. This should appear as a well-demarcated anechoic shape directly above the pubic symphysis. Evaluate in both transverse

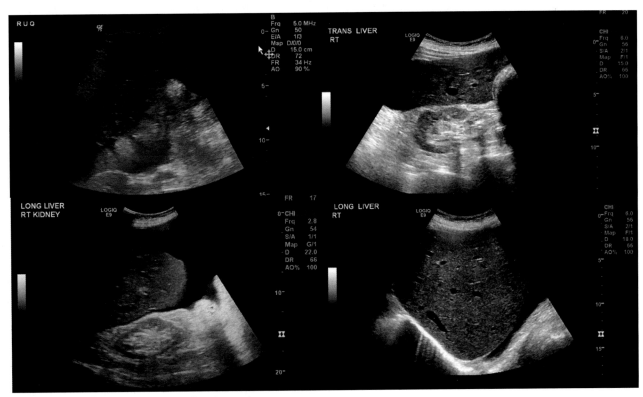

FIGURE 21-5. Right upper quadrant views showing ascites.

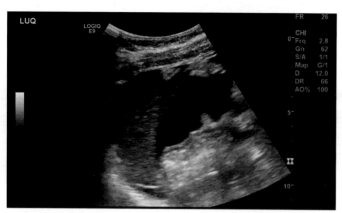

FIGURE 21-7. Peri-splenic ascites in the left upper quadrant.

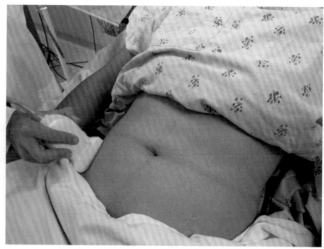

FIGURE 21-8. Probe placement for right lower quadrant evaluation.

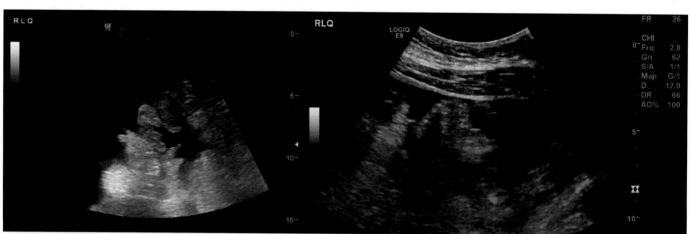

FIGURE 21-9. Examples of ascites in the right lower quadrant.

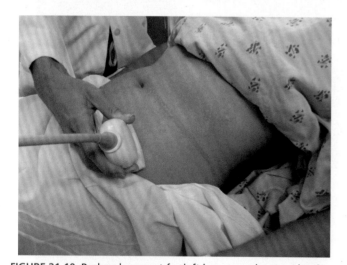

FIGURE 21-10. Probe placement for left lower quadrant evaluation.

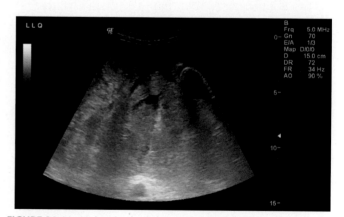

FIGURE 21-11. Ascites in the left lower quadrant.

and sagittal planes **(Figure 21-13)**. If the patient has recently voided, it may be too contracted to see **(Figure 21-14)**. In females, identify the uterus, and look for fluid behind the uterus, in the rectouterine space. Fluid in this area may appear near the bladder **(Figure 21-15)** or may be identified without clear visualization of the bladder **(Figure 21-16)**.

7. **Evaluate depth of fluid.** If ascitic fluid is visualized, evaluate depth using the centimeter marker on the side of the screen **(Figure 21-17)**. Exact distances can also be measured by selecting the CALIPER function **(Figure 21-18)**. Evaluate in centimeters the distance between ascitic fluid and the underlying structures such as bowel. Scan the abdomen and locate where the unobstructed pocket of ascitic fluid is deepest. This is typically the preferred site for a paracentesis (see Chapter 71 for further details). Be careful of areas where bowel may be floating near the surface **(Figure 21-19)**.

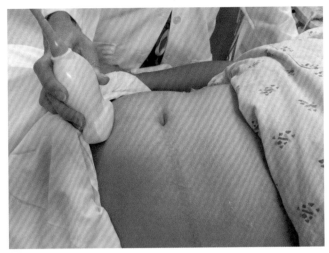

FIGURE 21-12. Probe placement for suprapubic evaluation.

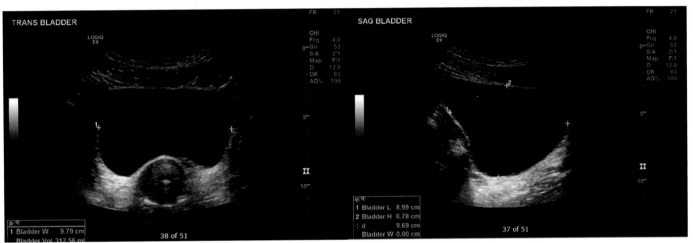

FIGURE 21-13. Images of normal bladder in transverse and sagittal planes. Note the cervix inferior to the bladder in the transverse image.

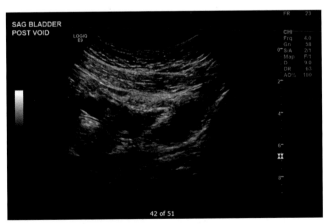

FIGURE 21-14. Image of bladder in the same patient after voiding. It is now contracted and difficult to visualize. This patient does not have ascites, but the contracted bladder can be confused for free fluid.

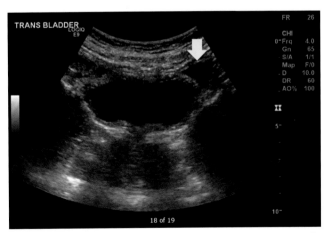

FIGURE 21-15. Transverse view of a bladder with a thickened wall. A small amount of free fluid can be seen outside the bladder on the patient's left (arrow).

PART 2

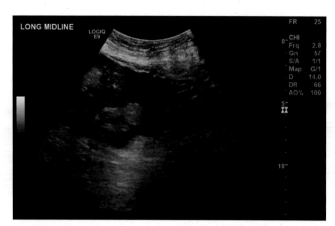

FIGURE 21-16. Ascites along the midline. In this example, the bladder is not visualized.

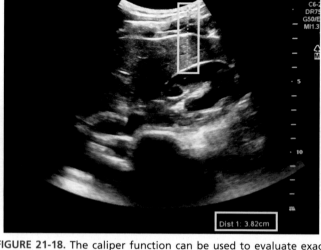

FIGURE 21-18. The caliper function can be used to evaluate exact distance between structures, such as depth from skin.

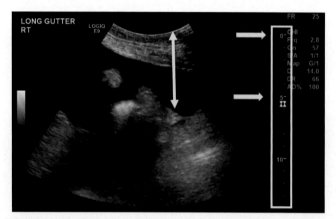

FIGURE 21-17. The side panel shows measurement in centimeters. Arrows point to 0 and 5 cm depth, respectively. In this example, distance from the skin to the bowel is approximately 5 to 6 cm.

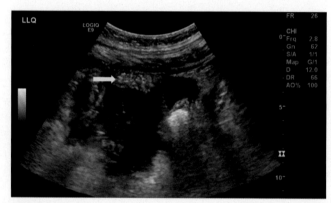

FIGURE 21-19. Notice that although there is ascitic fluid, areas of bowel are floating (arrow), making it a potentially dangerous site for paracentesis.

PATIENT MANAGEMENT

Patient management of ascites varies depending on several key questions, which can be used to determine how to treat these patients in the clinical setting (**Figure 21-20**).

First, consider if this is a new diagnosis. Because nonhepatic causes of ascites are identified in 15% of cases, diagnostic paracentesis is essential in a patient with a new diagnosis of ascites.[12] Fluid analysis and culture can determine etiology of the ascites and guide further management. Routine tests include culture and gram stain, cell count, total protein, and albumin. Cytology, lactate dehydrogenase, bilirubin, and tuberculosis testing can be sent on the basis of history and risk factors. Patients with signs of hemodynamic instability, infection, hyponatremia, decreased glomerular filtration rate (GFR), respiratory distress, or confusion should be hospitalized.

Second, consider whether or not the patient is symptomatic. If it is not a new diagnosis of ascites, management depends on symptoms and clinical suspicion. If the patient is asymptomatic with stable vitals and laboratory values, paracentesis is not necessary. Treatment

for these patients often focuses on reversing the cause of ascites, such as alcohol abstinence, treatment of hepatitis, salt restriction, and diuretics (spironolactone and/or furosemide).[12] These patients can often be managed in the ambulatory setting. Even if the patient is asymptomatic, the clinician should monitor for signs of decompensation that may require inpatient medical treatment, such as a drop in serum sodium, elevation in serum creatinine, unstable vital signs, or altered mental status.

Next, consider if the patient's cirrhosis is refractory or decompensated. Unfortunately, development of ascites is an indicator of morbidity and mortality. Patients with ascites have a 15% mortality at 1 year, and 44% at 5 years.[13] Therefore, many patients will at some point develop signs or symptoms of decompensation. In these patients, a paracentesis is typically indicated, for either diagnostic or therapeutic purposes, and frequently hospitalization is necessary. The paracentesis gives vital diagnostic information and often immediately alleviates symptoms by removing excess fluid. Some patients can be effectively managed in the outpatient setting with routine large volume paracentesis (LVP) to alleviate their symptoms, if no other complications are present. Other patients may develop

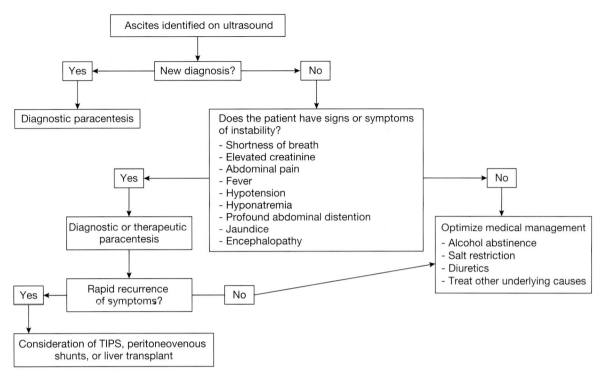

FIGURE 21-20. Treatment algorithm. TIPS, transjugular intrahepatic portosystemic shunts.

complications of decompensated cirrhosis, such as spontaneous bacterial peritonitis (SBP) or hepatorenal syndrome (HRS).

Patients with cirrhosis can develop a dangerous and life-threatening infection called SBP. Because of this, clinicians should have a low threshold to perform diagnostic paracentesis in patients with known or suspected cirrhosis and ascites on examination. Symptoms of SBP can be mild but can include fever, abdominal pain, and mental status changes. A neutrophil count in ascitic fluid of greater than >250 cells/mm^3, in the setting of positive body fluid cultures, is diagnostic for SBP and requires prompt treatment with IV antibiotics.[12] Antibiotics should be chosen on the basis of susceptibility from fluid cultures. Once a patient has been diagnosed with SBP, he or she requires prophylactic antibiotics to prevent the risk of recurrence.

Hepatorenal syndrome should be suspected in patients with cirrhosis and an elevation in serum creatinine >1.5, or an acute worsening from their baseline creatinine.[14] These patients often need therapeutic paracentesis, followed by medical therapy with albumin, octreotide, and a vasopressor such as midodrine.

Lastly, ultrasound has a critical role in following patients diagnosed with ascites over time. Rapid reaccumulation of fluid despite frequent LVP and optimal medical management is a poor prognostic indicator. Ultrasound can be used by clinicians to determine when medical therapy and paracentesis is no longer sufficient. At this point, many patients will need to be referred for consideration of transjugular intrahepatic portosystemic shunts (TIPS), peritoneovenous shunts, or liver transplantation.[12,15]

PEARLS AND PITFALLS

Pearls

- When assessing for intra-abdominal fluid, consider repositioning the patient slightly, make sure to get several views in each location, and do not be afraid to apply firm pressure to enhance the view.
- Ensure the patient is in a position of comfort. Patients with severe ascites often have dyspnea and will be uncomfortable, and potentially unsafe, lying flat on their backs.
- When assessing for an adequate pocket for paracentesis, it can be helpful to rotate that patient slightly to either left or right lateral decubitus to allow fluid to accumulate in the most dependent area.
- The abdominal wall contains the inferior epigastric vessels, which must be identified, prior to paracentesis. Patients with

advanced cirrhosis may also have distended superficial veins (caput medusae), which need to be identified and avoided.

- Obtain views both before and after voiding, to ensure adequate visualization of bladder and pelvic organs, and to distinguish them from ascitic fluid.

Pitfalls

- Not all fluid in the abdomen is ascites. Patient history and a thorough physical examination prior to performing ultrasound evaluation can narrow the differential diagnosis and help focus the examination.
- Make sure to distinguish bladder from ascitic fluid: When looking in the suprapubic view, if you see a hypoechoic area, fan

Pearls and Pitfalls, Continued

through it carefully and assess in multiple planes to determine whether it has a defined border consistent with the bladder or whether it is truly free flowing posterior to the bladder and consistent with intraperitoneal fluid (Figures 21-13 to 21-16).

- Remember that ultrasound can only identify the presence of fluid in the abdomen and cannot determine the type of fluid. If there is a history of trauma, anechoic free fluid in the abdomen is blood until proven otherwise. Clinical correlation is key.
- Especially in females, presence of free fluid prompts investigation for gynecologic causes of fluid, such as an ectopic pregnancy or a ruptured ovarian cyst.

- Obesity, with a thick abdominal wall, can make evaluation for ascites more difficult. Clinical correlation, and obtaining multiple images of different depths, can increase accuracy.
- Gaseous distention of the bowel is commonly mistaken for ascites and needs to be ruled out with a thorough patient history and physical examination, including percussion. If the patient has signs of bowel obstruction, this should be appropriately evaluated and ruled out prior to attempting paracentesis.
- A history of abdominal surgery can make adhesions a possibility, which can be difficult to visualize on ultrasound and may complicate a paracentesis.

BILLING

CPT Code	Description	Global Payment	Professional Component	Technical Component
76705	Echo Examination of Abdomen	$92.73	$30.08	$62.66

CPT codes and average national reimbursement for Medicare in 2016. Payment data are from https://www.cms.gov/apps/physician-fee-schedule/search/search-criteria.aspx. See Chapter 2 for details on ultrasound billing.

References

1. Hou W, Sanyal AJ. Ascites: diagnosis and management. *Med Clin North Am.* 2009;93:801-817.
2. Runyon BA. Ascites and spontaneous bacterial peritonitis. In Sleisenger MH, Feldman S, Friedman LS, Brandt LJ, eds. *Sleisenger and Fordtran's Gastrointestinal and Liver Disease Pathophysiology/Diagnosis/Management.* 10th ed. Philadelphia, PA: Saunders/Elsevier; 2016:1554.
3. Ginés P, Quintero E, Arroyo V, et al. Compensated cirrhosis: natural history and prognostic factors. *Hepatology.* 1987;7:122-128.
4. Golberg BB, Clearfield HR, Goodman GA, Morales JO. Ultrasonic determination of ascites. *Radiology.* 1970;96:15-22.
5. Garcia de Casasola Sanchez G, Torres Macho J, Casas Rojo JM, et al.; Working Group SEMI Clinical Ultrasound. Abdominal ultrasound and medical education. *Rev Clin Esp.* 2014;3:131-136.
6. Todsen T, Jensen ML, Tolsgaard MG, et al. Transfer from point-of-care Ultrasonography training to diagnostic performace on patients—a randomized controlled trial. *Am J Surg.* 2016;211:40-45.
7. Keil-Rios D, Terrazas-Solis H, Gonzalez-Garay A, Sanchez-Avila JF, Garcia-Juarez I. Pocket ultrasound device as a complement to physical examination for ascites evaluation and guided paracentesis. *Intern Emerg Med.* 2016;11:461-466.
8. Nazeer SR, Dewbre H, Millder A. Ultrasound-assisted paracentesis performed by emergency physicians vs the traditional technique: a prospective randomized study. *Am J Emerg Med.* 2005;23:363-367.
9. Mercaldi CJ, Lanes SF. Ultrasound guidance decreases complications and improves cost of care among patients undergoing thoracentesis and paracentesis. *Chest.* 2013;143:532-538.
10. Soni NJ, Lucas BP. Diagnostic point-of-care ultrasound for hospitalists. *J Hosp Med.* 2015;10:120-124.
11. Gishen F, Trotman I. Bedside Ultrasound—experience in a palliative care unit. *Eur J Cancer Care.* 2009;18:642-644.
12. Biecker E. Diagnosis and therapy of ascites in liver cirrhosis. *World J Gastroenterol.* 2011;17(10):1237-1248.
13. Planas R, Montoliu S, Ballesté B, et al. Natural history of patients hospitalized for management of cirrhotic ascites. *Clin Gastroenterol Hepatol.* 2006;4:1385-1394.
14. Arroyo V, Ginès P, Gerbes AL, et al. Definition and diagnostic criteria of refractory ascites and hepatorenal syndrome in cirrhosis. International Ascites Club. *Hepatology.* 1996;23:164-176.
15. Runyon BA. Care of patients with ascites. *N Engl J Med.* 1994;330(5):337-342.

CHAPTER 22

Does the Patient Have Cholelithiasis or Cholecystitis?

Matthew Fentress, MD, MSc, DTM&H

● Clinical Vignette

A 45-year-old overweight female presents to the clinic with 2 days of worsening right upper quadrant pain and nausea. The pain started 1 hour after a fatty meal and has gradually worsened. She reports subjective fevers. She has had a history of similar symptoms in the past that resolved without specific treatment, although they usually stopped in less than a day. She has no known past medical history and takes no medications. Does the patient have cholelithiasis or cholecystitis?

LITERATURE REVIEW

Over 20 million people in the United States are estimated to have gallbladder disease.[1] The prevalence of gallstones varies widely across ethnic and gender lines ranging from a low of 5.3% among non-Hispanic black men, up to a high of 26.7% among Mexican American women.[1] Large studies from Europe have shown similar burden of disease, with an overall prevalence of 18.8% in women and 9.5% in men.[2] In those with cholelithiasis, 1% to 4% will develop biliary colic every year, and of this symptomatic group, approximately 20% will develop acute cholecystitis if left untreated.[3] Overall, almost 1 in 10 people with asymptomatic gallstones can be expected to require treatment within 5 years.[4]

Abdominal ultrasound, which can be performed rapidly without exposing the patient to radiation, is widely recognized as the first-line imaging modality for the assessment of suspected gallbladder disease.[5] In a large meta-analysis spanning articles from 1966 to 1992, formal ultrasound of the right upper quadrant had a sensitivity and specificity of 84% and 99%, respectively, for the diagnosis of cholelithiasis.[6] For acute cholecystitis, formal ultrasound also performs well, with sensitivity ranging from 81% to 88% and specificity from 80% to 83%.[6,7] Although cholescintigraphy is more accurate for the diagnosis of acute cholecystitis than ultrasound, with a sensitivity of 97% and a specificity of 90%,[6] it is more time intensive and involves radiation exposure, and is usually reserved for cases when high suspicion for cholecystitis remains despite equivocal ultrasound findings.

Numerous studies demonstrate that the diagnostic accuracy for cholelithiasis and cholecystitis is similar when comparing formal imaging in a radiology suite with focused point-of-care ultrasound performed by a nonradiologist physician.[8-12] For instance, a recent systematic review of 8 articles and 710 subjects by Ross et al showed emergency physician-performed point-of-care ultrasound had a pooled sensitivity and a specificity of 89.8% and 88%, respectively, for symptomatic cholelithiasis. Some literature even suggests that certain aspects of the examination, such as the sonographic Murphy's, may have higher sensitivity in the hands of trained bedside ultrasonographers compared with a formal ultrasound.[10,12] Taken as a whole, these studies and others like them provide a strong evidence base to support the use of point-of-care ultrasound by nonradiologist physicians to diagnose suspected gallbladder disease.

The single most important question in any point-of-care ultrasound examination of the gallbladder is whether or not the patient has cholelithiasis. Gallstones appear on ultrasound as hyperechoic, mobile, gravity-dependent masses in the gallbladder lumen with posterior shadowing. The vast majority of patients with acute cholecystitis have cholelithiasis; acalculous cholecystitis accounts for only 5% to 10% of cases and is often associated with severe illness.[13] However, most patients with cholelithiasis do not have cholecystitis. Therefore, the diagnosis of acute cholecystitis by ultrasound requires the recognition of not just one ultrasonographic finding, but a constellation of such findings.

Four additional findings can be helpful if present: the sonographic Murphy's sign, gallbladder wall thickening, pericholecystic fluid, and dilation of the common bile duct (CBD). The test characteristics of these signs individually are generally weak,[12] but in combination they can be a powerful diagnostic tool. For instance, the combination of a positive sonographic Murphy's sign with cholelithiasis has a 92.2% positive predictive valuate (PPV) for acute cholecystitis, whereas the absence of both has 95% negative predictive value (NPV).[14] The addition of gallbladder wall thickening to cholelithiasis and sonographic Murphy's sign increases the PPV only modestly, to 93.8%.[14] It is important to note that a sonographic Murphy's sign is defined as the presence of maximal abdominal tenderness elicited by pressure of the ultrasound probe over a sonographically localized gallbladder.[7,15] This is different from the physical examination Murphy's sign, which is the arrest of inspiration with a deep palpation of the right upper quadrant.

The three remaining findings should be part of every examination, but they have somewhat lower sensitivity then cholelithiasis and sonographic Murphy's sign for cholecystitis. They do, however, remain highly specific. For instance, the sensitivity and specificity of gallbladder wall thickening is 65% and 91%, respectively. Pericholecystic fluid is even less sensitive, with a sensitivity and specificity of 26% and 94%, respectively.[12] Evaluation of the CBD is perhaps the most difficult part of a bedside ultrasound examination, especially for physicians with limited experience. It may also be the least helpful information for the bedside ultrasonographer. A recent retrospective review showed that isolated CBD dilation, without either coexisting gallbladder wall thickening, sonographic Murphys, pericholecystic fluid, or abnormal laboratory values, occurred in less than 1% of patients with confirmed cholecystitis or choledocholithiasis.[16] This raises the possibility that CBD measurement may add very little to an otherwise complete point-of-care ultrasound study for gallbladder disease. We do still recommend assessing the CBD when feasible because if it is dilated it may suggest other disease such as choledocholithiasis and should prompt further evaluation, which is outside the scope of this chapter.

A point-of-care ultrasound examination of the right upper quadrant for suspected biliary disease should address each of the five specific findings discussed earlier. A summary of some of these findings' test parameters is detailed in Table 22-1.

TABLE 22-1 Point-of-Care Ultrasound Examination Test Characteristics for Diagnosis of Acute Cholecystitis				
Ultrasound Finding	Sensitivity (%)	Specificity (%)	Negative Likelihood Ratio	Positive Likelihood Ratio
Gallstones	100	54	<0.01	2.2
Sonographic Murphy's sign	65	82	0.43	3.5
Gallbladder wall thickening	65	91	0.38	7.2
Pericholecystic fluid	26	94	0.78	4.6
Combination of gallstones and sonographic Murphy's sign *(both present for positive or both absent for negative)*	93	95	0.08	17
Combination of gallstones and wall thickening *(both present for positive or both absent for negative)*	96	97	0.05	28

TABLE 22-2 Recommendations for Use of Point-of-Care Ultrasound in Clinical Practice		
Recommendation	Rating	References
A clinician-performed point-of-care gallbladder ultrasound has similar diagnostic accuracy to that of formal ultrasound for the diagnosis of cholelithiasis and acute cholecystitis, and can reduce the time to diagnosis.	B	8-12, 18
A normal ultrasound of the gallbladder can be used to effectively rule out acute calculous cholecystitis and expedite workup.	B	8, 12, 14, 16-18

A = consistent, good-quality patient-oriented evidence; B = inconsistent or limited-quality patient-oriented evidence; C = consensus, disease-oriented evidence, usual practice, expert opinion, or case series. For information about the SORT evidence rating system, go to http://www.aafp.org/afpsort.

PERFORMING THE SCAN

1. **Preparation.** Place the patient in the supine position to start the examination. Position the ultrasound equipment to the right of the patient and select a low-frequency (2.5-5 mHz) curvilinear probe with an "abdomen" preset. Occasionally, a low-frequency phased array probe with a small footprint may be needed to image in between the ribs. If the gallbladder is not easily visualized in the supine position, the patient may be turned to the left lateral decubitus position. This will bring the gallbladder closer to the abdominal wall, change the position of the overlying air-filled bowel, and may make it easier to obtain the desired images.

2. **Identify the gallbladder in a long-axis view.** Start with the "subcostal sweep" technique. Place the probe inferior to the xiphoid process, with the probe marker oriented toward the patient's head or right shoulder (**Figure 22-1**). Move the probe laterally in a sweeping motion, following the oblique line of the costal margin, until an image of the gallbladder is obtained (**Figure 22-2**). It is often helpful to ask the patient to take and hold a deep breath. This pushes the gallbladder down below the costal margin and improves visualization. The gallbladder will appear as a hypoechoic tubular or circular structure lying posterior to the parenchyma of the liver. If you have difficulty locating the gallbladder with this approach, move on to the "X-7" technique (Figure 22-1). Place the probe inferior to the xiphoid process and slide laterally across the ribs approximately 7 cm, so that you are obtaining a window between the rib spaces (ie, an intercostal window). Regardless of which technique is used, once the gallbladder is identified, stop large movements and make only small adjustments in the probe angle or rotation to

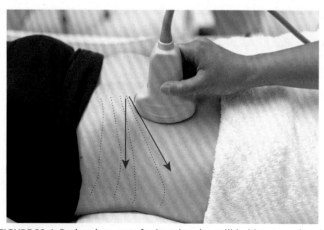

FIGURE 22-1. Probe placement for imaging the gallbladder. Arrowheads show probe movement for the subcostal sweep and the X-7 techniques.

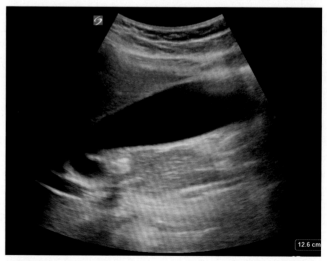

FIGURE 22-2. Normal gallbladder in long-axis view. Note the fold in the gallbladder wall near the neck.

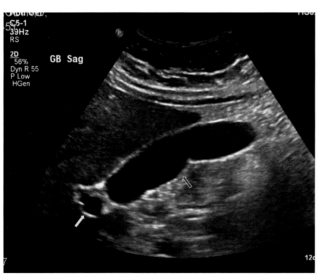

FIGURE 22-3. Gallbladder and portal vein, connected by the main lobar fissure, form an easily recognizable exclamation point. Solid arrow, portal vein; void arrow, gallbladder.

obtain a true long-axis view. The gallbladder in true long-axis view will look like the top of an exclamation point, with the median lobar fissure running between the portal triad and the gallbladder (**Figure 22-3**).

3. **Evaluate for cholelithiasis.** Once you have identified the gallbladder, fan through the entire organ, from end to end, in both long-axis and short-axis views. To obtain the short-axis view, simply center the long-axis view on the ultrasound screen and then rotate the probe 90°. As you fan through the organ in long- and short axis, look for gallstones within the lumen. Gallstones will appear as gravity-dependent, usually mobile hyperechoic masses with posterior shadowing (**Figure 22-4**). Occasionally, the stones may be difficult to visualize, especially if lodged in the neck, and the shadow may be the main finding identified (Figure 22-4C). Other abnormalities that may be seen and confused with gallstones include polyps and sludge. Polyps are hyperechoic, nonmobile, and do not cast a shadow (**Figure 22-5**). Gallbladder sludge is gravity-dependent material, of variable echogenicity, and also does not cast a shadow.

4. **Evaluate for sonographic Murphy's sign.** Bring the fundus of the gallbladder into the center of the ultrasound screen and press down on the gallbladder while asking the patient about the pain that he or she is experiencing. You may need to test multiple points in the right upper quadrant or epigastrium to confirm your findings in some cases. A true sonographic Murphy's sign elicits pain only over the gall bladder. If there is pain over the gallbladder and multiple other points or if there is no pain elicited, then the

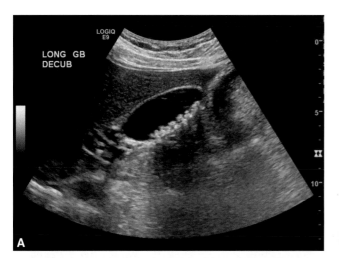

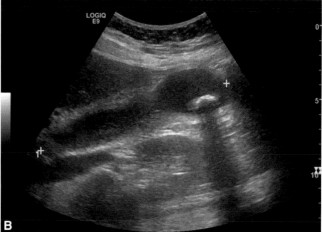

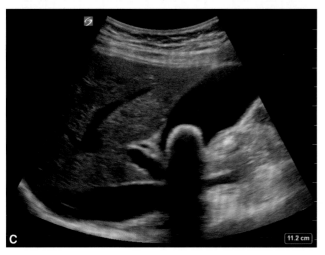

FIGURE 22-4. A, Multiple gallstones with posterior shadowing, without other signs of cholecystitis. B, Large gallstone with posterior shadowing and gallbladder wall thickening in acute cholecystitis. C, Gallstone in the neck of a gallbladder.

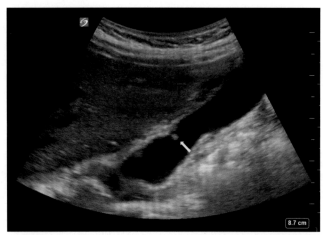

FIGURE 22-5. Gallbladder polyp in the anterior wall of a gallbladder. Arrow, polyp.

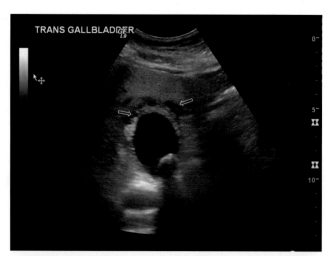

FIGURE 22-7. Transverse view of a gallbladder with pericholecystic fluid, gallbladder wall thickening, and cholelithiasis in a patient with acute cholecystitis. Arrows, pericholecystic fluid.

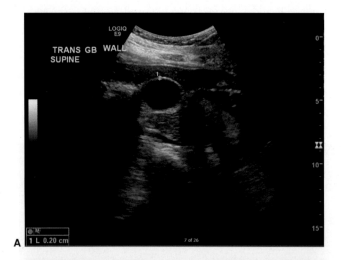

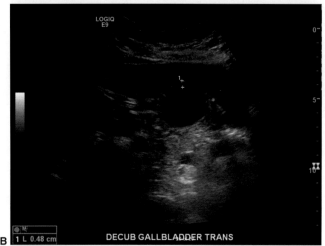

FIGURE 22-6. A, Normal gallbladder wall. B, Thickened gallbladder wall.

sonographic Murphy's sign is negative. This test is not always reliable when done through an intercostal window (such as that obtained by the "X-7" technique). If you have asked the patient to hold the breath during the examination, you can have him or her raise a finger to signal the point of maximal tenderness when testing for a sonographic Murphy's sign.

5. **Measure the thickness of the anterior gallbladder wall.** Normal gallbladder wall thickness is less than or equal to 3 mm. This measurement should always be performed on the anterior wall, as the posterior wall can appear artificially thickened because of acoustic enhancement. Obtain an image of the gallbladder in long or short axis, and measure the most anterior portion of the gallbladder wall (**Figure 22-6**). An anterior gallbladder wall greater than 3 mm, along with other suggestive findings, can be a predictor of acute cholecystitis.[12] However, there are many other causes of gallbladder wall thickening, including postprandial contraction and illnesses that cause systemic or local edema (eg, congestive heart failure, ascites, hepatitis, HIV, pancreatitis, chronic kidney disease).

6. **Evaluate for pericholecystic fluid.** Interrogate the entire organ in two dimensions as described earlier when searching for cholelithiasis. Pericholecystic fluid can usually be seen as a slender, hypoechoic wedge of fluid that collects around the wall of an inflamed gallbladder (**Figure 22-7**). If a suspected fluid collection is identified, evaluate it carefully to differentiate pericholecystic fluid from an edge artifact or ascites.

7. **Measure the diameter of the common bile duct.** The CBD is an echogenic walled tubular structure that courses superficial and parallel to the portal vein. Measured from inner wall to inner wall, it typically measures 2 to 6 mm in diameter. The size of the CBD can increase with age, so another rule of thumb is that the diameter should be less than one-tenth of the patient's age. Identify the portal triad in short-axis view as the "point" of the exclamation mark described earlier. This creates a Mickey Mouse sign, with the portal vein as the head, and the CBD and hepatic artery as the two ears (**Figure 22-8**). Use color flow to distinguish the two if in doubt—the hepatic artery will have pulsatile flow, whereas the CBD will have no flow. The CBD may also be imaged in the long-axis view, running parallel to the portal vein (**Figure 22-9**).

PATIENT MANAGEMENT

Bedside ultrasound of the right upper quadrant should be performed in any patient with suspected biliary disease. In the patient who presents to primary care with a history suggestive of symptomatic cholelithiasis, with no acute symptoms or physical examination findings, isolated cholelithiasis on ultrasound rules in the diagnosis. The patient can be referred directly to a general surgeon for

PART 2

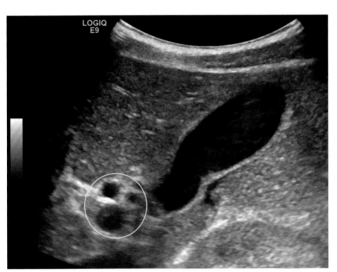

FIGURE 22-8. Common bile duct short axis with a Mickey Mouse sign

outpatient cholecystectomy. A formal ultrasound may be simultaneously ordered at the discretion of the performing provider and consulting surgeon. In clinic systems where the wait for outpatient imaging and specialty services is lengthy, the patient's care can be substantially expedited with this approach. If the bedside ultrasound examination is completely normal, then an alternate diagnosis should generally be considered.

In the patient who presents to primary care with acute symptoms or positive physical examination findings suggestive of biliary disease, bedside ultrasound may be most useful to rule out the diagnosis of acute cholecystitis. A suggested algorithm is presented in **Figure 22-10**. If the ultrasound examination is negative in a patient with low-moderate suspicion—no cholelithiasis, sonographic Murphy's sign, gallbladder wall thickening, pericholecystic fluid or CBD dilation—the likelihood of cholecystitis is exceedingly low and the diagnosis can effectively be ruled out in a nontoxic, ambulatory patient. If the ultrasound examination in a patient with moderate-high clinical suspicion is positive for any of the findings described earlier, particularly with highly suggestive signs such as the combination of cholelithiasis and sonographic Murphy's, surgical consultation is indicated. If high suspicion remains despite a negative examination, or the findings are equivocal, then further evaluation may be needed to clarify the diagnosis, such as cholescintigraphy, formal radiology ultrasound, and/or laboratory studies. The algorithm presented here, if strictly interpreted, may be overly sensitive for acute cholecystitis, but is a good starting point and should be considered an adjunct to the history and physical examination. For instance, recall that the absence of both cholelithiasis and sonographic Murphy's sign makes acute cholecystitis very unlikely, with a combined NPV of 95%.[14] Therefore, in the correct clinical context, the absence of these two findings alone could be sufficient to rule out the diagnosis in the outpatient setting.

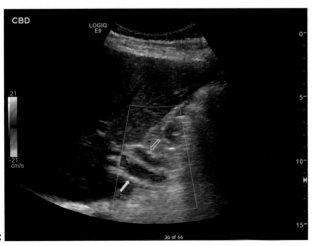

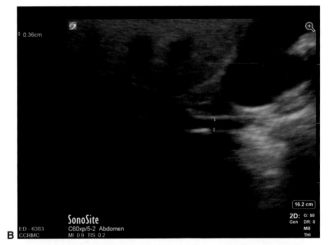

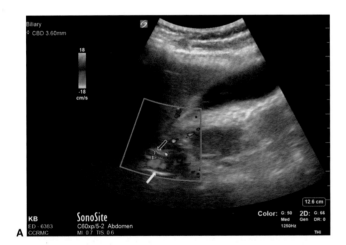

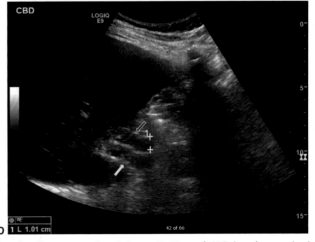

FIGURE 22-9. A, Normal common bile duct (CBD) in a long-axis view with color flow measuring 3.6 mm. B, Normal CBD in a long-axis view measuring 3.6 mm without color flow. C, Dilated CBD in a long-axis view with color flow. D, Dilated CBD in a long-axis view without color flow measuring 10.1 mm. Void arrow, CBD; solid arrow, portal vein.

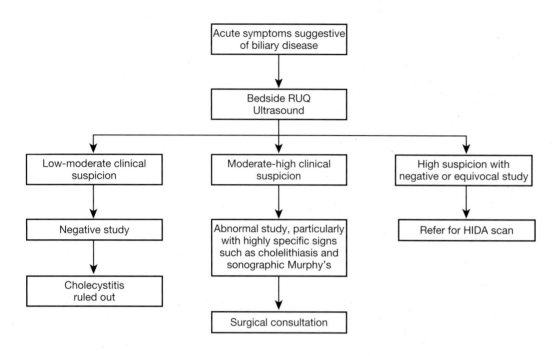

FIGURE 22-10. Algorithm for incorporating point-of-care ultrasound into the management of a patient with suspected biliary disease in an outpatient clinic. HIDA scan, hepatobiliary iminodiacetic acid scan; RUQ, right upper quadrant.

PEARLS AND PITFALLS

Pearls

- Do not spend too much time looking for the gallbladder in the supine position. If you have not visualized the gallbladder within the first 60 seconds of scanning in the supine position, move on to the left lateral decubitus position in a cooperative patient. This drops the liver and gallbladder beneath the costal margin and moves interfering loops of gas-filled bowel out of the way.
- Always examine the neck of the gallbladder closely. A gallstone lodged in the neck can cause significant symptoms but may be difficult to visualize on ultrasound. Look closely for posterior shadowing.

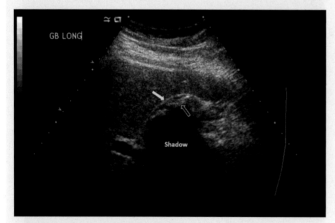

FIGURE 22-11. The Wall-Echo-Shadow-sign. The gallbladder is full of small stones and all that can be visualized is the gallbladder wall, a small amount of intracystic fluid, and the surface of the stones. A shadow artifact is produced below. Solid arrow, gallbladder wall; void arrow, surface of stones.

- Always measure the *anterior* gallbladder wall. The posterior gallbladder wall will often appear artificially thickened because of posterior acoustic enhancement.
- A gallbladder packed full of gallstones may appear on ultrasound as only a curved echogenic gallbladder wall with dense posterior shadowing, known as a Wall-Echo-Shadow sign (**Figure 22-11**).
- Use color flow to help distinguish between the hepatic artery and the CBD.

Pitfalls

- Polyps are easily mistaken for stones. Polyps are nonmobile and will not cast a shadow. If in doubt, you can roll the patient into different positions. Stones are gravity-dependent and will often move within the gallbladder lumen, whereas polyps will remain in a fixed position.
- Acalculous cholecystitis accounts for 5% to 10% of all cases of cholecystitis, usually in the context of severe illness. If the patient has no cholelithiasis but high concern remains for biliary disease, always obtain formal imaging.
- Both the duodenum and the inferior vena cava can be mistaken for the gallbladder. Always try to obtain the "exclamation point" view (Figure 22-3) to ensure you are looking at the gallbladder and not at another organ.
- Be careful not to mistake a fold in the gallbladder wall for a gallstone.
- Free peritoneal fluid in the right upper quadrant can occasionally be mistaken for pericholecystic fluid.
- Edge artifact can be misinterpreted as cholelithiasis or even pericholecystic fluid. Always image in two dimensions, and if still in doubt, change the patient's position to see if the abnormality remains.

BILLING

CPT Code	Description	Global Payment	Professional Component	Technical Component
76705	Abdominal ultrasound—limited	$182.96	$30.08	$152.88

CPT codes and average national reimbursement for Medicare in 2016. Payment data are from https://www.cms.gov/apps/physician-fee-schedule/search/search-criteria.aspx. See Chapter 2 for details on ultrasound billing.

References

1. Everhart JE, Kare M, Hill M, Maurer KR. Prevalence and ethnic differences in gallbladder disease in the United States. *Gastroenterology*. 1999;117:632.

2. Attili AF, Carulli N, Roda E, et al. Epidemiology of gallstone disease in Italy: prevalence data of the Multicenter Italian Study on Chlolelithiasis (MICOL). *Am J Epidemiol*. 1995;141:158-165.

3. Strasberg, SM. Acute calculous cholecystitis. *N Engl J Med*. 2008;358:2804-2811.

4. Halldestam I, Enell E-L, Kullman E, Borch K. Development of symptoms and complications in individuals with asymptomatic gallstones. *Br J Surg*. 2004;91:734-738. doi:10.1002/bjs.4547.

5. Bree RL, Ralls PW, Balfe DM, et al. Evaluation of patients with acute right upper quadrant pain. American College of Radiology. ACR Appropriateness Criteria. *Radiology*. 2000;215(suppl):153-157.

6. Shea JA, Berlin JA, Escarce JJ, et al. Revised estimates of diagnostic test sensitivity and specificity in suspected biliary tract disease. *Arch Intern Med*. 1994;154(22):2573-2581.

7. Kiewiet JJS, Leeuwenburgh MMN, Bipat S, Bossuyt PMM, Stoker J, Boermeester MA. A systematic review and meta-analysis of diagnostic performance of imaging in acute cholecystitis. *Radiology*. 2012;5(3):708-720. doi:10.1148/radiol.12111561.

8. Ross M, Brown M, McLaughlin K, et al. Emergency physician-performed ultrasound to diagnose cholelithiasis: a systematic review. *Acad Emerg Med*. 2011;18(3):227-235.

9. Scruggs W, Fox JC, Potts B, et al. Accuracy of ED bedside ultrasound for identification of gallstones: retrospective analysis of 575 studies. *West J Emerg Med*. 2008;9(1):1-5.

10. Kendall JL, Shimp RJ. Performance and interpretation of focused right upper quadrant ultrasound by emergency physicians. *J Emerg Med*. 2001;21(1):7-13.

11. Rosen CL, Brown DFM, Chang Y, et al. Ultrasonography by emergency physicians in patients with suspected cholecystitis. *Am J Emerg Med*. 2001;19:32-36.

12. Summers SM, Scruggs W, Menchine MD, et al. A prospective evaluation of emergency department bedside ultrasonography for the detection of acute cholecystitis. *Ann Emerg Med*. 2010;56:114-122.

13. Huffman JL, Schenker S. Acute acalculous cholecystitis: a review. *Clin Gastroenterol Hepatol*. 2010;8:15-22.

14. Ralls PW, Colletti PM, Lapin SA, et al. Real-time sonography in suspected cholecystitis: prospective evaluation of primary and secondary signs. *Radiology*. 1985;155:767-771.

15. Bree RL. Further observations on the usefulness of the sonographic Murphy sign in the evaluation of suspected acute cholecystitis. *J Clin Ultrasound*. 1995;23:169-172.

16. Becker BA, Chin E, Mervis E, Anderson CL, Oshita MH, Fox JC. Emergency biliary sonography: utility of common bile duct measurement in the diagnosis of cholecystitis and choledocholithiasis. *J Emerg Med*. 2014;46(1):54-60.

17. Villar J, Summers SM, Menchine MD, Fox JC, Wang R. The absence of gallstones on point-of-care ultrasound rules out acute cholecystitis. *J Emerg Med*. 2015;49(4):475-480. doi:10.1016/j.jemermed.2015.04.037.

18. Blaivas M, Harwood RA, Lambert MJ. Decreasing length of stay with emergency ultrasound examination of the gallbladder. *Acad Emerg Med*. 1999;6(10):1020-1023.

PART 2

SECTION 3

BOWEL

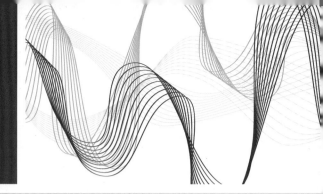

CHAPTER 23

Does the Patient Have a Bowel Obstruction?

Margaret R. Lewis, MD and Vivek S. Tayal, MD

● **Clinical Vignette**

A 52-year-old woman presents to clinic with sudden-onset abdominal pain. Symptoms started 3 hours prior to arrival. Patient describes pain as diffuse, severe, and with associated bilious emesis. Patient's medical history includes hypertension, controlled on medication, and prior appendectomy and removal of right ovarian teratoma. Does the patient have a bowel obstruction?

TABLE 23-1	Likelihood Ratios of Imaging for Small Bowel Obstruction	
Imaging Modality	+ Likelihood Ratio	− Likelihood Ratio
Abdominal x-ray	1.64	0.43
CT scan	3.6	0.18
MRI	6.77	0.12
Ultrasound (radiology)	14.1	0.13
Ultrasound (point-of-care)	9.55	0.04

From Taylor MR, Lalani N. Adult small bowel obstruction. *Acad Emerg Med.* 2013;20(6):528-544.

LITERATURE REVIEW

Bowel obstruction and associated abdominal pain are common presenting complaints to emergency departments (EDs), with abdominal pain representing 6.5% of all ED visits in one calendar year and small bowel obstruction (SBO) representing 2% of all ED visits.[1] An estimated 300 000 hospitalizations annually are thought to be the result of SBO.[2] Risk factors for SBO are prior abdominal surgery, constipation, abnormal bowel sounds, and/or abdominal distention.[3] SBOs are associated with a high risk of complications, including strangulation in up to 30% and bowel necrosis in up to 15%.[4] This may lead to bowel perforation, sepsis, and death.[5] Complications are more likely with advanced age, comorbid illness, or delay in diagnosis longer than 24 hours.[4] SBO may require surgical management in up to 24% of patients including lysis of adhesions, hernia repair, small bowel resection with lysis of adhesions, and small bowel resection with hernia repair.[6]

Given the complication risks, early diagnosis is key. X-ray, CT, MRI, and ultrasound are all imaging modalities used in the evaluation of the patient with suspected SBO. Of these imaging studies, x-ray has the least utility, with lower pooled positive likelihood ratio when compared to CT and MRI for SBO. CT is considered the definitive test for evaluation of SBO in the ED, but does have associated risks of serious allergic reaction to contrast[3] as well as radiation exposure. Although the use of ultrasound for SBO has only been evaluated in a few select studies, ultrasound was associated with more accurate positive likelihood ratios for both radiology-performed and point-of-care ultrasound when compared to other imaging modalities (**Table 23-1**).[3] When compared with abdominal x-ray

for the detection of bowel obstruction, ultrasonography was found to be just as sensitive, but more specific.[7] Furthermore, ultrasound for SBO assessment seems to be relatively easy to learn. Emergency medicine residents with 6 hours of training were shown to be as accurate as radiologists with an interrater kappa of 0.81 in one study.[8]

Sonographic findings associated with bowel obstruction include dilated, fluid-filled loops of bowel, with hyperechoic particles representing gas within the fluid-filled lumen. Other associated findings may include thickened bowel wall (greater than 3 mm), thickened valvulae conniventes (normally up to 2 mm), and to-and-fro motion of the bowel contents.[9] Findings that may indicate a need for early surgery include intraperitoneal free fluid, bowel wall thickness greater than 4 mm, and decreased or absent peristalsis with previously documented mechanical obstruction.[9] Also, the presence of an increasing amount of free fluid between loops of small bowel is associated with a worsening mechanical obstruction.[10]

Adjunctive Ultrasound Techniques

In addition to looking at the bowel directly for sonographic evidence of bowel obstruction, other ultrasound techniques such as looking at the groin, ventral abdomen, large bowel, and mesentery for signs of hernias, intussusception, internal hernia, and masses may be an adjunct. Regarding internal hernias and midgut volvulus, the whirlpool sign is mentioned as a sign that shows the mesentery twisted, causing the appearance of a "whirlpool."[11] See Chapters 25 and 44.

TABLE 23-2	Recommendations for Use of Point-of-Care Ultrasound in Clinical Practice		
Recommendation		**Rating**	**References**
Abdominal ultrasound can effectively rule in or rule out an SBO		C	3, 7
Point-of-care abdominal ultrasound for detection of SBO can be performed by practitioners following a brief training period		C	8

A = consistent, good-quality patient-oriented evidence; B = inconsistent or limited-quality patient-oriented evidence; C = consensus, disease-oriented evidence, usual practice, expert opinion, or case series. For information about the SORT evidence rating system, go to http://www.aafp.org/afpsort.

PERFORMING THE SCAN

1. **Preparation**. The patient should be positioned in the supine position.[12] If the patient has difficulty tolerating lying supine, they may be placed in the semi-recumbent position with abdomen exposed. Position the ultrasound machine accordingly and select a 3.5 to 5 MHz probe (curvilinear probe) with an abdominal preset (**Figure 23-1**).

Evaluation of four abdominal quadrants. Begin the ultrasound examination by placing the curvilinear probe in epigastric region in the transverse orientation. Using gentle compression to disperse any gas, evaluate for any dilated loops of bowel. After evaluating the epigastric region, place the probe in the longitudinal position in both the right and left paracolic gutters and assess for any dilated loops of bowel. Finally, place the probe in the suprapubic region in the transverse orientation to assess for any dilated loops of bowel. See **Figure 23-2** for

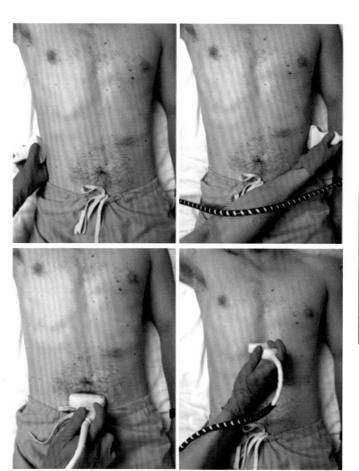

FIGURE 23-2. Ultrasound probe placement for the 4-quadrant evaluation for bowel obstruction.

probe placement. Evaluate for normal bowel by looking for alternating hyperechoic and hypoechoic lines as well as peristalsis (**Figure 23-3** and ▶ **Video 23-1**). Normal bowel is also compressible when using graded compression with the ultrasound probe. Evaluate for bowel obstruction by assessing for dilated loops of bowel greater than 2.5 cm (**Figure 23-4**), to-and-fro movement of bowel contents (**Figure 23-5** and ▶ **Video 23-2**), and identification of the plicae circulares projecting into the bowel lumen. This is also known as the keyboard sign as it resembles the alternating white and black keys of a piano keyboard (**Figure 23-6**). Assess also for late finding of bowel obstruction including decreased or absent peristalsis (**Figure 23-7** and ▶ **Video 23-3**) and free fluid between loops of small bowel (**Figure 23-8** and ▶ **Video 23-4**).

2. **Evaluation of entire abdomen**. If bowel obstruction was not noted on the initial 4-quadrant ultrasound, then the entire abdomen should be evaluated for potential bowel obstruction. The curvilinear probe should be placed in the right lower quadrant in the transverse position and then moved proximally and distally across the anterior abdomen using graded compression until the probe reaches the left lower quadrant, in a pattern akin to mowing-the-lawn (**Figure 23-9**). Assess for normal bowel and signs of bowel obstruction as listed in Step 2.

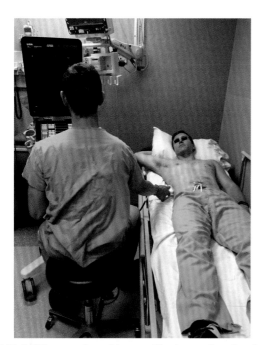

FIGURE 23-1. Ultrasound machine positioning and probe choice for abdominal ultrasound evaluation.

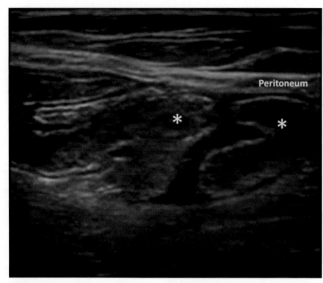

FIGURE 23-3. Image depicting alternating hyper- and hypoechoic lines of normal bowel (asterisk).

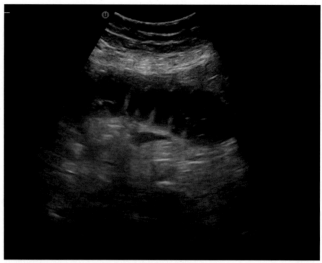

FIGURE 23-6. The keyboard sign: plicae circulares projecting into lumen of small bowel in small bowel obstruction.

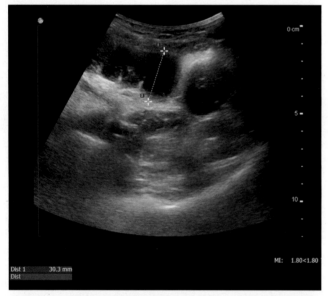

FIGURE 23-4. Dilated loop of small bowel greater than 2.5 cm consistent with a small bowel obstruction.

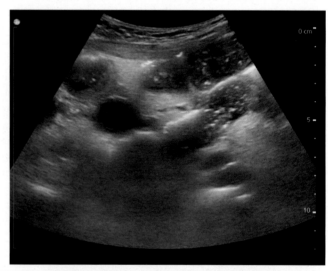

FIGURE 23-7. Dilated loop of small bowel with intraluminal contents. Recommend watching for peristalsis for 5 to 10 s in this view.

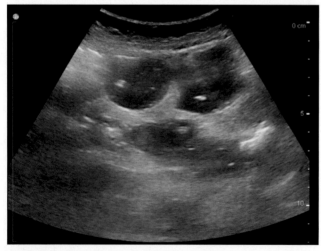

FIGURE 23-5. Dilated loop of small bowel with intraluminal contents.

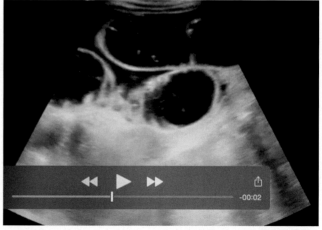

FIGURE 23-8. Free fluid between loops of small bowel, a late finding in small bowel obstruction. Still image courtesy of Claire Abramoff, MD.

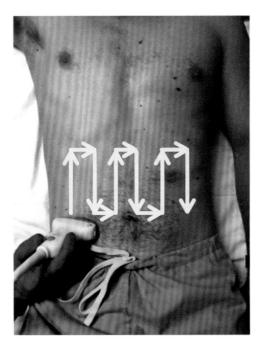

FIGURE 23-9. Evaluation of the anterior abdomen for small bowel obstruction.

PATIENT MANAGEMENT

In evaluating the patient who presents with abdominal pain, one must first consider whether the patient may have a bowel obstruction. Elements within the history and physical that are associated with SBO include prior abdominal surgery, constipation, abdominal distention, and/or abnormal bowel sounds. In patients who are high risk for complicated SBO such as those with peritoneal signs, unstable vital signs, or other significant risk factors, immediate triage to the ED for further evaluation and treatment is prudent. If ultrasound can be performed without delaying transfer of the patient, findings can be helpful in deciding to initiate early treatment of the patient including intravenous fluids, bowel rest, and decompression with nasogastric tube.

In patients who are low risk for SBO, other causes of abdominal pain should be considered. If the pretest probability for SBO is felt to be below 1.5%, then testing specifically for SBO is likely to be more harmful than beneficial.[3] However, the need for further testing for other conditions should be considered.

In the patient in whom SBO is suspected with an intermediate level of risk, a point-of-care ultrasound may help determine the need for initiation of treatment and referral to the ED for further testing and admission. If point-of-care ultrasound is negative for SBO, one may consider the patient's risks for SBO such as age, vital signs, and prior abdominal surgery as well as the presence of peritonitis to determine if patient needs further imaging versus close follow-up. If they are otherwise healthy, and with a benign abdominal examination, the patient may be appropriate for discharge with close follow-up and reexamination. If a SBO with dilated loops of bowel and to-and-fro peristalsis is detected on ultrasound, then one may begin bowel rest, intravenous fluid resuscitation, and consider decompression of the gastrointestinal tract with a nasogastric tube as well as referral to the ED for initiation or continued treatment, further imaging including CT evaluation, and surgical consultation (**Figure 23-10**).

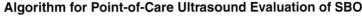

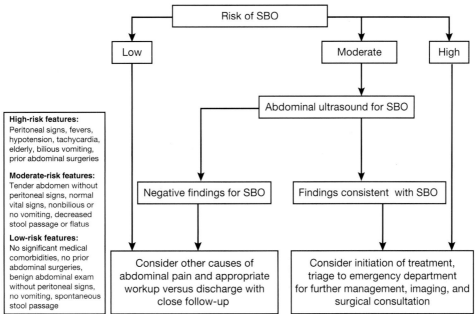

FIGURE 23-10. Management decision tree using point-of-care ultrasound in the evaluation of patient with suspected bowel obstruction (SBO).

PEARLS AND PITFALLS

Pearls

- Consider the patient's body habitus when selecting a probe. Consider a lower frequency probe in a patient with large abdominal girth and a higher frequency probe in thin patients or pediatric patients.
- Use compression when evaluating the bowel. Dilated, obstructed bowel should not be compressible.
- Watch for peristalsis for 5 to 10 seconds before continuing to scan.
- Treat patient's pain and nausea prior to scanning if patient is in severe pain. Patient may initially have difficulty lying still and supine and they may have continued nausea and vomiting, so treat these symptoms first.
- Look to see if transition point can be seen (dilated loops of bowel with adjacent decompressed bowel loops).
- Evaluate for plicae circulares to confirm small bowel. Plicae will appear as finger-like projections into small bowel lumen.
- Use landmarks such as iliac crest to identify locations in the abdomen.

Pitfalls

- Not treating patient's pain and nausea initially may make obtaining images difficult.
- Not using compression to gently displace abdominal gas for better evaluation of the abdomen
- Scan entire abdomen (all 4 quadrants) in a systematic approach to fully evaluate for SBO.
- Consider other causes of a dilated bowel such as ileus.

BILLING

CPT Code	Description	Global Payment	Professional Component	Technical Component
76705	Limited echo (ultrasound) of the abdomen	$93.31	$30.15	$63.16

CPT codes and average national reimbursement for Medicare in 2016. Payment data are from https://www.cms.gov/apps/physician-fee-schedule/search/search-criteria.aspx. See Chapter 2 for details on ultrasound billing.

References

1. Hastings RS, Powers RD. Abdominal pain in the ED: a 35 year retrospective. *Am J Emerg Med*. 2011;29(7):711-716.
2. Irvin TT. Abdominal pain: a surgical audit of 1190 emergency admissions. *Br J Surg*. 1989;76(11):1121-1125.
3. Taylor MR, Lalani N. Adult small bowel obstruction. *Acad Emerg Med*. 2013;20(6):528-544.
4. Fevang BT, Fevang J, Stangeland L, et al. Complications and death after surgical treatment of small bowel obstruction: a 35-year institutional experience. *Ann Surg*. 2000;231(4):529-537.
5. Cheadle WG, Garr EE, Richardson JD. The importance of early diagnosis of small bowel obstruction. *Am Surg*. 1988;54(9):565-569.
6. Foster NM, McGory ML, Zingmond DS, Ko CY. Small bowel obstruction: a population-based appraisal. *J Am Coll Surg*. 2006;203(2):170-176.
7. Ogata M, Mateer JR, Condon RE. Prospective evaluation of abdominal sonography for the diagnosis of bowel obstruction. *Ann Surg*. 1996;223(3):237-241.
8. Unlüer EE, Yavaşi O, Eroğlu O, Yilmaz C, Akarca FK. Ultrasonography by emergency medicine and radiology residents for the diagnosis of small bowel obstruction. *Eur J Emerg Med*. 2010;17(5):260-264.
9. Hefny AF, Corr P, Abu-Zidan FM. The role of ultrasound in the management of intestinal obstruction. *J Emerg Trauma Shock*. 2012;5(1):84-86.
10. Grassi R, Romano S, D'Amario F, et al. The relevance of free fluid between intestinal loops detected by sonography in the clinical assessment of small bowel obstruction in adults. *Eur J Radiol*. 2004;50(1):5-14.
11. Zhou H, Yan Y, Li C. The whirlpool sign: midgut volvulus. *Emerg Med J*. 2014;31(12):1015.
12. Nylund K, Ødegaard S, Hausken T, et al. Sonography of the small intestine. *World J Gastroenterol*. 2009;15(11):1319-1330.

Does the Patient Have Appendicitis?

David Flick, MD, Maria G. Valdez, MD, RDMS, and Aaron C. Jannings, MD

Clinical Vignette

A 14-year-old previously healthy boy presents to the outpatient clinic. He has had 3 days of progressive anorexia accompanied by nausea and vomiting. His mother reports an oral temperature at home of 101.1°F that does not seem to abate with acetaminophen. The boy has no significant medical history. On examination, he does not appear ill but is lying very still. His abdomen is somewhat firm with positive rebound and guarding and is very tender in the right lower quadrant half-way between the umbilicus and the anterior superior iliac spine. Does the patient have appendicitis?

TABLE 24-1	Alvarado Score
Symptoms	Score
Migratory right iliac fossa pain	1
Nausea/vomiting	1
Anorexia	1
Signs	
Tenderness in right iliac fossa	2
Rebound tenderness in right iliac fossa	1
Elevated temperature	1
Laboratory findings	
Leukocytosis	2
Neutrophil left shift	1
Total	10

A score of 5 to 6 is considered possible appendicitis, 7 to 8 as probable, and >9 very probable.

LITERATURE REVIEW

Acute appendicitis has long been recognized as a life-threatening emergency requiring early surgical intervention. It is currently the most common cause of emergency abdominal surgery.[1] Prevalence is higher in whites, males, and the 10- to 19-year age range. There is a lifetime risk of appendicitis of 8.6% for males and 6.7% for females.[2] In the pediatric population, appendicitis has been responsible for more hospital stays (greater than 5 days) than any other cause and accounts for the second most bed-days of all causes of pediatric admissions second only to congenital anomalies.[3] In pregnancy, appendicitis is the most common surgical emergency, with an incidence of 1 in 766 births. The risk of significant obstetric complications is also increased, with 33% of appendectomies performed in the first trimester resulting in spontaneous abortions and 14% of those performed in the second trimester resulting in premature delivery.[4]

Expedient diagnosis of acute appendicitis is key to ensuring timely intervention, and over the years techniques for diagnosis have evolved. The physical examination remained the basis of diagnosis for more than 100 years but lacked sensitivity, with many surgeries performed on patients with normal appendixes.[5] Clinical diagnostic scores were developed to help improve the accuracy of the clinical assessment of acute appendicitis. The most well-known is the Alvarado score that was first published in 1986 (Table 24-1). The Alvarado score uses three elements of the history: migration of pain to the right lower quadrant (RLQ) (1), anorexia (1), and nausea with vomiting; three physical examination findings: RLQ tenderness (2), rebound pain (1), and elevated temperature (1); and two laboratory findings: leukocytosis (2) and left shift of the white blood cell (WBC) differential (1). The maximum possible score is 10.[5] A score of 0 to 4 has been shown to be 99% sensitive at ruling out appendicitis.[6]

Additionally, similar scoring systems were developed for the pediatric patient population. The Pediatric Appendicitis Score (PAS) assigns the following point for each element in pediatric patients: RLQ tenderness with cough, percussion, or hopping (2), anorexia (1), fever (1), nausea or vomiting (1), tenderness over the right iliac fossa (2), leukocytosis with WBC >10 000 (1), left shift (1), and migration of pain to the RLQ (1). Studies report varying percentages of likelihood of appendicitis based on scores, but many agree that a score less than or equal to 3 represents low risk for discharge to home with parental observation and a score greater than or equal to 7 or 8 warrants surgical consultation and/or urgent imaging.[7-9]

Although these scoring systems are useful in improving the clinical assessment for acute appendicitis, computed tomography (CT) imaging has replaced clinical assessment as the gold standard for diagnosis. Increasing utilization of CT has led to decreased rates of negative appendectomies without increased risk of perforations.[10] However, concerns over the safety of CT and risks of radiation exposure have spurred further inquiries into alternative diagnostic modalities to include the use of ultrasound. This is especially true in the pediatric and obstetric patient populations.[11]

Ultrasound provides an alternative to CT that can be performed rapidly at the bedside and is free of radiation. The ultrasound technique most commonly used is the graded compression technique. Puylaert first described this technique in 1986 and since then it has been extensively studied and improved.[12] The graded compression technique uses the probe to apply gradual pressure in order to displace gas-filled loops of bowel and bring the appendix closer to the abdominal wall and transducer for improved visualization. In effect, the appendix becomes "sandwiched" between the anterior abdominal wall and the psoas muscle.

Radiology-performed ultrasound for appendicitis has a sensitivity of 85% and a specificity of 90% compared with 95% and 96%, respectively, for CT.[13-15] A limitation of ultrasound is the high rate of nonvisualization of the appendix, leading to inconclusive examinations. This is especially likely when the appendix is normal. Additionally, the accuracy of the ultrasound examination is operator dependent and is improved in the hands of more experienced practitioners.[16] It appears that sensitivity may be lower in less experienced providers, although specificity remains high. A meta-analysis found that point-of-care ultrasound for evaluation of acute appendicitis in children was accurate in the hands of emergency medicine physicians (sensitivity = 80%, specificity = 92%), although sensitivity was lower than in specialist performed examinations (sensitivity = 91%, specificity = 97%).[16,17] Despite this limitation, there is evidence that with focused training followed by supervised scanning, nonspecialists can achieve acceptable diagnostic results. A small study followed novice emergency medicine residents after a 1-day focused training course. In the emergency department, they performed ultrasound examinations that were compared with radiologist-performed imaging. Initially accuracy was poor, but after the first 20 examinations, they were able to perform examinations with a sensitivity of 90% and a specificity of 93% when compared to the radiologists as the gold standard.[18]

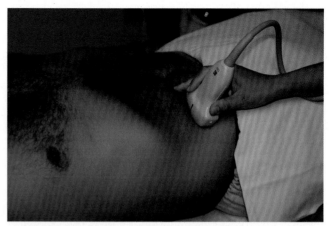

FIGURE 24-1. Proper probe placement for scanning near McBurney's point.

TABLE 24-2	Recommendations for Use of Point-of-Care Ultrasound in Clinical Practice		
Recommendation		Rating	References
Bedside ultrasound can be used as an accurate diagnostic tool in the evaluation of acute appendicitis		A	16-18
Bedside ultrasound for acute appendicitis can be accurate after limited, focused training by nonspecialists		B	18

A = consistent, good-quality patient-oriented evidence; B = inconsistent or limited-quality patient-oriented evidence; C = consensus, disease-oriented evidence, usual practice, expert opinion, or case series. For information about the SORT evidence rating system, go to http://www.aafp.org/afpsort.

PERFORMING THE SCAN

1. **Preparation.** Provide adequate analgesia to reduce patient discomfort during the examination. The pressure applied to the abdomen by the transducer in order to displace the bowel is significant and will cause pain in the patient with pathology. Place the patient in a supine position with the knees flexed to relax the abdominal muscles. Both a curvilinear (2-5 MHz) and linear (5-10 MHz) transducer can be used to image the appendix.[19] In general, the probe of choice will depend on the patient's body habitus. A linear probe will provide the best resolution at the expense of depth. Thus, it is best used in thin, young patients. A curvilinear abdominal probe will provide greater depth and a larger footprint and is thus used most often in patients with a greater proportion of soft tissue.[20]

2. **Transducer position.** The appendix is located in the RLQ at McBurney's point, which is the midpoint of an imaginary line drawn between the umbilicus and the right anterosuperior iliac spine[21] (**Figure 24-1**). The location of the appendix is variable and not always located at McBurney's point. If a patient has pain localized elsewhere, an alternative starting option is to place the probe at the patient's maximal point of tenderness. If the patient has generalized right lower abdominal pain, start by placing the probe in the right upper quadrant below the inferior border of the right costal margin with the transducer indicator toward the patient's right.

3. **Scan through the abdomen.** Move the probe inferiorly or laterally, scan areas in both the longitudinal and transverse views every 1 cm. Once you recognize the haustra of the ascending colon, apply firm, steady pressure on the transducer in order to displace the compressible small bowel until the anterior abdominal wall makes contact with the psoas muscle. Take care to not lift the probe off the patient as the bowel and bowel gas will again obscure the window once pressure is released. Slide the probe inferiorly along the abdominal wall and visualize the pulsatile iliac vessels in the right iliac fossa (**Figure 24-2**).

4. **Visualize the appendix** (**Figure 24-3A**). The cecum should give rise to the tubular, blind-ending appendix. Follow the appendix to its blind end. To improve visualization, place the patient in a left posterior oblique (LPO) position and scan coronally along the right flank with the beam aimed posteriorly (**Figure 24-3B**). An LPO position can displace the cecum or terminal ileum laterally, avoiding the interfering colonic gas. This can help visualize a retrocecal appendix.[22] Provide posterior compression

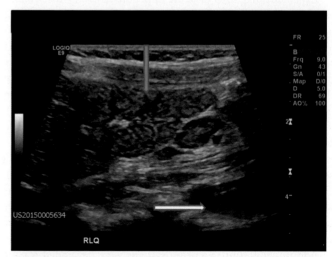

FIGURE 24-2. The right lower quadrant with compression. Note the absence of bowel gas. The rectus abdominis (blue arrow) is compressed down to the level of the psoas muscle (white arrow).

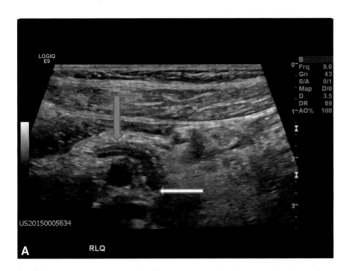

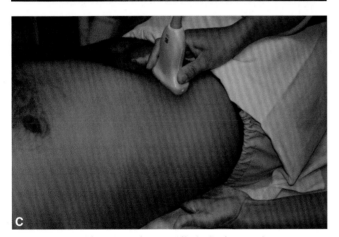

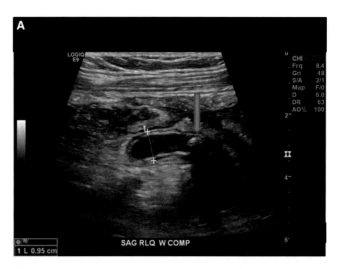

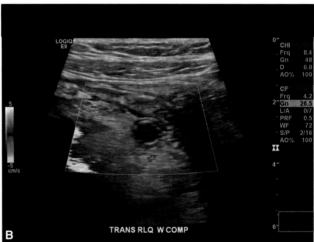

FIGURE 24-4. A, The pathologic appendix in its long axis. Note the appendix measures greater than 6 mm with compression. There is minimal periappendiceal edema and a frank appendicolith (blue arrow). Image credit: Meghan Smith, RDMS. B, The pathologic appendix in short axis. Note the noncompressible, target-like appearance of the appendix. Image credit: Meghan Smith, RDMS.

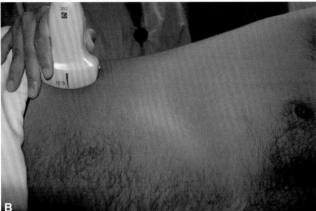

FIGURE 24-3. A, The normal appendix in its long axis appears as a tubular structure (blue arrow). Note the presence of the wall of the structure as well as the blind end (white arrow). B, A left posterior oblique position can help visualize the appendix, especially one in the retrocecal position. C, Addition of posterior pressure can help bring the appendix closer to the ultrasound probe.

in addition to the usual anterior abdominal wall pressure to improve visualization[23] (**Figure 24-3C**).

5. **Assess the appendix** (**Figure 24-4**). A normal appendix is, on average, 5 to 10 cm in length, compressible, and gas, fluid, or fecal-filled and without evidence of hyper-vascularization.

An inflamed appendix is defined as a noncompressible, tubular, blind-ending structure, greater than 6 mm in diameter. Secondary signs of an abnormal appendix include hyperemia (the classic "ring of fire" sign when Doppler ultrasonography is applied), single-wall thickness greater than 3 mm, and a target sign appearance with a fluid-filled hypoechoic center surrounded by a hyperechoic muscular layer.

6. **Assess for secondary findings of appendicitis.** When the appendix is not visualized, it is important to actively assess for secondary features of inflammation. These nonspecific findings include periappendiceal fluid or the presence of an appendicolith, which will appear as an echogenic focus with a posterior acoustic shadow. A perforated or ruptured appendix will exhibit loss of echogenic submucosal structure or mixed echogenic fluid in the iliac fossa.[24] A mass-like lesion with mixed echogenicity may represent a phlegmon or abscess. See Table 24-3 for abnormal findings in appendicitis.

TABLE 24-3	Abnormal Ultrasound Features in Appendicitis
Noncompressible appendix with a single-wall thickness of >3 mm or double-wall thickness of >6 mm	
Hyperemia of the appendix	
Periappendiceal fluid	
Appendicolith	
Pain over the appendix with probe compression	

TABLE 24-4 Pediatric Appendicitis Score	
Variable	**Score**
Migratory right lower quadrant pain	1
Anorexia	1
Nausea/vomiting	1
Fever >38°C	1
Right iliac fossa tenderness	2
Pain with cough/percussion/hopping	2
White blood cell count >10 000 cells/mL	1
Neutrophils >7500 cells/mL	1
Total	10

A score <5 is considered unlikely to be appendicitis, 5 as possible appendicitis, and ≥6 as likely appendicitis.

PATIENT MANAGEMENT

Ultrasound is the imaging modality of choice for suspected appendicitis in children and pregnant women[25] (**Figure 24-5**). Additionally, sonography may be used as first-line imaging modality in all patients with suspected appendicitis as it is easily available, avoids exposure to nonionizing radiation, requires no contrast media, and is cost-efficient.[26] If after completing a thorough history, examination, and labs and calculating an Alvarado score (see Table 24-1) or PAS (**Table 24-4**) there is suspicion for acute appendicitis, one can proceed with ultrasonography.[27] If a normal appendix is visualized in conjunction with an otherwise normal workup, discharging the patient home with close outpatient follow-up in less than 24 hours may be considered. If a pathologic appendix is visualized (noncompressible tubular structure, greater than 6 mm in diameter), consulting surgery for evaluation and disposition is recommended. If the appendix is not visualized or the ultrasound examination is nondiagnostic with secondary signs or nonspecific signs of appendicitis, a complete reevaluation in less than 24 hours or sooner as clinically indicated, or admission for observation may be considered. If the appendix is not visualized or the ultrasound examination is nondiagnostic, one can also consider CT of the abdomen and pelvis. If the CT of the abdomen and pelvis confirms appendicitis, a surgical consult is warranted. If the appendix is normal on CT, discharging the patient home with close outpatient follow-up within 24 hours is appropriate. If the CT abdomen/pelvis is inconclusive, one can reevaluate the patient in less than 24 hours or admit for observation.[25,28,29]

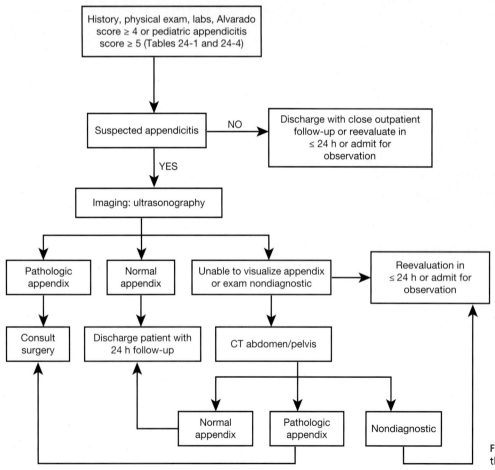

FIGURE 24-5. Algorithm for management of the patient with right lower quadrant pain.

PEARLS AND PITFALLS

Pearls

- The appendix often lies superior to the iliac vessels. Follow the iliac vessels from the aortic bifurcation to the inguinal ligament when having difficulty visualizing the appendix.
- If unable to visualize the appendix with the patient supine with knees flexed, have the patient place the right leg over the left leg without rolling the hip off the table to bring the appendix closer to the abdominal wall.
- A left oblique lateral decubitus position can displace the cecum or terminal ileum laterally, which can help visualize a retrocecal appendix.
- If a RLQ fails to reveal an appendix, consider endovaginal sonography for a pelvic appendix in a female.

Pitfalls

- Take care not to confuse the terminal ileum with the appendix. Although the terminal ileum is tubular, it will exhibit peristalsis and is not blind ended.
- An enlarged appendix can measure up to 2 in and can be confused with the small bowel. Make sure to follow along its whole length to reach a blind end.
- Many clinicians tend to reposition the probe by lifting it off the patient or stopping to apply more gel. Apply plenty of gel and maintain firm, constant pressure to maximize displacement of the bowel and bowel gas to visualize the appendix.
- Failure to visualize the distal appendiceal tip can be a missed appendicitis. Additionally, the appendiceal tip may be the initial site of appendicitis while the rest of the appendix remains unaffected.

BILLING

CPT Code	Description	Global Payment	Professional Component	Technical Component
76705	Limited abdominal ultrasound	$182.96	$152.88	$30.08

CPT codes and average national reimbursement for Medicare in 2016. Payment data are from https://www.cms.gov/apps/physician-fee-schedule/search/search-criteria.aspx. See Chapter 2 for details on ultrasound billing.

References

1. Brown MA. Imaging acute appendicitis. *Semin Ultrasound CT MRI.* 2008;29:293-307.
2. Addiss DG, Shaffer N, Fowler BS, et al. The epidemiology of appendicitis and appendectomy in the United States. *Am J Epidemiol.* 1990;132(5):910-925.
3. Henderson J, Goldacre MJ, Fairweather JM. Conditions accounting for substantial time spent in hospital in children aged 1-14 years. *Arch Disease Childhood.* 1992;67:83-86.
4. Andersen B, Nielsen TF. Appendicitis in pregnancy: diagnosis, management and complications. *Acta Obstet Gynecol Scand.* 1999;78(9):758-762.
5. Alverado A. A practical score for the early diagnosis of acute appendicitis. *Ann Emerg Med.* 1986;15:557-564.
6. Ohle R, O'Reilly F, O'Brien KK, et al. The Alvarado score for predicting acute appendicitis: a systematic review. *BMC Med.* 2011;9:139
7. Goldman RD, Carter S, Stephens D, et al. Prospective validation of the pediatric appendicitis score. *J Pediatr.* 2008;153(2):278-282.
8. Hatcher-Ross K. Sensitivity and specificity of the pediatric appendicitis score. *J Pediatr.* 2009;154(2):308.
9. Zuniga RV, Arribas JL, Montes SP, et al. Application of pediatric appendicitis score on the emergency department of a secondary level hospital. *Pediatr Emerg Care.* 2012;28(6):489-492.
10. Drake FT, Flum DR. Improvement in the diagnosis of appendicitis. *Adv Surg.* 2013;47:299-328.
11. Rosen MP, Ding A, Blak MA, et al. ACR appropriateness criteria right lower quadrant pain—suspected appendicitis. *J Am Coll Radiol.* 2011;8:749-755.
12. Puylaert JB. Acute appendicitis: US evaluation using graded compression. *Radiology.* 1986;158(2):355-360.
13. Dahabreh IJ, Adam GP, Halladay CW, Steele DW, Daiello LA. *Diagnosis of right lower quadrant pain and suspected acute appendicitis.* AHRQ Comparative Effectiveness Reviews. Rockville (MD): Agency for Healthcare Research and Quality (US); 2015. Report No.: 15(16)-EHC025-EF.
14. Keyzer C, Zalcman M, De Maertelaer V, et al. Comparison of US and unenhanced multi-detector row CT in patients suspected of having acute appendicitis. *Radiology.* 2005;236(2):527-534.
15. Kaewlai R, Lertlumsakulsub W, Srichareon P. Body mass index, pain score and Alvarado score are useful predictors of appendix visualization at ultrasound in adults. *Ultrasound Med Biol.* 2015;41(6):1605-1611.
16. Benabbas R, Hanna M, Shah J, Sinert R. Diagnostic accuracy of history, physical examination, laboratory tests, and point-of-care ultrasound for pediatric acute appendicitis in the emergency department: a systematic review and meta-analysis. *Acad Emerg Med.* 2017;24(5):523-551.
17. Matthew Fields J, Davis J, Alsup C, et al. Accuracy of point-of-care ultrasonography for diagnosing acute appendicitis: a systematic review and meta-analysis. *Acad Emerg Med.* 2017;24(9):1124-1136.
18. Kim J, Kim K, Kim J, et al. The learning curve in diagnosing acute appendicitis with emergency sonography among novice emergency medicine residents. *J Clin Ultrasound.* 2018;46(5):305-310.
19. Quigley AJ, Stafrace SS. Ultrasound assessment of acute appendicitis in paediatric patients: methodology and pictorial overview of findings seen. *Insights Imaging.* 2013;4(6):741-751.
20. Mallin M, Craven P, Ockerse P, et al. Diagnosis of appendicitis by bedside ultrasound in the ED. *Am J Emerg Med.* 2015;33:430-432.
21. Hagen-Ansert SL. The gastrointestinal tract. In *Textbook of Diagnostic Ultrasonography,* vol 1, 6th ed. Mosby; 2006:chap 9.
22. Ung C, Chang ST, Jeffrey RB, Patel BN, Olcott EW. Sonography of the normal appendix: its varied appearance and techniques to improve its visualization. *Ultrasound Q.* 2013;29(4):333-341.
23. Lee JH, Jeong YK, Park KB, et al. Operator-dependent techniques for graded compression sonography to detect the appendix and diagnose acute appendicitis. *AJR Am J Roentgenol.* 2005;184(1):91-97.
24. Sanchez TR, Corwin MT, Davoodian A, Stein-Wexler R. Sonography of abdominal pain in children: appendicitis and its common mimics. *J Ultrasound Med.* 2016;35(3):627-635.

25. Old JL, Dusing RW, Yap W, Dirks J. Imaging for suspected appendicitis. *Am Fam Phys*. 2005;71(1):71-78.

26. Pinto F, Pinto A, Russo A, et al. Accuracy of ultrasonography in the diagnosis of acute appendicitis in adult patients: review of the literature. *Crit Ultrasound J*. 2013;5 Suppl 1:S2.

27. Wagenaar AE, Tashiro J, Wang B, et al. Protocol for suspected pediatric appendicitis limits computed tomography utilization. *J Surg Res*. 2015;199(1):153-158.

28. Toorenvliet BR, Wiersma F, Bakker RF, et al. Routine ultrasound and limited computed tomography for the diagnosis of acute appendicitis. *World J Surg*. 2010;34(10):2278-2285.

29. Mostbeck G, Adam EJ, Nielsen MB, et al. How to diagnose acute appendicitis: ultrasound first. *Insights Imaging*. 2016;7(2):255-263.

Does the Patient Have Intussusception?

Aun Woon (Cindy) Soon, MD, FAAP, FRACP and Peter James Snelling, BSc, MBBS (Hons), MPHTM, GCHS, CCPU, FRACP, FACEM

● Clinical Vignette

A 10-month-old male infant presents to the clinic with a 6-hour history of intermittent abdominal pain and drawing his legs up every 10 to 15 minutes. He has had three episodes of nonbilious vomiting today. He is otherwise well with an unremarkable past medical history. Given that his 6-year-old brother has similar symptoms, you deduce that he most likely has a viral illness. You plan to send him home with a close follow-up but would like to be reassured first that he does not have intussusception. Does the patient have intussusception?

LITERATURE REVIEW

Intussusception is the invagination, or telescoping, of a proximal segment of intestine (intussusceptum) into the lumen of a more distal segment (intussuscipiens).[1] It is a common cause of gastrointestinal obstruction and acute abdomen in the pediatric population.[2] This diagnosis is more frequent in males and typically presents in patients 3 months to 6 years of age, with the majority presenting before 2 years of age. It has an estimated incidence of about 56 cases per 100 000 per year in the United States.[3]

The pathogenesis of intussusception is predominately idiopathic and is assumed to be secondary to lymphoid hyperplasia acting as a lead point.[4] Viral illnesses have been implicated as the cause of hypertrophy of the lymphoid tissue. A lead point is identified only in approximately 10% of cases (eg, Meckel's diverticulum, lymphoma).[5] Ileocolic intussusception represents greater than 90% of all pediatric intussusceptions, arising in the distal ileum and passing through the ileocecal valve into the cecum.[1,4] Intussusception creates a bowel obstruction, which leads to ischemia and necrosis of the incarcerated intestine. Although spontaneous reduction can occur, the natural history is progression to intestinal perforation, sepsis, and death.[2,4]

In the typical cases of intussusception, there is an acute onset of colicky abdominal pain that recurs at frequent intervals. However, it remains an elusive diagnosis, given that the classically taught findings of intermittent abdominal pain, red currant jelly stool (a late sign), vomiting, and a palpable abdominal mass occur only in up to 40% of patients.[6] Therefore, radiologic imaging is usually necessary to confirm the diagnosis in patients for which there is a clinical suspicion.[7] Although readily available, the use of abdominal radiographs has variable degrees of accuracy and exposes children to ionizing radiation.[8-10] Ultrasound has been demonstrated to be a superior modality to diagnose intussusception, with reported sensitivities of 98% to 100% and specificities of 88% to 100% for experienced sonographers.[4,6,11,12] Therefore, intussusception presents itself as an ideal point-of-care ultrasound (POCUS) application for primary care physicians to expedite the care of these patients,

particularly given the adverse outcomes associated with a delayed reduction.[13,14]

POCUS for intussusception is showing great promise, even in the hands of those with limited experience.[15,16] In a prospective study by Riera et al, physician novice sonographers were able to diagnose ileocolic intussusceptions using POCUS with a sensitivity of 85% (95% confidence interval [CI] 54%-97%) and a specificity of 97% (95% CI 89%-99%) after a 1-hour training session.[17] On the basis of evidence in current literature, POCUS should be used as a rule-in rather than a rule-out test among inexperienced sonographers in order not to miss this important diagnosis. Larger-scale trials are required to evaluate the diagnostic accuracy and efficacy of POCUS for intussusception.

TABLE 25-1	Recommendations for Use of Point-of-Care Ultrasound in Clinical Practice	
Recommendation	Rating	Reference
Point-of-care ultrasound for the evaluation of ileocolic intussusception can be performed at the point-of-care effectively by practitioners with only brief training.	B	17

A = consistent, good-quality patient-oriented evidence; B = inconsistent or limited-quality patient-oriented evidence; C = consensus, disease-oriented evidence, usual practice, expert opinion, or case series. For information about the SORT evidence rating system, go to http://www.aafp.org/afpsort.

PERFORMING THE SCAN

1. **Preparation.** The patient should be lying in the supine position. Scanning a patient in this age group may be challenging, and measures should be taken to ensure the patient's comfort in order to perform a successful scan. Select the high-frequency, linear array transducer, and choose the appropriate depth setting according to the patient's size.
2. **Evaluate the large bowel.**
   a. **Ileocolic and ascending colon.** Place the probe in the transverse orientation in the right lower quadrant (RLQ) region with the probe marker pointing to the patient's right. Find the psoas muscle; this would be the starting landmark of the scan (**Figure 25-1**). Once you have identified the psoas muscle, slowly move the transducer cranially toward the patient's right upper quadrant (RUQ) until you see the liver and gallbladder (**Figures 25-2 and 25-3A**). It is important to use graded compression to move out bowel gas and compress overlying soft tissue.
   b. **Transverse colon.** When you visualize the liver at the RUQ, rotate the probe 90° clockwise, with the indicator pointing to the patient's head. Slowly move the transducer in the longitudinal orientation toward the patient's left upper quadrant (LUQ) to evaluate the transverse colon (**Figure 25-3B**).

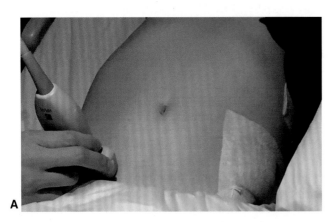

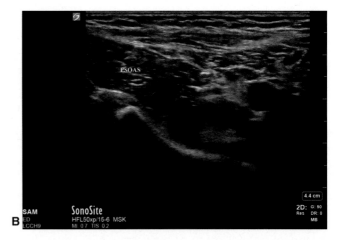

FIGURE 25-1. A, Probe on the right lower quadrant in transverse orientation. B, Image of the psoas muscle; this is the starting landmark of the scan.

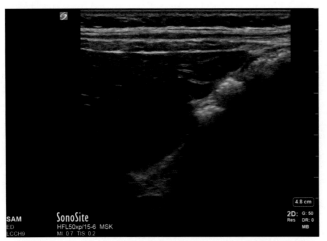

FIGURE 25-2. Image of liver and gallbladder in the right upper quadrant.

c. **Descending colon.** Once you reach the LUQ, rotate the transducer 90° counterclockwise, with the indicator pointing to the patient's right. Slowly move the transducer caudally, evaluating the descending colon before completing the scan at the left lower quadrant (LLQ) region (**Figure 25-3C**).

3. **Ileocolic intussusception.** Ileocolic intussusceptions are commonly found in the RUQ or subhepatic region. They are often described as a "target" or "pseudo-kidney" sign with concentric hypoechoic and echogenic layers where the intussusceptum is lodged within the intussuscipiens (**Figure 25-4**). Ileocolic intussusceptions are larger than small bowel intussusceptions with an anterior-posterior diameter of at least 2.5 cm (**Figure 25-5**).[18,19] Once an intussusception is identified, color Doppler imaging can be used to assess for bowel perfusion.

PATIENT MANAGEMENT

In the past decade, the use of ultrasound to diagnose intussusception has largely replaced other diagnostic modalities, given evidence of its high sensitivity and specificity in detecting ileocolic intussusception.[11] The availability of after-hours ultrasound in community and rural hospitals is often limited, resulting in physicians often having to base their decisions in regard to the patients' disposition on clinical suspicion alone. POCUS is able to not only assist the physician in the clinical decision-making process but also potentially reduce the time to diagnosis and appropriate treatment.[13]

It is important, however, to recognize how inexperience affects the accuracy of POCUS. A positive POCUS ultrasound scan for intussusception is extremely helpful in the clinical decision-making process, but an inexperienced sonographer with a high index of suspicion should consider further imaging despite a negative scan.

When planning patient management, it is important to determine the availability of radiology ultrasound and the level of clinical concern. Weihmiller et al developed a clinical decision tree to risk-stratify patients with possible intussusception.[20] Patients older than 5 months with a negative abdominal x-ray, the absence of bilious emesis, and the presence of diarrhea were determined to be at low risk for intussusception with a sensitivity of 97% (95% CI: 86-100) and negative predictive value of 99% (95% CI: 93-100). A patient with a moderate to high clinical suspicion of intussusception would require further imaging and workup despite a negative POCUS scan. To date, POCUS has yet to be studied as part of a management process for pediatric patients with possible intussusception, however, based on best available evidence we propose a patient management algorithm here (see **Figure 25-6**).

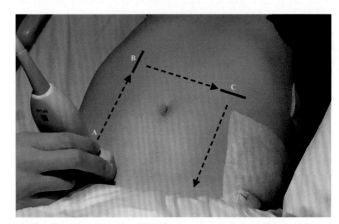

FIGURE 25-3. A, Probe on the right lower quadrant in transverse orientation. B, Probe on the right upper quadrant in longitudinal orientation. C, Probe on the left upper quadrant in transverse orientation.

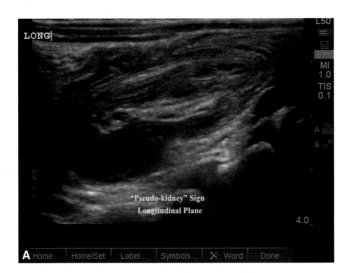

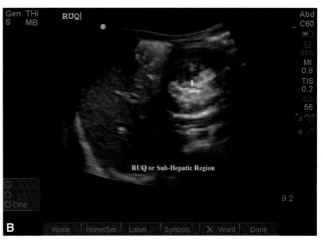

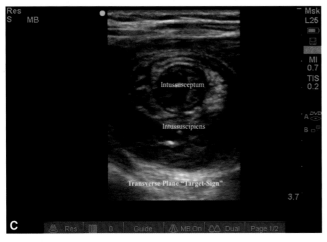

FIGURE 25-4. Images of intussusception. Longitudinal plane "pseudo-kidney" sign (A), intussusception in the RUQ or subhepatic region (B), and transverse plane "target-sign" (C). I, intussusception; RUQ, right upper quadrant.

If an intussusception is diagnosed, pediatric radiology and surgery should be consulted. Enema (air or contrast) is the treatment of choice to reduce intussusception in many institutions. Surgical intervention is required if the procedure is unsuccessful or if there is a complication of bowel perforation.

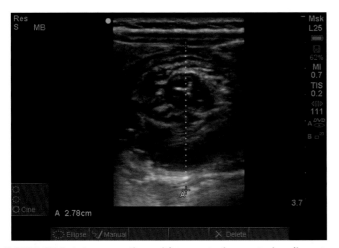

FIGURE 25-5. Intussusception with an anterior-posterior diameter of 2.78 cm.

PEARLS AND PITFALLS

Pearls

- Ensure the comfort of the patient by laying the patient supine on a parent's lap and using warmed ultrasound gel.
- Use distraction techniques and consult a child life specialist if available.
- Use a starting depth between 4 and 7 cm.
- Use graded compression to displace bowel gas from the field of view.

Pitfalls

- Suboptimal imaging can occur when using a low-frequency curvilinear probe or when scanning at depths that are too shallow or deep.
- False positives have been reported because of fecal matter, thickened bowel wall (eg, enterocolitis), volvulus, mesenteric adenopathy, or misidentification of the kidney or psoas muscle.[13,16,21]
- A negative POCUS for intussusception should be met with caution, given the reported lower sensitivity among inexperienced users.[17]

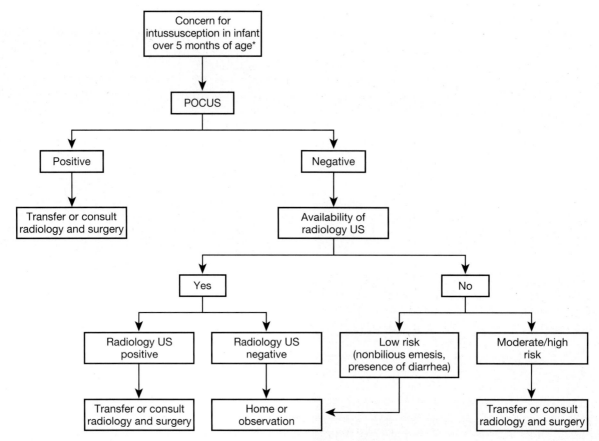

FIGURE 25-6. Algorithm for the management of intussusception. POCUS, point-of-care ultrasound; US, ultrasound.
*Infants less than 5 months of age almost never develop intussusception.

BILLING

CPT Code	Description	Global Payment	Professional Component	Technical Component
76705	Limited abdominal ultrasound including a specific study of a single organ, a limited area of the abdomen or a follow-up study	$92.73	$30.08	$62.66

CPT codes and average national reimbursement for Medicare in 2016. Payment data are from https://www.cms.gov/apps/physician-fee-schedule/search/search-criteria.aspx. See Chapter 2 for details on ultrasound billing.

ACKNOWLEDGMENT

We would like to thank Dr Russ Horowitz for his contribution to this chapter.

References

1. Lopes J, Huddart SN. Intussusception. *Surgery (Oxford)*. 2013;31(12):626-630.
2. Fischer TK, Bihrmann K, Perch M, et al. Intussusception in early childhood: a cohort study of 1.7 million children. *Pediatrics*. 2004;114:782-785.
3. Parashar UD, Holman RC, Cummings KC, et al. Trends in intussusception-associated hospitalizations and deaths among US infants. *Pediatrics*. 2000;106:1413-1421.
4. Mandeville K, Chien M, Willyerd A, Mandell G, Hostetler MA, Bulloch B. Intussusception; clinical presentations and imaging characteristics. *Pediatr Emerg Care*. 2012;28(9):842-844.
5. Justice FA, Nguyen LT, Tran SN, et al. Recurrent intussusception in infants. *J Paediatr Child Health*. 2011;47(11):802-805.
6. Waseem M, Rosenberg HK. Intussusception. *Pediatr Emerg Care*. 2008;24:793-800.
7. Territo HM, Wrotniak BH, Qiao H, Lillis K. Clinical signs and symptoms associated with intussusception in young children undergoing ultrasound in the emergency room. *Pediatr Emerg Care*. 2014;30:718-722.
8. Klein EJ, Kapoor D, Shugerman RP. The diagnosis of intussusception. *Clin Pediatr (Phila)*. 2004;43:343-347.
9. Hernandez JA, Swischuk LE, Angel CA. Validity of plain films in intussusception. *Emerg Radiol*. 2004;10:323-326.
10. Roskind CG, Ruzal-Shapiro CB, Dowd EK, Dayan PS. Test characteristics of the 3-view abdominal radiograph series in the diagnostics of intussusception. *Pediatr Emerg Care*. 2007;23:785-789.
11. Hryhorczuk AL, Strouse PJ. Validation of US as a first-line diagnostic test for assessment of pediatric ileocolic intussusception. *Pediatr Radiol*. 2009;39(10):1075-1079.

12. Bhisitkul DM, Listernick R, Shkolnik A, et al. Clinical application of ultrasonography in the diagnosis of intussusceptions. *J Pediatr*. 1992;121:182-186.

13. Chang YJ, Hsia SH, Chao HC. Emergency medicine physicians performed ultrasound for pediatric intussusceptions. *Biomed J*. 2013;36(4):175-178.

14. Losek JD. Intussusception: don't miss the diagnosis. *Pediatr Emerg Care*. 1993;9:46-51.

15. Doniger SJ, Salmon M. Point-of-care ultrasonography for the rapid diagnosis of intussusception. A case series. *Pediatr Emerg Care*. 2016;32(5):340-342.

16. Alletag MJ, Riera A, Langhan ML, Chen L. Use of emergency ultrasound in the diagnostic evaluation of an infant with vomiting. *Pediatr Emerg Care*. 2011;27(10):986-989.

17. Riera A, Hsiao AL, Langhan ML, Goodman TR, Chen L. Diagnosis of intussusception by physician novice sonographers in the emergency department. *Ann Emerg Med*. 2012;60:264-268.

18. Park NH, Park SI, Park CS, et al. Ultrasonographic findings of small bowel intussusception, focusing on differentiation from ileocolic intussusception. *Br J Radiol*. 2007;80(958):798-802.

19. Lioubashevsky N, Hiller N, Rozovsky K, Segev L, Simanovsky N. Ileocolic versus small-bowel intussusception in children: can US enable reliable differentiation? *Radiology*. 2013;269(1):266-271.

20. Weihmiller SN, Buonomo C, Bachur R. Risk stratification of children being evaluated for intussusception. *Pediatrics*. 2011;127(2)e296-e303.

21. Dean AJ, Lafferty K, Villanueva TC. Emergency medicine bedside ultrasound diagnosis of intussusception in a patient with chronic abdominal pain and unrecognized Peutz-Jeghers syndrome. *J Emerg Med*. 2003;24:203-210.

PART 2

Does the Patient Have Pyloric Stenosis?

Aun Woon (Cindy) Soon, MD, FAAP, FRACP and Peter James Snelling, BSc, MBBS (Hons), MPHTM, GCHS, CCPU, FRACP, FACEM

● **Clinical Vignette**

A 5-week-old infant is brought into the clinic with 1 week of nonbilious projectile vomiting, associated with lethargy and poor weight gain. He otherwise has an unremarkable perinatal history. On examination, he appears mildly dehydrated and has a small palpable mass in the right upper quadrant of the abdomen. Does the patient have pyloric stenosis?

LITERATURE REVIEW

Infantile hypertrophic pyloric stenosis (IHPS) is the pathologic thickening of the pyloric muscle, leading to progressive gastric outlet obstruction. It typically occurs in 2 to 8 weeks of life, with an approximate incidence of 2 to 3.5 per 1000 live births.[1,2] It is more common in males, first-born children, and preterm infants, but its etiology is largely unknown.[2,3]

The typical presentation of IHPS is the infant who develops nonbilious, forceful vomiting immediately after feeding with persistent hunger. They are usually described as dehydrated with a palpable "olive" mass in the right upper quadrant of the abdomen, but this is not a consistent finding. They can also have visible reverse peristalsis and poor weight gain. The classical laboratory finding is hypochloremic hypokalemic metabolic alkalosis from gastric acid loss.[4]

Transabdominal ultrasound is the investigation of choice for the diagnosis of IHPS, given the limitation of clinical examination.[5] Ultrasonography for IHPS has demonstrated sensitivities of 98% to 100% and specificities of 99% to 100% in experienced hands.[6] Pyloric muscle thickness of greater than 3 mm and pyloric muscle length greater than 14 mm are indicative of IHPS.[7,8] Failure of gastric contents to pass through the pylorus is also supportive of the diagnosis.

In a prospective study by Sivitz et al, physician novice sonographers were able to diagnose IHPS using point-of-care ultrasound (POCUS) with a sensitivity of 100% (95% confidence interval [CI] 62%-100%) and a specificity of 100% (95% CI of 92%-100%) after a 45-minute training session.[9] In other studies, although emergency physicians and resident surgeons who performed POCUS were unable to report test performance characteristics, they demonstrated it to be feasible and adequately performed.[10,11] Although highly promising, larger-scale trials are required to validate these conclusions.

TABLE 26-1	Recommendations for Use of Point-of-Care Ultrasound in Clinical Practice		
Recommendation		Rating	Reference
Usage of point-of-care ultrasound for evaluation of idiopathic hypertrophic pyloric stenosis can be performed effectively by novice physician sonographers.		B	9

A = consistent, good-quality patient-oriented evidence; B = inconsistent or limited-quality patient-oriented evidence; C = consensus, disease-oriented evidence, usual practice, expert opinion, or case series. For information about the SORT evidence rating system, go to http://www.aafp.org/afpsort.

PERFORMING THE SCAN

1. **Preparation.** The patient should ideally be lying in the right decubitus position (left side elevated), although a supine position is acceptable as well. Scanning a patient in this age group may be challenging, and measures should be taken to ensure the patient's comfort in order to perform a successful scan. Select the high-frequency, linear array transducer, and choose the appropriate depth setting according to the patient's size. Ensure that the mother has either glucose-water solution or milk ready to feed the child during the scan.

2. **Locate the pylorus.**[9] Place the transducer on the subxiphoid region in the transverse orientation (**Figure 26-1**). Locate the liver edge and the anterior gastric wall (**Figure 26-2**). Trace the wall laterally toward the patient's right and caudally until you locate the pylorus. Once the pylorus is visualized, measure the width of the muscle wall and the length of the pyloric channel (**Figures 26-3 and 26-4**). Observe the pylorus for about 5 to 10 minutes to visualize the passage of gastric contents through the pyloric channel (**Figure 26-5** and ▶ **Video 26-1**). Also observe for changes in muscle width during this time as the width may appear falsely thickened during pylorospasm.

3. **Pyloric stenosis.** A hypertrophied pylorus can sometimes be located subjacent to the gallbladder.[12] A muscle width of greater than 3 mm and channel length greater than 14 mm is considered

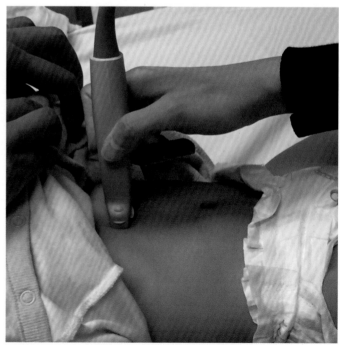

FIGURE 26-1. Transducer on the subxiphoid/epigastric region in the transverse orientation.

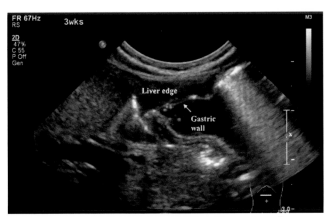

FIGURE 26-2. Image of liver edge and anterior gastric wall.

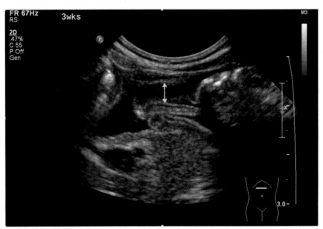

FIGURE 26-3. Measuring the width of the pyloric muscle wall (longitudinal view).

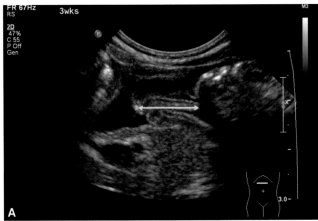

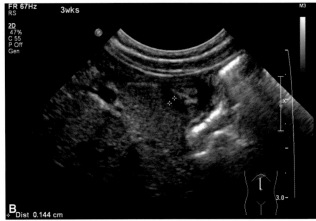

FIGURE 26-4. A, Measuring the length of the pyloric channel (longitudinal view). B, Measuring the width of the pyloric muscle wall (transverse view).

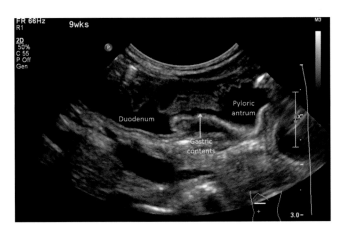

FIGURE 26-5. Gastric contents in the pyloric channel.

FIGURE 26-6. Pyloric stenosis in longitudinal view.

positive (**Figures 26-6 and 26-7**). Preference should be given to the width measurement should there be discrepancies in the width and length measurements.[8] The study is considered negative if gastric contents are visualized passing through a relaxed, dilated pylorus during the period of observation.

PATIENT MANAGEMENT

When planning patient management, it is important to determine the availability of radiology ultrasound and level of clinical concern. Evidence to date has shown that novice

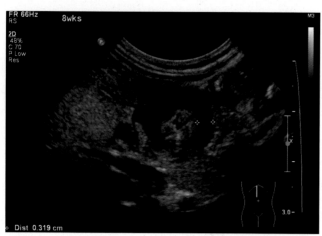

FIGURE 26-7. Pyloric stenosis in transverse view.

physician sonographers are able to detect IHPS using POCUS with a high specificity, making it an acceptable "rule-in" test.[9] However, it is important to recognize the limitations of novice physician sonographers, especially when a "negative" result is obtained. A high clinical suspicion should prompt further imaging and/or consult despite a negative scan. There are no known studies to date incorporating POCUS as part of a management process of a pediatric patient with possible HPS. One possible management strategy, based on expert opinion, is illustrated in **Figure 26-8**.

If HPS is diagnosed, pediatric surgery should be consulted. Surgical pyloromyotomy is the standard treatment of choice. The decision to perform an open procedure or laparoscopy lies in the discretion of the surgeon because there is no strong evidence currently supporting one procedure over the other.[13] A majority of infants are usually discharged about 2 days after the surgery.

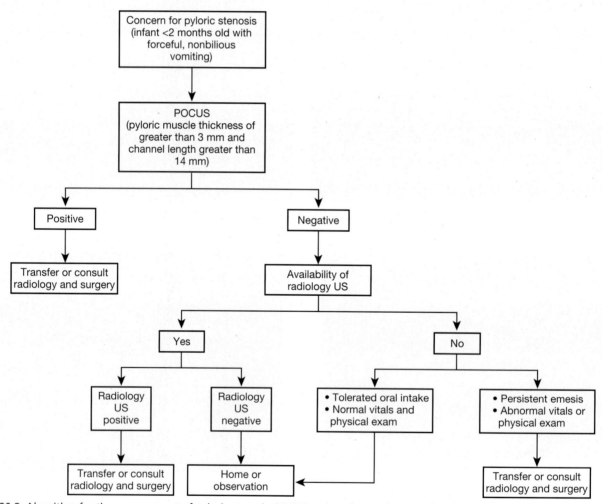

FIGURE 26-8. Algorithm for the management of pyloric stenosis. POCUS, point-of-care ultrasound; US, ultrasound.

PEARLS AND PITFALLS

Pearls

- To ensure the patient's comfort, measures such as using warmed gel, warmed room, glucose-water solution, and parental presence may be helpful.
- If palpable, the probe can be placed directly over the "olive" mass.[10]
- Gastric air or bowel gas may cause shadowing artifact that obscures the view of the pylorus. Feeding the child and having the child in the right decubitus position allows the fluid to displace gastric air, enabling better visualization of the pylorus.

Pitfalls

- Beware of transient thickening of the pyloric muscle due to peristalsis or pylorospasm, which can mimic IHPS.[14] In cases of suspected pylorospasm, the pylorus should be visualized for 3 minutes, or measurements can be repeated within 5 to 10 minutes.[15]
- A false negative examination can occur because the gastric or duodenal wall can be mistaken for the pylorus.
- Inadequate depth settings can result in nonvisualization of the pylorus.[9]

BILLING

CPT Code	Description	Global Payment	Professional Component	Technical Component
76705	Limited abdominal ultrasound including a specific study of a single organ, a limited area of the abdomen or a follow-up study	$92.73	$30.08	$62.66

CPT codes and average national reimbursement for Medicare in 2016. Payment data are from https://www.cms.gov/apps/physician-fee-schedule/search/search-criteria.aspx. See Chapter 2 for details on ultrasound billing.

ACKNOWLEDGMENT

We would like to thank Roger Gent, Head Sonographer in Paediatric Ultrasound at Women's and Children's Hospital in Adelaide, South Australia, for his contribution to this chapter.

References

1. To T, Wajja A, Wales PW, Langer JC. Population demographic indicators associated with incidence of pyloric stenosis. *Arch Pediatr Adolesc Med.* 2005;159(6):520-525.
2. Krogh C, Fischer TK, Skotte L, et al. Familial aggregation and heritability of pyloric stenosis. *JAMA.* 2010;303(23):2393-2399.
3. Zhu J, Zhu T, Lin Z, Mu D. Perinatal risk factors for infantile hypertrophic pyloric stenosis: a meta-analysis. *J Pediatr Surg.* 2017;52:1389-1397.
4. Touloukian RJ, Higgins E. The spectrum of serum electrolytes in hypertrophic pyloric stenosis. *J Pediatr Surg.* 1983;18(4):394-397.
5. Godbole P, Sprigg A, Dickson JA, Lin PC. Ultrasound compared with clinical examination in infantile hypertrophic pyloric stenosis. *Arch Dis Child.* 1996;75:335-337.
6. Hernanz-Schulman M. Pyloric stenosis: role of imaging. *Pediatr Radiol.* 2009;39(2):S134-S139.
7. Kofoed PE, Høst A, Elle B, Larsen C. Hypertrophic pyloric stenosis: determination of muscle dimensions by ultrasound. *Br J Radiol.* 1988;61:19.
8. Rohrschneider WK, Mittnacht H, Darge K, Tröger J. Pyloric muscle in asymptomatic infants: sonographic evaluation and discrimination from idiopathic hypertrophic pyloric stenosis. *Pediatr Radiol.* 1998;28:429.
9. Sivitz AB, Tejani C, Cohen SG. Evaluation of hypertrophic pyloric stenosis by pediatric emergency physician sonography. *Acad Emerg Med.* 2013;20: 646-651.
10. Malcom GE III, Raio CC, Rios MD, Blaivas M, Tsung JW. Feasibility of emergency physician diagnosis of hypertrophic pyloric stenosis using point-of-care ultrasound: a multi-center case series. *J Emerg Med.* 2009;37(3):283-286.
11. McVay MR, Copeland DR, McMahon LE, et al. Surgeon-performed ultrasound for diagnosis of pyloric stenosis is accurate, reproducible, and clinically valuable. *J Pediatr Surg.* 2009;44:169-171.
12. Levine D, Wilkes DC, Filly RA. Pylorus subjacent to the gallbladder: an additional finding in hypertrophic pyloric stenosis. *J Clin Ultrasound.* 1995;23(7):425-428.
13. Sathya C, Wayne C, Gotsch A, Vincent J, Sullivan KJ, Nasr A. Laparoscopic versus open pyloromyotomy in infants: a systematic review and meta-analysis. *Pediatr Surg Int.* 2017;33(3):325-333. doi:10.1007/s00383-016-4030-y.
14. Dias SC, Swinson S, Torrao H, et al. Hypertrophic pyloric stenosis: tips and tricks for ultrasound diagnosis. *Insights Imaging.* 2012;3:247-250.
15. Blumer SL, Zucconi WB, Cohen HL, Scriven RJ, Lee TK. The vomiting neonate: a review of the ACR appropriateness criteria and ultrasound's role in the workup of such patients. *Ultrasound Q.* 2004;20:79-89.

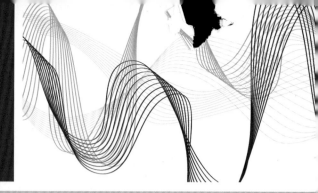

CHAPTER

27

Does the Patient Have a Viable Intrauterine Pregnancy?

Benjamin J. F. Huntley, MD, FAAFP, Francis M. Goldshmid, MD, FAAFP, and Erin S. L. Huntley, DO

● Clinical Vignette

A 23-year-old G4 P3003 with 2 to 3 months of amenorrhea and a positive pregnancy test presents for her first prenatal visit with complaints of new-onset vaginal bleeding. Her hemoglobin is normal, her blood type is O+, and her cervix is visibly closed without evidence of active bleeding on speculum examination. Does the patient have a viable intrauterine pregnancy?

LITERATURE REVIEW

Vaginal bleeding in the first trimester of pregnancy is a common complaint. The bleeding may be painless or painful and may range from spotting to frank bleeding with or without clot and tissue passage. Underlying causes can be benign or life threatening (Table 27-1). Regardless of the presenting symptoms, it is important to always initially consider it an emergency until proven otherwise. Ultrasound is extremely useful in these cases because of its ability to quickly determine the location of the pregnancy and to evaluate viability.

Ectopic Pregnancy

An ectopic pregnancy occurs when a fertilized egg implants outside the normal intrauterine environment. Most commonly,

TABLE 27-1 Differential Diagnosis of First Trimester Vaginal Bleeding

Ectopic pregnancy

Pregnancy loss (see Table 27-3)

Threatened abortion

Vaginitis/sexually transmitted infections

Postcoital bleeding

Cervical and endometrial polyps

Fibroids

Trauma

this occurs in the fallopian tube but may also occur in the uterine cornua, the cervix, the ovary, a prior hysterotomy scar, or the abdomen.[1]

Ectopic pregnancy occurs in 2% of all pregnancies in the United States. Among women presenting in the first trimester with abdominal pain, vaginal bleeding, or both, the prevalence is as high as 18%.[2] It is the leading cause of first trimester mortality, causing 6% of all pregnancy-related deaths.[3,4] The major risk factors for ectopic pregnancy include prior ectopic pregnancy, history of pelvic inflammatory disease, prior pelvic surgery (especially previous tubal ligation, interruption, or occlusion), and a history of pregnancy with concurrent intrauterine device (IUD) use.[5-8] It is important to note, however, that at least half of all women presenting with ectopic pregnancy have no identifiable risk factors or definitive physical findings on presentation, and therefore it is paramount to have a high index of suspicion in the first trimester patient presenting with bleeding or abdominal pain.[9] Evaluation with ultrasonography should be performed as soon as possible.

Definitive Intrauterine Pregnancy

If an intrauterine pregnancy (IUP) is visualized on ultrasonography, then an ectopic pregnancy is unlikely. A heterotopic pregnancy, in which an intrauterine and ectopic pregnancy coexist, is extremely rare with an incidence of less than 1/30,000 confirmed pregnancies.[10] Definitive diagnosis of an IUP requires visualization of either a fetal pole or a yolk sac within a gestational sac. Visualization of an empty gestational sac suggests an IUP but does not confirm it. This is because an ectopic pregnancy may present with a pseudogestational sac—a nonspecific collection of fluid within the uterine cavity. The frequency of pseudogestational sacs in women with ectopic pregnancies is approximately 10%.[3] Free fluid in the posterior cul-de-sac is another nonspecific finding. Although it can be a sign of a ruptured ectopic pregnancy, it also be seen in healthy women through all phases of the menstrual cycle.[11]

Normal, early IUPs are frequently impossible to confirm via ultrasonography as the yolk sac or fetal pole may not yet be visible. In these cases, quantitative serum beta human chorionic

TABLE 27-2	**Diagnosis of Definitively Failed First Trimester Pregnancy**

CRL ≥7 mm and no heartbeat

MSD ≥25 mm and no fetal pole

Still no fetal pole with heartbeat ≥2 wk after ultrasound showed gestational sac without a yolk sac

Still no fetal pole with heartbeat ≥11 d after ultrasound showed gestational sac with a yolk sac

Abbreviations: CRL, crown-rump length; MSD, mean gestational sac diameter.

Modified from Doublet PM, Benson CB, Bourne, T. Diagnostic criteria for nonviable pregnancy in first trimester. *N Engl J Med.* 2013;369:1443-1451.

gonadotropin (beta-hCG) can be a useful adjunctive test. The beta-hCG threshold above which an IUP should be visible on transvaginal ultrasound is called the discriminatory zone. Above a beta-hCG level of 1500 mIU/mL, 80% of viable pregnancies can be detected. Sensitivity improves to 91% when using a beta-hCG cutoff of 2000 mIU/mL. Multiple-gestation pregnancies and rarely normal singleton pregnancies may not be visible at a beta-hCG level of 2000 mIU/mL. The best evidence-based approach establishes the discriminatory zone at 3510, at which point 99% of intrauterine pregnancies are visualized.[12] Patients with pregnancies of unknown location whose quantitative beta-hCG is greater than 3510 mIU/mL should generally be considered to have an abnormal pregnancy until proven otherwise.

Once confirmed as intrauterine in location, IUPs are further subclassified as viable, nonviable, or of indeterminate viability. Viability is determined by the presence of fetal cardiac activity, which should be visualized in all fetuses with a crown-rump length (CRL) of at least 7 mm.[13,14] Until viability is confirmed, the pregnancy is referred to as an IUP of unknown viability.

If a fetus does not have cardiac activity and the CRL measures less than 7 mm, viability is indeterminate, and a repeat ultrasound is warranted in 7 to 14 days. If there is still no heartbeat 11 days after the first ultrasound, then the fetus is confirmed to be nonviable. Additionally, other ultrasonographic features can be used to confirm nonviability and are listed in Table 27-2.

If the fetus is nonviable, the pregnancy is then diagnosed as a spontaneous abortion, or, as it is more familiarly known by most

patients, a miscarriage. The main risk factors for spontaneous abortion include previous history of spontaneous abortion, advanced maternal age, smoking, abdominal or pelvic trauma, infection, and elevated preconception maternal blood pressure.[15-19] The most common reasons for spontaneous abortion are chromosomal abnormalities such as aneuploidy, congenital anomalies, teratogenic exposures, and trauma.

First trimester spontaneous abortions can be grouped into one of four categories: missed abortions, incomplete abortions, complete abortions, and inevitable abortions (Table 27-3).

a. Inevitable Abortion

An inevitable abortion is diagnosed when the cervix is open but no products of conception can be seen at the os. There is no history of passage of any tissue, although there will usually be a history of vaginal bleeding (possibly with clots) with or without pelvic pain. Although there is often no detectable fetal cardiac activity, technically the diagnosis of inevitable abortion is independent of heartbeat, which could be present despite the cervical os being open and the products of conception not having yet been expelled. In such cases, it is not possible to prevent an impending loss.

b. Incomplete Abortion

An incomplete abortion is diagnosed when there is a nonviable IUP, and there is either a history of expelled partial tissue or partial tissue present in the vagina or at the os on sterile speculum examination. The cervix may be open or closed, but in either case, there is still tissue remaining within the uterus. On ultrasound, there will be evidence of a nonviable IUP that is distorting the endometrial space and that has the appearance of debris with heterogeneous echogenicity. This may cause the endometrial stripe to appear thickened (**Figure 27-1**). The patient will usually complain of vaginal bleeding and may have ongoing pelvic pain.

c. Complete Abortion

When the uterus has completely expelled the nonviable IUP and the cervix is subsequently closed, a complete abortion is diagnosed. The patient will still have a positive pregnancy test because of

TABLE 27-3	**Definitions of Abortion Subtypes**

Term	Definition
Spontaneous abortion	Natural occurring pregnancy loss
Induced abortion	Intentional medical or surgical termination of pregnancy
Elective abortion	Induced abortion at patient's request
Therapeutic abortion	Induced abortion for medical reasons
Threatened abortion	Any bleeding associated with an intrauterine pregnancy
Inevitable abortion	Vaginal bleeding, open cervix, expulsion of products of conception has not yet begun
Incomplete abortion	Vaginal bleeding, open cervix, expulsion of products of conception has not begun
Complete abortion	Vaginal bleeding, cervix variable, completed expulsion of products of conception
Missed abortion	Fetal or embryonic demise remains in uterus, cervix closed
Septic abortion	Fetal or embryonic demise that is infected

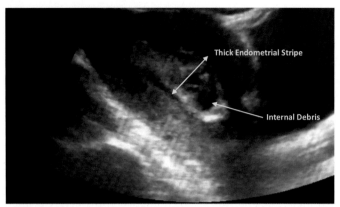

FIGURE 27-1. Incomplete abortion with debris and thickened endometrial stripe.

TABLE 27-4	Recommendations for Use of Point-of-Care Ultrasound in Clinical Practice		
Recommendation		Rating	References
A normal pregnancy should exhibit a gestational sac when beta subunit of human chorionic gonadotropin levels reach 3510 mIU/mL (3510 IU/L) and cardiac activity when the embryonic crown-rump length is ≥7 mm.		C	12-14
Nonsurgical treatments for incomplete abortion of an embryo have a high likelihood of success; however, misoprostol or surgical treatment is more effective than expectant management.		A	36

A = consistent, good-quality patient-oriented evidence; B = inconsistent or limited-quality patient-oriented evidence; C = consensus, disease-oriented evidence, usual practice, expert opinion, or case series. For information about the SORT evidence rating system, go to http://www.aafp.org/afpsort.

temporally downtrending beta-hCG values. She will also complain of vaginal bleeding and report a history of passage of clots or tissue. Transvaginal ultrasound will show a thin endometrial stripe with minimal, if any, debris within the uterus. Vaginal examination may demonstrate light vaginal bleeding.

d. Threatened Abortion

Threatened abortion is diagnosed in patients who present with vaginal bleeding wherein a viable IUP is diagnosed on ultrasound. The cervix is found to be closed, and there must also be no alternative explanation for the bleeding such as cervicitis, trauma, cervical polyps, or cancer. Viewing a subchorionic hematoma (**Figure 27-2**) can also help identify the etiology of bleeding. Vaginal bleeding occurs in 25% of all pregnancies and is a risk factor for subsequent pregnancy loss.[20] However, in the majority of patients presenting with threatened abortion, pregnancy will continue without complications.[21] At 8 weeks postbleed, pregnancies that have continued successfully will have loss rates drop to 3%.[22]

Pregnancy of Unknown Location

Pregnancy of unknown location describes episodes of vaginal bleeding in pregnancies where ultrasound fails to definitively visualize either an IUP or ectopic pregnancy. Clinical possibilities include: (1) a nonvisualized ectopic, (2) an early gestation that is not yet able to be sonographically visualized, or (3) a nonviable pregnancy that did not advance beyond a gestational sac without yolk sac or fetal pole.

PERFORMING THE SCAN

Transabdominal Ultrasound

Step 1: Position the patient. Ensure the patient is lying comfortably on the examination table with the head of the bed elevated to 30° or to the patient's preferred height (**Figure 27-3**).

Step 2: Find the basic landmarks. The first step is point-of-care transabdominal ultrasound using a curvilinear probe, which has a probe marker on the transducer's side that corresponds with an indicator dot on the ultrasound monitor. Hold the probe in the patient's transverse body plane so the probe marker is on the patient's right side (**Figure 27-4**). Rotate the probe marker cephalad to change to a sagittal body plane. Place the probe just superior to the pubic symphysis and systematically scan the entire pelvis to identify key structures: the uterus, the bladder, the cervix, and the adnexa. The uterus, when viewed midline in the sagittal maternal plane, will appear like the magnified end of a cotton swab, with a narrow neck proximal to the cervix and a wider fundus that appears to bow out to the left of the screen (**Figure 27-5**). The narrow neck dives into the pelvis and leads to the anterior and posterior lips of the cervix. It is often difficult to see the cervix on transabdominal ultrasound because of shadowing from the pubic symphysis.

If the pregnancy is unexpectedly found to be in the second or third trimester, evaluate the fetal lie, amniotic fluid, fetal cardiac activity, placental location, and fetal number. For more details, see

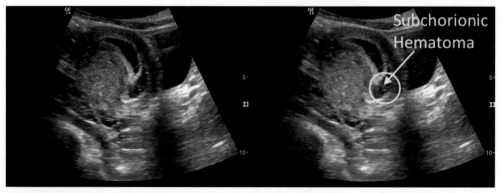

FIGURE 27-2. Subchorionic hematoma visualized posteriorly on transabdominal ultrasound.

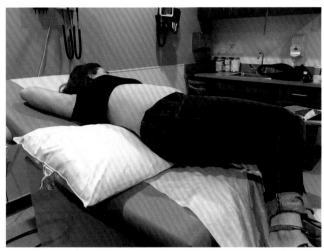

FIGURE 27-3. Patient positioning for transabdominal ultrasound.

The Big Five in Chapter 28. However, other than fetal number and possibly cardiac activity, most of these features will not develop or become clinically important until later in pregnancy.

Step 3: Evaluate for pelvic free fluid. In the sagittal view, pay close attention to the space inferior to the uterine fundus. This is the rectouterine pouch, or posterior cul-de-sac, and free

fluid will be seen here. If present, have increased suspicion of an ectopic pregnancy. When a patient is prone, any fluid in the pelvis will accumulate here because of gravity, and the presence of fluid may be a helpful diagnostic tool depending on the patient presentation. There is an example of a small amount of free fluid in Figure 27-5. See Chapter 50 for further examples of free pelvic fluid.

Step 4: Identify the intrauterine contents. Evaluate the intrauterine contents next. If an IUP is identified, document the total number of gestational sacs, total number of embryos, and presence or absence of a heartbeat, and comment on any abnormal implantation. See "Performing the Transvaginal Ultrasound" section for more details.

Transvaginal Ultrasound

Step 1: Position the patient. Have the patient empty her bladder prior to the start of the examination. Ensure the patient is properly positioned in the dorsal lithotomy position with a drape covering the lower half of her body (**Figure 27-6**).

Cover the transvaginal probe in a sterile sheath filled with gel. Add sterile gel to the tip of the external portion of the sheathed probe. Have the patient rest her lower buttocks on the very edge of the examination table to allow for maximal mobility of the probe. Insert the probe gently into the vagina, or have the patient insert the probe herself. Point the probe marker upward to the ceiling, showing a sagittal plane at the start of the examination. Use the tip of the empty

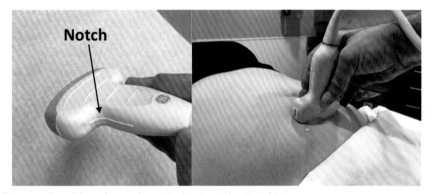

FIGURE 27-4. Photo of curvilinear probe with probe marker pointing to patient's right.

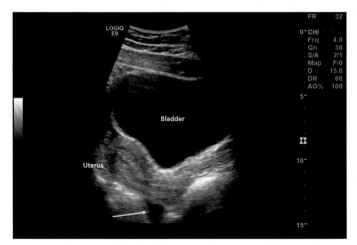

FIGURE 27-5. Transabdominal image of the uterus. The uterus and bladder are labeled. The arrow points to a small pocket of free fluid.

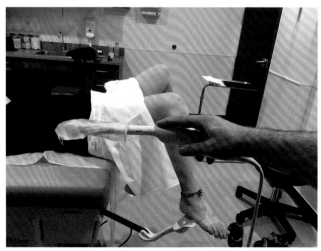

FIGURE 27-6. Patient positioning for transvaginal ultrasound.

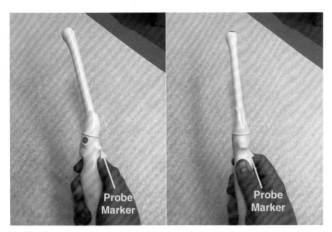

FIGURE 27-7. Transvaginal probe with probe marker labeled.

bladder as a landmark. It is easily visualized and sits just anterior to the uterine cervix. In the sagittal plane, it will appear as an almost anechoic triangular structure, where one of the apices points inferiorly toward the uterocervical junction. Use varying levels of pressure and depth to help acquire the ideal images and identification of important structures, such as the adnexa, the ovaries, and the cervix.

Step 2: Find the basic landmarks. Once inserted, rotate the endovaginal probe 90° counterclockwise to obtain images in the sagittal and coronal planes (**Figure 27-7**).

Locate the midline of the uterus in the sagittal plane and find the cornua at either superolateral pole of the fundus. Scan laterally to identify the corresponding adnexa. The ovaries appear oval shaped with a thin capsule and are usually filled with multiple hypoechoic

follicles, surrounded by a ring of blood vessels seen on color Doppler as having a "chocolate chip cookie" appearance (**Figure 27-8**). The ovaries are often overlying the external iliac vein. Document whether ovaries were or were not identified. An adnexal mass in the setting of a pregnancy of unknown location, especially in conjunction with pelvic free fluid, is an ectopic pregnancy until proven otherwise.[23]

In the sagittal view, the uterus will appear like the end of a Q-Tip, similar to the aforementioned findings on transabdominal ultrasound but with greater resolution and detail (**Figure 27-9**). Identify the cervix; if obtaining a cervical length is clinically indicated, note this tissue easily deforms with excessive transducer pressure, leading to a falsely appearing longer and thinner cervix (**Figure 27-10**). Make fanlike sweeps through the body of the uterus—from sidewall to sidewall and from cervix to fundus—and through the adnexae, looking for an IUP or evidence of an extrauterine pregnancy or mass.

Step 3: Evaluate for pelvic free fluid. When using a transvaginal probe to assess for free fluid in the posterior cul-de-sac (**Figure 27-11**), both the coronal and the sagittal views prove helpful. Start in the midline sagittal plane and scan through the entire uterus. On the screen, pay attention to the potential hypoechoic space that exists inferior to the uterus, usually just below the neck of the uterus. This is where the posterior cul-de-sac lies. If this space appears to have a large amount of anechoic free fluid, turn the probe 90° counterclockwise while holding the cul-de-sac in view, and evaluate the same space in the coronal view. In this view, the uterus will appear at the superior portion of the screen, and any free fluid will come into view inferiorly. By measuring the height, width, and depth of fluid in both the coronal and the sagittal planes, quantify the amount of fluid present. If clotted blood is present in this space, it will settle on the inferior portion of the screen (on top of the

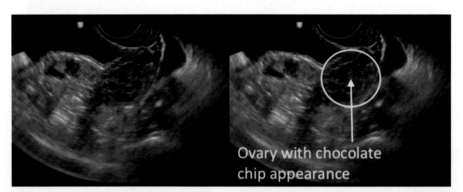

FIGURE 27-8. Transvaginal image of a normal ovary. Notice classic "chocolate chip" appearance.

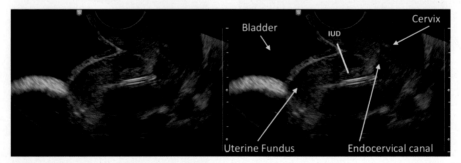

FIGURE 27-9. Transvaginal image of a normal uterus in the sagittal plane. Incidentally, an intrauterine device (IUD) with reverberation artifact can be seen in the lower fundus (see Chapter 34). The IUD, fundus, cervix, and bladder are labeled.

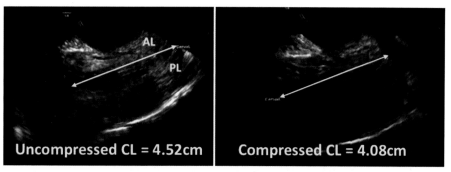

FIGURE 27-10. Transvaginal view of cervix compressed and relaxed with anterior and posterior (AP) lips noted. AL, anterior cervical lip, PL, posterior cervical lip.

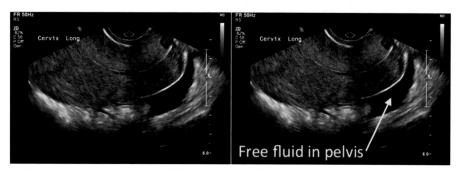

FIGURE 27-11. Free fluid in the pelvis seen on transvaginal ultrasound. This fluid appears to be located in the posterior vaginal vault as it can be seen near the tip of the cervix.

rectum) and will have a hyperechoic debris-like appearance when compared to fresh blood, which would be above it but below the posterior uterine wall.

Step 4: Identify the intrauterine contents. Evaluate the contents of the uterus. Identify the anechoic round- or oval-shaped fluid collection of a gestational sac,[24,25] if present. Note the gestational sac is usually visible by 5 weeks.[26,27] Scan the gestational sac and identify the yolk sac, a hypoechoic ring asymmetrically located within the uterus with respect to the midline that develops within the gestational sac by 5 to 6 weeks and is usually 3 to 5 mm in

diameter[14]; the yolk sac is often circumscribed by a smooth, thick band of homogeneous hyperechoic tissue called the decidual ring. Lastly, scan the intrauterine contents to assess for a fetal pole, which appears around 6 weeks of gestational age and is usually abutting the yolk sac in early pregnancy[26] (**Figure 27-12**). Note the presence or absence of fetal cardiac activity, as identified by the fluttering visible in the midline of the fetal pole. M-mode can be used to document static images of cardiac activity[27] (**Figure 27-13** and ▶ **Video 27-1**). See The Big Five in Chapter 28 for more details on performing M-mode.

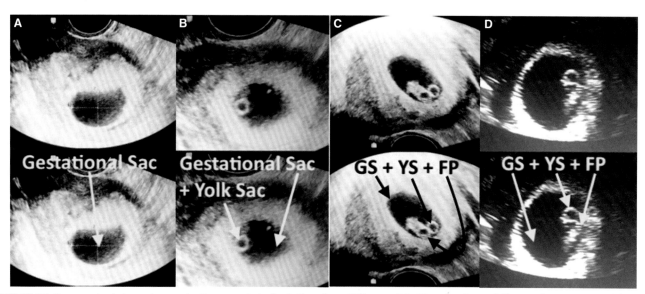

FIGURE 27-12. Transvaginal views demonstrating panel. A, Gestational sac (GS), panel B, GS and yolk sac (YS), panel C, GS, YS, and fetal pole (FP). Note that panel D demonstrates how a static image of a YS adjacent to an FP can be mistaken for a fetal head.

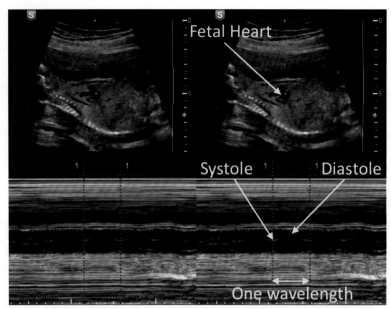

FIGURE 27-13. In the two-dimensional image of the fetus (top window), M-mode is used to display a dynamic wave form of the fetal heart (bottom window).

PATIENT MANAGEMENT

Any patient with vaginal bleeding who is known to be in the first trimester of pregnancy or who has a newly positive pregnancy test should be considered to have first trimester bleeding. The first goal in evaluating the patient is to determine whether they are hemodynamically stable. Any patient who is tachycardic, hypotensive, or showing other signs of shock should immediately have two large-bore intravenous catheters placed and be resuscitated with isotonic fluid boluses. Emergency medical services should be contacted, and the patient should be moved to the closest location where definitive emergency medical and surgical care can be provided. In hemodynamically stable patients, the goal is to determine pregnancy location and viability. They should initially be evaluated with transabdominal ultrasonography, and followed by assessment with transvaginal sonography if the pregnancy location cannot be determined. Quantitative beta-hCG should be obtained if it is available. Diagnosis of IUP requires visualization of a gestational sac containing either a yolk sac or a fetal pole, and when this is not visualized, a high suspicion for an abnormal pregnancy should be maintained. This is especially true if the beta-hCG is above the discriminatory zone (3510 mIU/mL). The most concerning diagnosis to consider is that of an ectopic pregnancy, although the possibility of failed IUP or early IUP of undetermined viability remains in the differential as well.

In all cases of first trimester bleeding—and with bleeding during pregnancy in general—maternal blood type evaluation should be performed to evaluate for the potential need for Rho(D) immunoglobulin administration.

Diagnosis of Ectopic Pregnancy

A patient who has a nondiagnostic transvaginal ultrasound can be followed in the outpatient setting if hemodynamically stable, has

guaranteed follow-up, and has no signs or symptoms highly suspicious for ectopic pregnancy. If these criteria are not all met, then monitoring in the inpatient setting should be considered. Repeat ultrasonography in 2 to 3 days is warranted with appropriate patient counseling regarding the possibility of an ectopic pregnancy. Repeat quantitative beta-hCG should be obtained when repeat ultrasound fails to identify a visualized ectopic or an IUP. In a normal IUP, beta-hCG levels should increase by at least 80% every 48 hours.[23] A falling beta-hCG is consistent with a failed pregnancy that could either be a spontaneous abortion or a spontaneously resolving ectopic pregnancy. These patients can be followed with serial beta-hCGs as described later.

Some patients will have neither a normally rising nor a falling beta-hCG level. In these instances, an increase in beta-hCG of less than 53% in 48 hours confirms an abnormal pregnancy with a sensitivity of 99%[28] but does not provide information regarding whether this is an ectopic pregnancy or a failed IUP. These patients can be treated empirically for presumed ectopic; however, concerns about possible unnecessary exposure to methotrexate have led to guidelines that call for consideration of uterine aspiration in order to look for chorionic villi.[29] Providers should have a discussion with the patient regarding the risks and benefits of such a procedure, along with those of empiric treatment.

If aspiration is performed and chorionic villi are present, then failed IUP is confirmed and no further diagnostic workup is required. These patients can then be treated for spontaneous abortion, as described later. If, however, no chorionic villi are found, then close follow-up and repeat beta-hCG testing in 12 to 24 hours is warranted. If the beta-hCG increases or plateaus (ie, shows a decrease of only 10%-15%), then this may be due to either incomplete evacuation of a failed IUP or the presence of a persistent ectopic pregnancy.[29] Given the risk of allowing a persistent ectopic to go untreated, definitive ectopic treatment should be provided.[29] If the beta-hCG levels drop more than 50%, however, this is most likely a failed IUP, and these patients can be closely monitored clinically with serial beta-hCGs.[29-31] For patients in whom the beta-hCG drops between 15% to 50%, close follow-up with serial beta-hCGs is imperative. Although the majority of these patients will be determined to have failed IUPs, there is still a moderate risk for a nonvisualized ectopic pregnancy being present.[29,30]

Management of Ectopic Pregnancy

Ectopic pregnancy can be treated medically or surgically, although most patients will meet criteria for medical management with methotrexate. Criteria include absent or mild symptoms, quantitative beta-hCG < 5000 mIU/mL (some experts recommend <2000 mIU/mL),[32] absent fetal cardiac activity, and gestational sac < 3.5 to 4 cm.[11,29,32,33] Prior to initiating treatment, the patient should have a baseline beta-hCG, complete blood count (CBC) with differential, liver function panel, kidney function panel, blood type, and antibody screen performed.[33]

Methotrexate is dosed as follows[29]:

- A single dose of methotrexate is given intramuscularly on day 1 at a dosage of 50 mg/m^2 body surface area. Beta-hCG levels are checked on day 4 and again on day 7.
- If the beta-hCG level between day 4 and day 7 decreases by more than 15%, continue to check beta-hCG levels weekly until they are no longer detectible.
- If the decrease in beta-hCG between day 4 and day 7 is less than 15%, a second dose of methotrexate at the same dosage may be readministered with subsequent serial beta-hCG measurement.
- If the beta-hCG level does not decrease 15% from day 4 to day 7 postsecond dose, surgical management is recommended.
- Note that it is normal to see a rise in beta-hCG to above pretreatment levels between day 1 and day 4 of treatment, but levels should then begin to fall predictably thereafter.[29] Resolution of beta-hCG levels to nonpregnant levels usually takes 2 to 4 weeks but can take as long as 8 weeks.[29]

Methotrexate should not be used in cases of hemodynamic instability, ruptured ectopic pregnancy, or in patients with medical contraindications. Contraindications include active pulmonary or peptic ulcer disease, breastfeeding patients, or patients with clinically important hematologic, renal, or liver baseline laboratory abnormalities.[29,33] In these cases and in patients who have failed initial attempts at medical therapy, surgical consultation should be considered.

Rarely stable patients with suspected ectopic pregnancy can be treated with expectant management alone. This should be considered only for cases where the following criteria are met and only after the patient has been counseled extensively on the risks of tubal rupture, hemorrhage, and the possibility of emergency surgery. Criteria include absence of fetal cardiac activity, gestational sac, and extrauterine mass on transvaginal ultrasound; absence of signs of possible tubal rupture; low and decreasing beta-hCG levels; and guaranteed close follow-up.

Diagnosing Spontaneous Abortion

When an IUP is confirmed on ultrasound, the next step is to determine viability. Historically, three broad criteria have been used to diagnose a spontaneous abortion on transvaginal ultrasound: (1) the absence of cardiac activity once the embryo has reached a certain CRL; (2) the absence of an embryo in a gestational sac above a mean sac diameter threshold; and (3) the absence of an embryo with a heartbeat after a certain passage of time from the initial ultrasound.[14]

A recent systematic review in the *New England Journal of Medicine* by the Society of Radiologists in Ultrasound Multispecialty Panel on Early First Trimester Diagnosis of Miscarriage and Exclusion of a Viable IUP has recommended using a cutoff of 7 mm for CRL without associated cardiac activity as a diagnostic criterion for spontaneous abortion, which would lead to a specificity of 100% and a positive predictive value as close to 100% as could be measured.[14]

Recommendations for diagnosing definitively failed pregnancy use a cutoff of 25 mm for the mean sac diameter of a gestational sac without a yolk sac or fetal pole present in order to capture a specificity of 100% and a positive predictive value as close to 100% as could be measured.[14]

Some spontaneous abortions may never develop a gestational sac that would reach 25 mm in size or develop an embryo that would reach 7 mm in length. For this reason, a third and final set of criteria for diagnosing nonviability were recommended by the same systematic review. These criteria are as follows: definitively failed first trimester pregnancy can be diagnosed if either (1) the initial scan showed a gestational sac without a yolk sac and a follow-up scan at least 14 days later failed to show an embryo with a heartbeat or if (2) the initial scan showed a gestational sac with a yolk sac and a follow-up scan at least 11 days later failed to detect an embryo with a heartbeat.[14] Note that these two criteria exist independently of the measured CRL or mean sac diameter at either scan time.

Management of Spontaneous Abortion

Missed abortions are managed expectantly, medically, or surgically. Most missed abortions will get expelled with minimal harm to the patient within 1 to 2 weeks. After 4 weeks, the concern for infection and conversion to a septic abortion grows significant, and if the patient continues to desire conservative management, close follow-up should be scheduled. Should the patient desire a more expedient solution, medical management with misoprostol may be offered, or surgical management with either vacuum aspiration or suction curettage can be considered.

The dosing of misoprostol per the American College of Obstetricians and Gynecologists' guidelines for inevitable, incomplete, and missed abortions is as follows[34]:

- Misoprostol 800 µg is given vaginally.
- A second dose may be considered up to 7 days later if expulsion has not yet occurred.

The World Health Organization also has published a set of guidelines for misoprostol administration[35]:

- For missed abortions, 800 µg may be given once vaginally or 600 µg may be given once orally;
- For incomplete abortions, 600 µg is given once orally.

These dosing regimens may be completed in the home setting with appropriate and adequate patient counseling about hemorrhage, worsening or changing symptoms, and other possible complications (**Figure 27-14**).

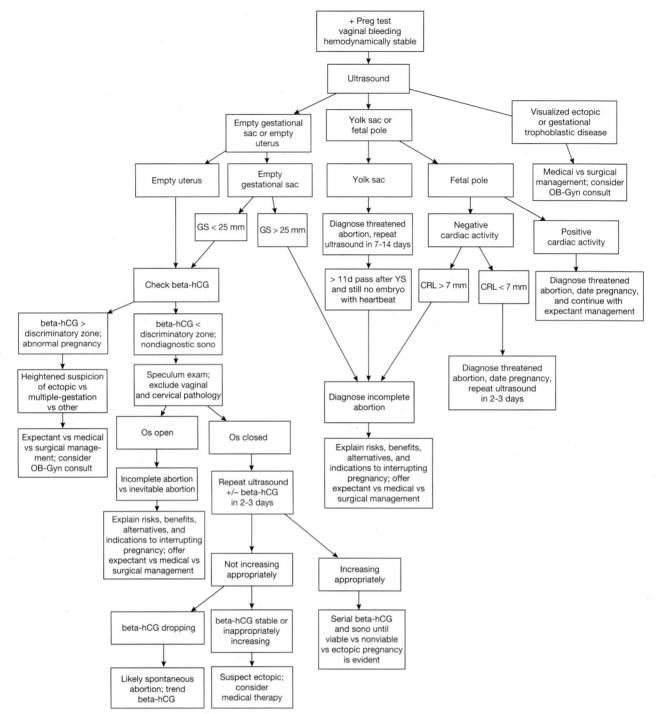

FIGURE 27-14. Management flow chart of hemodynamically stable patients. CRL, crown–rump length; GS, gestational sac; hCG, human chorionic gonadotropin.

PEARLS AND PITFALLS

Pearls

- Have the patient place her buttocks on the very edge of the examination table to allow for maximal mobility of the transvaginal probe and improved comfort.
- During transvaginal sonogram, varying pressure and depth of the probe will help identify structures, particularly the cervix and adnexa/ovaries.
- Use the bladder for a reference point, as it will be anterior to the uterus in all planes.
- Failed intrauterine pregnancies require delicate, thoughtful, and compassionate conversation with the patient, and emotional support is equally as important as medical support, if not more so. Most patients will want to know if they did anything to cause the pregnancy loss. It is important to reassure them that this is almost never the case.

Pitfalls

- If the yolk and fetal pole are both present, be sure not to mistake a yolk sac that is abutting a small fetal pole for the fetal cranium. Be sure to exclude this from the CRL measurement. If you are unsure, have the patient return in 1 week for a repeat scan.
- Do not mistake the pseudosac of an ectopic pregnancy for the gestational sac of an IUP.
- Do not fail to scan the entire contents of the uterus and adnexa.
- Do not mistake the intestines for adnexae or ovaries. An easy way to distinguish between the two is to apply downward pressure with the transducer; tissues that compress easily and are filled with grainy, slow-moving particles are likely to be bowel with fecal matter, whereas an ovary will be noncompressible.
- The incidence of heterotopic pregnancy is increased in patients who have undergone assisted fertility treatments, and a visualized IUP is less able to rule out a concurrent ectopic pregnancy.

BILLING

CPT Code	Description	Global Payment	Professional Component	Technical Component
76801	Ultrasound, pregnant uterus, real time with image documentation, fetal and maternal evaluation, first trimester (14 wk 0 d), transabdominal approach; single or first gestation	$126.33	$51.32	$75.01
76805	Ultrasound, pregnant uterus, fetal and maternal evaluation, > first trimester—transabdominal; single or first gestation	$145.71	$51.68	$94.03
76815	Ultrasound, pregnant uterus, limited (fetal heartbeat, placental location, fetal position and/or qualitative amniotic fluid volume), one or more fetuses	$86.85	$33.74	$53.12
76816	Ultrasound, pregnant uterus, follow-up (reevaluation of fetal size by measuring standard growth parameters and amniotic fluid volume, reevaluation of organ system(s)) suspected or confirmed to be abnormal on previous scan, transabdominal approach, per fetus	$118.79	$45.22	$73.57
76817	Limited transvaginal ultrasound of pregnant uterus	$99.77	$39.12	$60.65

CPT codes and average national reimbursement for Medicare in 2016. Payment data are from https://www.cms.gov/apps/physician-fee-schedule/search/search-criteria.aspx. See Chapter 2 for details on ultrasound billing.

References

1. Bouyer J, Coste J, Fernandez H, Pouly JL, Job-Spira N. Sites of ectopic pregnancy: a 10 year population-based study of 1800 cases. *Hum Reprod.* 2002;17(12):3224-3230.
2. Barnhart KT, Sammel MD, Gracia CR, Chittams J, Hummel AC, Shaunik A. Risk factors for ectopic pregnancy in women with symptomatic first-trimester pregnancies. *Fertil Steril.* 2006;86:36-43.
3. Doubilet PM, Benson CB. First, do no harm…to early pregnancies. *J Ultrasound Med.* 2010;29:685-689.
4. Chang J, Elam-Evans LD, Berg CJ, et al. Pregnancy-related mortality surveillance—United States, 1991-1999. *MMWR Surveill Summ.* 2003;52:1-8.
5. Bouyer J, Coste J, Shojaei T, et al. Risk factors for ectopic pregnancy: a comprehensive analysis based on a large case-control, population-based study in France. *Am J Epidemiol.* 2003;157:185.
6. Ankum WM, Mol BW, Van der Veen F, Bossuyt PM. Risk factors for ectopic pregnancy: a meta-analysis. *Fertil Steril.* 1996;65:1093.
7. Cheng L, Zhao WH, Meng CX, et al. Contraceptive use and the risk of ectopic pregnancy: a multicenter case-control study. *PLoS One.* 2014; 9:e115031.
8. Li C, Zhao WH, Zhu Q, et al. Risk factors for ectopic pregnancy: a multicenter case-control study. *BMC Pregnancy Childbirth.* 2015;15:187.
9. American College of Obstetricians and Gynecologists. ACOG practice bulletin no. 94: medical management of ectopic pregnancy. *Obstet Gynecol.* 2008;111:1479-1485.
10. De Voe RW, Pratt JH. Simultaneous intrauterine and extrauterine pregnancy. *Am J Obstet Gynecol.* 1948;56:1119-1126.
11. Davis JA, Gosink BB. Fluid in the female pelvis: cyclic patterns. *J Ultrasound Med.* 1986;5(2):75-79.

PART 2

12. Connolly A, Ryan DH, Stieber AM, Wolfe HM. Reevaluation of discriminatory and threshold levels for serum beta-hCG in early pregnancy. *Obstet Gynecol.* 2013;121(1):65-70.

13. American College of Obstetricians and Gynecologists. ACOG practice bulletin no. 175: ultrasound in pregnancy. *Obstet Gynecol.* 2016;128:e241-e256.

14. Doubilet PM, Benson CB, Bourne T. Diagnostic criteria for nonviable pregnancy in first trimester. *N Engl J Med.* 2013;369:1443-1451.

15. Nobles CJ, Mendola P, Mumford SL, Naimi AI, Yeung EH. Preconception blood pressure levels and reproductive outcomes in a prospective cohort of women attempting pregnancy. *Hypertension.* 2018;71:904-910.

16. Nybo Andersen AM, Wohlfahrt J, Christens P, Olsen J, Melbye M. Maternal age and fetal loss: population based register linkage study. *BMJ.* 2000;320(7251):1708.

17. Regan L, Braude PR, Trembath PL. Influence of past reproductive performance on risk of spontaneous abortion. *BMJ.* 1989;299(6698):541.

18. Chatenoud L, Parazzini F, di Cintio E, et al. Paternal and maternal smoking habits before conception and during the first trimester: relation to spontaneous abortion. *Ann Epidemiol.* 1998;8(8):520.

19. Kline J, Levin B, Kinney A, Stein Z, Susser M, Warburton D. Cigarette smoking and spontaneous abortion of known karyotype. Precise data but uncertain inferences. *Am J Epidemiol.* 1995;141(5):417.

20. Paspulati RM, Bhatt S, Nour SG. Sonographic evaluation of first-trimester bleeding. *Radiol Clin North Am.* 2008;46(2):437.

21. Deaton JL, Honoré GM, Huffman CS, Bauguess P. Early transvaginal ultrasound following an accurately dated pregnancy: the importance of finding a yolk sac or fetal heart motion. *Hum Reprod.* 1997;12(12):2820.

22. Simpson JL, Mills JL, Holmes LB, et al. Low fetal loss rates after ultrasound-proved viability in early pregnancy. *JAMA.* 1987;258:2555.

23. Deutchman M, Tubay AT, Turok DK. First trimester bleeding. *Am Fam Physician.* 2009;79(11):985-992.

24. Benson CB, Doubilet PM, Peters HE, Frates MC. Intrauterine fluid with ectopic pregnancy: a reappraisal. *J Ultrasound Med.* 2013;32:389-393.

25. Barnhart K, van Mello NM, Bourne T, et al. Pregnancy of unknown location: a consensus statement of nomenclature, definitions, and outcome. *Fertil Steril.* 2011;95:857-866.

26. Bree RL, Edwards M, Böhm-Velez M, Beyler S, Roberts J, Mendelson EB. Transvaginal sonography in the evaluation of normal early pregnancy: correlation with hCG level. *AJR Am J Roentgenol.* 1989;153:75-79.

27. Goldstein I, Zimmer EA, Tamir A, Peretz BA, Paldi E. Evaluation of normal gestational sac growth: appearance of embryonic heartbeat and embryo body movements using the transvaginal technique. *Obstet Gynecol.* 1991;77:885-888.

28. Barnhart KT, Sammel MD, Rinaudo PF, Zhou L, Hummel AC, Guo W. Symptomatic patients with an early viable intrauterine pregnancy: HCG curves redefined. *Obstet Gynecol.* 2004;104:50-55.

29. American College of Obstetricians and Gynecologists. ACOG practice bulletin no. 193: tubal ectopic pregnancy. *Obstet Gynecol.* 2018;131:e91-e103.

30. Shaunik A, Kulp J, Appleby DH, Sammel MD, Barnhart KT. Utility of dilation and curettage in the diagnosis of pregnancy of unknown location. *Am J Obstet Gynecol.* 2011;204:130.e1-130.e6.

31. Rivera V, Nguyen PH, Sit A. Change in quantitative human chorionic gonadotropin after manual vacuum aspiration in women with pregnancy of unknown location. *Am J Obstet Gynecol.* 2009;200:e56-e59.

32. Barash JH, Buchanan EM, Hillson C. Diagnosis and management of ectopic pregnancy. *Am Fam Physician.* 2014;90(1):34-40.

33. Practice Committee of American Society for Reproductive Medicine. Medical treatment of ectopic pregnancy: a committee opinion. *Fertil Steril.* 2013;100(3):638-644. doi:10.1016/j.fertnstert.2013.06.013.

34. Committee on Practice Bulletins—Gynecology. The American College of Obstetricians and Gynecologists Practice Bulletin no. 150. Early pregnancy loss. *Obstet Gynecol.* 2015;125(5):1258.

35. Weeks A, Faúndes A. Misoprostol in obstetrics and gynecology. *Int J Gynaecol Obstet.* 2007;99 (suppl 2):S156-S159.

36. American College of Obstetricians and Gynecologists. Medical management of first-trimester abortion. Practice Bulletin No. 143. *Obstet Gynecol* 2014;123:676-692.

What Is the Gestational Age?

Erin S. L. Huntley, DO and Benjamin J. F. Huntley, MD, FAAFP

● Clinical Vignette

A 32-year-old gravida 4, para 2-0-1-2 with a history of obesity and oligomenorrhea presents to clinic to establish care as a new patient. She had a positive home pregnancy test that is confirmed by repeating in the office, but she does not recall her last menstrual period. What is the gestational age?

TABLE 28-1	Factors Associated With Inaccurate Dating

1. Younger age
2. Lower education
3. Publicly insured
4. Nonwhite ethnicity
5. Unmarried
6. Late to prenatal care or no prenatal care

Pearl M, Weir ML, Kharrazi M. Assessing the quality of last menstrual period date on California birth records. *Pediatr Perinat Epidemiol.* 2007;21(suppl 2):50-61. Buekens P, Delvoye P, Wollast E, Robyn C. Epidemiology of pregnancies with unknown last menstrual period. *J Epidemiol Community Health.* 1984;38:79-80.

LITERATURE REVIEW

Traditionally, the estimated date of delivery (EDD) is calculated by adding 280 days to the date of the first day of the last menstrual period (LMP). This assumes a regular 28-day cycle with ovulation occurring on the 14th day. However, up to 29% of women have at least one short or long menstrual cycle per year, which leads to inaccuracy in reported LMP and EDD calculation.[1] Additionally, there are many factors that are associated with inaccurate LMP dating (Table 28-1).[2,3] For these reasons, it is important to verify EDD with sonographic measurements as early in pregnancy as possible. Ultrasound measurement of the embryo or fetus in the first trimester is the most accurate method for establishing or confirming gestational age and should be done in each pregnancy.[4] The later a dating ultrasound is performed in pregnancy, the less accurate it is. This is especially true beyond 22 weeks of gestation. Therefore,

when a patient initially presents later than the first trimester, it is prudent to perform a sonogram at the first prenatal visit to decrease inaccuracy.

Ultrasonographic markers of development appear in a predictable timeline in the first trimester and can be reliably used for estimating gestational age. The gestational sac can be seen at approximately 4 weeks and will grow 1 mm/day in mean sac diameter (MSD) until the 9th week. By 5.5 weeks, the yolk sac appears, and by 6 weeks the fetal pole is evident. Fetal cardiac activity should be seen by 6.5 weeks or with a crown-rump length (CRL) measuring 7 mm. Using these markers will help define gestational age very early in pregnancy (**Figure 28-1**).

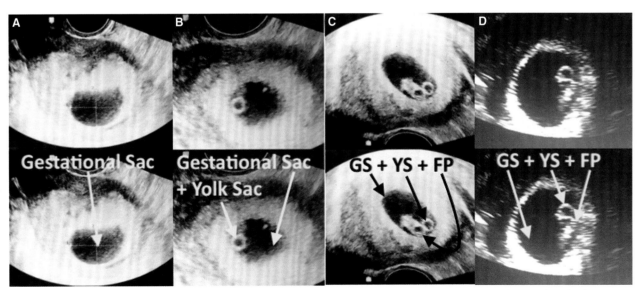

FIGURE 28-1. Transvaginal views demonstrating progression of fetal developmental markers. A, An empty gestational sac (GS) corresponding to a gestational age of 4 to 5 weeks. B, GS and yolk sac (YS) without fetal pole (FP) corresponding to 5 to 5.5 weeks of gestational age. C, GS, YS, and FP corresponding to 6 weeks of gestational age, although crown-rump length (CRL) measurement would be the most accurate way to date this pregnancy. D, GS, YS, and FP. Note how the YS could be mistaken for a fetal head and mistakenly incorporated into the CRL if care were not taken.

When the fetal pole is visible, the most accurate method of estimating the gestational age is by incorporating the CRL measurement. The earlier the CRL is performed, the more accurate it is, and the gestational age can be estimated within 5 days in early pregnancy and within 7 days later in the first trimester. In very early pregnancies, the fetal pole may not be accurately visualized via transabdominal ultrasonography, and transvaginal imaging may be necessary. However, as long as a fetal pole can be seen via the transabdominal route, the estimates of gestational age calculated from it are just as accurate as those obtained transvaginally.[5] Later in pregnancy, estimates of gestational age based on CRL become unacceptably inaccurate, regardless of the method used to obtain them. Therefore, the CRL should be used only up to a gestational age of 14 weeks or a corresponding CRL of 84 mm.[6]

Beyond 14 weeks of gestational age, calculation using complete fetal biometry is more accurate. There are four standard measurements currently recommended by the American Institute of Ultrasound in Medicine (**Table 28-2**): biparietal diameter (BPD), head circumference (HC), femur length (FL), and abdominal circumference (AC).[7] Biometric measurements are typically measured via a transabdominal approach owing to larger fetal size and marked anatomic detail seen after 14 weeks. Fetal biometry is most easily measured before the fetus presents deeper in the pelvis. Therefore, 18 to 20 weeks is the ideal gestational age for initial biometric assessment.

Early in the second trimester, HC is the most reliable independent parameter of age estimation. It is accurate to within 1 week between the gestational ages of 14 and 20 weeks. As gestation advances into the third trimester, accuracy wanes to plus or minus 3 weeks. The FL is often the easiest value to obtain and is accurate in the early second trimester to ±1 week but becomes increasingly less accurate as gestational age advances. Late third trimester FL measurements are accurate only within 3.5 weeks of the true gestational age. The AC has the largest variability of the four measurements. The accuracy of this measure wanes significantly as gestational age advances and in the late third trimester has the poorest reliability at 4.5 weeks. However, this measurement most accurately reflects fetal weight. Historically, multiple formulas have been employed to estimate fetal weight based; however, the most common formula used in the United States is the Hadlock formula, which is accurate to within 15% of actual birth weight.[7]

Although each of these biometric parameters has its own benefits and limitations, the collective use of all four together to obtain a calculated ultrasound age results in the greatest accuracy and is the recommended approach. Most ultrasounds commercially available today can perform this calculation after biometric measurements are obtained. The result of the calculation that incorporates all the biometric parameters is generally referred to as the average ultrasound age (AUA). Because confidence intervals widen as gestational age advances, once gestational age is confirmed by the first ultrasound, the estimated due date should not change—every subsequent biometric measurement becomes simply an index of fetal growth.

The Big Five

Every time an obstetric ultrasound is performed, there are five key components that should be assessed, if possible. These components all play an important role in management of pregnancy and can be rapidly and easily assessed by ultrasonography. We refer to these as The Big Five. The Big Five consists of fetal lie, amniotic fluid, fetal cardiac activity, placental location, and fetal number (**Table 28-3**). Fetal lie is defined by the fetal part that lies directly over the pelvic inlet. This is most important in the later third trimester as breech presentations require planning prior to delivery. Cardiac activity is best documented by video or M-mode. It is important to evaluate presence of cardiac activity to determine fetal health and viability. Amniotic fluid can be quantified via single deepest pocket or amniotic fluid index or qualitatively reported as adequate or inadequate by experienced evaluators and is a good indicator of fetal health. Placental location should be assessed to assure it does not come near to the internal os of the cervix. Low-lying placenta or placenta previa will require monitoring and potentially c-section if persistent into the third trimester. Finally, singleton or multiple fetus is reported by fetal number and independent placental, amniotic fluid, fetal cardiac activity, and fetal lie should be reported for each as appropriate.

TABLE 28-2 **Summary of Biometric Scan Planes**

Crown-rump length (CRL)
- True midsagittal plane
- Fetal spine longitudinally in view
- Fetus in neutral flexed position
- Maximum length from cranium to caudal rump measured as a straight line

Biparietal diameter (BPD) and head circumference (HC)
- Through third ventricle and thalami
- Perpendicular to parietal bones
- Calvaria should be symmetrical
- BPD measured from outer edge of anterior bone to inner edge of posterior bone
- HC measured with ellipse around outer edge of entirety of fetal cranium

Abdominal circumference (AC)
- Axial plane of fetus
- Above the kidneys
- Below the heart
- Stomach is visible
- Umbilical vein/portal sinus "hockey stick"
- Ellipse around skin

Femur length (FL)
- Align the transducer with the long axis of the bone
- Ideally, femur is parallel to probe

Adapted from AIUM practice guideline for the performance of obstetric ultrasound examinations.

TABLE 28-3 **Basic Components of Point-of-Care Obstetric Ultrasound**

The Big Five:
1. Fetal lie
2. Amniotic fluid
3. Fetal cardiac activity
4. Placenta location
5. Fetal number

Adapted from AIUM practice guideline for the performance of obstetric ultrasound examinations.

TABLE 28-4	Recommendations for Use of Point-of-Care Ultrasound in Clinical Practice		
Recommendation		**Rating**	**Rating**
The first trimester of pregnancy is the most accurate timing of determining gestational age and should be the goal of each pregnancy.		A	6
Ultrasound examination is recommended in every pregnancy. At all gestational ages, it is an accurate method of determining gestational age, fetal number, viability, and placental location.		A	13
A conversation detailing the limitations and benefits of ultrasound should be had with each patient.		C	14
18-22 weeks of gestation is the optimal timing for a single ultrasound examination without other specific indications.		C	14

A = consistent, good-quality patient-oriented evidence; B = inconsistent or limited-quality patient-oriented evidence; C = consensus, disease-oriented evidence, usual practice, expert opinion, or case series. For information about the SORT evidence rating system, go to http://www.aafp.org/afpsort.

PERFORMING THE SCAN

Step 1: Positioning. Begin with a transabdominal transducer. Have the patient lie supine with left lateral tilt, displacing the uterus off the maternal vena cava, which allows for adequate maternal right-sided return, maintained cardiac output, and uteroplacental perfusion. For a transabdominal approach keep a full bladder to move bowel out of the pelvis, and utilize this fluid window for viewing the uterus. If structures are poorly visualized because of small size and cannot be accurately measured, a transvaginal probe can be used. For a transvaginal approach, have the patient empty her bladder to prevent displacement of the uterus away from the probe.

Step 2: Probe and image orientation. In order to maximize the likelihood of accurate image acquisition and interpretation, arrange the ultrasound on the same side of the bed, and conduct scanning in the same fashion every time to facilitate linking hand-eye coordination with basal ganglion learned motor movements.

Traditionally, a curvilinear abdominal probe with machine settings set to obstetric mode is used to acquire transabdominal obstetric ultrasonographic images. By convention, when imaging maternal structures, the probe is held in the sagittal plane with the indicator toward the maternal cranium or in an orthogonal plane so as to capture an axial scan plane with the indicator toward the maternal right side (**Figure 28-2**). However, deviation from these planes is often necessary to image fetal structures. Adjust depth and gain accordingly.

Step 3: Measuring the embryo or fetus. Begin with a transabdominal probe and make large sweeping translational motions across the maternal abdomen just superior to the pubic symphysis to identify the uterus. Systematically evaluate the intrauterine contents in a gridlike pattern. For the experienced sonographer, this should take no more than 10 seconds. Decide which method will be most accurate

for dating the pregnancy. CRL should be chosen if the gestational age appears to be less than 14 weeks or a corresponding CRL of 84 mm. If the pregnancy appears more advanced, then perform full biometry without CRL measurement.

Crown-Rump Length

Identify the gestational sac within the uterus. Rotation of the probe marker 90° counterclockwise or clockwise will change the scan plane to a transverse plane or coronal view of the pelvis (**Figures 28-3 and 28-4**). If a fetal pole is seen, align with its long axis using these methods of alternating probe orientation and then freeze the screen. This measurement should be obtained in a true midsagittal plane, with the fetal spine longitudinally in view and the maximum length from cranium to caudal rump measured as a straight line (**Figure 28-5**).

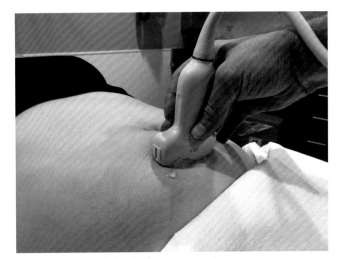

FIGURE 28-2. Transabdominal sonogram setup.

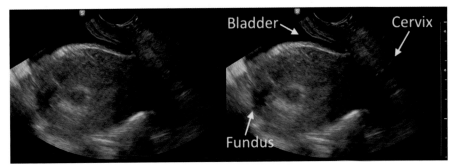

FIGURE 28-3. Pelvic transvaginal sagittal scan plane (sono pic).

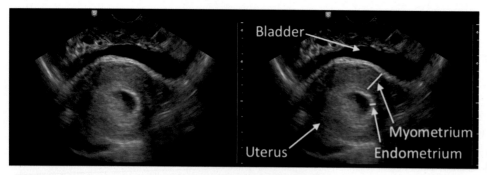

FIGURE 28-4. Pelvic transvaginal transverse scan plane (sono pic).

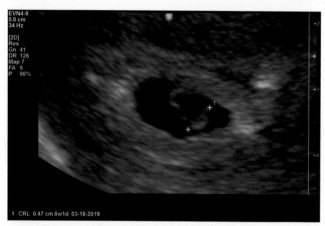

FIGURE 28-5. Crown-rump length markers (sono pic).

The measurement should be obtained when the fetus is in a resting, flexed position. Measure the CRL on three separately acquired images. Choose the report function to view a gestational age calculated from the measurements.

Full Biometry Without CRL Measurement

Head Circumference

If intrauterine fetal structures are clearly seen transabdominally, continue fetal biometry via the transabdominal approach. Find the appropriate scan plane for obtaining both the HC and the BPD by identifying the thalami in a plane parallel to the base of the skull. The cavum septum pellucidi (CSP) should be seen anterior to the thalamai (**Figure 28-6**). In the appropriate scan plane, the fetal skull should appear smooth and symmetrical bilaterally and be oval in shape.[8] With the image frozen, place an ellipse around the outer edge of the fetal skull but take care not to include cranial skin (**Figure 28-7**).

Biparietal Diameter

Use the identical scan plane to identify the BPD as that used for the HC—the plane must transverse the third ventricle and thalami, and the calvaria must be smooth and symmetric bilaterally (**Figure 28-8**). Once this view is achieved, freeze the image and place the cursors from the outer edge of the near calvarium to the inner edge of the far calvarium (**Figure 28-9**).

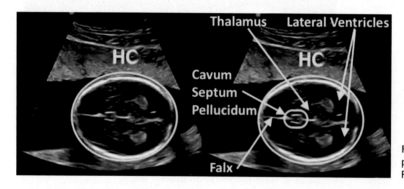

FIGURE 28-6. Head circumference (HC) with annotated scan plane landmarks. Courtesy of Kevin Bergman, Contra Costa Regional Medical Center.

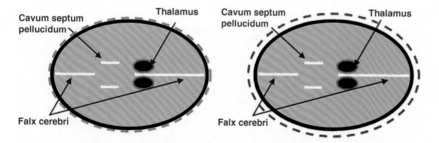

Yes   No

FIGURE 28-7. Diagram of inappropriate ellipse placement in head circumference.

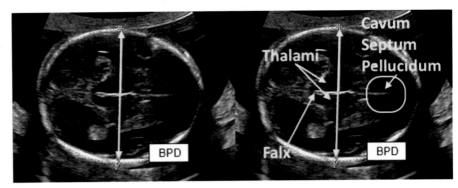

FIGURE 28-8. Biparietal diameter (BPD) with annotated scan plane landmarks. Courtesy of Kevin Bergman, Contra Costa Regional Medical Center.

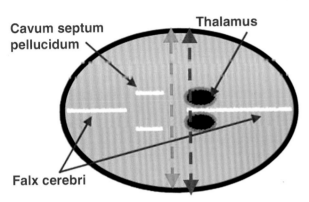

FIGURE 28-9. Diagram of inappropriate caliper placement in biparietal diameter measurement. The green hashed arrow indicates proper placement from outer table of the leading cranial edge to the inner table of the distant cranial edge, and the red hashed arrow indicates incorrect placement.

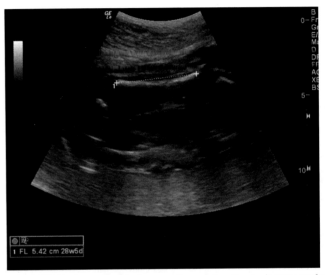

FIGURE 28-10. Sonographic image of correct caliper placement for femur length measurement.

Femur Length

To obtain the FL, align the transducer parallel to the axis of the femur so as to capture the longest possible measurement. Be sure to obtain an image in which the femur is perpendicular to the ultrasound beam, and only measure the femur closest to the transducer that will appear at the top of the screen (**Figure 28-10**). Be sure to only measure the blunt ends of the ossified femur. Do not include any "spines" protruding from the femur, and do not include the hypoechoic diaphysis (**Figure 28-11**).[9]

Abdominal Circumference

Obtain the proper scan plane with an axial image through the fetal abdomen, coursing transversely through the liver at its widest part. It should be caudal to the fetal heart but cranial to the fetal kidneys. The stomach should be visualized as an anechoic circular structure. The spine should be visualized with one rib coming off both sides. The umbilical vein should have a "hockey stick" appearance (**Figure 28-12**). Freeze the image and place the ellipse measurement around the circumference. The correct measurement is fitted to the skin edges (**Figure 28-13**).

Calculate Average Ultrasound Age and Estimated Fetal Weight

Once HC, BPD, FL, and AC values have been collected and saved, choose the report function on the sonogram machine, and the calculated AUA and estimated fetal weight (EFW) will be displayed.

Step 4: The Big Five. Take note of the fetal lie. Start with the transducer transverse just above the pubic bone and then scan

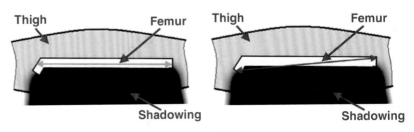

FIGURE 28-11. Diagram of incorrect measurement of femur length.

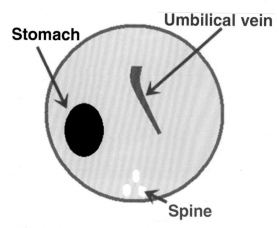

FIGURE 28-12. Diagram of correct orientation of umbilical and hepatic vasculature in abdominal circumference measurement. Courtesy of Kevin Bergman, Contra Costa Regional Medical Center.

superiorly on the mother's abdomen. Notice the order of appearance of the head, thorax, and abdomen. Examples of fetal lie include cephalic, breech, transverse and cord. In noncephalic fetal lie, it may be beneficial to find the fetal cranium and follow its corresponding spine until the point closest to the cervical os is reached. Turn the probe into a sagittal plane to confirm the findings.

Assess the amniotic fluid. Divide the abdomen into four equal quadrants and the ultrasound transducer applied perpendicular to the floor. The largest pocket of amniotic fluid without fetal parts or umbilical cord, measuring at least 1 cm in width at the narrowest point of each quadrant, is identified and the image is frozen. Calipers are used to measure vertical pockets of amniotic fluid perpendicular to the floor, and the sum of these four values yields the amniotic fluid index (**Figure 28-14**). In the case of a multiple pregnancy, amniotic fluid values should be recorded separately for each amniotic sac. See Chapter 29 for more details.

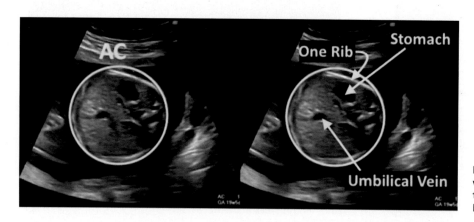

FIGURE 28-13. Abdominal circumference (AC) with annotated scan plane landmarks. Courtesy of Kevin Bergman, Contra Costa Regional Medical Center.

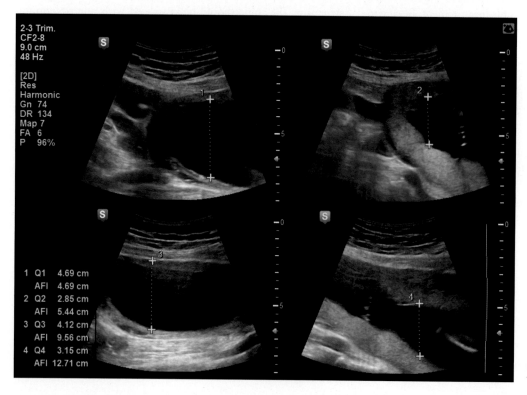

1	Q1	4.69 cm
	AFI	4.69 cm
2	Q2	2.85 cm
	AFI	5.44 cm
3	Q3	4.12 cm
	AFI	9.56 cm
4	Q4	3.15 cm
	AFI	12.71 cm

FIGURE 28-14. Normal amniotic fluid index.

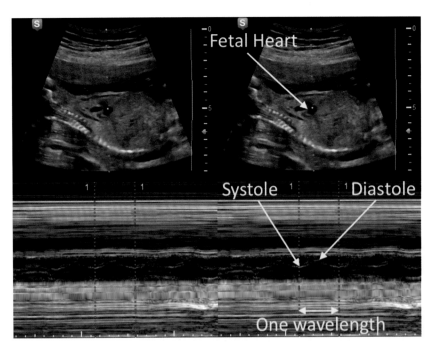

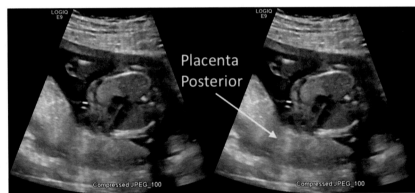

FIGURE 28-15. In the two-dimensional image of the fetus (top window), M-mode is used to display a dynamic waveform of the fetal heart (bottom window) to calculate fetal heart rate.

FIGURE 28-16. Normal posterior placenta. Note the surrounding hypoechoic myometrium. The internal cervical os is not in view in this image.

Assess fetal cardiac activity using M-mode. To acquire M-mode data on most ultrasound machines, tap the M-mode button once to superimpose a linear vector over the two-dimensional display and ensure that the line passes through the area of interest. Click the M-mode button again to acquire the proper image. Hit freeze and use the ultrasound's calculator function to place the crosshairs on identical locations of offset wave points to calculate the fetal heart rate (**Figure 28-15**).

Assess placental location. Sweep the abdomen with the curvilinear probe in transverse plane and identify the placental location. The placenta will appear as a hyperechoic structure attached internally to the myometrium. It will be homogeneous early in pregnancy and may develop areas of hyperechoic calcifications later in pregnancy (**Figure 28-16**). Take note of proximity to the cervix. It is important to scan fully from one side of the placenta to the other in the transverse and sagittal planes because there may be areas that protrude from the main structure. If the closest part of the placenta appears to be within 2 cm of the internal os, a confirmatory transvaginal examination is warranted.

Assess for multiple gestations. Sweep fully through the entire uterus in the transverse and sagittal planes. If multiples are suspected, find a fetal cranium and follow its corresponding spine to be convinced of that fetus's position and corresponding small parts before trying to identify any subsequent unique fetus. Capture a screenshot of two fetal craniums in the same scan plane, if possible. By convention, fetus A is designated as the fetus closest to the internal cervical os.

PATIENT MANAGEMENT

Once sonographic gestational age is obtained, it is compared to that calculated from the LMP. The decision to change the working EDD of the pregnancy is very important and should be done only on the basis of strict guidelines as the implications for future management of the pregnancy, such as future sonograms to evaluate growth and timing of delivery, are directly dependent on this. Changing the working EDD for the pregnancy should occur only on the basis of the first ultrasound performed and only if the AUA is outside the margin of error, which is increasingly broad later in the pregnancy (Table 28-5 and **Figure 28-17**).

In addition to assessment of gestational age, assessment of the EFW may be necessary in pregnancies at risk for growth restriction or macrosomia. Furthermore, if at any point the fundal height deviates more than 3 cm from the gestational age, concern for abnormal fetal growth should stimulate sonographic growth evaluation.

Intrauterine growth restriction (IUGR) is defined as an EFW of less than the 10th percentile. Hypertensive diseases affecting pregnancy increase the risk, and it is recommended that the assessment of EFW occur every 4 weeks in the third trimester. IUGR is important to identify

TABLE 28-5	Guidelines for Redating Based on Ultrasonography		
Gestational Age Range[a]	**Method of Measurement**	**Discrepancy Between Ultrasound Dating and LMP Dating That Supports Redating**	
≤13 6/7 wk	CRL		
• ≤8 6/7 wk		More than 5 d	
• 9 0/7 wk to 13 6/7 wk		More than 7 d	
14 0/7 wk to 15 6/7 wk	BPD, HC, AC, FL	More than 7 d	
16 0/7 wk to 21 6/7 wk	BPD, HC, AC, FL	More than 10 d	
22 0/7 wk to 27 6/7 wk	BPD, HC, AC, FL	More than 14 d	
28 0/7 wk and beyond[b]	BPD, HC, AC, FL	More than 21 d	

[a]Based on LMP.
[b]Because of the risk of redating a small fetus that may be growth restricted, management decisions based on third-trimester ultrasonography alone are especially problematic and need to be guided by careful consideration of the entire clinical picture and close surveillance.

Abbreviations: AC, abdominal circumference; BPD, biparietal diameter; CRL, crown-rump length; FL, femur length; HC, head circumference; LMP, last menstrual period.

Reprinted with permission from Committee on Obstetric Practice, the American Institute of Ultrasound in Medicine, and the Society for Maternal-Fetal Medicine. Committee Opinion No 700: methods for estimating the due date. *Obstet Gynecol.* 2017;129(5):e150-e154. Copyright © 2017 by The American College of Obstetricians and Gynecologists.

because affected pregnancies are at increased risk of stillbirth and neonatal morbidity and mortality. The risk is even higher for pregnancies affected early or with severe IUGR with EFW below the 3rd percentile. Because of the risk, serial assessment of fetal well-being is important once IUGR is diagnosed. Frequent nonstress testing, amniotic fluid index measurements, and biophysical profiles are all methods of evaluating fetal well-being; however, Doppler velocimetry is the only testing that will reflect abnormalities prior to the onset of fetal acidemia and thus facilitate interventions and potential delivery prior to perinatal mortality.

A challenge exists in identifying those fetuses who are constitutionally small versus those pathologically underachieving their growth potential. This is especially difficult in patients that presented late to prenatal care without an early determination of fetal age. In these instances, it can be impossible to know whether a pregnancy measuring small for expected dates is due to IUGR or inaccurate dating. In every case, it is important to track serial growth measurements every 3 to 4 weeks to assess whether growth percentile is consistent. The interval for growth assessment should never be less than 2 weeks, because this would increase the risk of false-positive diagnosis of abnormal fetal growth because of intrinsic variability of measurements. If growth is consistent along percentile lines at follow-up assessment, then it is most likely a normal pregnancy that was dated incorrectly or that is constitutionally small. If, however, growth percentiles are dropping, IUGR is the most likely cause.

Fetal macrosomia describes a fetus overachieving its growth potential greater than EFW of 4500 g per the American Congress of Obstetricians and Gynecologists (ACOG). Common risk factors include maternal obesity, pregestational and gestational diabetes, postdates pregnancy, and prior macrocosmic pregnancy. Such pregnancies are at elevated risk of adverse events surrounding delivery, such as shoulder dystocia, fetal injury, postpartum hemorrhage, and sphincter lacerations. The ACOG recommends screening for macrosomia with ultrasound assessment of EFW at 36 weeks and consideration of planned cesarean delivery for EFW >4500 g in women with diabetes and EFW >5000 g in women without diabetes.[10]

The absolute error of assessment of fetal growth increases as pregnancy advances, with only 50% of fetuses estimated to be larger than 4500 g achieving a birth weight within 10% of the sonographically estimated weight. However marginal, it remains the best predictor of fetal weight and the best tool in the management of potential birth complications.

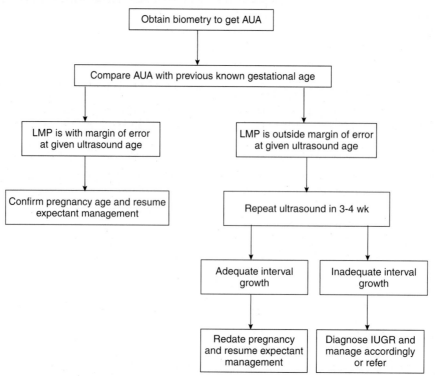

FIGURE 28-17. Algorithm for determining gestational age by last menstrual period (LMP) or ultrasound. AUA, average ultrasound age; IUGR, intrauterine growth restriction.

PEARLS AND PITFALLS

Pearls

- If no fetal pole is seen, measure the MSD by measuring the sac height and width in the sagittal plane and then measure the sac width in the transverse plane. Find the mean of these measurements to find the MSD. The MSD plus 30 estimates the number of days of gestational age. This can be divided by 7 to find the gestational age in weeks. Although this can provide an estimate of gestational age, the patient should still follow up for a CRL measurement because this is the most accurate method of dating.
- When patients present late for prenatal care and EFW is measuring small for expected gestational age, it can be difficult to differentiate IUGR from incorrect dating. As mentioned earlier, the patient should be followed with serial growth scans to help differentiate between the two. However, additional measurements performed at that time can be helpful. The cerebellum grows at a predictable and constant rate even in the presence of IUGR. The transcerebellar diameter to AC ratio is therefore constant (0.14 + 0.01; mean + standard deviation [SD]) throughout normal pregnancy, and a ratio exceeding 2 SD above the mean is predictive of growth restriction[11] (**Figure 28-18**).

Pitfalls

- When measuring the CRL, take care not to accidentally include the yolk sac or a fetal limb in the measurement (Figure 28-1D).
- When measuring the FL, it is possible to confuse other fetal long bones, such as the tibia or humerus, with the femur. It is best to be sure that both ends of the suspected femur articulate with the correct structures—the pelvis and a second long bone, the tibia.
- When obtaining the image for HC and BPD, be sure the plane of cut is correct. The thalami and CSP should be visualized. The orbits and cerebellum should not be in the image. The shape should be oval and not circular.
- When measuring the BPD, be sure to measure from the outside to the inside of the skull when going from top to bottom of the screen. A common mistake is placing the calipers incorrectly, resulting in incorrect measurement, that is, outer to outer, inner to inner.
- When measuring the AC, be sure to trace around the outer skin edges, including all subcutaneous tissue. Otherwise, the measurements will underestimate fetal weight.
- Be sure to isolate the umbilical vein so that it is not touching the outer AC. If it is, the transducer is angled too inferiorly rather than perpendicularly to the midline.[12]
- Attempt to insonate the abdomen from an angle that places the fetal spine at the sides or bottom of the screen. This will help prevent shadow artifact from obscuring the other abdominal structures.

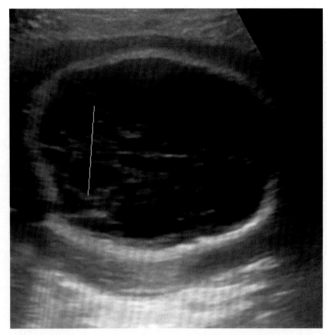

FIGURE 28-18. A sonographic image of the cerebellum with a caliper marking the transverse cerebellar diameter. This plane is obtained by finding the plane used for the head circumference (HC) and biparietal diameter (BPD) measurements and slightly rotating the probe inferiorly over the posterior brain until the cerebellum comes into view.

BILLING

CPT Code	Description	Global Payment	Professional Component	Technical Component
76801	Ultrasound, pregnant uterus, real time with image documentation, fetal and maternal evaluation, first trimester (14 wk 0 d), single or first gestation	$126.33	$51.32	$75.01
76805	Ultrasound, pregnant uterus, fetal and maternal evaluation, > first trimester; single or first gestation	$145.71	$51.68	$94.03

CPT codes and average national reimbursement for Medicare in 2016. Payment data are from https://www.cms.gov/apps/physician-fee-schedule/search/search-criteria.aspx. See Chapter 2 for details on ultrasound billing.

References

1. Munster K, Schmidt L, Helm P. Length and variation in the menstrual cycle—a cross section study. *Br J Obstet Gynecol*. 1992;99:422-429.

2. Pearl M, Weir ML, Kharrazi M. Assessing the quality of last menstrual period date on California birth records. *Pediatr Perinat Epidemiol*. 2007;21(suppl 2):50-61.

3. Buekens P, Delvoye P, Wollast E, Robyn C. Epidemiology of pregnancies with unknown last menstrual period. *J Epidemiol Community Health*. 1984;38:79-80.

4. Moorthy RS. Transvaginal sonography. *Med J Armed Forces*. 2000;56(3):181-183.

5. Grisolia G, Milano K, Pilu G, et al. Biometry of early pregnancy with transvaginal sonography. *Ultrasound Obstet Gynecol*. 1993;3(6):403-411.

6. American College of Obstetricians and Gynecologists. *ACOG Committee Opinion #700: Methods for Estimating Due Date*. Washington, DC: American College of Obstetricians and Gynecologists; 2017.

7. Hadlock FP. Sonographic estimation of fetal age and weight. *Radiol Clin North Am*. 1990;28:39.

8. Shepard M, Filly RA. A standardized plane for biparietal diameter measurement. *J Ultrasound Med*. 1982;1:145.

9. Goldstein RB, Filly RA, Simpson G. Pitfalls in femur length measurements. *J Ultrasound Med*. 1987;6:203.

10. American College of Obstetricians and Gynecologists' Committee on Practice Bulletins—Obstetrics. Practice Bulletin No. 173: fetal macrosomia. *Obstet Gynecol*. 2016;128(5):e195-e209.

11. Dilmen G, Toppare MF, Turhan NO, Oztürk M, Işik S. Transverse cerebellar diameter and transverse cerebellar diameter/abdominal circumference index for assessing fetal growth. *Fetal Diagn Ther*. 1996;11(1):50-56.

12. Chinn DH, Filly RA, Callen PW. Ultrasound evaluation of fetal umbilical and hepatic vascular anatomy. *Radiology*. 1982;144:153.

13. American Institute of Ultrasound in Medicine. AIUM practice guideline for the performance of obstetric ultrasound examinations. *J Ultrasound Med*. 2013;32:1083–1101. doi:10.7863/ultra.32.6.1083.

14. American College of Obstetricians and Gynecologists. ACOG Practice Bulletin no. 175: Ultrasound in Pregnancy. *Obstet Gynecol*. 2016;128:e241-e256.

What Is the Status of Fetal Well-Being?

Benjamin J. F. Huntley, MD, FAAFP and Brandon Williamson, MD

● Clinical Vignette

A 19-year-old primigravida at 34 weeks 6 days presents to the outpatient clinic with a complaint of decreased fetal movement since the previous night. Thus far, she has had an uncomplicated pregnancy. Her vitals and physical examination are normal, but nonstress testing (NST) is not available in the clinic. What is the status of fetal well-being?

LITERATURE REVIEW

The goal of antepartum fetal testing is to identify pregnancies at increased risk for morbidity or mortality. It is important to identify pregnancies that may require intervention while avoiding inappropriate intervention in healthy pregnancies. Antepartum fetal surveillance is performed for a variety of maternal or pregnancy-related conditions.[1] The most common indication is decreased fetal movement (Table 29-1).

Antepartum testing takes advantage of the fact that fetuses respond to hypoxemia in a predictable fashion. Pathophysiologic changes manifest in a stepwise fashion and include heart rate decelerations, loss of variability in the fetal heart tracing, reduction in fetal activity, and decrease in amniotic fluid levels. Different methods of antepartum testing incorporate aspects of these changes and include the NST, the contraction stress test, the biophysical profile (BPP), and the modified biophysical profile (mBPP) (see summary of test properties in Table 29-2[1]). Of these different methods, the BPP and mBPP can be performed with ultrasound in the primary care setting.

Appropriate interpretation of antenatal testing requires an appreciation of fetal neurologic function. Near term, a fetus spends approximately 60% to 70% of its time in an *active* sleep state, lasting

TABLE 29-1 Indications for Antepartum Testing

Indication	Starting Gestational Age	Frequency of Biophysical Profile
A2 gestational diabetes mellitus (DM)	32 wk	Weekly
Type 1 or 2 DM	28-32 wk depending upon glycemic control and complications	Weekly, biweekly beginning at 32 wk
High-risk chronic hypertension (HTN; medications/comorbidity)	32 wk	Weekly, with consideration of biweekly at 36 wk
Gestational HTN (mild)	At diagnosis	Weekly
Gestational HTN (severe)	At diagnosis	Weekly, with consideration of biweekly at 36 wk
Preeclampsia without severe features	At diagnosis	Biweekly
Preeclampsia with severe features	At diagnosis	Biweekly
Antiphospholipid syndrome	32 wk	Weekly
Cholestasis	At diagnosis	Weekly
Hemoglobinopathies	32 wk	Weekly, biweekly at 36 wk
Hyperthyroidism	37 wk	Weekly
Renal disease	32 wk	Weekly
Systemic lupus erythematosus (SLE)	32 wk	Weekly, with consideration of earlier and more frequent testing in active disease
AMA (over 40 y old)	36 wk	Weekly
Major fetal anomalies	32 wk	Weekly
Fetal growth restriction	At diagnosis ≥28 wk	Weekly with umbilical artery Doppler
Multifetal gestation	28-36 wk depending upon chorionicity, amnionicity, and complications	Weekly vs. biweekly depending on chorionicity, amnionicity, and complications
Oligohydramnios	At diagnosis ≥28 wk	Weekly
Late term or postterm pregnancy	41 wk 0 d	Weekly
Previous intrauterine fetal demise	32 wk (or 2 wk prior to past loss)	Weekly
Decreased fetal movement	At diagnosis	Once

Indications, mode of testing, start dates, and frequency of testing are variable by region and practice. Antepartum testing for an individual patient must take into account these factors as well as appropriate referral.

Abbreviation: AMA, advanced maternal age.

TABLE 29-2	Summary of Antepartum Fetal Surveillance Modalities		
Test Name	**Description**	**Results**	**Interpretation**
Maternal Movement Assessment	Subjective perception of changes in fetal movement or objective tally of fetal movement over a set period of time ("Fetal kick counts")	No evidence-based recommendations to define optimal number of movements or time duration	Subjective decreased fetal movement confers increased risk of adverse perinatal outcomes; however, effectiveness in preventing stillbirth is uncertain
Contraction Stress Test (CST)	Monitor response of fetal heart rate to uterine contractions. Three contractions ≥40 s/10 min period required; oxytocin augmentation or nipple stimulation if parameters not met spontaneously. Assess for presence or absence of late fetal decelerations	Negative: no late decelerations Positive: late decelerations with ≥50% of contractions Equivocal-suspicious: variable decelerations, or late decelerations with <50% of contractions Equivocal: decelerations >q2 min or lasting >90 s Unsatisfactory: <3 contractions in 10 min or an uninterpretable tracing	Stillbirth rate 0.3 per 1000 in negative CST
Nonstress Test (NST)	Assess for spontaneous fetal heart rate accelerations (duration >15 s, with achieved peak > 15 bpm above baseline if >32 wk gestational age (GA), or >10 bpm if <32 wk GA) over 20 min sample; may extend to 40 min or include vibroacoustic stimulation if nonreactive	Reactive: ≥2 accelerations/20 min Nonreactive: <2 accelerations/20 min	Stillbirth rate 1.9 per 1000 in reactive NST If nonreactive, stillbirth rate is variable: pursue CST or BPP
Modified Biophysical Profile (mBPP)	NST and amniotic fluid assessment	Normal: Reactive NST and single deepest pocket (SDP) >2 cm Abnormal: either nonreactive NST or SDP <2 cm	Stillbirth rate for normal mBPP: 0.8 per 1000 If abnormal, stillbirth rate is variable: pursue CST or BPP
Biophysical Profile (BPP)	NST, sonographic assessment of: amniotic fluid volume, fetal breathing, fetal movement, and fetal tone	8 or 10: normal 6: equivocal 4, 2, or 0: abnormal Regardless of score, oligohydramnios warrants further evaluation at any GA	BPP 8 or 10: stillbirth rate 0.8 per 1000 BPP of 6 or less, stillbirth rate variable: further evaluation or delivery as indicated

Note there is a lack of high-quality evidence from randomized controlled trials (RCTs) that antepartum fetal surveillance decreases the risk of fetal death. These tests do not predict acute changes such as placental abruption or umbilical cord accidents. In general, these tests have high false-positive rates, low positive predictive values, and high negative predictive values. Note that whenever oligohydramnios is present, delivery is typically indicated between 36 and 37 weeks; at <36 weeks, if expectantly managed, then follow antepartum testing and fetal growth ultrasounds.

around 40 minutes at a time and associated with regular breathing movements, intermittent head, limb and trunk movements, increased fetal heart rate, variability, and frequency of accelerations detected on continuous fetal monitoring. Fetuses spend approximately 25% of their time in *quiet* sleep states, which last around 20 minutes at a time in duration and are associated with a slowing of the fetal heart rate and decreased variability.[2]

In addition to physiologic cycles, fetal movements are affected by external factors such as maternal activity, nutrition, and ingestion of drugs or medications. Steroids, tobacco, sedatives, and opioids are all associated with decreased fetal movement and low BPP scores.[3] As gestational age progresses, the range of normal fetal inactivity lengthens, with upper limits of normal reaching 75 minutes without detectable fetal movement.[4]

In a normally developing fetus, certain characteristics develop in a stepwise fashion and can be observed on ultrasonography. In order of appearance these are tone, gross movement, breathing movements, and heart rate variability. When asphyxia develops, compromised fetuses lose these characteristics in reverse order.[5] Given that variability of fetal heart rate is the last of the findings to develop, the earliest sign of compromise may be detected by a nonreactive NST (less than two fetal heart rate accelerations from baseline). The loss of fetal tone, which is associated with a 14-fold increased risk of fetal death,[6] is the last finding to be lost as the fetal condition deteriorates.

The BPP assesses five biophysical characteristics in the fetus: heart rate variability, breathing movements, gross movements, tone, and amniotic fluid levels (Table 29-3).

TABLE 29-3	Components of Biophysical Profile	
Biophysical Variable	**Normal (2-points)**	**Abnormal (0-points)**
Fetal breathing movements	≥1 episode of continuous fetal breathing movements for ≥30 s	No episodes of ≥30 s
Gross body/limb movements	≥3 distinct limb or body movements (episodes of active continuous movement are considered a single movement)	<3 distinct limb or body movements
Fetal tone	≥1 episode of extension of a fetal trunk or extremity with return to flexion, or opening and closing of a hand	Slow extension with return to partial flexion, movement of limb in full extension, or absent fetal movement
Reactive fetal heart rate	≥2 accelerations in 20 minutes	<2 accelerations in 20 minutes
Amniotic fluid volume	Single deepest vertical pocket of ≥2 cm in two perpendicular planes	Single deepest pocket <2 cm

Modified from Manning FA. Biophysical profile scoring. In Nijhuis J, ed. *Fetal Behaviour*. New York, NY: Oxford University Press; 1992:241.

Amniotic fluid assessment is added as it is a good predictor of chronic placental sufficiency, whereas the other components are good predictors of acute asphyxia and acidemia. Components that are normal are awarded 2 points; those that are abnormal or insufficient earn 0 points. The BPP is scored by the cumulative total of the individual component scores, with a maximum of 10 if all five components are normal. The BPP is a 30-minute study, although the examination can be terminated early if all findings are documented. Most studies only take 10 minutes to complete. Normal BPPs are associated with a stillbirth rate of only 0.8 per 1000.[7] Studies show that evaluating with the BPP in high-risk patients enables obstetric care providers to predict the likelihood of ensuing fetal demise and make management interventions that decrease perinatal morbidity and mortality.[8-10] Failure to respond appropriately to abnormal test results constitutes a large portion of perinatal deaths with avoidable risk factors.[11]

Using different cutoff scores yields different levels of sensitivity and specificity. Lower BPP scores correlate with lower false-positive rates and are inversely associated with increasing rates of poor outcomes such as intrauterine growth restriction, low Apgar scores, and fetal distress. Alternatively, higher scores of 8 to 10 are associated with a less than 1:1000 chance of poor pregnancy outcomes.[12] Therefore, the recommended cutoff to provide the ideal balance of sensitivity and specificity is a score of <8. The predictive value for antenatal testing is generally over the course of 3 to 7 days and if the underlying condition continues, serial testing is recommended.

Full BPPs may not need to be completed in all patients and several abbreviated versions have been described. When all components of the abbreviated versions are normal, they have been found to have similar predictive values as the full BPP.[13] One version, referred to as the mBPP, includes only the NST and amniotic fluid assessment. The other version includes only the four ultrasound components without the NST.[14] The BPP is therefore the only option for antenatal testing that can be completed with ultrasound alone when fetal heart rate monitoring is not available. However, both versions of the abbreviated BPPs have lower positive predictive value with more false positives. If an abbreviated version of the BPP remains abnormal, a full BPP should be performed.

TABLE 29-4	Recommendations for Use of Point-of-Care Ultrasound in Clinical Practice		
Recommendation		**Rating**	**Definition**
Women at high risk for stillbirth should undergo antepartum fetal surveillance		B	1
An abnormal nonstress test or modified biophysical profile should be further evaluated by a full biophysical profile; further management depends on the results of the biophysical profile, the gestational age, the quantity of amniotic fluid, and the maternal condition.		B	1
In the absence of contraindications, management of abnormal antepartum testing may include induction of labor with continuous monitoring		C	1

A = consistent, good-quality patient-oriented evidence; B = inconsistent or limited-quality patient-oriented evidence; C = consensus, disease-oriented evidence, usual practice, expert opinion, or case series. For information about the SORT evidence rating system, go to http://www.aafp.org/afpsort.

PERFORMING THE SCAN

Step 1: Setup and The Big Five. Have the patient lie in the dorsal supine position with left lateral tilt (**Figure 29-1**), and instruct her to notify the examiner in case of any discomfort. A curvilinear probe, between 2 and 5 MHz, is selected. Note the time the examination is started. The examiner begins with a brief survey of the fetal lie, amniotic fluid, fetal cardiac activity, placental location, and fetal number, that is, The Big Five (see Chapter 28 for details).

Step 2: Amniotic fluid assessment. Measure the single deepest pocket. While keeping the transducer parallel to the floor rather than perpendicular to the gravid abdomen, sweep across all four quadrants of the maternal abdomen to locate the quadrant that has the single deepest pocket of amniotic fluid. Using calipers, measure the vertical distance between the anterior wall of the uterus (or posterior edge of an anterior placenta) and the first fetal part. This pocket of fluid should be at least 1 cm wide and should not include any umbilical cord, as demonstrated in **Figure 29-2**.

Step 3: Assess fetal breathing. Obtain a midline sagittal view of the fetus such that fetal lungs, diaphragm, and abdominal contents are clearly visualized on the screen and assess for fetal breathing movements. Fetal breathing movements are seen as downward movement of the diaphragm often with inward collapse of the chest. Continuous breathing for at least 30 seconds is required for a positive score (**Figure 29-3** and ▶ **Video 29-1**).

Note that if fetal breathing motions are not readily apparent, consider searching for other BPP components listed below while intermittently returning to the diaphragm view to note any fetal breathing movements.

Step 4: Assess fetal tone. Intermittently depart from the midline sagittal scan plane and identify fetal extremities to assess for fetal tone. Fetal tone is defined as spine or extremity extension that returns to flexion. At least one example of fetal tone is required for a positive score (**Figure 29-4**).

Note that visualizing the opening and closing of a fetal hand is sufficient to fulfill this component of the BPP.

Step 5: Assess fetal movement. Fetal movements are defined as gross movements of a limb or torso. Continuous movement is only counted as one movement. At least three distinct movements are required for a positive score (**Figures 29-5 and 29-6**).

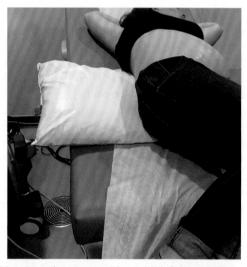

FIGURE 29-1. Dorsal supine position with left lateral tilt.

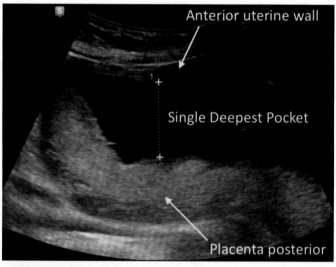

FIGURE 29-2. Single deepest pocket assessment of amniotic fluid.

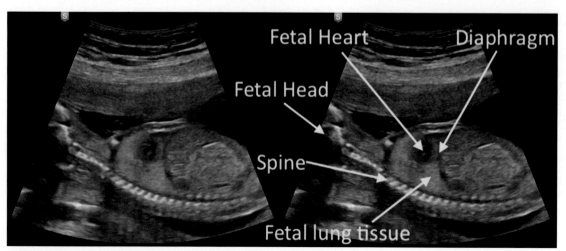

FIGURE 29-3. The fetal diaphragm is identified at which point fetal breathing can be easily observed.

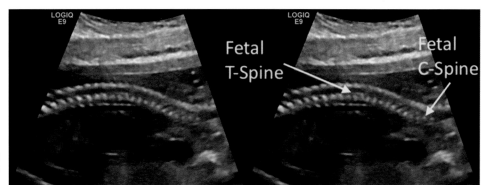

FIGURE 29-4. The fetal spine is identified at which point truncal extension and flexion of the fetus can be easily observed.

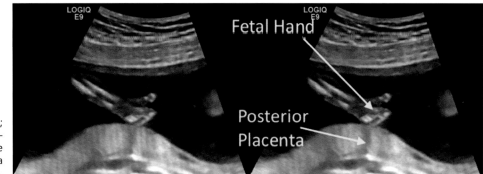

FIGURE 29-5. The fetal hands are identified; this view enables the sonographer to document components of movement or tone by visualizing the opening and closing of a fetal hand, or the distinct limb movements.

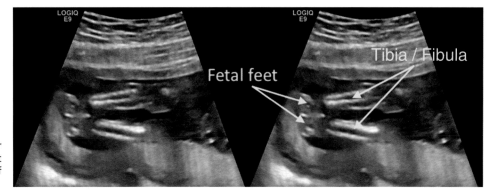

FIGURE 29-6. Similar to visualizing the upper extremities, identification of the fetal feet can also be used to aid in the detection of distinct limb movements.

PATIENT MANAGEMENT

The workup for decreased fetal movement (**Figure 29-7**) or other at-risk fetal situations traditionally starts with an mBPP. If the NST is nonreactive over a 20-minute window, extend the study an additional 20 minutes and consider the use of vibroacoustic stimulation. Because of the high false-positive rate and low positive predictive value of mBPP, persistent abnormal results should be followed with further testing to minimize the rate of unnecessary delivery and iatrogenic adverse outcomes. If either the NST is nonreactive or if oligohydramnios/polyhydramnios exists, the next step in the workup is to perform a complete BPP.

The BPP is used as a clinical decision tool. Interpretation and management of BPP scores are outlined in **Table 29-5**. A score of 8

or 10 with normal amniotic fluid implies a low risk for fetal demise within 1 week. An exception is made if the score is 8 but oligohydramnios is present. The American College of Obstetricians and Gynecologists (ACOG) recommends delivery for oligohydramnios at the time of diagnosis once gestational age is greater than 36 weeks 0 days.[15] A score of 6 with normal amniotic fluid is an equivocal test result and requires retesting 24 hours later to observe if one of the absent components returns to normal. A fetus at term with a BPP of 6 may be considered for delivery. BPP scores ≤4 typically warrant delivery.

If an NST is unavailable, a BPP without NST with a score of 8 is considered equivalent to a score of 8 or 10 on a full BPP. If a score of less than 8 is found, appropriate referral must be made for a full BPP including NST or contraction stress testing.

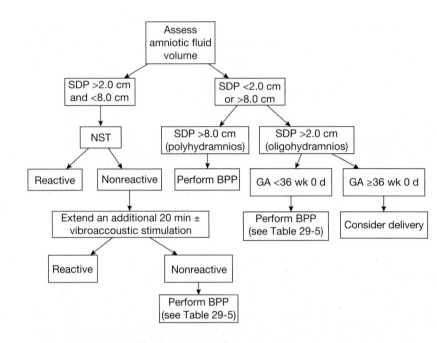

FIGURE 29-7. Recommended evaluation for patient presenting with the complaint of decreased fetal movements. BPP, biophysical profile; GA, gestational age; NST, nonstress test; SDP, single deepest pocket.

TABLE 29-5	Interpretation and Management of Biophysical Profile (BPP) Score	
Score	**Interpretation**	**Management**
8-10	Normal; low risk for chronic asphyxia	Repeat testing at weekly to twice-weekly intervals
6	Equivocal; suspect chronic asphyxia	If ≥36 wk gestation, or <36 wk with known fetal lung maturity, consider delivery; else, repeat BPP in 4-6 h and deliver if oligohydramnios is present
4	Abnormal; suspect chronic asphyxia	Delivery usually indicated; if <32 wk, consider individualized management (extended monitoring)
0-2	Abnormal; strongly suspect chronic asphyxia	Extend testing time to 120 min; if persistently <4, deliver regardless of gestational age

Modified from Manning FA, Harman CR, Morrison I, et al. Fetal assessment based on fetal biophysical profile scoring. Am J Obstet Gynecol. 1990;162(2):398-402. Copyright © 1990 Elsevier. With permission; Manning FA. Biophysical profile scoring. In: Nijhuis J, ed. *Fetal Behaviour*. New York, NY: Oxford University Press; 1992:241. Reproduced with permission of Oxford Publishing Limited through PLSclear.

PEARLS AND PITFALLS

Pearl

- Have a clock with a second hand or timer available when you assess fetal breathing.

Pitfalls

- Be careful not to mistake maternal breathing for fetal breathing. During maternal breathing the entire fetus will move up and down on the monitor corresponding with maternal breaths; however, during fetal breathing the fetal thoracic cavity expands and contracts.

- Be careful not to mistake absent findings because of fetal sleep cycles or maternal ingestion of sedatives or opioids for signs of chronic fetal asphyxia warranting delivery.

- It should still be remembered that fetal surveillance cannot predict the occurrence of intrauterine catastrophes such as an umbilical cord accidents or placental abruption.

BILLING

CPT Code	Description	Global Payment	Professional Component	Technical Component
76818	Fetal biophysical profile with nonstress testing	$123.88	$55.50	$68.39
76819	Fetal biophysical profile without nonstress testing	$90.23	$40.46	$49.77

CPT codes and average national reimbursement for Medicare in 2016. Payment data are from https://www.cms.gov/apps/physician-fee-schedule/search/search-criteria.aspx. See Chapter 2 for details on ultrasound billing.

References

1. American College of Obstetricians and Gynecologists. ACOG Practice Bulletin no. 145: antepartum fetal surveillance. *Obstet Gynecol.* 2014;124(1):182-192.

2. Van Woerden EE, VanGeijn HP. Heart-rate patterns and fetal movements. In Nijhuis J, ed. *Fetal Behaviour.* New York, NY: Oxford University Press; 1992:41.

3. Hijazi ZR, East CE. Factors affecting maternal perception of fetal movement. *Obstet Gynecol Surv.* 2009;64:489.

4. Patrick J, Campbell K, Carmichael L, Natale R, Richardson B. Patterns of gross fetal body movements over 24-hour observation intervals during the last 10 weeks of pregnancy. *Am J Obstet Gynecol.* 1982;142:363.

5. Vintzileos AM, Gaffney SE, Salinger LM, Campbell WA, Nochimson DJ. The relationship between fetal biophysical profile and cord pH in patients undergoing cesarean section before the onset of labor. *Obstet Gynecol.* 1987;70:196.

6. Maning FA, Platt L, Sipos L. Antepartum fetal evaluation: development of a fetal biophysical profile. *Am J Obstet Gynecol.* 1980;136:737.

7. Manning FA, Morrison I, Harman CR, Lange IR, Menticoglou S. Fetal assessment based on fetal biophysical profile scoring: experience in 19,221 referred high risk pregnancies. II. An analysis of false-negative fetal deaths. *Am J Obstet Gynecol.* 1987;157:880-884.

8. Manning FA, Platt LD. Maternal hypoxemia and fetal breathing movements. *Obstet Gynecol.* 1979;53:758-760.

9. Manning FA, Snijders R, Harman CR, Nicolaides K, Menticoglou S, Morrison I. Fetal biophysical profile score. VI. Correlation with antepartum umbilical venous fetal pH. *Am J Obstet Gynecol.* 1993;169:755-763.

10. Manning FA. Fetal biophysical profile: a critical appraisal. *Clin Obstet Gynecol.* 2002;45:975.

11. Mersey Region Working Party on Perinatal Mortality. Perinatal health. *Lancet.* 1982;1:491.

12. Greenberg ML. Chapter 12: Antepartum fetal evaluation. In Gabbe SG, ed. *Obstetrics Normal and Problem Pregnancies.* 7th ed. Philadelphia, PA: Elsevier; 2016:253.

13. Graham N, Harman C. Chapter 56: Antepartum testing. In Berghella V, ed. *Maternal-Fetal Evidence Based Guidelines.* 3rd ed. Boca Raton, FL: CRC Press; 2017.

14. Manning FA, Morrison I, Lange IR, Harman CR, Chamberlain PF. Fetal biophysical profile scoring: selective use of the nonstress test. *Am J Obstet Gynecol.* 1987;156(3):709-712.

15. American College of Obstetricians and Gynecologists. ACOG Committee Opinion no. 560: medically indicated late-preterm and early-term deliveries. *Obstet Gynecol.* 2013;121(4):908-910.

PART 2

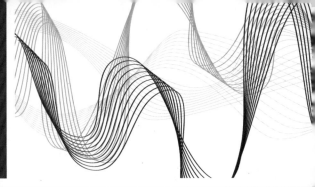

Charisse W. Kwan, MD, FRCPC

Clinical Vignette

An otherwise healthy 14-year-old boy presents to your office with a 3-hour history of swelling and pain to his right scrotum. He sustained minor trauma to the groin 2 days ago during football practice, but denies fever, dysuria, or hematuria. He also denies any sexual history. On physical examination, his right scrotum is slightly reddened, with swelling below the testicle. He complains of tenderness. The left scrotum is normal. There is no inguinal lymphadenopathy and cremasteric reflexes are present bilaterally. Does this patient have testicular torsion?

LITERATURE REVIEW

Although the most common causes of acute scrotal pain are benign, rare and serious causes can result in the loss of the testicle if not diagnosed and treated early. Unfortunately, the history and physical examination cannot always differentiate pathologies that require acute management in pediatric patients, many of whom are unable to articulate their symptoms. Of particular concern is the differentiation of testicular torsion from less acute causes of testicular pain, such as epididymitis, orchitis, or torsion of the appendix testes. There is evidence that an abnormal ipsilateral cremasteric reflex, nausea/vomiting, sudden onset of symptoms, high position of testes, and scrotal skin changes may be highly predictive of pediatric testicular torsion.[1-4] However, even in adult

patients, testicular torsion rarely presents with all the classic textbook symptoms, often making it difficult to diagnose on history and physical examination alone.

Augmentation of the physical examination with ultrasound can be of great value, particularly in nonverbal patients. In adults, ultrasound of the scrotum performed by emergency physicians with adequate training has been reported to have a sensitivity and specificity of 94% and 95%, respectively, in diagnosing testicular torsion, epididymitis, orchitis, hernia, hydrocele, testicular rupture, testicular mass, or no pathology in the adult population.[5,6]

PERFORMING THE SCAN

1. Place the patient in a supine frog leg position with exposure of the inguinal region and testes only (**Figure 30-1**).
2. Use a linear high-frequency transducer in the transverse plane (**Figure 30-2**). Examine the asymptomatic testis first, looking at the spermatic cord, epididymis, and testicle. Pay particular attention to the testicular size, echogenicity, and vascularity. Then, examine the testis in the long axis (**Figure 30-3**). Use continuous clips, if possible. The appendix testis is difficult to find unless it is torsed and edematous (**Figure 30-9**).
3. Color Doppler or power Doppler should be used to examine flow to the testicle and surrounding structures. Infection can manifest as an increased Doppler flow such as in epididymitis (**Figure 30-4**).
4. Carefully repeat the examination on the affected testis both in short and long axis.

TABLE 30-1	Recommendations for Use of Point-of-Care Ultrasound in Clinical Practice		
Recommendation		Rating	References
In children with high pretest probability of testicular torsion, trauma, or incarcerated hernia, ultrasound should be performed without delaying referral to help expedite the diagnosis and care. It may also rule in a more benign condition.		C	5-8, 10
In children with low-to-moderate probability of testicular torsion, trauma, or incarcerated hernia, ultrasound should be performed to rule in a more benign condition and catch the atypical presentations of more critical diagnosis.		C	5, 9

A = consistent, good-quality patient-oriented evidence; B = inconsistent or limited-quality patient-oriented evidence; C = consensus, disease-oriented evidence, usual practice, expert opinion, or case series. For information about the SORT evidence rating system, go to http://www.aafp.org/afpsort.

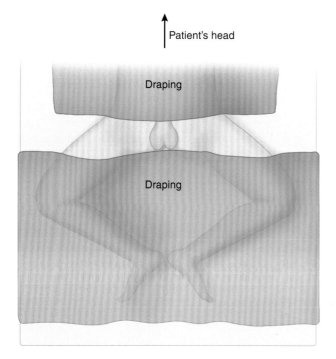

FIGURE 30-1. Place the patient in a supine frog leg position. Drape bedsheets over the penis, abdomen, and legs. Expose only the scrotum and inguinal canal.

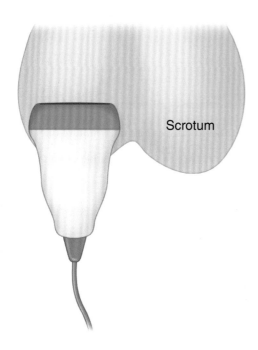

FIGURE 30-2. Scan in transverse.

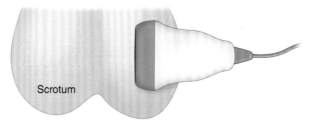

FIGURE 30-3. Scan in long axis (oriented to the axis of the testicle).

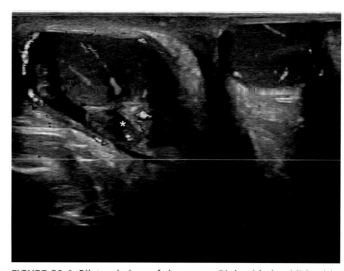

FIGURE 30-4. Bilateral view of the testes. Right-sided epididymitis. (Asterisk) Enlarged epididymis with increased flow. Note that there is color flow to both testes.

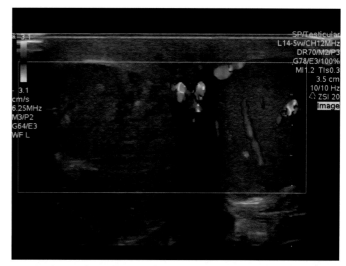

FIGURE 30-5. Bilateral view of the testes. Symptomatic right testicle. The right testicle has a change in echotexture and no color flow compared to the left testicle.

5. A view with both testes in transverse orientation can compare size, echogenicity, and vascularity side by side. Notice the difference in size and echogenicity. Decreased flow of the affected testis suggests testicular torsion (**Figure 30-5**).

PATIENT MANAGEMENT

When a pediatric patient presents with scrotal pain, the most time-sensitive pathologies to rule out are testicular torsion, incarcerated hernia, and traumatic testicular rupture. Other pathologies may include: epididymitis, epididymo-orchitis, torsion of the appendix testes, hydrocele, varicocele, testicular mass/tumor, or inguinal hernia.

Testicular torsion requires immediate urologic consultation for surgical management. Decreased or absent flow on ultrasound in the symptomatic testicle is indicative of testicular torsion. If the testicle has detorsed, there may be increased flow to the affected testicle and this testicle is at high risk or torsion again in the future.[7,8] Urologic consultation is indicated but may not be required emergently. A comprehensive ultrasound should be done to examine for torsion-detorsion or partial torsion. Ultrasound findings of a twisted spermatic cord is 100% sensitive and specific[9] for testicular torsion (**Figure 30-6**). There can also be an accompanying reactive hydrocele.

A child with scrotal pain may also have an incarcerated hernia containing bowel (**Figure 30-7**). There is a lack of peristalsis in the bowel, with air and fluid within the bowel loops. If the patient has signs of bowel obstruction and/or the hernia is irreducible, then prompt surgical consultation is required. If there is swelling of the inguinal canal, it is important to examine this with ultrasound as well. There may be a testis that has retracted and become caught within the canal.

Following trauma, a child with scrotal pain may have a ruptured testis (**Figure 30-8**). Ultrasound should be used to determine whether this is present as antibodies to sperm may form and cause sterility in these patients. Urologic consultation is, again, required promptly.[10,11]

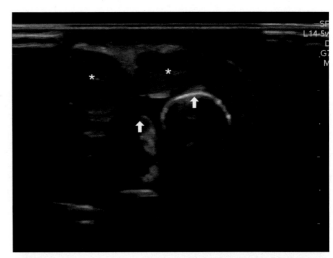

FIGURE 30-7. Bilateral view of the testes. Incarcerated hernia with bowel gas within the bowel loops (upward arrows). There is a dirty shadow from the bowel gas. (Asterisk) indicates both testicles.

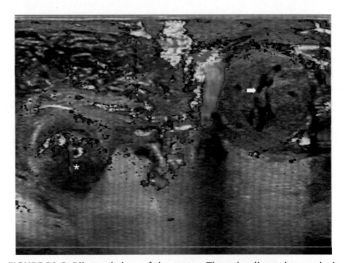

FIGURE 30-8. Bilateral view of the testes. There is a linear hypoechoic collection (rightward arrow) indicating rupture or fracture of left testicle (right side of the image), no flow centrally, and increased flow to surrounding traumatized tissue. (Asterisk) indicates right testicle with normal color flow.

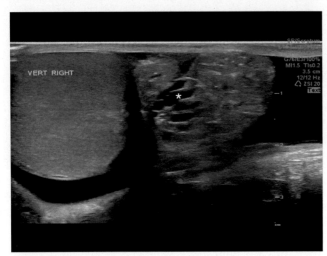

FIGURE 30-6. Long-axis view of the right testicle with the twisted spermatic cord (asterisk, whirlpool) on the right of the image. Patient head is oriented to the right of the image. Note the reactive hydrocele.

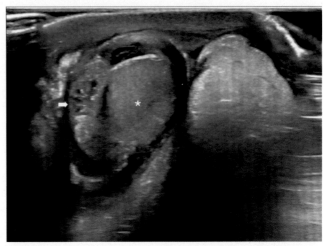

FIGURE 30-9. Transverse view of right testicle (asterisk) with enlarged testicular appendix (rightward arrow) of mixed echogenicity.

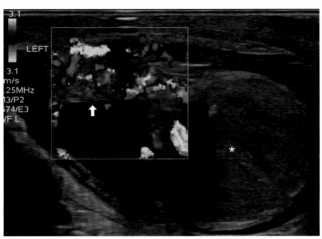

FIGURE 30-10. Transverse view of left testicle (asterisk) with enlarged epididymis (upward arrow) of mixed echogenicity. Note the increased flow to both the epididymis and the testes indicating epididymo-orchitis. There is also a hydrocele.

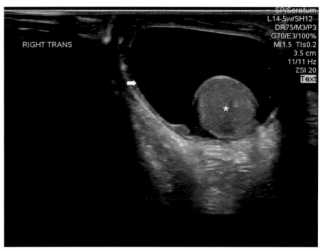

FIGURE 30-13. Transverse view of the right testicle (asterisk). The large hydrocele appears as a hypoechoic collection surrounding the testicle (rightward arrow).

A torsed appendix testis can also mimic the pain of a testicular torsion. It appears as a round appendage with increased flow surrounding it and no flow within the appendage (Figure 30-9).

Epididymitis, epididymo-orchitis (**Figure 30-10**), and orchitis all present with pain to the scrotum. It is a common cause of

acute scrotal pain. In these cases, there are changes in echotexture; increased size and increased flow are seen in the affected structure (epididymis, testis, or both).

A varicocele can occur in adolescents (**Figure 30-11**). This is sometimes described as having the appearance of a "bag of worms." In the supine resting patient, a vessel diameter size larger than 2 to 3 mm defines a varicocele.[12] When the patient performs a Valsalva, the movement of blood can be seen in the low-flow varicose vein on ultrasound. If the patient has difficulty with pain, urology consultation may be necessary for long-term management.

Rarely, in children, a testicular mass is seen (**Figure 30-12**). Atypical structures that are not easily identified as an obvious pathology should be sent for further comprehensive imaging with possible urologic consultation.[13]

Hydroceles are extremely common in children (**Figure 30-13**). They can be congenital and benign or because of a reactive process to any nonspecific inflammatory process in the area. Clinical history and physical examination provide the context and aid in differentiating benign versus reactive etiologies.

Table 30-2 summarizes the ultrasound characteristics of the above-mentioned differential for the pediatric acute scrotum. **Figure 30-14** is a diagram suggesting a possible management strategy for the pediatric patient presenting with acute testicular pain. Management pathways should always be in consultation with the local urology team and their endorsement of the pathway is essential.

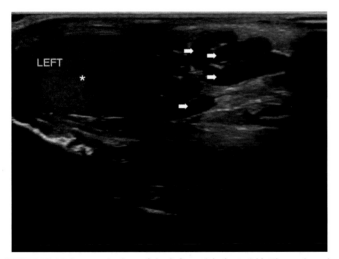

FIGURE 30-11. Long-axis view of the left testicle (asterisk). The varicocele is demonstrated as hypoechoic long tubular structures at the bottom of the scrotum that resemble a "bag of worms" (rightward arrows).

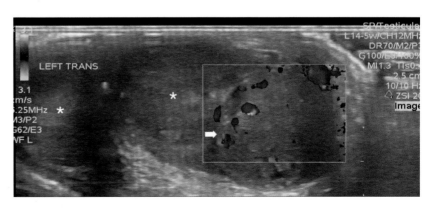

FIGURE 30-12. Bilateral view of the testes (asterisks). The round mass appears beside the left testicle (rightward arrow). It appears to be about the same size as the left testicle, has color flow and mixed echogenicity.

TABLE 30-2	Differential Diagnosis and Ultrasound Characteristics				
	Abnormal Testicular Echotexture	Increased Testicular Size	Decreased Testicular Flow	Increased Testicular Flow	Abnormal Surrounding Structures
Testicular torsion	Yes	Yes	Yes	Torsion/detorsion*	±hydrocele
Inguinal hernia	No	No	No	No	Yes—bowel loops seen
Ruptured testicle	Yes	Yes	Possible	Possible	Yes—hematoma
Epididymitis	No	No	No	No—but increased flow to the epididymis	±hydrocele
Epididymo-orchitis	Yes	Yes	No	Yes	±hydrocele
Torsion of the appendix testis	No	No	No	Yes	Yes—round appendage with no flow
Tumor	Possible	Possible	No	Possible	Mass within testis or outside
Varicocele	No	No	No	No	Yes—"bag of worms"
Congenital hydrocele	No	No	No	No	Fluid—hydrocele

*Pain decreased from initial onset of symptoms.

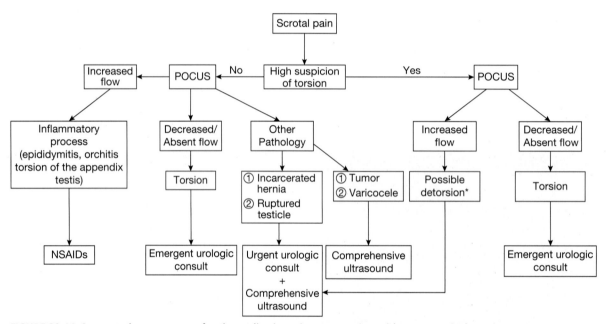

FIGURE 30-14. Suggested management for the pediatric patient presenting with acute testicular pain.

PEARLS AND PITFALLS

Pearls

- Flow can be difficult to assess in children because of the small vessels and vasoconstriction. Applying a warm compress underneath both testes while performing the scan can increase blood flow to the area and increased visibility on color Doppler. Power Doppler may be necessary.
- Set the color Doppler gain when examining the asymptomatic testis before applying it to the symptomatic testis. Do not adjust the gain setting again when examining the symptomatic testis, or else it is difficult to compare flow.
- Testes can be retractile and sometimes be found very high in the scrotal sac, or even in the inguinal canal.

Pitfalls

- Do not mistake extratesticular blood flow for intratesticular blood flow. Ensure that you see consistent blood flow to the center of the testes in question.
- Always assess for blood flow even when other pathology is seen. Otherwise, it may lead to a false-negative result for testicular torsion.
- Detorsion of a testis can result in increased blood flow to that testis. If this is suspected based on the clinical presentation and ultrasound demonstrates increased flow to the symptomatic testis, refer to urology.

BILLING

CPT Code	Description	Global Payment	Professional Component	Technical Component
76870	Ultrasound examination scrotum	$68.39	$32.58	$35.80

CPT codes and average national reimbursement for Medicare in 2016. Payment data are from https://www.cms.gov/apps/physician-fee-schedule/search/search-criteria.aspx. See Chapter 2 for details on ultrasound billing.

References

1. Srinivasan A, Cinman N, Feber KM, Gitlin J, Palmer LS. History and physical examination findings predictive of testicular torsion: an attempt to promote clinical diagnosis by house staff. *J Pediatr Urol.* 2011;7(4):470-474.

2. Boettcher M, Bergholz R, Krebs TF, Wenke K, Aronson DC. Clinical predictors of testicular torsion in children. *Urology.* 2012;79(3):670-674.

3. Liang T, Metcalfe P, Sevcik W, Noga M. Retrospective review of diagnosis and treatment in children presenting to the pediatric department with acute scrotum. *AJR Am J Roentgenol.* 2013;200(5):W444-W449.

4. Boettcher M, Bergholz R, Krebs TF, et al. Differentiation of epididymitis and appendix testis torsion by clinical and ultrasound signs in children. *Urology.* 2013;82(4):899-904.

5. Blaivas M, Sierzenski P, Lambert M. Emergency evaluation of patients presenting with acute scrotum using bedside ultrasonography. *Acad Emerg Med.* 2001;8(1):90-93.

6. Blaivas M, Batts M, Lambert M. Ultrasonographic diagnosis of testicular torsion by emergency physicians. *Am J Emerg Med.* 2000;18(2):198-200.

7. Bomann JS, Moore C. Bedside ultrasound of a painful testicle: before and after manual detorsion by an emergency physician. *Acad Emerg Med.* 2009;16(4):366.

8. Smith RJ, Horrow MM. Ultrasonographic evaluation of acute urinary tract and male genitourinary pathology. *Ultrasound Clinics.* 2011;6(2):195-213.

9. Vijayaraghavan SB. Sonographic differential diagnosis of acute scrotum: real-time whirlpool sign, a key sign of torsion. *J Ultrasound Med.* 2006;25(5):563-574.

10. Cannis M, Mailhot T, Perera P. Bedside ultrasound in a case of blunt scrotal trauma. *West J Emerg Med.* 2013;14(2):127-129.

11. Matzek BA, Linklater DR. Traumatic testicular dislocation after minor trauma in a pediatric patient. *J Emerg Med.* 2013;45(4):537-540.

12. Kim ED, Lipshultz LI. Role of ultrasound in the assessment of male infertility. *J Clin Ultrasound.* 1996;24(8):437-453.

13. Thimann D, Badawy M. 7-month-old male with scrotal swelling. *Emerg Med J.* 2014;31(6):521-522.

How Thick Is the Patient's Endometrial Stripe?

Lauren Castleberry, MD, FACOG and Joy Shen-Wagner, MD, FAAFP

● Clinical Vignette

A 55-year-old postmenopausal patient presents with complaints of vaginal bleeding. Her medical history is complicated by hypertension, diabetes mellitus type II, and morbid obesity with a body mass index (BMI) of 45. She has a history of a bilateral tubal ligation but, no other gynecologic surgeries. Her family history is non-contributory. She does not smoke, drink alcohol, or use any illicit drugs. She has had three prior vaginal deliveries and denies a history of uterine fibroids. Her last Pap smear was within the past year and was negative, with negative high-risk human papillomavirus testing. Physical examination demonstrates a normal-sized uterus and no appreciable adnexal masses. Her cervix appears normal and no lacerations, polyps, or other anatomic abnormalities are visible within the vaginal vault. You want to rule out endometrial cancer with a bedside ultrasound. How thick is the patient's endometrial stripe?

LITERATURE REVIEW

Endometrial cancer is the most common gynecologic malignancy in the United States.[1] The most common presentation is post-menopausal bleeding, occurring in more than 90% of patients with endometrial carcinoma. However, most often, the underlying cause of postmenopausal bleeding is benign disease including polyps or endometrial atrophy (Tables 31-1 and 31-2).[2,3] Because of the risk for underlying malignancy, it is imperative that an efficient and decisive workup is performed to determine the cause of postmeno-pausal bleeding. Dilation and curettage in the operating room was the standard method of evaluation for many years, but in-office endometrial biopsy has been shown to have a similar sensitivity and specificity in the postmenopausal patient population—99.6% and 98% to 100%, respectively.[4]

Unfortunately, both procedures are uncomfortable and are accompanied with additional cost. Furthermore, the anesthesia required for curettage can lead to increased morbidity for the pa-tient. Although less invasive and not requiring general anesthesia, all too frequently, endometrial biopsies are insufficient to make a definitive diagnosis. In a study of 97 consecutive patients with postmenopausal bleeding, attempts to obtain adequate endometrial tissue failed in 47% of the patients. Initial biopsy attempts were

more likely to fail in patients with an endometrial thickness of <5 mm, although that group was also found to have a lower risk of cancer or atypia.[5]

Other studies have supported this endometrial thickness cutoff to determine who should undergo endometrial sampling. In a multicenter study by Karlsson et al. involving 1168 women with postmenopausal bleeding scheduled for curettage, no cases of malignancy were identified in patients who had a transvaginal endometrial thickness of <5 mm on ultrasound.[6] Given these findings, transvaginal ultrasound (TVUS) has become first line in the evaluation of postmenopausal bleeding as a means of triaging those patients who require tissue biopsy.

Finally, studies have also been performed to evaluate the endometrial thickness and its accuracy in detecting endometrial disease in women on hormone replacement therapy (HRT). In a meta-analysis that evaluated the accuracy of TVUS in diagnosing endometrial pathologic conditions in postmenopausal women with vaginal bleeding, patients using HRT were compared to those who were not.[7] Using a 5 mm endometrial thickness threshold, TVUS identified 95% of endometrial disease among women not using HRT and 91% among women who were using HRT. Among women with normal histologic findings, 8% of women not using HRT had an abnormal TVUS compared with 23% of women who were. Hence, the specificity was better in women who did not use HRT. Because the sensitivity of TVUS did not vary significantly with hormone use, TVUS was reliable in excluding endometrial disease whether the patient was on HRT or not. Using a 5 mm threshold, the negative likelihood ratio for women who did not use HRT was 0.05 and in women who did use HRT it was 0.12. However, because the specificity of the TVUS did vary based on the use of HRT, the positive likelihood ratio was 11.9 among non-HRT users and 4.0 among those who did use HRT. Hence, a woman with a pretest probability of any endometrial disease of 5% has a 39% chance of having endometrial disease after an abnormal TVUS result if she is not on HRT but a 17% chance if she is on HRT.

In conclusion, a transvaginal endometrial thickness mea-surement of ≥5 mm may be used reliably to triage *symptomatic* postmenopausal patients for endometrial sampling. Although data do not support using the endometrial thickness to screen for endometrial pathology, there is support in the literature to use the same threshold of 5 mm to perform sampling on patients with postmenopausal bleeding who are on HRT.

TABLE 31-1	Risk Factors for Type 1 Uterine Corpus Cancer	
Factors Influencing Risk		**Estimated Relative Risk**
Older age		2-3
Residency in North America or Northern Europe		3-18
Higher level of education or income		1.5-2
White race		2
Nulliparity		3
History of infertility		2-3
Menstrual irregularities		1.5
Late age at natural menopause		2-3
Early age at menarche		1.5-2
Long-term use of unopposed estrogen		10-20
Tamoxifen use		2-3
Obesity		2-5
Estrogen-producing tumor		>5
History of type 2 diabetes, hypertension, gallbladder disease, or thyroid disease		1.3-3
Lynch syndrome		6-20

Modified from Gershenson DM, McGuire WP, Gore M, et al., ed. Gynecologic cancer: controversies in management. Philadelphia, PA: Churchill Livingstone; 2004. Copyright © 2004 Elsevier. With permission.

TABLE 31-2	Etiologies of Postmenopausal Bleeding
Cause of Bleeding	**Frequency**
Endometrial atrophy	60-80
Exogenous estrogens	15-25
Endometrial or cervical polyps	2-12
Endometrial hyperplasia	5-10
Endometrial cancer	10
Miscellaneous (eg, cervical cancer, uterine sarcoma, trauma)	10

Reprinted from Hsu C, Chen C, Wang K. Assessment of postmenopausal bleeding. *Int J Gerontol*. 2008;2(2):55-59. Copyright © 2008 Elsevier. With permission.

TABLE 31-3	Recommendations for Use of Point-of-Care Ultrasound in Clinical Practice		
Recommendation		**Rating**	**References**
In a patient with postmenopausal bleeding and an endometrial stripe measuring ≤4 mm on transvaginal ultrasound, initial tissue biopsy is not required.		A	5, 6
The significance of an incidentally found thickened endometrial stripe of >4 mm in a postmenopausal patient is unknown and routine endometrial biopsy (EMB) is not indicated. In the same way, transvaginal ultrasound (TVUS) should not be used to screen for endometrial cancer in the postmenopausal patient.		B	9, 10
In patients on hormone replacement therapy with postmenopausal bleeding and an endometrial thickness of ≥5 mm, tissue sampling is indicated.		A	7

A = consistent, good-quality patient-oriented evidence; B = inconsistent or limited-quality patient-oriented evidence; C = consensus, disease-oriented evidence, usual practice, expert opinion, or case series. For information about the SORT evidence rating system, go to http://www.aafp.org/afpsort.

PERFORMING THE SCAN

Because the studies reporting the utility of the endometrial stripe thickness in detecting endometrial abnormalities were performed using TVUS, only the transvaginal approach will be discussed here.

1. **Patient preparation.** Have the patient void prior to starting the examination. After voiding, place her in the dorsal lithotomy position with her legs in stirrups. If stirrups are not available, then place a covered pillow or bedpan under the buttocks to elevate the pelvis and allow the operator full mobility of the transvaginal probe. Use a transvaginal probe with a frequency of 5 MHz or higher (**Figure 31-1**).

2. **Identifying the uterus.** Locate the uterus in the sagittal view, taking care to identify the anterior and posterior borders. Perform a quick sweep from left to right in the sagittal plane and inferior to superior in the coronal view to visualize the uterus in its entirety (**Figures 31-2 and 31-3**).

3. **Evaluating and measuring the endometrium.** Evaluate the endometrium for any thickness or focal abnormalities, as well as the presence of fluid. With the midline image of the uterus in the sagittal plane, measure the anterior and posterior portions of the basal endometrium and exclude endometrial fluid

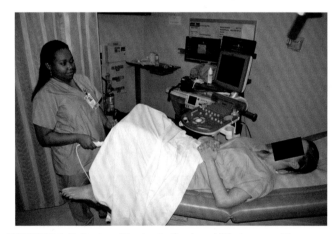

FIGURE 31-1. Patient positioning in the dorsal lithotomy position.

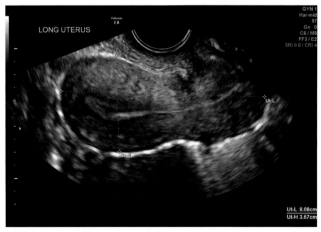

FIGURE 31-2. An image of the long axis of a uterus on transvaginal ultrasound imaging. The uterine length is measured in the long axis from the fundus to the external os of the cervix. The depth is also measured, from the anterior to the posterior walls, perpendicular to the length of the uterus.

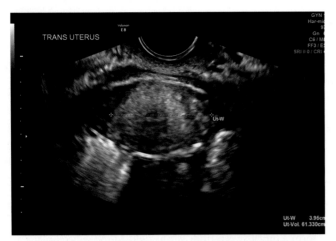

FIGURE 31-3. The uterine width is measured in the coronal view.

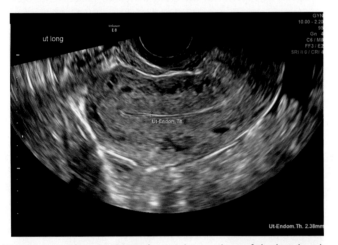

FIGURE 31-4. The anterior and posterior portions of the basal endometrium are measured in this image of a normal endometrial stripe.

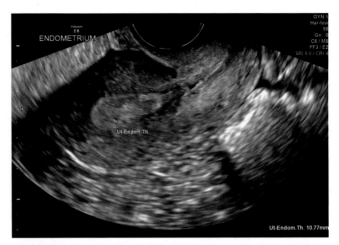

FIGURE 31-5. This image depicts a thickened and homogeneous endometrial stripe.

or adjacent hypoechoic myometrium. If imaging is difficult to obtain because of poor visualization or obstructing masses, state this on the report. In these cases, sonohysterography may be useful to further delineate the endometrial lining and evaluate for endocavitary masses.[8] Additionally, 3D ultrasound may be useful to further evaluate intracavitary masses (**Figures 31-4 to 31-6**).

4. **Evaluate the adnexa.** Perform a cursory evaluation of the adnexa, checking the adnexa for any obvious abnormalities or pathology. The fallopian tubes are often not visible when normal and postmenopausal ovaries are typically small and can be hard to identify; if any obvious abnormalities of either the ovaries or fallopian tubes are noted, document these findings along with their relationship to the uterus, size, and sonographic characteristics if present (**Figures 31-7 to 31-9**).

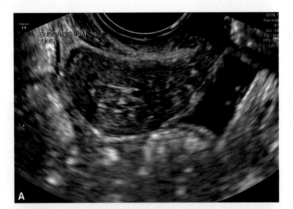

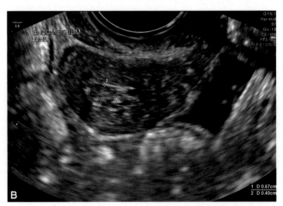

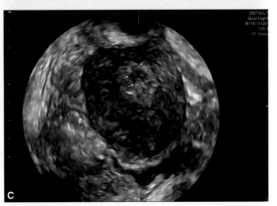

FIGURE 31-6. A, The endometrium is heterogeneous and distorted by a relatively hypoechoic intracavitary lesion. B, The more hypoechoic intracavitary lesion is measured in the sagittal plane. C, 3-D imaging can also help to define the borders of any intracavitary lesions that are found.

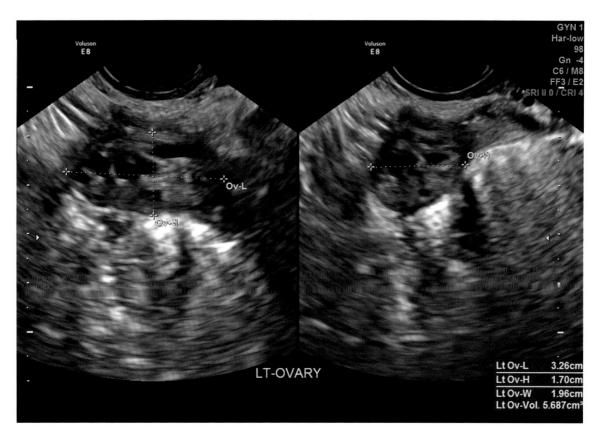

FIGURE 31-7. A normal-appearing left ovary.

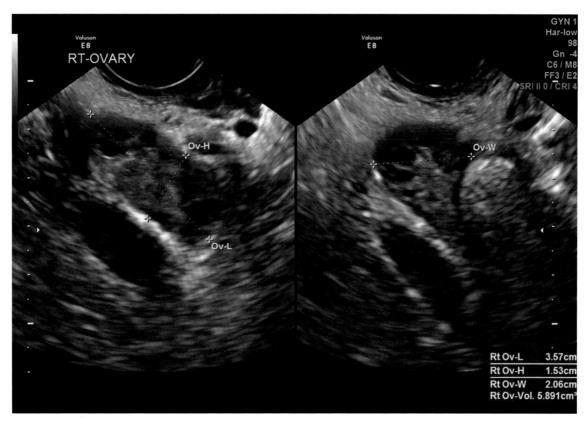

FIGURE 31-8. A normal-appearing right ovary.

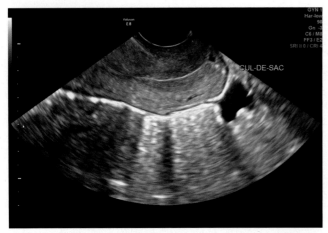

FIGURE 31-9. The cul-de-sac should be evaluated for free fluid.

PATIENT MANAGEMENT

After obtaining the endometrial stripe measurement, reassurance can be given to the postmenopausal patient whose stripe measures <5 mm in thickness. Her symptoms can be monitored for recurrence or worsening; if her symptoms do persist, then an outpatient endometrial biopsy should be performed.

However, in the postmenopausal patient whose endometrial thickness measures ≥5 mm, endometrial sampling should be performed before any additional therapeutic interventions are offered. If the endometrial stripe appears heterogeneous and suspicious for intracavitary pathology, a saline infusion sonogram (SIS) may be helpful to further characterize the lesions prior to developing a management plan. In such cases, a hysteroscopy with dilation and curettage, polypectomy, or myomectomy may be of greater utility for both diagnosis and treatment (**Figure 31-10**).

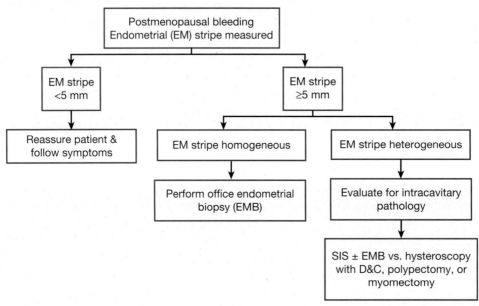

FIGURE 31-10. Treatment algorithm for postmenopausal bleeding. D&C, dilation and curettage; SIS, saline infusion sonogram.

PEARLS AND PITFALLS

Pearls

- One way to ensure that you are truly measuring the endometrial stripe and not an area that *looks* like the endometrial stripe is to make sure you can see the endometrial stripe along the long axis of the uterus all the way inferior to the cervical canal. These two lines should connect.
- If the endometrial stripe is difficult to visualize, try placing color Doppler over the area; this often helps to delineate the borders.
- The postmenopausal endometrium is not always easy to identify. If you find that you are struggling to clearly see the borders, then this is a patient that will require further evaluation with either SIS or hysteroscopy.

Pitfalls

- Routine screening of asymptomatic postmenopausal patients using endometrial stripe measurements is not recommended. In the event of an incidental finding of a thickened endometrial stripe, individualized assessment and care is suggested, taking into account the patient's personal characteristics and risks for endometrial cancer.[1]
- There are insufficient data to support the use of endometrial thickness measurements in a premenopausal patient for the evaluation of uterine cancer. This is in large part because the endometrial thickness changes in response to the various hormone levels during a normal menstrual cycle.

BILLING

CPT Code	Description	Global Payment	Professional Component	Technical Component
76830	Ultrasound, pelvic, transvaginal	$123.89	$35.45	$88.44

CPT codes and average national reimbursement for Medicare in 2016. Payment data are from https://www.cms.gov/apps/physician-fee-schedule/search/search-criteria.aspx. See Chapter 2 for details on ultrasound billing.

References

1. American College of Obstetricians and Gynecologists. ACOG Committee Opinion No. 440. The role of transvaginal ultrasonography in the evaluation of post-menopausal bleeding. *Obstet Gynecol.* 2009;114:409-411.
2. Goldstein RB, Bree RL, Benson CB, et al. Evaluation of the woman with postmenopausal bleeding: society of Radiologists in Ultrasound-Sponsored Consensus Conference statement. *J Ultrasound Med.* 2001;20:1025-1036.
3. Van den Bosch T, Ameye L, Van Schoubroeck D, Bourne T, Timmerman D. Intra-cavitary uterine pathology in women with abnormal uterine bleeding: a prospective study of 1220 women. *Facts Views Vis Obgyn.* 2015;7(1):17-24.
4. Dijkhuizen FP, Mol BW, Brolmann HA, Heintz AP. The accuracy of endometrial sampling in the diagnosis of patients with endometrial carcinoma and hyperplasia: a meta-analysis. *Cancer.* 2000;89(8):1765-1772.
5. Elsandabesee D, Greenwood P. The performance of Pipelle endometrial sampling in a dedicated postmenopausal bleeding clinic. *J Obstet Gynaecol.* 2005;25:32-34.
6. Karlsson B, Granberg S, Wikland M, et al. Transvaginal ultrasonography of the endometrium in women with postmenopausal bleeding—a Nordic multi-centre study. *Am J Obstet Gynecol.* 1995;172:1488-1494.
7. Smith-Bindman R, Kerlikowske K, Feldstein V, et al. Endovaginal ultrasound to exclude endometrial cancer and other endometrial abnormalities. *JAMA.* 1998;280:1510-1517.
8. American Institute for Ultrasound in Medicine. AIUM practice guideline for the performance of pelvic ultrasound examinations. *J Ultrasound Med.* 2010;29(1):166-172.
9. Fleischer AC, Wheeler JE, Lindsay I, et al. An assessment of the value of ultrasonographic screening for endometrial disease in postmenopausal women without symptoms. *Am J Obstet Gynecol.* 2001;184:70-75.
10. Yasa C, Dural O, Bastu E, Ugurlucan F, Nehir A, Iyibozkurt A. Evaluation of the diagnostic role of transvaginal ultrasound measurements of endometrial thickness to detect endometrial malignancy in asymptomatic postmenopausal women. *Arch Gynecol Obstet.* 2016;294:311-316.

PART 2

Does the Patient Have an Adnexal Mass?

Joshua N. Splinter, MD, William MacMillan Rodney, MD, FAAFP, FACEP,
Gary Paul Willers, II, DO, and John Rocco MacMillan Rodney, MD, FAAFP, RDMS

● Clinical Vignette

A 38-year-old Caucasian female presents with 3 months of intermittent pelvic pain. Her pain is described as a colicky ache. She tried taking nonsteroidal anti-inflammatory drugs (NSAIDs) without relief. Her medical history and family history are otherwise unremarkable. On examination, she is mildly tender to palpation in her suprapubic region. On bimanual examination, she is tender in the region of her left adnexa, and there is palpable fullness in that area. Her urinalysis and urine pregnancy test are both negative. Does the patient have an adnexal mass?

LITERATURE REVIEW

The term "adnexa" describe the ovaries, fallopian tubes, and supporting tissues.[1] Adnexal masses are relatively common. In a study of more than 39,000 women, ovarian masses were identified in 15.3% of premenopausal women and 8.2% of postmenopausal women.[2] Adnexal masses have a broad differential, but fortunately, most are benign and will spontaneously resolve.[3,4] Several of the most common types of masses along with their typical ultrasound findings can be found in Table 32-1.

The primary goal of the evaluation of an adnexal mass is to differentiate benign, self-resolving conditions from the rare life-threatening conditions, such as ovarian malignancies. Ultrasound is an excellent tool for this purpose. It has long been known that some ultrasonographic features such as a simple unilocular cyst are highly associated with benign pathology, whereas other findings, such as ascites, are highly suggestive of malignancy.[5] Over 90% of adnexal masses can be accurately stratified by subjective evaluation from experienced ultrasonographers.[6] Thus, the American College of Radiology (ACR) recommends a transvaginal ultrasound (TVUS) as the initial step in all women with suspected adnexal masses.[7] Transabdominal ultrasound can be helpful as an adjunct to TVUS or when the transvaginal method is not available. Optimal ovarian lesion characterization appears to be obtained through the combination of grayscale ultrasound morphology and color Doppler flow imaging information.[8-10]

TABLE 32-1 The Most Common Types of Masses, Along With Their Typical Ultrasound Findings

Adnexal Mass	Common Ultrasound Findings
Physiologic follicle	Anechoic, smooth, well-circumscribed cyst with posterior acoustic enhancement and without blood flow. This is a common finding in premenopausal women as well as the first few years of menopause. See Figure 32-1
Corpus luteum	Homogeneous cyst with "ring of fire" appearance on Doppler due to circumferential vascularity. No internal vascularity. See Figure 32-2
Hemorrhagic cysts	Varied in appearance with circumferential vascularity and varied wall thickness. Fibrin strands and clots may mimic septations or solid components. These are less concerning in a young low-risk patient with good follow-up, but such findings should cause high suspicion in the postmenopausal patient. See Figure 32-3
Endometriomas	The ovaries are the most common site of endometriosis. The classic finding is a homogeneous, hypoechoic cyst, and diffuse low-level echoes. Although septations are possible, such a finding should expand your differential. Small wall nodules are sometimes noted and these, and the entire cyst, should be explored with Doppler to confirm absence of blood flow. See Figure 32-4.
Polycystic ovaries	10 or more simple cysts in a "string of pearls" appearance is the classic finding. There are no cysts larger than 10 mm. The ovaries themselves are often enlarged at over 10 mL of volume each. See Figure 32-5.
Cystic teratoma (dermoid cyst)	Varied appearance. High suspicion if hyperechoic nodule and distal shadowing (Figure 32-6), regionally bright echoes, hyperechoic lines and dots (Figure 32-7), or fluid-fluid level (Figure 32-8) noted. Any two of these is associated with a high predictive value for cystic teratoma.[15]
Hydrosalpinx	Noted fluid-filled dilation of the fallopian tube with a "waist sign" (opposing indentations) seen on ultrasound. See Figure 32-9.
PID w/tubo-ovarian cyst	A febrile patient with pelvic pain or a positive gonorrhea/chlamydia panel shows cystic, thick-walled lesions with high internal blood flow. Additional findings may include a notably thickened endometrium and fallopian tubes. See Figure 32-10.
Pedunculated uterine fibroid	May be difficult to distinguish if unable to visualize the entirety of the pedicle. Emphasis should be on identifying ovaries as this is a common mimic. See Figure 32-11 and ▶ Video 32-1.
Cystadenoma	Cystadenomas appear as an anechoic simple cyst on cursory examination, but septations or nodules may be noted on careful imaging. Follow-up ultrasound or additional imaging would be warranted to rule out cystadenocarcinoma. See Figure 32-12.
Malignancy	There is a broad presentation for malignancy, which is most commonly cystadenocarcinoma in the ovaries. The most worrisome findings are ascites, solid components, and increased vascularity. See Figures 32-13 and 32-14.

Abbreviation: PID, pelvic inflammatory disease.

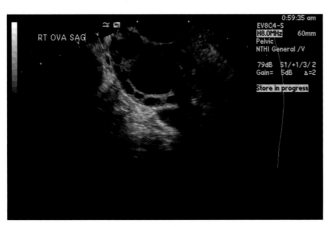

FIGURE 32-1. Normal follicles. Intraovarian simple cysts that are less than 3 cm in diameter are considered normal follicles.

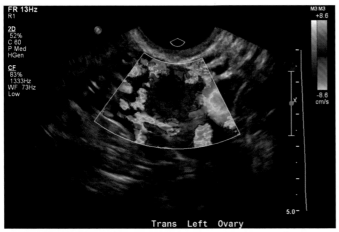

FIGURE 32-2. A corpus luteum cyst with increased Doppler flow surrounding, which is also known as the "ring of fire."

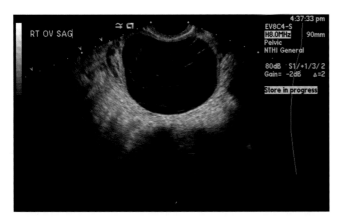

FIGURE 32-3. A hemorrhagic cyst appears as a complex cyst with internal septations and mixed solid and cystic components. In this cyst, areas of reabsorption can be seen as anechoic areas in the periphery. Solid components of hemorrhagic cysts tend to have concave borders as opposed to the convex borders of malignant solid components.

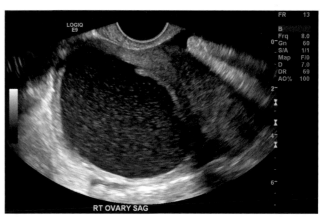

FIGURE 32-4. An endometrioma with classic appearance of a homogeneous, hypoechoic cyst, with diffuse low-level echoes.

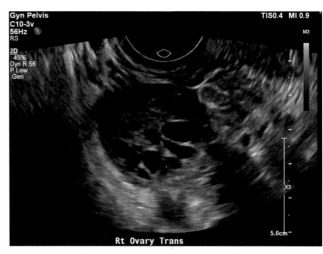

FIGURE 32-5. A polycystic ovary with classic "string of pearls" appearance.

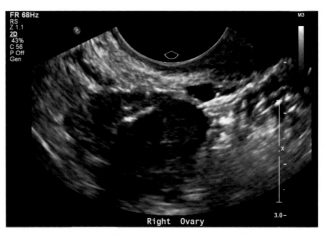

FIGURE 32-6. A dermoid cyst containing a hyperechoic nodule with posterior shadowing. This classic finding is also known as a Rokitansky nodule.

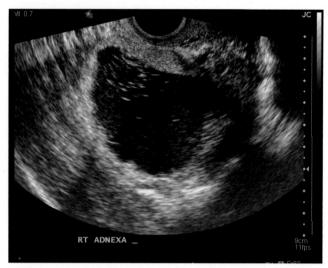

FIGURE 32-7. A dermoid cyst with the classic finding of hyperechoic foci appearing as "lines and dots."

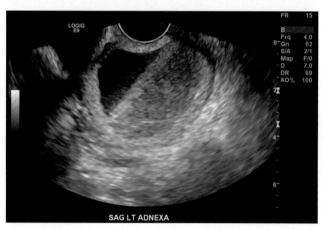

FIGURE 32-8. A dermoid cyst with a fluid-fluid level, which may be caused by fat layering on top of water.

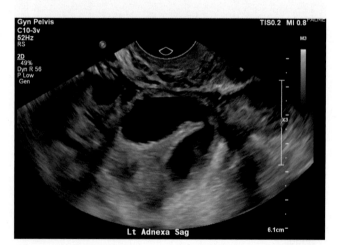

FIGURE 32-9. A hydrosalpinx. Note the anechoic tubular structure with areas of narrowing on both sides of the tube known as the "waist sign."

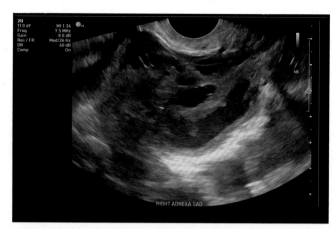

FIGURE 32-10. A tubo-ovarian abscess. Note a tubular structure with thickened walls and complex fluid inside. There is overall a heterogeneous appearance of the adnexa. Clinical context is helpful in these instances as patients will often have risk factors along with tenderness on examination.

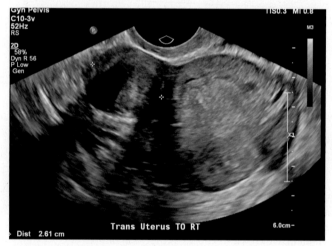

FIGURE 32-11. A pedunculated fibroid in the right adnexa. The fibroid is noted to be continuous with the myometrium and separate from the ovary. This can be seen better in the accompanying video (Video 32-1).

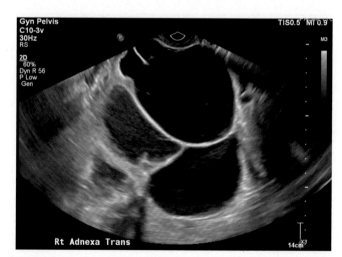

FIGURE 32-12. A cystadenoma appearing as a multilocular cyst with some areas of solid thickening of the septa that appears to be more than 7 mm in thickness. No blood flow was noted on Doppler (not shown). The cyst appears to be 14 cm in largest diameter when compared to the scale to the right of the image. This mass had no benign or malignant findings per the International Ovarian Tumor Analysis (IOTA) Simple Rules and would be designated indeterminant.

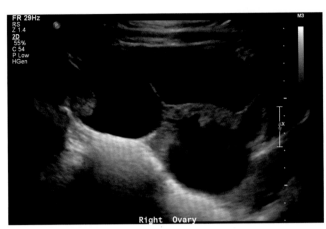

FIGURE 32-13. A cystadenocarcinoma appearing as a multilocular cyst with some areas of solid thickening of the septa and greater than four papillary projections, which were not all visualized on this image. Significant blood flow was noted on Doppler (Figure 32-14) in the solid components. This mass had no benign findings and several malignant findings per the International Ovarian Tumor Analysis (IOTA) Simple Rules and would be designated malignant.

Intending to create a simple, reproducible, and objective system for the evaluation of adnexal masses, the International Ovarian Tumor Analysis (IOTA) study group described the "Simple Rules" in 2008. The Simple Rules are split into evidence-based features of benign masses (B-Features) and those of malignant masses (M-Features). A list of these features can be found in **Table 32-2**. If any B-Features are present in the absence of M-Features, the mass is considered benign. When any M-Features are present in the absence of B-Features, the mass is deemed to be malignant. If no B- or M-Features are present, or if there is a combination of the two, the mass is considered inconclusive. Because of a high incidence of malignancies, inconclusive tumors are often treated as if they are malignant. The Simple Rules have been validated in large data sets and have a 93% sensitivity and 81% specificity when all inconclusive tumors are assumed to be malignant.[5,11] When multiple B-Features are present in the absence of M-Features, the sensitivity improves to >99%.[5] When multiple M-Features are present in the absence of B-Features, the specificity improves to >98%.[5]

Other imaging modalities have been considered in addition to, and independent of, ultrasound. Magnetic resonance imaging (MRI)

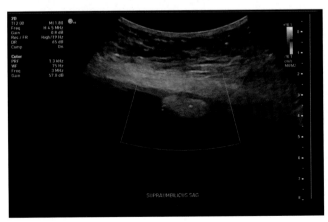

FIGURE 32-14. A close-up view of a papillary projection from the mass in Figure 32-13. Note the increased Doppler flow in the solid component.

TABLE 32-2	The International Ovarian Tumor Analysis (IOTA) "Simple Rules" Stratify Ovarian Masses by Benign and Malignant Features

B-Features	M-Features
Unilocular cyst	Irregular solid tumor
<7 mm or absent solid components	4+ papillary structures
Presence of acoustic shadowing	Ascites
No blood flow	Strong color flow
Smooth multilocular cyst less than 10 cm in diameter	Irregular solid multilocular tumor

Only B-Features suggest a benign lesion. Only M-Features suggest a malignancy. If neither or a combination of features, the mass is indeterminate and further imaging or consult should be obtained.

is a valuable secondary adjunct to ultrasound findings concerning for malignancy, with a specificity approximately three times that of ultrasound.[12,13] MRI is highly accurate in assessing masses that are inconclusive on initial TVUS assessment and therefore is the imaging modality of choice in these situations.

Computed tomography (CT) with intravenous contrast also shows a much higher specificity than ultrasound, and close to that of MRI, making it an appropriate option if MRI is unavailable or contraindicated.[12,14]

TABLE 32-3	Recommendations for Use of Point-of-Care Ultrasound in Clinical Practice

Recommendation	Rating	References
Two-dimensional grayscale ultrasound with additional color flow Doppler evaluation is the recommended first-line imaging study to evaluate an adnexal mass	A	6, 12, 13

A = consistent, good-quality patient-oriented evidence; B = inconsistent or limited-quality patient-oriented evidence; C = consensus, disease-oriented evidence, usual practice, expert opinion, or case series. For information about the SORT evidence rating system, go to http://www.aafp.org/afpsort.

PERFORMING THE SCAN

1. **Prepare for the examination.** Prior to beginning, review the patient's personal and family medical history. Document the patient's last menstrual period and the use of any hormones, such as birth control or hormone replacement therapy (HRT). Place the patient in a lithotomy position, which allows abdominal and TVUS approaches. The urinary bladder is best emptied for TVUS examinations, but most examinations can be performed adequately with some urine in the bladder. Both the curvilinear and transvaginal probes should be available (**Figure 32-15**).

2. **Perform a brief transabdominal ultrasound of the pelvis.** Start with the transabdominal approach. Place the curvilinear probe in the midline of the pelvis in a sagittal plane over the uterus. Scan through the entire uterus and adnexa in sagittal and transverse planes. The insertion of fallopian tubes at the cornua is challenging to see transabdominally. If the fallopian

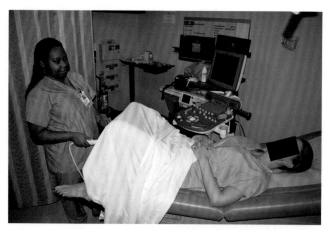

FIGURE 32-15. Patient positioning in the dorsal lithotomy position. Image courtesy of Lauren Castelberry, MD.

tubes are visible, note any areas of irregularity compared to the general appearance of the tube. When seen, fallopian tubes should be measured in both transverse and sagittal planes, and color flow Doppler images should be obtained. If located, the ovaries should be measured in three orthogonal planes. Examine the surrounding adnexal region for free fluid (**Figure 32-16**).

3. **Perform a transvaginal ultrasound of the uterus.** Using a clean transvaginal sheath, apply gel inside the sheath, cover the probe, and apply ultrasound gel to probe tip. Insert the probe to a depth where the entire fundus is visualized. Visualize the position of the uterus and cervix. Examine the uterus in both sagittal and coronal planes, describing the presentation, length, width, and an estimated uterine volume. The space between the posterior wall of the uterus and rectum is called the pouch of Douglas, or the rectouterine pouch or posterior cul-de-sac. Note any fluid present within this area. Note if it extends out of the pelvis and into the abdomen (**Figure 32-17**).

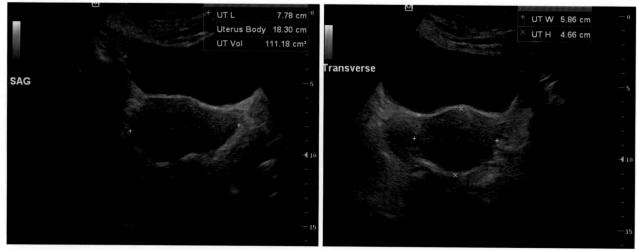

FIGURE 32-16. An image of the long (left) and short (right) axis of a normal uterus on transabdominal ultrasound imaging.

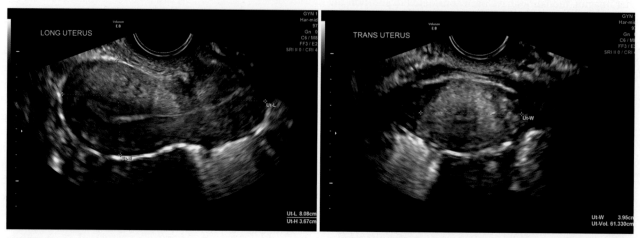

FIGURE 32-17. An image of the long (left) and short (right) axis of a normal uterus on transvaginal ultrasound imaging. Image courtesy of Lauren Castelberry, MD.

4. **Evaluate the fallopian tube.** After locating the fundus, angle the probe to locate the insertion site of the fallopian tube at the interstitium. Scan the area of the typical anatomic location of the fallopian tube, and, if possible, follow it until reaching the ovary. In the absence of pathology, the fallopian tubes are not visible via transabdominal or transvaginal approaches. Pregnancies can occur anywhere within the tube as well as extrauterine. Fluid present within the tube, or hydrosalpinx, most commonly represents pelvic inflammatory disease, but can be related to other causes ranging from endometriosis to appendicitis.

5. **Evaluate the ovaries.** Distal to the fimbria is the location of the ovary. Because the ovary is hormonally responsive, its appearance will vary. The normal premenopausal ovary will have multiple, small nondominant follicles measuring less than 1 cm in diameter early in the menstrual cycle and develop a dominant follicle typically measuring 1 to 3 cm near midcycle. Measure the ovary in three perpendicular (orthogonal) planes, utilizing two measurements in the sagittal plane and the third measurement in the coronal plane. Cysts may be present within the ovary. These should be measured at the location of the largest diameter and described as either simple or complex. Simple cysts contain only fluid, whereas complex cysts contain both fluid and solid contents. See **Figure 32-18B**. Document whether septations are present or absent. Color flow Doppler can be used to further evaluate and differentiate cysts likely benign versus malignant. Simple cysts less than 3 cm in diameter are considered normal follicles.

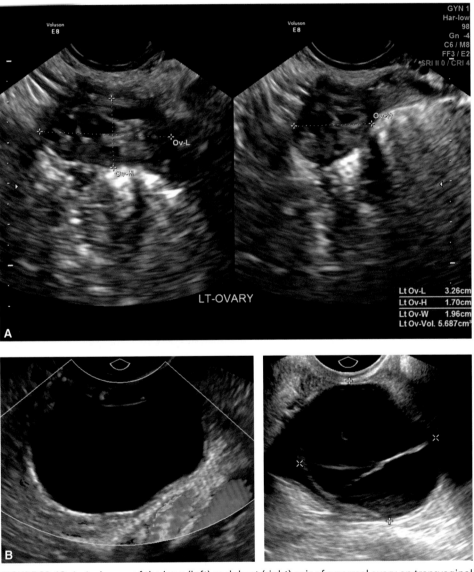

FIGURE 32-18. A, An image of the long (left) and short (right) axis of a normal ovary on transvaginal ultrasound imaging. Image courtesy of Lauren Castelberry, MD. B, A simple cyst is anechoic, without internal Doppler flow and normal posterior acoustic enhancement (left). A complex cyst may contain septations or internal solid components (right). Both of these cysts have benign features without malignant features per the International Ovarian Tumor Analysis (IOTA) Simple Rules and would be classified as benign.

PATIENT MANAGEMENT

The importance of ultrasound in adnexal mass is risk stratification that answers the question, "Is this mass benign?" If the mass is not almost definitely benign, further evaluation will be needed.

Acute patients should be managed in an appropriately emergent manner. These cases might include an adnexal mass with a positive pregnancy test suggesting ectopic pregnancy. Findings of acute pelvic pain, large cysts, and lack of flow on Doppler might indicate torsion. Acute pelvic pain and fever would give suspicion of tubo-ovarian abscess.

Begin the evaluation with an evidence-based approach such as the IOTA Simple Rules. If the mass is likely benign, further management can be guided via subjective interpretation and serial examinations as described later. If the mass is deemed high risk for malignancy, immediate request for a consultation for surgery or gynecologic oncology should be made. Other cases may require consultation from radiology for additional ultrasound or secondary imaging, such as MRI.

Beyond the Simple Rules, a stepwise approach to pattern recognition can be performed. Table 32-2 provides a description of common findings.

If the adnexal mass has the appearance of a simple cyst, follow-up may be guided on history and patient comfort. This may include no further study in the premenopausal patient. If follow-up ultrasound is chosen, it is common to schedule 2, 6, or 10 weeks later so the repeat study is at a different stage in the patient's menstrual cycle. If the mass is not a simple cyst, consider if only physiologic processes may have caused it, as this will also assist in follow-up considerations.

If the differential includes pathologic processes, consider if they are all benign. In these cases, serial ultrasound is likely appropriate.

The inconclusive mass is a clinical dilemma. The choice of further evaluation will be determined by differential and patient history. For instance, the clots in a suspected hemorrhagic cyst in a stable patient may mimic some solid components of a malignancy. In an otherwise low-risk patient, such a finding would be appropriate for serial ultrasound in 2 weeks. In higher risk patients, or differentials that are less likely to declare themselves in such a short follow-up period, MRI would be an appropriate study.

A lower threshold for additional workup should be had in postmenopausal women, in whom ovarian cancer is 3.5-fold more prevalent than in premenopausal women.[10]

The clinical role of CA-125, and other tumor markers, remains unclear and likely only provides an obvious stratification if markedly elevated (>300 u/mL), indicating a malignancy. A normal CA-125 should not give reassurance that the mass is benign. An indeterminate mass with a persistently mildly elevated CA-125 should prompt consideration of expert referral (**Figure 32-19**).

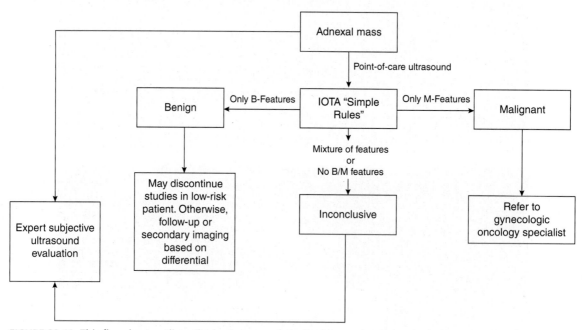

FIGURE 32-19. This flowchart outlines the basic approach to the International Ovarian Tumor Analysis (IOTA) Simple Rules using benign and malignant features of the adnexal mass to stratify risk and clinical approach. Experienced ultrasonographers may apply a purely subjective approach to the evaluation of adnexal masses.

PEARLS AND PITFALLS

Pearls

- Obtain a thorough history and perform a detailed physical examination prior to performing the ultrasound. One of the major benefits of providing point-of-care ultrasound in the primary care setting is the ability to perform a service for a patient who is known to you. Rather than looking at a limited set of static images obtained by a technologist, you can view these images in real time and obtain additional views as needed, which may not be part of the standard set of images obtained by a technologist. This is an invaluable resource present only with point-of-care ultrasound.

- Have the patient appropriately gowned prior to beginning the scan. It is inefficient use of time to have the patient undress between transabdominal and transvaginal scans. Transitioning between both scans should be seamless.

- Often the patient can assist you in finding the pathology if present. Use their descriptions of pain, fullness, etc., when scanning to localize areas of concern.

Pitfall

- Whenever possible, perform a transabdominal ultrasound before the transvaginal examination. Some large cystic masses may be impossible to differentiate from free fluid with only transvaginal examination. The "bird's-eye" view of the transabdominal examination is often helpful to develop context of the "zoomed-in" view provided by transvaginal scanning.

BILLING

CPT Code	Description	Global Payment	Professional Component	Technical Component
76856	Ultrasound, pelvic (nonobstetric), real time with image documentation; complete	$111.35	$35.09	$76.26
76857	Ultrasound, pelvic (nonobstetric), real time with image documentation; limited or follow-up (eg, for follicles)	$48.34	$25.42	$22.91
76830	Transvaginal ultrasound non-obstetric	$123.88	$35.45	$88.44

CPT codes and average national reimbursement for Medicare in 2016. Payment data are from https://www.cms.gov/apps/physician-fee-schedule/search/search-criteria.aspx. See Chapter 2 for details on ultrasound billing.

References

1. Ramsden I, Welsby P. *Clinical History Taking and Examination: An Illustrated Color Text*. Edinburgh, London: Churchill Livingstone; 2002:65.
2. Pavlik EJ, Ueland FR, Miller RW, et al. Frequency and disposition of ovarian abnormalities followed with serial transvaginal ultrasonography. *Obstet Gynecol*. 2013;122(2 pt 1):210-217.
3. Borgfeldt C, Andolf E. Transvaginal sonographic ovarian findings in a random sample of women 25-40 years old. *Ultrasound Obstet Gynecol*. 1999;13(5):345-350.
4. Castillo G, Alcázar JL, Jurado M. Natural history of sonographically detected simple unilocular adnexal cysts in asymptomatic postmenopausal women. *Gynecol Oncol*. 2004;92(3):965-969.
5. Timmerman D, Van Calster B, Testa A, et al. Predicting the risk of malignancy in adnexal masses based on the Simple Rules from the International Ovarian Tumor Analysis group. *Am J Obstet Gynecol*. 2016;214(4):424-437.
6. Valentin L, Ameye L, Jurkovic D, et al. Which extrauterine pelvic masses are difficult to correctly classify as benign or malignant on the basis of ultrasound findings and is there a way of making a correct diagnosis? *Ultrasound Obstet Gynecol*. 2006;27(4):438-444.
7. Harris RD, Javitt MC, Glanc P, et al.; American College of Radiology. ACR Appropriateness Criteria® clinically suspected adnexal mass. *Ultrasound Q*. 2013;29(1):79-86.
8. Buy JN, Ghossain MA, Hugol D, et al. Characterization of adnexal masses: combination of color Doppler and conventional sonography compared with spectral Doppler analysis alone and conventional sonography alone. *AJR Am J Roentgenol*. 1996;166(2):385-393.
9. Kinkel K, Hricak H, Lu Y, Tsuda K, Filly RA. US characterization of ovarian masses: a meta-analysis. *Radiology*. 2000;217(3):803-811.
10. Kinkel K, Lu Y, Mehdizade A, Pelte MF, Hricak H. Indeterminate ovarian mass at US: incremental value of second imaging test for characterization—meta-analysis and Bayesian analysis. *Radiology*. 2005;236(1):85-94.
11. Kaijser J. Towards an evidence-based approach for diagnosis and management of adnexal masses: findings of the International Ovarian Tumour Analysis (IOTA) studies. *Facts Views Vis Obgyn*. 2015;7(1):42-59.
12. Fan X, Zhang H, Meng S, Zhang J, Zhang C. Role of diffusion-weighted magnetic resonance imaging in differentiating malignancies from benign ovarian tumors. *Int J Clin Exp Med*. 2015;8(11):19928-19937.
13. Sohaib SA, Mills TD, Sahdev A, et al. The role of magnetic resonance imaging and ultrasound in patients with adnexal masses. *Clin Radiol*. 2005;60(3):340-348.
14. Gatreh-Samani F, Tarzamni MK, Olad-Sahebmadarek E, Dastranj A, Afrough A. Accuracy of 64-multidetector computed tomography in diagnosis of adnexal tumors. *J Ovarian Res*. 2011;4:15.
15. Patel MD, Feldstein VA, Lipson SD, Chen DC, Filly RA. Cystic teratomas of the ovary: diagnostic value of sonography. *AJR Am J Roentgenol*. 1998;171(4):1061-1065.

PART 2

What Is the Patient's Postvoid Residual Bladder Volume?

John Doughton, MD

● **Clinical Vignette**

A 54-year-old woman presents to clinic with the chief complaint of involuntary loss of urine. She reports that in between voids she will have continuous dribbling of urine and has the feeling that her bladder is not completely empty after urinating. She is embarrassed and does not want to leave the house or be far from a restroom as a result. What is the patient's postvoid residual bladder volume?

TABLE 33-1	Recommendations for Use of Point-of-Care Ultrasound in Clinical Practice		
Recommendation		**Rating**	**References**
Physician-performed bedside ultrasound is accurate and reliable for determining a postvoid residual bladder volume.		A	5-12

A = consistent, good-quality patient-oriented evidence; B = inconsistent or limited-quality patient-oriented evidence; C = consensus, disease-oriented evidence, usual practice, expert opinion, or case series. For information about the SORT evidence rating system, go to http://www.aafp.org/afpsort.

LITERATURE REVIEW

Measurement of postvoid residual (PVR) bladder volume or the amount of urine remaining in the bladder after a voluntary void has significant diagnostic utility for the primary care provider. Determining a PVR is helpful to evaluate common clinical presentations such as: urinary incontinence, concern for acute or chronic urinary retention, chronic urinary tract infections, and acute kidney injury.[1] In the pediatric population, bladder ultrasound can reduce catheterization attempts when urinalysis and culture are needed as part of an infectious workup.[2]

In patients with urinary incontinence, measuring a PVR is helpful to distinguish overflow incontinence and/or urinary retention from stress incontinence or overactive bladder.[3] In the case of overactive bladder, a PVR is recommended prior to initiating anticholinergic therapy, as overactive bladder and bladder outlet obstruction are commonly seen together.[4] Asymptomatic urinary retention or obstruction can also contribute to recurrent urinary tract infections and impaired renal function.[5] The above scenarios are but a few of the examples of the clinical utility of measuring a bedside PVR.

Previously, a PVR was measured only by bladder catheterization, which is still regarded as the gold standard.[1] However, bladder catheterization is an invasive procedure that brings risk of trauma and introducing infection. Bedside ultrasound offers a noninvasive alternative with accuracy that is supported by scientific evidence. With the emergence of three-dimensional (3D) portable bedside bladder ultrasound, several studies were published looking at ultrasound accuracy as compared to bladder catheterization. A 1993 study in the *Journal of Neuroscience Nursing* by Chan demonstrated that noninvasive bladder ultrasound provided a reliable PVR measurement with the added benefit of being safe and inexpensive.[6] These results have been confirmed in subsequent studies,[5,7-9] and a 2006 systematic review determined based on four separate studies that bedside ultrasound was an effective and cost-saving alternative to bladder catheterization, with a mean voided volume deviation of <10%.[5]

A recent review by the *Journal of International Nephrology* proposes that beside ultrasound evaluation should be a part of the physical examination for evaluating acute urinary obstruction or retention, citing the studies above among others in support of the accuracy and efficiency of this examination.[10] Although the majority of studies to this point evaluate the accuracy of 3D bladder scanners, a 2015 article in *Anesthesia and Analgesia* demonstrated that a simple handheld bedside ultrasound was useful for diagnosing postoperative urinary retention and performed well compared to both 3D bladder scanners and bladder catheterization.[11] In regard to physician versus sonographer performed studies, a recent study in *International Urology and Nephrology* compared the two groups and showed no statistically significant difference in PVR volumes measured.[12]

PERFORMING THE SCAN

1. **Preparation.** As in any bedside ultrasound application, understanding the anatomy is critical to the success of the examination. The bladder is an extraperitoneal organ located cephalad to the pubic symphysis (**Figure 33-1**). In females, the bladder is positioned anterior to the uterus. In males, the prostate is located inferior to the bladder and surrounds the bladder neck. The patient should be positioned supine, with the head of the bed elevated to 30 degrees. Select the lower frequency (2-5 MHz) curvilinear transducer. Though a linear probe has higher resolution, the combination of deeper tissue penetration and a broader ultrasound beam makes the curvilinear transducer ideal for imaging the entirety of the bladder.[13]

2. **Imaging the bladder.** Utilize a suprapubic approach. Palpate the pubic symphysis and place the curvilinear transducer just superior to that point (**Figure 33-2**). Orient the transducer in a transverse plane, with the probe marker to the patient's right. Aim the ultrasound beam posterior and inferior to the pubic symphysis. A full bladder will often be easily visualized (**Figure 33-3**).

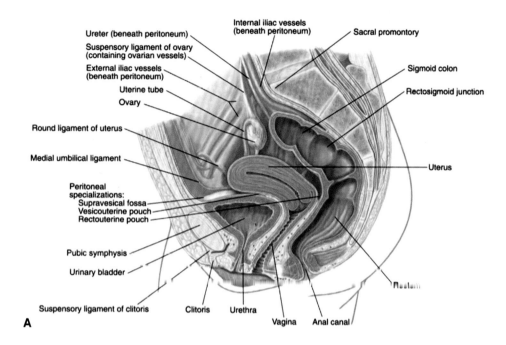

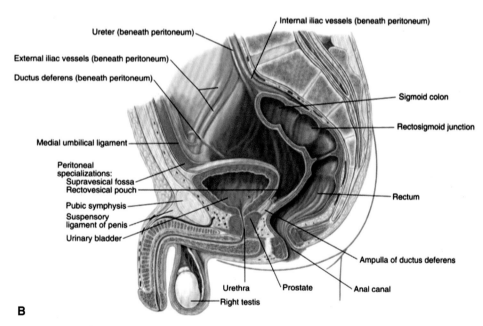

FIGURE 33-1. Anatomic diagram of the female (A) and male (B) bladder.

However, if the bladder does not come immediately into view, slide the transducer superiorly and fan inferiorly. Increase the depth so that the entirety of the posterior wall is visualized and adjust the gain so that the urine is anechoic. Fan superiorly and inferiorly to visualize the bladder in its entirety. Capture the image in which the bladder is the largest. Once the transverse image is captured, rotate the transducer 90 degrees clockwise to obtain a sagittal view (**Figure 33-4**). Fan the transducer left and right to again visualize the entirety of the bladder and capture the largest bladder image (**Figure 33-5**).

3. **Calculating bladder volume.** Bladder volume requires measurements of the bladder width, depth, and length. The width

and depth are obtained in the transverse plane (**Figure 33-6**), and the length is obtained in the sagittal plane (**Figure 33-7**). In order to calculate the volume of a cube, every bladder volume formula contains **width × depth × length.** However, as the bladder is not a perfect cube, a correction factor must be included. There is some disagreement as to which correction factor to use. Some advocate for a correction factor of 0.53 to represent an ellipsoid.[14] However, based on Chan's 1993 study,[6] the majority of point-of-care ultrasound experts prefer to use a correction factor of 0.75. We suggest the following formula:

$$\text{Width} \times \text{Depth} \times \text{Length} \times 0.75$$

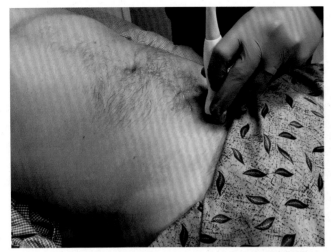

FIGURE 33-2. Transducer position to obtain the transverse view of the bladder. Probe marker positioned to patient's right.

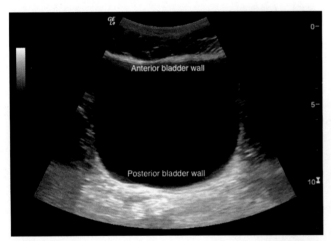

FIGURE 33-3. Transverse view of the male bladder, with anterior and posterior portions labeled. Note acoustic enhancement posterior to the bladder.

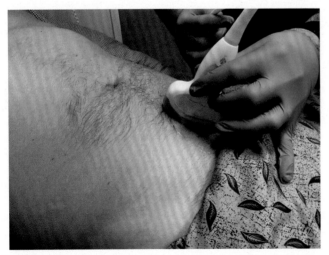

FIGURE 33-4. Transducer position to obtain the longitudinal, or sagittal, view of the bladder. Probe marker positioned toward the patient's head.

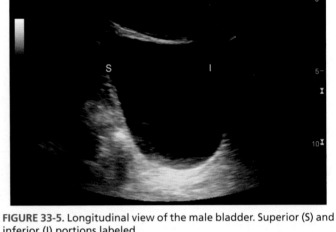

FIGURE 33-5. Longitudinal view of the male bladder. Superior (S) and inferior (I) portions labeled.

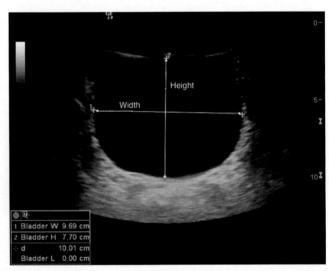

FIGURE 33-6. Measurement of bladder width and height demonstrated in the transverse view.

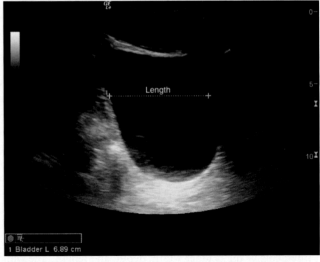

FIGURE 33-7. Measurement of bladder length demonstrated in the longitudinal view.

TABLE 33-2 **Incontinence Classification and Treatment**

Incontinence Type	Symptoms	Objective Findings	First-Line Treatment
Stress	Small volume, provoked by cough, sneezing, laughing	Normal postvoid residual (PVR) Positive cough stress test	Pelvic floor muscle strengthening (Kegel's exercises)
Urge	Urgency prior to voiding, variable volume	Normal PVR Negative cough stress test, though can have delayed leakage	Bladder training exercises Antimuscarinic agent
Overflow	Variable volume, symptoms not brought on by stress and no urgency prior to void	Elevated PVR (>200 mL)	Variable depending on etiology (obstruction vs detrusor underactivity)
Functional	Cognitive or physical impairments to voiding	Normal PVR Negative cough stress test	Treatment of underlying functional impairment
Mixed	Frequently combination of stress and urge symptoms	Variable	Begin with pelvic floor muscle strengthening Can then trial antimuscarinic agent

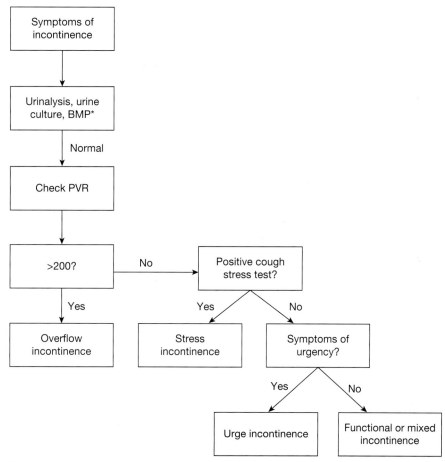

*Important to rule out underlying infection, hyperglycemia, or constipation

FIGURE 33-8. Undifferentiated urinary incontinence algorithm. BMP, basic metabolic panel; PVR, postvoid residual.

However, in cases of very full bladders that more closely resemble ellipsoids, it is reasonable to use the correction factor of 0.53.

PATIENT MANAGEMENT

PVR measurements are used in many different clinical contexts. A PVR >100 is abnormal, and PVRs >300 can be associated with the risk of renal dysfunction and upper urinary tract dilatation.[1]

Over time, this can lead to "bladder stretch injuries" or cellular changes that cause impaired storage and voiding.[15]

In the patient with concern for acute urinary retention, an elevated PVR is an indication for urinary catheter placement for decompression. In the patient with overactive bladder, an elevated PVR at baseline would be a contraindication to starting anticholinergic therapy. For the patient with undifferentiated urinary incontinence, an elevated PVR supports a diagnosis of overflow incontinence rather than stress, urge, or functional incontinence. The "cough stress test," or having patients with a full bladder cough in the supine and standing positions and evaluating for urinary leakage, is used to differentiate stress incontinence from urge or functional incontinence in patients with a normal PVR. It is important to understand that in many cases patients will have mixed incontinence or components of various etiologies. The following algorithm aids in differentiating types of incontinence. Please also see Table 33-2 for a summary of incontinence type and first-line treatment.[16] The following algorithm (**Figure 33-8**) aids in differentiating types of incontinence.

PEARLS AND PITFALLS

Pearls

- Make sure to visualize the largest view of each dimension for measurement (width, depth, and length) when performing your calculations.
- Understand which correction factor your machine uses, as many have built-in formulas. Remember that a larger bladder more closely resembling an ellipse can be more accurately calculated using the correction factor of 0.53.

Pitfalls

- Ascites can be confused for the bladder. Complete scanning in multiple planes can help identify ascites and clarify the picture. If you are still not sure in the inpatient setting, a Foley catheter can be placed.
- Contracted abdominal muscles will make it more difficult to visualize depth well. As such, have patient in a relaxed position.
- A common pitfall is measuring the anteroposterior diameter twice and missing the caudal-cephalad diameter. To avoid this, as demonstrated in the images obtain two measurements in the transverse view (width and depth) and ensure you are measuring length while in the sagittal view (see **Figure 33-7**).

BILLING

CPT Code	Description	Global Payment	Professional Component	Technical Component
76705	Ultrasound, abdominal, real time with image documentation; limited (e.g., single organ, quadrant, follow-up)	$92.44	$30.10	$62.34

CPT codes and average national reimbursement for Medicare in 2016. Payment data are from https://www.cms.gov/apps/physician-fee-schedule/search/search-criteria.aspx. See Chapter 2 for details on ultrasound billing.

References

1. Kelly CE. Evaluation of voiding dysfunction and measurement of bladder volume. *Rev Urol.* 2004;6 Suppl 1:S32-S37.
2. Chen L, Hsiao AL, Moore CL, Dziura JD, Santucci KA. Utility of bedside bladder ultrasound before urethral catheterization in young children. *Pediatrics.* 2005;115(1):108-111.
3. Ng CK, Gonzalez RR, Te AE. Refractory overactive bladder in men: update on novel therapies. *Curr Urol Rep.* 2006;7(6):456-461.
4. Culligan PJ, Heit M. Urinary incontinence in women: evaluation and management. *Am Fam Physician.* 2000;62(11):2433-2444, 2447, 2452.
5. Medical Advisory Secretariat. Portable bladder ultrasound: an evidence-based analysis. *Ont Health Technol Assess Ser.* 2006;6(11):1-51.
6. Chan H. Noninvasive bladder volume measurement. *J Neurosci Nurs.* 1993;25(5):309-312.
7. Jalbani IK, Ather MH. The accuracy of three-dimensional bladder ultrasonography in determining the residual urinary volume compared with conventional catheterisation. *Arab J Urol.* 2014;12(3):209-213.
8. Hvarness H, Skjoldbye B, Jakobsen H. Urinary bladder volume measurements: comparison of three ultrasound calculation methods. *Scand J Urol Nephrol.* 2002;36(3):177-181.
9. Griffiths CJ, Murray A, Ramsden PD. Accuracy and repeatability of bladder volume measurement using ultrasonic imaging. *J Urol.* 1986;136(4):808-812.
10. Kaptein MJ, Kaptein EM. Focused real-time ultrasonography for nephrologists. *Int J Nephrol.* 2017;2017:3756857.
11. Daurat A, Choquet O, Bringuier S, Charbit J, Egan M, Capdevila X. Diagnosis of postoperative urinary retention using a simplified ultrasound bladder measurement. *Anesth Analg.* 2015;120(5):1033-1038.
12. Lavi A, Tzemah S, Hussein A, et al. A urologic stethoscope? Urologist performed sonography using a pocket-size ultrasound device in the point-of-care setting. *Int Urol Nephrol.* 2017;49(9):1513-1518.
13. Soni N, Arntfield R, Pierre K. Chapter 21: Bladder. In *Point-of-Care Ultrasound.* 1st ed. Philadelphia, PA: Elsevier Saunders; 2015:162-166.
14. *Bladder and Pelvis.* Minneapolis, MN: Abbott Northwestern Hospital, IM Residency; 2016-2017. http://imbus.anwresidency.com/txtbook/23_bladderpelvis.html. Accessed August 8, 2017.
15. Halachmi S. The molecular pathways behind bladder stretch injury. *J Pediatr Urol.* 2009;5(1):13-16.
16. Khandelwal C, Kistler C. Diagnosis of urinary incontinence. *Am Fam Physician.* 2013;87(8):543-550.

CHAPTER 34

Is the Patient's Intrauterine Device in the Proper Location?

Joy Shen-Wagner, MD, FAAFP and Lauren Castleberry, MD, FACOG

Clinical Vignette

A 34-year-old healthy woman presents with inability to feel her intrauterine device (IUD) strings. Six months ago, she had an uncomplicated vaginal delivery and underwent 6-week postpartum placement of a levonorgestrel (LNG) secreting IUD. She denies symptoms of pain or abnormal bleeding. In fact, she has not had a menstrual cycle and asks about the possibility of pregnancy. Physical examination demonstrates a normal-sized uterus, and on speculum examination, her cervix appears normal; however, the IUD strings cannot be visualized. A urine pregnancy test is negative. Is the patient's intrauterine device in the proper location?

LITERATURE REVIEW

IUDs are used in hundreds of millions of women worldwide. In 2015, 13.7% of surveyed women aged 15 to 49 reported using them, with the lowest utilization in Africa 3.8% of surveyed women and highest in Asia 17.4% (up to 40% in China).[1] Since 2001, with the introduction of newer and safer IUDs, there has been an increase in the United States, with up to 11.1% among women aged 25 to 34 reporting using them.[2,3] Other factors affecting the increase in IUD use include the removal of nulliparity as a contraindication from the copper T IUD package insert in 2005 and the Food and Drug Administration (FDA) approval of the Mirena IUD to treat dysmenorrhea and dysfunctional uterine bleeding. In 2009 and 2015, the American Congress of Obstetricians and Gynecologists (ACOG) recommended that long-acting reversible contraception (LARC), implants, and IUDs should be offered as first-line contraception to most women.[4,5] Given the rise in IUD prevalence in the United States, primary care practitioners need to be familiar with how to manage IUD complications, including missing IUD strings, amenorrhea, pain, and bleeding. Pelvic ultrasound is both a vital and an inexpensive bedside tool that aids in the workup, decision-making, and management process associated with these complaints.

Missing IUD strings is one of the most common IUD complications and raises the possibility of IUD malposition. Anywhere from 4.5% to 18.1% of IUD users have missing strings on string checks or at the time of removal.[6] The majority of IUD strings are retracted in the uterus or in the cervical canal (possibly from tension after upward IUD migration), and reassurance can be easily obtained by bedside ultrasound. Amenorrhea, which is seen in 20% of LNG IUD users,[7] cannot be a reliable indicator of IUD presence, and pregnancy should be ruled out.[8] A protocol to rule out expulsion or perforation is necessary.

There are five general ways that an IUD can be malpositioned: *expulsion*, *perforation*, *displacement* in the lower uterine segment, *malrotation*, and *embedment* of the crossbars or main stem into the endometrium or myometrium. Conventional 2D ultrasound is an excellent tool to triage for expulsion, perforation, or displacement but is less capable than 3D ultrasound of identifying IUD malrotation and embedment. In an ultrasound study by Braaten et al., 10.4% of 1748 women with IUDs were identified as malpositioned. The majority of malpositioned IUDs, 73.1%, were *displaced* (low-lying) in the lower uterine segment or cervix, and 11.5% were *embedded* or *rotated*.[9] Although displacement and embedment can be associated with increased pelvic pain, dyspareunia, abnormal bleeding, difficult removals, and possibly decreased contraceptive efficacy, it can also be asymptomatic.[10] *Expulsion* (loss of the IUD via the cervix) is a less common complication, with rates ranging from 2% to 10% in the first year.[11] Usually, it occurs within the first month of placement and carries the risk of unintended pregnancy. *Perforation* (either partial or full) is the most serious complication and requires surgical removal. Fortunately, perforation rates are low (0.3-2.6 in 1000) and are associated with a short pregnancy-to-placement time interval, a patient that is currently breastfeeding, and practitioner inexperience.[12] IUD perforations were historically thought to be associated with complications such as pelvic adhesions, abscesses, and bowel perforations. The latest data show a more benign profile. From 2006 to 2013, a prospective cohort study in seven European countries followed over 60,000 women with IUDs (30% copper and 70% LNG IUD). Perforation rates were similar, but surprisingly, none of the 81 patients with perforations suffered from serious complications (peritonitis, bowel, bladder perforation) and required treatment beyond removal.[12]

When IUD strings are not visible on examination, ultrasound is the first step in determining the location. Ultrasound is widely available, low-cost, and effective. Additionally, it does not have the risk of radiation associated with other imaging modalities.[6,8,13,14] Most studies assessing ultrasound evaluation of IUD location used the transvaginal (TV) approach. In Finland, Palo et al. studied 20 women with Mirena IUDs comparing transvaginal ultrasound (TVUS) and transabdominal ultrasound (TABUS); it concluded that TVUS was preferred because TABUS relied on the patient having a full bladder. There was also more posterior shadowing from the LNG IUD in the TV studies, which helped IUD location.[15]

Alternate modes of imaging for IUD location include x-ray, CT, MRI, and hysteroscopy.[16] A two-view plain film can be helpful when expulsion is expected and the IUD cannot be confidently visualized on ultrasound.[13] CT scan is helpful in the presurgical planning for laparoscopic IUD removal. There is a paucity of studies comparing ultrasound to x-rays, CT scans, and MRIs as initial imaging tools,[17] although it has been shown that both LNG and copper IUDs are safe for up to 3T MRI.[18] With 3D ultrasound emerging as the new gold standard for evaluating the endometrial cavity, newer studies have compared 3D ultrasound to 2D ultrasound. It appears that although 3D can more precisely locate the LNG IUD and the crossbars in the endometrial cavity and myometrium, 2D is still able to locate IUDs in the fundal portion of the uterus, albeit with less detail.[19] Additionally, it appears that the type of IUD influences the clarity of visualization in 2D and 3D images. Moschos demonstrated that the LNG IUD is less conspicuous on 2D ultrasound than the copper IUD. The 3D ultrasound was able to increase the conspicuity score of the LNG IUD to the same level as the copper; however, there was no improvement in visualization of copper IUDs over 2D.[20]

In the past, some practitioners have advocated routine ultrasound to confirm placement after all IUD insertions. However, current recommendations are *against* this practice. Petta and Faundes conducted a 2-year prospective randomized controlled study of women who had a copper T IUD placed in Brazil from 1992 to 1994. They compared outcomes in two groups of women—235 women who received ultrasound 30 to 40 days after IUD placement to check for appropriate fundal location and a control group of 201 women who did not receive imaging. They concluded that there were 25 possible unnecessary removals. They hypothesized that even though ultrasound was helpful in identifying low-lying IUDs, these IUDs seem to retain some efficacy and that routine ultrasound after IUD placement leads to unnecessary removals.[21] Faundes's follow-up study found that the copper IUD had a tendency to shift positions within the first 3 months after placement.[22] Morales-Rosello described spontaneous upward movement of low-lying T-shaped IUDs, on average of 4.9 mm, within the first 3 months of placement.[23] These findings may be explained by the idea that there is a settling period after IUD placement and that initial postprocedural ultrasound results may not predict long-term IUD outcome.

Intrauterine Device Description

There are three types of IUD in use worldwide—inert, copper, and hormone secreting. The copper and hormone secreting IUDs both work by releasing chemicals into the uterus, either copper ions or

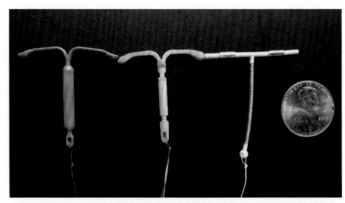

FIGURE 34-1. Mirena, Skyla, and ParaGard from left to right. Compared to the Mirena, the Skyla has a thinner stem and a silver ring added for increased ultrasound visibility. Penny is included for size reference.

LNG. Inert IUDs work only by physical interaction and are usually made of plastic or stainless steel. Inert IUDs were among the first IUDs, most notably the ring and the Lippes Loop. No inert IUDs are currently available in the United States, although they are commonly used in some other countries. A newer version of the stainless steel ring is still widely used in China. The ring is difficult to remove and is considered to be a permanent contraception.[24]

At the time of writing, there were five IUDs that were FDA approved for use in the United States, and they are described below (**Figure 34-1** and Table 34-1).

The copper TCu-380A (ParaGard, Teva Women's Health, Inc, North Wales, PA, USA) is a third-generation copper-containing IUD that has been used in the United States since 1988. It has the same polyethylene frame (32 mm horizontally and 36 mm vertically), with barium sulfate added for radiopacity, and two white polyethylene monofilament strings for retrieval.[25]

TABLE 34-1 | **IUD Descriptions**

	Copper TCu-380A	LNG IUD			
Brand	**ParaGard**	**Mirena**	**Skyla**	**Liletta**	**Kyleena**
Description	T-shaped polyethylene frame with 176 mg of copper wire coiled along the stem and a 68.7 mg collar on each cross bar	T-shaped polyethylene frame with a reservoir in the stem containing silicone mixture of 52 mg of LNG; releases approx. 20 µg/day, decreasing to half that value after 5 years	T-shaped polyethylene frame with a silver collar above the reservoir in the stem that contains silicone mixture of 13.5 mg of LNG; releases approx. 14 µg/day, decreasing to half that value after 3 years	T-shaped polyethylene frame with a reservoir in the stem containing silicone mixture of 13.5 mg of LNG; releases approx. 14 µg/day, decreasing to half that value after 3 years	T-shaped polyethylene frame with a reservoir in the stem containing silicone mixture of 19 mg of LNG; releases approx. 17.5 µg/day, decreasing to half that value after 5 years
Size of device	32 mm horizontally 36 mm vertically	32 mm horizontally 32 mm vertically	28 mm horizontally 30 mm vertically	32 mm horizontally 32 mm vertically	28 mm horizontally 30 mm vertically
Ultrasound qualities	Highly echogenic line with ringed down artifact with strong posterior shadowing	Two echogenic foci with posterior shadowing in between, may have ringed down artifact			
String description	White	Dark silver	Black	Blue	Blue

Abbreviations: IUD, intrauterine device; LNG, levonorgestrel.

Adapted from the Association of Reproductive Health Professionals, Washington, DC. http://www.arhp.org/Publications-and-Resources/Clinical-Fact-Sheets/The-Facts-About-Intrauterine-Contraception. Accessed December 2, 2016.[32]

TABLE 34-2	Recommendations for Use of Point-of-Care Ultrasound in Clinical Practice		
Recommendation		**Rating**	**References**
In the event of questionable intrauterine device (IUD) location (missing IUD strings, symptoms of bleeding and pelvic pain), ultrasound should be used to confirm intrauterine status and IUD position.		C	6, 13, 14, 28
Ultrasound is capable of establishing the location of a copper and levonorgestrel IUD.		B	14, 15, 19, [20-22]
Ultrasound should not be used routinely to check IUD position in an asymptomatic patient and in the setting of a normal clinical examination.		B	10, 14, 23
In the event of pregnancy, the IUD should be removed when possible without an invasive procedure.		C	11

A = consistent, good-quality patient-oriented evidence; B = inconsistent or limited-quality patient-oriented evidence; C = consensus, disease-oriented evidence, usual practice, expert opinion, or case series. For information about the SORT evidence rating system, go to http://www.aafp.org/afpsort.

The Mirena, developed in 2001 by Bayer Healthcare Pharmaceuticals Inc. (Pittsburgh, PA), is made of a 32×32 mm polyethylene frame, with barium sulfate added for radiopacity, and a silicone sleeve containing LNG and two silvery monofilament strings for retrieval. It releases 20 μg/day of LNG and is FDA approved for 5 years of use.[7]

Skyla (2013), Liletta (2015), and Kyleena (2016) are the newest LNG T-shaped IUDs on the market. Skyla and Liletta are both approved for 3 years of use, although clinical trials are still ongoing. Skyla's claimed advantage is its smaller size (28 mm horizontal and 30 mm vertical) and thinner insertion tube (3.8 mm vs. 4.4 mm in the case of Mirena). It was the first IUD approved for nulliparous women and releases 14 μg/day of LNG.[18] Kyleena is made by the same manufacturer as that of Mirena and Skyla. It is the same size as Skyla but releases a lower amount of hormone than Mirena; 17.5 μg/day but approved for a full 5 years. Liletta (32×32 mm) advertises a lower cost. It releases 18.6 μg/day of LNG.[26] Imaging for Skyla, Liletta, and Kyleena is theoretically similar to that of Mirena, except that the Skyla has a highly echogenic 99.9% silver ring (for easier ultrasound identification) on the stem just inferior to the crossbars.

PERFORMING THE SCAN

Identification of the copper IUD can be done using both transabdominal (TAB) and TV approaches; however, the TV approach is superior for identification of LNG IUDs, especially in a retroflexed uterus. Alternatively, if the uterus is enlarged or has many fibroids, TABUS is better at identification of the uterine fundus. The main advantage of the TAB approach is convenience, given the availability of abdominal probes, and easy patient setup.

Scanning protocols begin with the TAB approach requiring the patient to have a full bladder. This allows for a global view of the pelvis and structural identification. The patient is then asked to empty his or her bladder before moving onto the TV scan.

Transabdominal Pelvic Ultrasound

The patient should have a full bladder, which serves as an acoustic window for ultrasound of the uterus. If the patient has already emptied the bladder prior to scanning, move on to the TV or request the patient to drink 500 mL of water, and repeat the scan in 30 minutes.

1. Setup: Use the curvilinear (frequency of 3.5-5.0 MHz) probe on the GYN setting.
2. Patient position: Have the patient lying supine and the suprapubic region of the pelvis accessible for scanning (**Figure 34-2**).
3. Long axis (sagittal view): Hold the abdominal probe in the vertical position low in the pelvis, just above the pubic symphysis, with the probe marker pointing cephalad (and presumably toward the uterine fundus in an anteverted uterus). Scan through the patient's bladder and adjust the depth of view and focus point so that it captures the uterus below. Fan the probe from left to right to scan through the entire uterus. Tilt the probe back and forth on its longitudinal axis to show more of the fundus or the cervix (Figure 34-2C and D).
4. Short axis (transverse view): Rotate the abdominal probe 90° so that it is horizontal with the probe marker pointing to the patient's right. By fanning the handle vertically up and down, scan through the entire uterus (Figure 34-2E).
5. Locating the IUD: Follow the identification patterns outlined in the TV scanning section. If the IUD position is unclear, move on to the TV examination (**Figure 34-3**).

Transvaginal Pelvic Ultrasound

1. Setup: Place ultrasound gel on the distal end of the endocavitary transducer (frequency of 8.0-13.0 MHz), and place the latex cover over the top and roll the edge to cover the entire transducer. Eliminate any bubbles. Place additional gel on the cover (**Figure 34-4**).
2. Patient positioning: The patient should void before the examination and be placed in dorsal lithotomy position with her feet in stirrups and her pelvis at the edge of the examination table, allowing for ample space for ultrasound maneuvering.
3. Holding the transvaginal transducer: Start by holding the probe so that the ultrasound probe marker is pointing upward. Align the thumb with the probe marker, and curl the fingers along the underside of the handle (**Figure 34-5**).
4. Long axis (sagittal view): Introduce the transducer past the introitus about 4 to 5 cm in a downward sloping angle, to rest in front of the cervix. It is helpful to use the empty bladder on the screen as a landmark because the cervix usually sits just posterior to the bladder. This will bring the longitudinal axis of the uterus (cervix, isthmus, and uterine body) into the sagittal view (**Figure 34-6**).

Without rotation of the handle, scan through the entire uterus by fanning the handle to the right and left. Identify the uterine fundus, body, and isthmus; cervix; as well as the endometrial

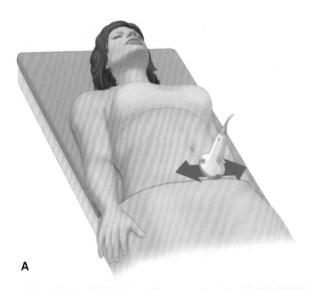

A

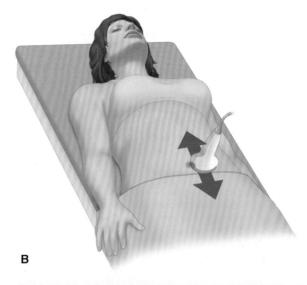

B

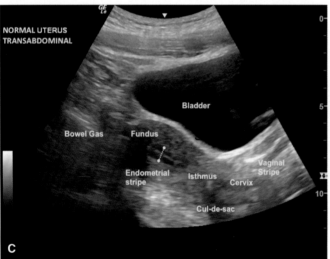

NORMAL UTERUS
TRANSABDOMINAL

Bladder

Bowel Gas   Fundus

Endometrial
stripe   Isthmus   Cervix

Vaginal
Stripe

Cul-de-sac

C

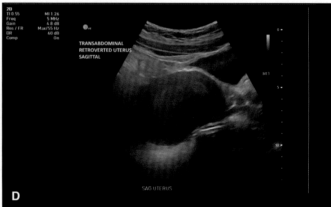

TRANSABDOMINAL
RETROVERTED UTERUS
SAGITTAL

SAG UTERUS

D

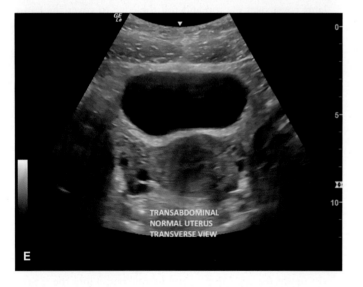

TRANSABDOMINAL
NORMAL UTERUS
TRANSVERSE VIEW

E

FIGURE 34-2. A, Patient positioning with probe in the sagittal plane. Fan through the structures in the direction of the green arrows. B, Patient positioning with probe in the transverse positioning. Fan through the structures in the direction of the green arrows. C, Transabdominal (TAB) sagittal view of normal anteverted uterus. D, TAB sagittal view of retroverted uterus. E, Transverse view of normal uterus (right ovary also visible).

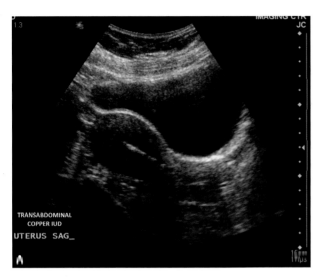

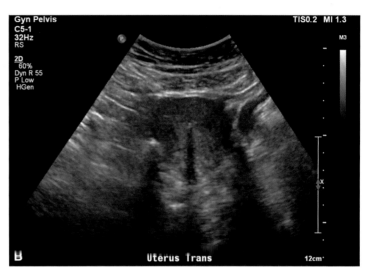

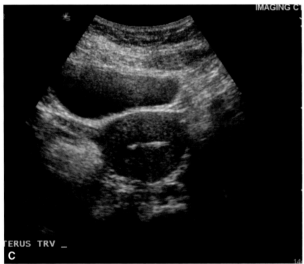

FIGURE 34-3. A, Transabdominal (TAB) sagittal view of the uterus with a copper intrauterine device (IUD). B, TAB transverse view of the uterus with a copper IUD at the stem. C, TAB transverse view of the uterus with a copper IUD at the crossbar.

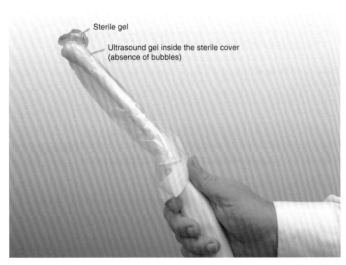

FIGURE 34-4. Hold the transvaginal transducer so that the thumb is aligned with the probe marker pointed upward, and curl the fingers along the underside of the handle.

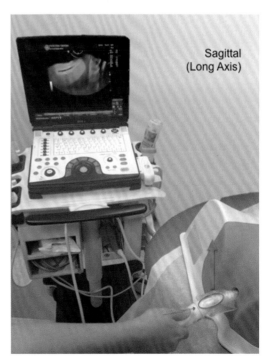

FIGURE 34-5. Transvaginal ultrasound (US) of simulated normal uterus in sagittal view on a laptop US with a pelvic simulator in the foreground. Small arrow points to probe marker. Large arrow indicates the orientation of the probe marker.

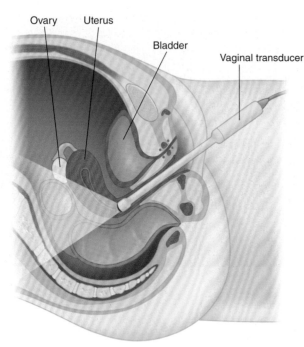

FIGURE 34-6. Sagittal plane produced by vertical ultrasound beam through the long axis of the uterus.

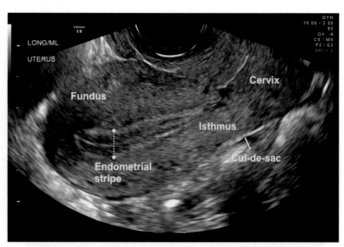

FIGURE 34-8. Transvaginal ultrasound of normal anteverted uterus. Identify the fundus, body, isthmus, cervix, endometrial stripe, and cul-de-sac.

stripe, internal and external os, and cul-de-sac (**Figures 34-7 and 34-8**).

Most women will have an anteverted uterus, but a minority of women will have a retroverted uterus. Additionally, the uterus can change positions depending on the distention of the surrounding bladder or rectosigmoid colon. In an anteverted uterus, to see more of the uterine fundus, depress the handle inferiorly, allowing the ultrasound beam to point upward toward the fundus (**Figures 34-9 to 34-11**).

In a retroverted uterus, move the handle more superiorly, pointing the ultrasound beam downward to see more of the uterine fundus. The image will seem flipped from right to left on the screen compared to an anteverted uterus.

5. Short axis (transverse view): Without changing hand position on the transducer, rotate the transducer 90° to the left (counter-clockwise), which points the probe marker to the patient's right side, and this will produce the transverse plane or short-axis view of the uterus (**Figures 34-12 and 34-13A**).

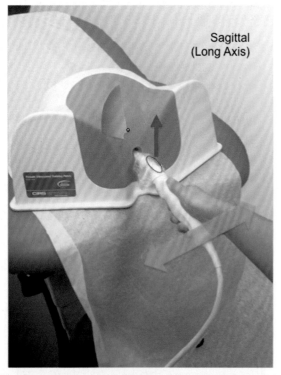

FIGURE 34-7. Without rotation of the handle, scan through the entire uterus by fanning the probe right and left. Red arrow indicates the upward orientation of the probe marker. Green arrow represents the horizontal movement of the handle.

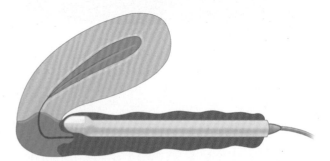

FIGURE 34-9. Drawing of ultrasound transducer relative to anteverted uterus.

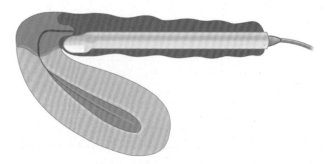

FIGURE 34-10. Drawing of ultrasound transducer relative to retroverted uterus.

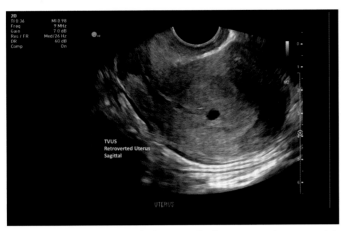

FIGURE 34-11. Transvaginal ultrasound of retroverted uterus with incidental small gestational sac.

By fanning the handle up and down, scan from the cervix (holding the handle in the neutral position) through the isthmus, body, and fundus of the uterus (scanning anteriorly by moving the handle posteriorly) (**Figure 34-13B**).

6. Locating the IUD: Levonorgestrel Secreting IUD

In the long-axis sagittal view, the Mirena has two echogenic regions—proximally at the T-arms and distally at the stem with 2 cm of acoustic shadowing in between. Look for a shadow cast downward from the endometrium, which may be the only recognizable sign for LNG IUD presence.[8,13,20] There may be a reverberation artifact from the stem (**Figures 34-14 and 34-15**).

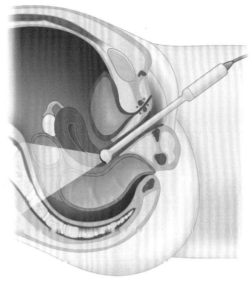

FIGURE 34-12. Transverse plane produced by horizontal ultrasound beam through the short axis of the uterus.

Take note that the distal tip of the IUD stem (where the stem intersects the T) should be at the fundal position within the endometrium and that the proximal end is above the level of the isthmus. The shadowing from the stem measures about 2 cm. Faundes et al. describe the appropriate distance between IUD and endometrium as being within 7 mm, IUD to myometrium distance within 11 mm, and IUD to fundus distance within 27 mm. Another

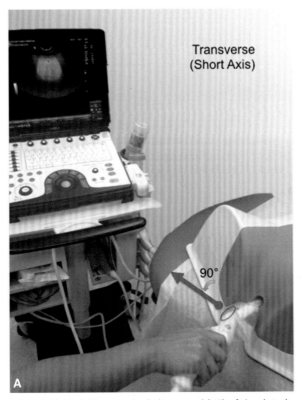

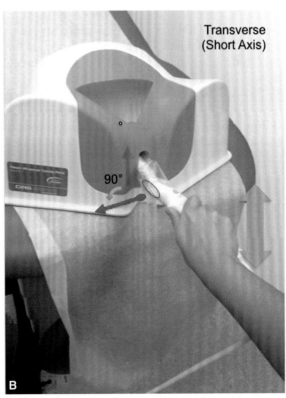

FIGURE 34-13. A, Transvaginal ultrasound (US) of simulated normal uterus in transverse view on a cart-based US with a pelvic simulator in the foreground. Red arrow indicates the orientation of the probe marker. B, With the probe marker pointed toward the patient's right, scan through the entire uterus by fanning the probe in the vertical plane. Red arrow indicates the orientation of the probe marker. Green arrow indicates the axis of fanning the probe during transverse scanning.

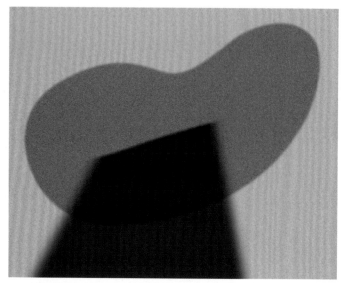

FIGURE 34-14. In the sagittal view, for the levonorgestrel secreting intrauterine device look for a broad shadow cast downward between two echogenic points, in the fundal region.

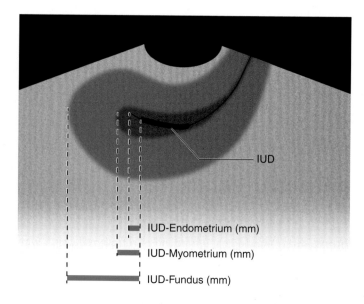

FIGURE 34-16. Intrauterine device (IUD) to endometrium distance ≤7 mm, IUD to myometrium distance ≤11 mm, IUD to fundus distance ≤27 mm. Another generally accepted measurement is ≤20 to 25 mm from the IUD to the fundus.

generally accepted measurement is 20 to 25 mm from the IUD to the fundus.[10] No part of the IUD should be within the cervical canal (**Figures 34-16 and 34-17**).

In the transverse view, identify the crossbars of the T at the fundus casting broad shadows or the shaft of the IUD as a narrow beam of shadow in the uterine body. For placement, check to see that the crossbars and stem are midline (**Figures 34-18 to 34-20**).

Ultrasound of the copper IUD: Its copper coils make the arms and the stem of the copper IUD bright with continuous echogenicity with strong posterior shadowing.[27] Because of the density of the shaft, there may be a reverberation artifact below the IUD appearing like multiple parallel lines.[13] These identifiers allow for easy location on both TABUS and TVUS. Follow the same scanning protocol used for the Mirena IUD. Once visualized, check that the IUD stem is midline and in the appropriate fundal position (**Figures 34-21 and 34-22** and ▶ Video **Video 34-1**).

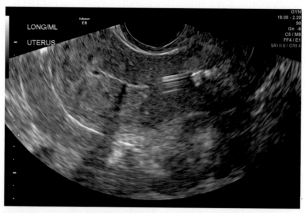

FIGURE 34-17. Transvaginal ultrasound sagittal view of uterus with Mirena intrauterine device in the lower uterine segment.

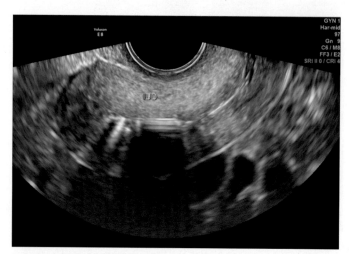

FIGURE 34-15. Transvaginal ultrasound sagittal view with Mirena intrauterine device in the correct fundal region of the uterus.

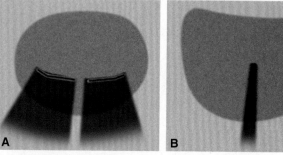

FIGURE 34-18. In the transverse view, identify the echogenic crossbars casting two broad shadows or the shaft of the intrauterine device as a narrow beam of shadow in the uterine body. To check positioning, confirm that the crossbars or shaft is midline in the uterus.

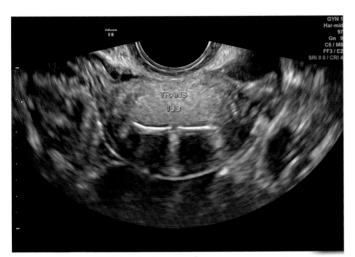

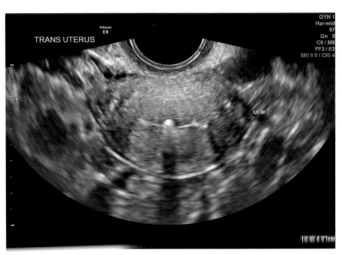

FIGURE 34-19. Transvaginal ultrasound transverse view of uterus with Mirena intrauterine device (IUD) at the level of the crossbars.

FIGURE 34-20. Transvaginal ultrasound transverse view of uterus with Mirena intrauterine device at the stem.

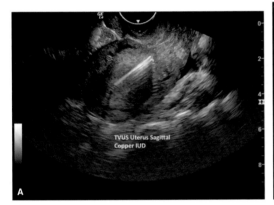

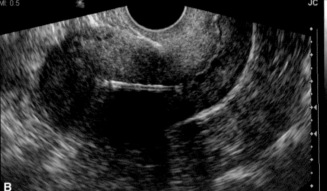

FIGURE 34-21. A, Transvaginal ultrasound (TVUS) sagittal view with copper intrauterine device (IUD) in the fundal region of the uterus. B, (Alternate) TVUS sagittal view with copper IUD in the fundal region of the uterus.

3D Ultrasound

3D ultrasound is highly effective at visualizing the IUD in the coronal plane and checking for malposition, embedment, failure of the crossbars to fully expand, and malrotation. It can be requested during a formal pelvic ultrasound study; however, its bedside availability is still currently limited and, hopefully, will be an adjunct in the future (**Figure 34-23**).[24]

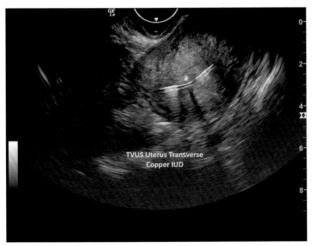

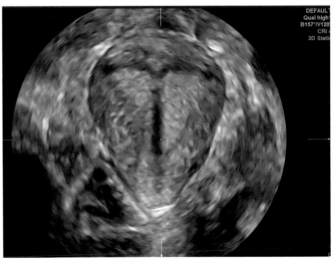

FIGURE 34-22. Transvaginal ultrasound (TVUS) transverse view with copper intrauterine device (IUD) at the level of the crossbars.

FIGURE 34-23. Three-dimensional reconstruction of the uterine coronal plane with a Mirena intrauterine device in the correct fundal location.

PATIENT MANAGEMENT

When a patient presents with missing IUD strings, a speculum examination should be performed and attempts made to coax the strings from the endocervical canal with a cytobrush (from a Pap smear kit). If the strings are still not visible, then expulsion and perforation should be ruled out by visualization of the IUD on ultrasound. A urine pregnancy test is also helpful for triage at this time if there are concerns for pregnancy.[28]

If the IUD is found in the lower uterine cavity, it is theorized that copper and LNG IUDs have differing levels of efficacy. It is likely that the hormonal effects of LNG IUDs are still maintained in these situations. Braaten and Goldberg recommend counseling an asymptomatic woman to keep a low-lying LNG IUD. On the other hand, low-lying copper IUDs should be replaced. For all IUDs, if any part is in the endocervical canal, removal is warranted.[9]

If the IUD is within the fundal region on US, then the patient can be reassured that the IUD is in proper position. The strings have likely migrated into the uterus. If the patient wishes to maintain the IUD, no further actions need to be taken until the time of removal. If the patient wishes for the IUD to be removed, the endocervix should be explored with a Kelly forceps, or Patterson alligators, in hopes of locating the IUD strings within the endocervical canal. If unsuccessful, then an in-office removal should be attempted with local anesthesia and thread retrievers, grasping forceps, hooks or suction curettes.[6] If this is unsuccessful, then a hysteroscopy is warranted (**Figures 34-24 to 34-26**).

If the patient is pregnant with an intrauterine pregnancy and desires to keep the pregnancy, then IUD removal is recommended by the American College of Obstetricians if it can be removed without invasive procedures. If the IUD string is *not* visible at the cervical os or easily retrievable from the endocervical canal, or if the gestational sac is between the IUD and the cervix on ultrasound, then retrieval should not be attempted. The patient should be advised that although retained LNG and copper IUDs have not been shown to be harmful to the fetus, leaving the IUD in situ in pregnancy is associated with increased intrauterine infections,

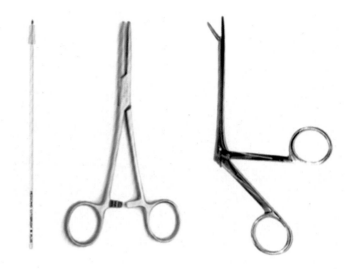

FIGURE 34-25. (From left to right) Cytobrush, Kelly forceps, Patterson Alligator.

preterm labor, and miscarriage and that medical attention for symptoms of vaginal bleeding, pelvic pain, vaginal discharge, and fever is advisable.[11]

If the patient is pregnant and does not desire to keep the pregnancy, then the IUD can be removed at the time of therapeutic abortion.

If the patient is pregnant and the IUD is *not* found on ultrasound, then documentation needs to be made in the chart for an exploration at the time of delivery or termination. The assumption is IUD expulsion; however, if an IUD is not found, than follow-up radiograph (after delivery) is warranted to rule out perforation.

If the patient is not pregnant and the IUD is not seen on ultrasound and there is no strong clinical evidence of a partial or full expulsion, a follow-up abdominal x-ray (making sure the apices of the diaphragm are included) should be ordered to rule out perforation.

An IUD in utero can be confirmed on abdominal x-ray if the IUD position is low in the pelvis, near midline, with the T-arms positioned superior to the stem.[27] If on x-ray the IUD appears to be outside the pelvis, then there is concern for perforation, and the recommendation is to have the patient undergo surgical removal (typically via diagnostic laparoscopy). CT or MRI may be completed for surgical planning purposes (**Table 34-3 and Figure 34-27**).[29-31]

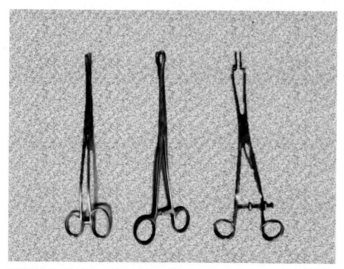

FIGURE 34-24. (From left to right) Curved grasping forceps, Ringed forceps, and endocervical speculum.

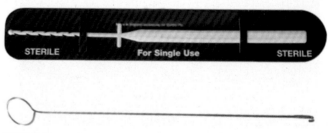

FIGURE 34-26. (Top) Intrauterine device (IUD) thread retriever, (bottom) IUD hook.

TABLE 34-3	Five Types of IUD Malposition and Their Ultrasound Findings		
Type of Malposition	Description	US Finding	X-ray
Expulsion	Missing IUD string and loss of IUD via the cervix and vagina.	Absence of IUD in situ	Absence of IUD
Perforation	Missing IUD string and partial or complete passage of IUD through the myometrium.	Absence of IUD in situ (or partially through the fundus in partial perforations)	IUD seen outside of the pelvis
Displacement	IUD in the uterine cavity but outside of the fundal position ± elongated IUD string.	IUD in the lower uterine segment, in the isthmus, or cervical canal on sagittal view	IUD in the pelvis
Malrotation	Crossbars of T-shaped IUD are outside of coronal plane.	Crossbars of copper IUD may be visualized off horizontal axis in the short-axis view. LNG IUD crossbars are difficult to visualize, and 3D US may be needed	IUD in the pelvis
Embedment	Crossbars or stem of IUD has entered the endometrium or myometrium.	In the short-axis view, the crossbars of copper IUD may be visualized entering the endometrium or myometrium, and the stem may appear off-center in the uterus. LNG IUD crossbars are difficult to visualize, and 3D US may be needed	IUD in the pelvis

Abbreviations: IUD, intrauterine device; LNG, levonorgestrel; US, ultrasound.

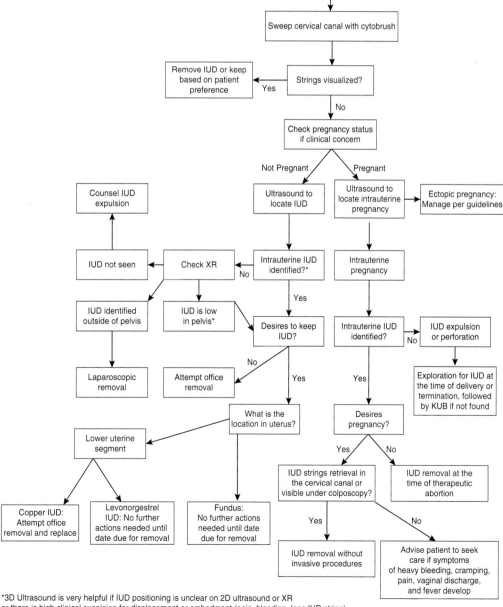

FIGURE 34-27. Suggested algorithm for intrauterine device location using ultrasound. Modified from Prabhakaran S, Chuang A. In-office retrieval of intrauterine contraceptive devices with missing strings. *Contraception.* 2011;83(2):102-106; Rivlin K, Westhoff C. Comprehensive gynecology. *Fam Plan.* 2017;13:237-257; Marchi NM, Castro S, Hidalgo MM, et al. Management of missing strings in users of intrauterine contraceptives. *Contraception.* 2012;86(4):354-358. ; Vilos GA, Di Cecco R, Marks J. Algorithm for nonvisible strings of levonorgestrel intrauterine system. *J Minim Invasive Gynecol.* 2010;17(6):805-806.

*3D Ultrasound is very helpful if IUD positioning is unclear on 2D ultrasound or XR or there is high clinical suspicion for displacement or embedment (pain, bleeding, long IUD string).

PEARLS AND PITFALLS

Pearls

- If the IUD string cannot be seen on a speculum examination, first attempt a sweep of the endocervical canal with the cytobrush (used in Papanicolaou smears).
- Look for a shadowing cast from the endometrium, which may be the only indication of the LNG IUD.
- A low-lying IUD will commonly migrate upward into place within the first 3 months of placement.

Pitfalls

- Amenorrhea does not automatically mean an LNG IUD is in place; pregnancy should be ruled out.
- Absence of IUD on ultrasound does not mean expulsion until perforation has been ruled out with a plain film x-ray. Be sure that the apices of the diaphragm are included because the IUDs can move with bowel peristalsis to the far regions of the abdomen.
- Mirena's strings can be very echogenic and can be seen in the cervical canal. This should not be confused with the IUD on ultrasound.

BILLING

CPT Code	Description	Global Payment	Professional Component	Technical Component
76857	Pelvic ultrasound (US), abdominal (nonobstetric), limited	$48.34	$25.42	$22.42
76830	Pelvic US, transvaginal (nonobstetric), complete	$123.88	$35.45	$88.44
No CPT code exists. Use Modifier −52 to indicate less than complete study	Pelvic US, transvaginal (nonobstetric), limited	Not available	Not available	Not available
58301	Removal of intrauterine device	$95.96	Not available	Not available

CPT codes and average national reimbursement for Medicare in 2016. Payment data are from https://www.cms.gov/apps/physician-fee-schedule/search/search-criteria.aspx. See Chapter 2 for details on ultrasound billing.

References

1. United Nations, Department of Economic and Social Affairs, Population Division. Trends in contraceptive use worldwide 2015 (ST/ESA/SER.A/349). 2015.
2. Branum A, Jones J. Trends in long-acting reversible contraception use among U.S. women aged 15–44. *NCHS Data Brief*. 2015;(188):1-8.
3. Braaten KP, Goldberg AB. Malpositioned IUDs: when you should intervene (and when you should not). *OBG Manag*. 2012;24:38-46.
4. American College of Obstetricians and Gynecologists. *Number 642. ACOG Committee Opinion*. Washington, DC: ACOG; 2015.
5. American College of Obstetricians and Gynecologists Committee on Gynecologic Practice; Long-Acting Reversible Contraception Working Group. ACOG committee opinion no. 450: increasing use of contraceptive implants and intrauterine devices to reduce unintended pregnancy. *Obstet Gynecol*. 2009;114(6):1434-1438.
6. Prabhakaran S, Chuang A. In-office retrieval of intrauterine contraceptive devices with missing strings. *Contraception*. 2011;83(2):102-106.
7. Bayer HealthCare Pharmaceuticals. Mirena prescribing information. www.mirena-us.com. Accessed December 2, 2016.
8. Van Schoubroeck D, Van Den Bosch T, Mortelman P, Timmerman D. Picture of the Month: sonographic determination of the position of a levonorgestrel intrauterine device. *Ultrasound Obstet Gynecol*. 2009;33:121-124.
9. Braaten KP, Benson CB, Maurer R, Goldberg AB. Malpositioned intrauterine contraceptive devices: risk factors, outcomes, and future pregnancies. *Obstet Gynecol*. 2011;118:1014-1020.
10. Faundes D, Bahamondes L, Faundes A, Petta C, Diaz J. No relationship between the IUD position evaluated by ultrasound and complaints of bleeding and pain. *Contraception*. 1997;56:43-47.
11. American College of Obstetricians and Gynecologists. ACOG practice bulletin no. 121: long-acting reversible contraception: implants and intrauterine devices. *Obstet Gynecol*. 2011;118(1):184-196.
12. Heinemann K, Reed S, Moehner S, Minh TD. Risk of uterine perforation with levonorgestrel-releasing and copper intrauterine devices in the European Active Surveillance Study on Intrauterine Devices. *Contraception*. 2015;91(4):274-279.
13. Peri N, Graham D, Levine D. Imaging of intrauterine contraceptive devices. *J Ultrasound Med*. 2007;26:1389-1401.
14. de Kroon CD, van Houwelingen JC, Trimbos JB, Jansen FW. The value of transvaginal ultrasound to monitor the position of an intrauterine device after insertion. A technology assessment study. *Hum Reprod*. 2003;18:2323-2327.
15. Palo P. Transabdominal and transvaginal ultrasound detection of levonorgestrel IUD in the uterus. *Acta Obstet Gynecol Scand*. 1997;76:244-247.
16. Bonilla-Musoles F, Pardo G, Simon C. How accurate is ultrasonography in monitoring IUD placement? *J Clin Ultrasound*. 1990;18(5):395-399.
17. Zhong LP, Huang LL, Zou Y, et al. Comparison of ultrasound plus radiography versus computed tomography in the diagnosis of ectopic intrauterine devices [in Chinese]. *Zhonghua Yi Xue Za Zhi*. 2012;92(1):5-8.
18. Bayer HealthCare Pharmaceuticals. Skyla prescribing information. http://labeling.bayerhealthcare.com/html/products/pi/Skyla_PI.pdf. Accessed December 2, 2016.
19. Kerr N, Dunham R, Wolstenhulme S, Wilson J. Comparison of two- and three-dimensional transvaginal ultrasound in the visualization of intrauterine devices. *Ultrasound*. 2014;22(3):141-147.
20. Moschos E, Twickler DM. Does the type of intrauterine device affect conspicuity on 2D and 3D ultrasound? *AJR Am J Roentgenol*. 2011;196:1439-1443.

21. Petta CA, Faundes D, Pimentel E, et al. The use of vaginal ultrasound to identify copper T IUDs at high risk of expulsion. *Contraception*. 1996;54(5):287-289.

22. Faundes D, Perdigao A, Faundes A, et al. T-shaped IUDs accommodate in their position during the first 3 months after insertion. *Contraception*. 2000;62(4):165-168.

23. Morales-Rosello J. Spontaneous upward movement of lowly placed T-shaped IUDs. *Contraception*. 2005;72:430-431.

24. Benacerraf B, Shipp T, Bromley B. Three-dimensional ultrasound detection of abnormally located intrauterine contraceptive devices which are a source of pelvic pain and abnormal bleeding. *Ultrasound Obstet Gynecol*. 2009;34(1): 110-115.

25. Reiner J, Brindle K, Khati N. Multimodality imaging of intrauterine devices with an emphasis on the emerging role of 3-dimensional ultrasound. *Ultrasound Q*. 2012;28:251-260.

26. Teva Women's Health, Inc., Website. ParaGard IUD prescribing information. www.paragard.com. Accessed December 2, 2016.

27. Allergan Specialty Pharmaceuticals Liletta prescribing information. www .allergan.com/assets/pdf/liletta_pi. Accessed December 2, 2016.

28. Nowitzki KM, Hoimes ML, Chen B, Zheng LZ, Kim YH. Ultrasonography of intrauterine devices. *Ultrasonography*. 2015;34(3):183-194.

29. Rivlin K, Westhoff C. Comprehensive gynecology. *Fam Plan*. 2017;13:237-257.

30. Marchi NM, Castro S, Hidalgo MM, et al. Management of missing strings in users of intrauterine contraceptives. *Contraception*. 2012;86(4):354-358.

31. Vilos GA, Di Cecco R, Marks J. Algorithm for nonvisible strings of levonorgestrel intrauterine system. *J Minim Invasive Gynecol*. 2010;17(6):805-806.

32. Association of Reproductive Health Professionals. Washington DC. http://www .arhp.org/Publications-and-Resources/Clinical-Fact-Sheets/The-Facts-About-Intrauterine-Contraception. Accessed December 2, 2016.

PART 2

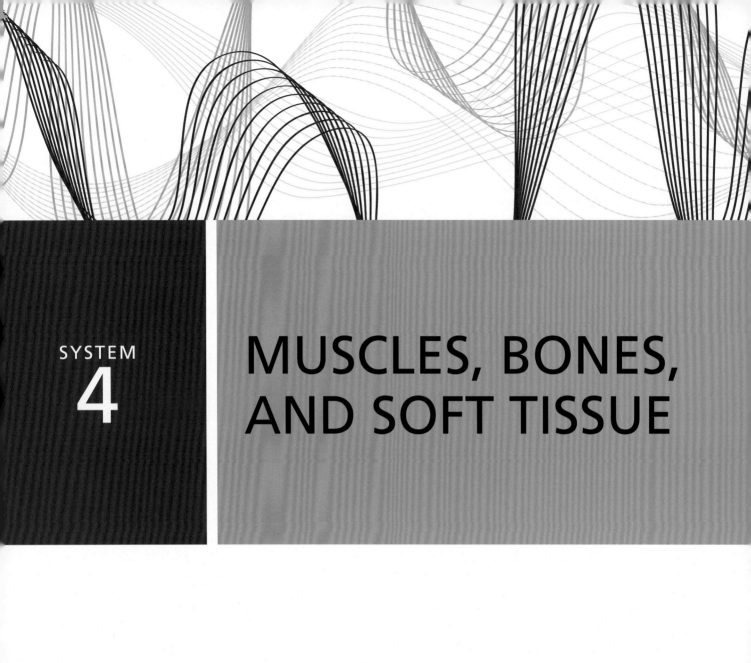

SYSTEM
4

MUSCLES, BONES, AND SOFT TISSUE

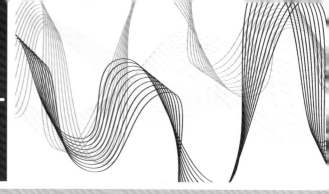

CHAPTER

35

Does the Patient Have a Joint Effusion?

Nicole T. Yedlinsky, MD, CAQSM, FAAFP, RMSK, Alex Mroszczyk-McDonald, MD, CAQSM, FAAFP, and Joshua R. Pfent, MD

Clinical Vignette

A 6-year-old previously healthy girl presents to clinic with the chief complaint of right hip pain and is walking with a limp. She plays outside frequently and has no known history of trauma. There are several small scrapes and bruises on her legs and a small bug bite on her upper right thigh. Her vital signs are within normal limits. The right hip is tender to palpation over the anterior joint space, and the hip has a decrease in active range of motion because of pain. You have concern for septic arthritis and want to rule it out at the bedside. Does the patient have a joint effusion?

LITERATURE REVIEW

Joint pain is ubiquitous in primary care, with over 20% of visits related to musculoskeletal conditions.[1] It can be a challenge to differentiate between intra-articular and other pathology such as contusions, sprains, and strains of the soft tissue surrounding a joint. Incorporating point-of-care ultrasound into the examination can help determine the presence or absence of a joint effusion. This can increase speed and accuracy when identifying intra-articular pathology, resulting in improved clinical care.

A joint effusion is defined as an increase in intra-articular fluid that causes expansion of the joint capsule. Physical examination may show a swollen appearance of the joint, as well as pain with joint movement, whereas effusion of the knee may cause suprapatellar or peripatellar swelling.[2] However, the physical examination alone has been shown to lack sensitivity. Specificity to detect knee effusion based on physical examination findings is near 90%, but sensitivity is only 10% to 40%.[3] Furthermore, it can be difficult to determine the presence of a joint effusion in patients with obesity, significant muscle hypertrophy, or pathologic changes from arthritis.

Multiple imaging modalities are available to evaluate for a joint effusion including ultrasound, radiographs, CT, and MRI. Ultrasound is the most clinically useful and expeditious imaging modality as it allows visualization of the joint capsule for expansion and presence of fluid and can evaluate for potential causes of an effusion. Point-of-care ultrasound can assist with needle guidance for therapeutic and diagnostic procedures.[4]

Ultrasound is the imaging modality of choice when evaluating for joint effusion of the hip[5,6] because as little as 1 mL of intra-articular fluid can be seen.[7,8] When evaluating the knee for effusion, ultrasound was found to have 81.3% sensitivity and 100% specificity[9] and can detect effusions less than 5 mL.[10,11] Although there are limited data regarding speed of ultrasound joint effusion skill acquisition specifically, there is information that this skill can be taught to medical students and more senior physicians, with statistically significant improvement in skill and confidence.[12]

Ultrasound may also be used to evaluate bony surfaces, muscles, tendons, ligaments, bursae, and the joint space. Ultrasound-guided needle aspiration and injection is portable, increases safety, and has no exposure to ionizing radiation. The needle can be guided from the surface of skin into the joint, and injection or aspiration can be performed under direct visualization.

Etiologies of joint effusion can be broadly categorized as noninflammatory, inflammatory, or hemorrhagic. Noninflammatory causes include osteoarthritis, osteonecrosis, and injuries, whereas inflammatory causes include septic arthritis, transient synovitis, and crystal-induced arthritis. Hemorrhagic causes include coagulopathies, trauma, and tumors. Careful consideration of the patient's age, history, and physical examination will help guide the differential diagnosis.[13] Synovial fluid analysis can aid in evaluating the etiology of an effusion including color, clarity, and viscosity and can also be used to obtain Gram stain, cell count, and crystal detection.

Septic arthritis requires urgent evaluation and treatment to preserve joint function. It has an incidence of 2 to 10 per 100,000 in the general population[14] and is most commonly the result of *Staphylococcus aureus*, with an incidence of 40% to 50%.[15] *Neisseria gonorrhoeae*, streptococci, and other gram-negative rods have an incidence of 10% to 20% each, whereas mycobacterium and fungi are less common causes.[16,17] Septic arthritis is most frequently caused by hematogenous spread, but can also occur by direct inoculation and local spread. Complications include joint destruction, growth arrest, and sepsis, so rapid assessment and treatment are very important.

Aspiration of a joint effusion should be performed urgently when the differential includes septic arthritis so that appropriate

TABLE 35-1	Recommendations for Use of Point-of-Care Ultrasound in Clinical Practice		
Recommendation		Rating	References
Ultrasonography is effective in evaluating for joint effusion.		A	6-9, 11

A = consistent, good-quality patient-oriented evidence; B = inconsistent or limited-quality patient-oriented evidence; C = consensus, disease-oriented evidence, usual practice, expert opinion, or case series. For information about the SORT evidence rating system, go to http://www.aafp.org/afpsort.

treatment can be initiated. Once obtained, synovial fluid analysis will guide treatment. The aspirate in septic arthritis has a white blood cell count greater than 50,000, with a predominance (>90%) of polymorphonuclear leukocytes. However, higher white blood cell counts increase the probability of septic arthritis. Though synovial fluid culture and susceptibility testing will guide antibiotic treatment for bacterial infections, this should not delay initiation of empiric antibiotics. If symptoms do not resolve with treatment, further imaging studies are indicated, and surgical intervention may be warranted.

PERFORMING THE SCAN

1. **Preparation.** The patient should be positioned in a manner that will allow them to remain still and comfortable for an extended period of time. The body part that is affected should be at a comfortable height to scan and be easily accessible. Position the ultrasound equipment appropriately, with the examiner, patient, and ultrasound image in a generally straight line. The ultrasound machine should generally be positioned on the contralateral side of the patient, with the operator standing on the side that needs to be examined.

   The transducer should be held gently low on the probe, close to the scanning surface. Select a curvilinear or linear probe with a soft tissue preset. Superficial joints may be easily visualized with a high-frequency linear probe, whereas deeper joints such as the hip may require a lower frequency curvilinear probe to adequately visualize the anatomy. Take into consideration the size of the patient and the amount of soft tissue that may be overlying the joint. Apply a liberal amount of ultrasound gel to the transducer surface.

2. **Localize the joint space using ultrasound.** KNEE: For evaluation of the knee, place the patient in a supine position with the knee flexed at 20° to 30° angle (**Figure 35-1**) and evaluate the joint using the high-frequency linear probe with the depth adjusted to about 3 cm.

   The probe should be placed longitudinally in the suprapatellar position, with the probe marker toward the patient's head and the inferior edge of the probe resting at the superior pole of the patella (**Figure 35-2**). Normally, there can be seen a small amount of fluid and synovial fold observed posterior to the quadriceps tendon (**Figure 35-3**). A joint effusion will cause distention of the suprapatellar recess deep to the quadriceps tendon, with anechoic fluid appearing black, separating the prefemoral and suprapatellar fat pads (**Figure 35-4**). In the transverse orientation (**Figure 35-5**), the compact fibrillar fibers of the quadriceps tendon will be seen in short axis and an effusion can be seen deep to this structure (**Figure 35-6**). Fluid may be seen tracking into the medial and

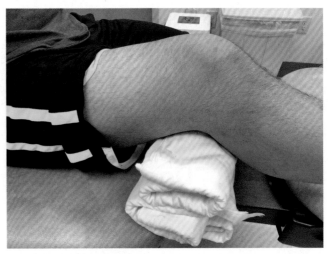

FIGURE 35-1. Patient position for scanning of the knee.

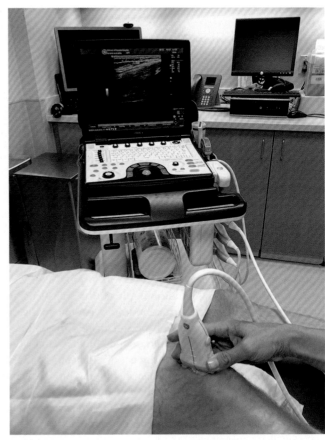

FIGURE 35-2. Probe placement for scanning of the knee in longitudinal axis.

lateral gutters of the suprapatellar recess. Lateral views can show extension of the effusion. Compressibility, changes in appearance with joint movement, and lack of internal flow with Doppler imaging suggest an effusion rather than synovitis.[9] If the examiner is unsure, examining the contralateral joint may help determine what is normal for the patient.[4]

If joint aspiration is performed under ultrasound guidance, the transverse axis is best utilized with an in-plane needle approach (**Figure 35-7**). The needle is presented from the lateral aspect of the knee and introduced into the anechoic fluid pocket under

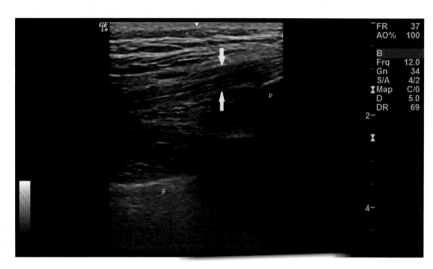

FIGURE 35-3. Normal knee. Longitudinal ultrasonography of the proximal normal knee. Labels show the patella (P), the femur (F), and the quadriceps tendon between the arrows.

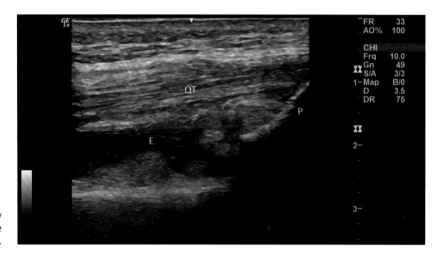

FIGURE 35-4. Knee effusion. Longitudinal ultrasonography of the proximal knee with effusion. Labels show the patella (P), the quadriceps tendon (QT), and effusion (E).

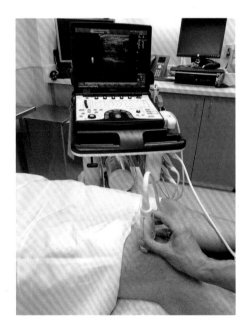

FIGURE 35-5. Probe placement for scanning of the knee in transverse axis.

direct visualization. This approach avoids traversing the quadriceps tendon and is better tolerated by patients. See Chapter 52 for additional information on aspiration and injection using ultrasound guidance.

HIP: For evaluation of the hip, place the patient supine with the hip in a slightly externally rotated position (**Figure 35-8**) and select a curvilinear low-frequency probe with the depth adjusted to about 6 cm. In younger patients or those with minimal soft tissue, a linear high-frequency probe may be adequate.

Find the inguinal crease and visualize a line between the pubic symphysis and the anterior superior iliac spine of the hip. Place the probe about halfway between these two landmarks, perpendicular to this line (**Figure 35-9**). Slide the probe superior and inferior in this orientation until the femoral head and convexity of the femoral neck is visualized (**Figure 35-10**). Normally there should be no anechoic fluid visualized in the joint or at the femoral neck. When present, a joint effusion will result in anechoic fluid visualized between the anterior and posterior layers of the anterior joint capsule and settle in the convexity of the femoral neck (Figure 35-10). The distance of the outer margin of the hip capsule and the surface of the femoral neck may be measured and compared to the contralateral hip (**Figure 35-11**).[18]

If hip joint aspiration is performed under ultrasound guidance, the needle should be introduced distal to the probe using an in-plane needle approach. The needle should be directed toward the convexity of the femoral neck and introduced into the anechoic fluid pocket under direct visualization. See Chapter 52 for additional information on aspiration and injection under ultrasound guidance.

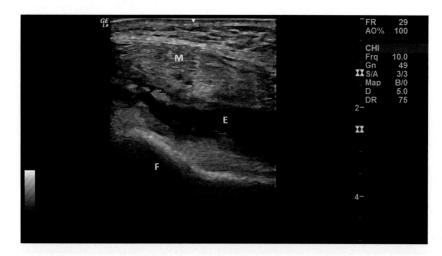

FIGURE 35-6. Knee effusion. Transverse ultrasonography of the proximal knee with effusion. Labels show the femur (F), quadriceps muscle and tendon (M), and the effusion (E).

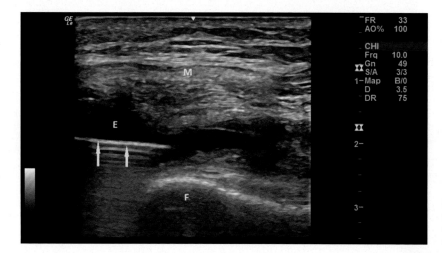

FIGURE 35-7. Knee effusion. Transverse ultrasonography of the proximal knee with effusion with guided needle aspiration. Labels show the femur (F), quadriceps muscle and tendon (M), effusion (E), and needle (arrows).

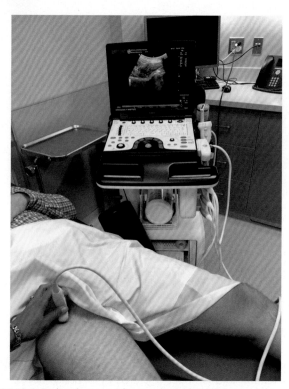

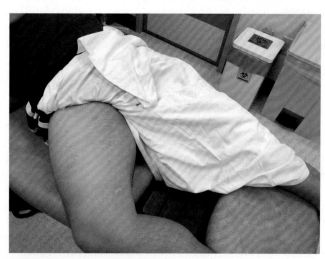

FIGURE 35-8. Patient position for scanning of the hip.

FIGURE 35-9. Probe placement for scanning of the hip.

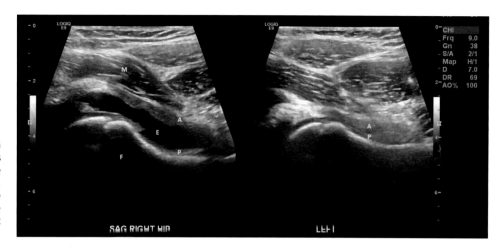

FIGURE 35-10. Normal hip and hip with effusion. Sagittal ultrasonography shows the left and right hip. Labels are the femoral head (F), iliopsoas muscle (M), anterior (A) and posterior (P) layers of the joint capsule, which on the right side are separated by effusion (E) and on the left side there is no effusion.

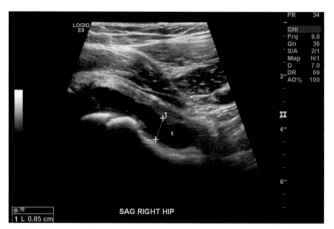

FIGURE 35-11. Hip effusion. Sagittal ultrasonography shows the right hip with an effusion (E). Measurement of the effusion shows it is 0.85 cm wide.

PATIENT MANAGEMENT

The morbidity associated with septic arthritis is high. If there is clinical suspicion, evaluation should begin promptly. Ultrasound should be utilized to determine if a hip or knee effusion is present. If there is no effusion, septic arthritis is unlikely. However, if the index of suspicion for a septic joint remains elevated, obtaining joint fluid for analysis as well as blood work with a complete blood count, erythrocyte sedimentation rate, C-reactive protein, and blood cultures may be appropriate.

If there is an effusion based on ultrasonographic findings, then the joint should be further examined and additional history obtained to determine risk for joint dislocation, bony erosion, or fracture. If there is suspicion, radiographs, CT, or MRI can be obtained. Bilateral imaging can be helpful to compare the contralateral unaffected joint as ossification centers or growth plates can often be difficult to assess.

If a joint effusion is present and there does not appear to be any other intra-articular joint abnormality, a joint aspiration should be urgently performed ideally with ultrasound guidance and before antibiotic administration. Synovial fluid studies obtained include culture with susceptibility testing, Gram stain, cell count, and differential. Laboratory evaluation with a complete blood count, erythrocyte sedimentation rate, C-reactive protein, and blood cultures can be helpful. Collecting samples for gonococcal infection may also help in diagnosis. Antistreptolysin-O (ASO) titers can be tested if group A streptococcus, rheumatic fever, or poststreptococcal arthritis is suspected. Further, coccidioidomycosis serology should be considered for patients who live in endemic areas of the western United States or Mexico.

The patient should be started on empiric intravenous antibiotics in the setting of septic arthritis. Joint drainage by needle aspiration, arthroscopic drainage, or open surgical drainage needs to be performed. An orthopedic surgeon should be urgently consulted (**Figure 35-12**).

PEARLS AND PITFALLS

Pearls

- Ensure optimal positioning for examiner and patient comfort.
- Apply copious amounts of gel and "float" the transducer to avoid pressure or contact on painful joints to reduce patient discomfort and improve image quality.
- When ultrasonographic or radiographic findings are equivocal, comparison to the unaffected contralateral joint will help identify subtle changes.

Pitfalls

- When evaluating for a joint effusion, avoid applying too much pressure as it may compress the effusion and result in a false-negative value.
- When performing ultrasonographic evaluation for a joint effusion, be careful not to mistake synovial hypertrophy or synovial folds for an effusion. Effusions will usually be compressible with probe pressure, whereas synovial hypertrophy is not. Additionally, synovial hypertrophy will usually demonstrate vascular flow with color Doppler, whereas an effusion will not.

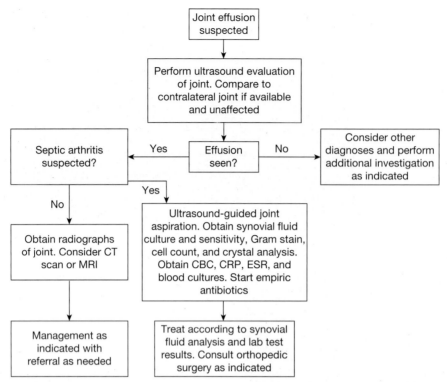

FIGURE 35-12. Treatment algorithm. CBC, complete blood count; CRP, C-reactive protein; ESR, erythrocyte sedimentation rate.

BILLING

CPT Code	Description	Global Payment	Professional Component	Technical Component
76882	Ultrasound, extremity, nonvascular, real time with image documentation; limited, anatomic specific	$36.61	$84.55	$121.16

CPT codes and average national reimbursement for Medicare in 2016. Payment data are from https://www.cms.gov/apps/physician-fee-schedule/search/search-criteria.aspx. See Chapter 2 for details on ultrasound billing.

References

1. Mackay C, Canizares M, Davis AM, Badley EM. Health care utilization for musculoskeletal disorders *Arthritis Care Res.* 2010;62(2):161-169.
2. Zuber T. Knee joint aspiration and injection. *Am Fam Physician.* 2002;66(8):1497-1501.
3. Berlinberg A, Ashbeck E, Roemer F, et al. Diagnostic performance of knee physical exam and participant-reported symptoms for MRI-detected effusion-synovitis among participants with early or late stage knee osteoarthritis: data from the Osteoarthritis Initiative. *Osteoarthritis Cartilage.* 2019;27(1):80-89.
4. Alves T, Girish G, Brigido M, Jacobson J. Ultrasound of the knee: scanning techniques, pitfalls, and pathologic conditions. *Radiographics.* 2016;36(6):1759-1775.
5. Nestorova R, Vlad V, Petranova T, et al. Ultrasonography of the hip. *Med Ultrason.* 2012;14(3):217-224.
6. Zeiger MM, Dor U, Schultz RD. Ultrasonography of the hip joint effusions. *Skelet Radiol.* 1987;16:607-611.
7. Moss SG, Schweitzer ME, Jacobson JA, et al. Hip joint fluid: detection and distribution at MR imaging and US with cadaveric correlation. *Radiology.* 1998;208:43-48.
8. Valley VT, Stanhmer SA. Targeted musculoarticular sonography in the detection of joint effusions. *Acad Emerg Med.* 2001;8:361-367.
9. Draghi F, Urciuoli L, Alessandrino F, Corti R, Scudeller L, Grassi R. Joint effusion of the knee: potentialities and limitations of ultrasonography. *J Ultrasound.* 2015;18(4):361-371.
10. Hauzeur JP, Mathy L, De Maertelaer V. Comparison between clinical evaluation and ultrasonography in detecting hydrarthrosis of the knee. *J Rheumatol.* 1999;26:2681.
11. Hong BY, Lee JI, Kim HW, et al. Detectable threshold of knee effusion by ultrasonography in osteoarthritis patients. *Am J Phys Med Rehabil.* 2011;90:112.
12. Yamada T, Minami T, Soni NJ, et al. Skills acquisition for novice learners after a point-of-care ultrasound course: does clinical rank matter? *BMC Med Educ.* 2018;18:202.
13. Safdar NM, Rigsby CK, Iyer RS, et al. ACR appropriateness criteria acutely limping child up to age 5. *J Am Coll Radiol.* 2018;15(11S):S252-S262.
14. Kaandorp CJ, van Schaardenburg D, Krijnen P, et al. Risk factors for septic arthritis in patients with joint disease: a prospective study. *Arthritis Rheum.* 1995;38:1819-1825.
15. Ryan MJ, Kavanagh R, Wall PG, Hazelman BL. Bacterial joint infections in England and Wales: analysis of bacterial isolates over a four year period. *Br J Rheumatol.* 1997;36:370-373.
16. Goldenberg DL. Septic arthritis [review]. *Lancet.* 1998;351:197-202.
17. Peters RH, Rasker JJ, Jacobs JW, et al. Bacterial arthritis in a district hospital. *Clin Rheumatol.* 1992;11:351-355.
18. Pauroso S, Di Martino A, Tarantino CC, Capone F. Transient synovitis of the hip: ultrasound appearance: mini-pictorial essay. *J Ultrasound.* 2011;14:92-94.

Does the Patient Have a Rotator Cuff Tear?

Michael J. Murphy, MD, CAQSM and Tenley E. Murphy, MD, FAAFP, CAQSM

● Clinical Vignette

A 70-year-old right-hand-dominant male with a past medical history of sick sinus syndrome s/p pacemaker placement comes into your office with 6 weeks of right shoulder pain. He states he remembers that he was cleaning his garage and felt a sharp pain after placing a box on a tall shelf. He has been taking acetaminophen, as well as using ice and heat as needed for pain, but he states that his pain has persisted. He denies numbness, tingling, or radicular symptoms. His pain is over his lateral shoulder and worse with overhead activities and when sleeping on the affected shoulder at night. On physical examination, the right shoulder has mildly decreased strength and decreased active range of motion in abduction. Jobe (empty can) test, Neer test, and Hawkins test are positive. Drop arm test is negative. Anteroposterior (AP), true AP (Grashey), scapular Y, and axillary radiographs show no fracture or dislocation, but he has moderate degenerative changes at the acromioclavicular (AC) joint and a type II to III acromion with osteophytes without significant glenohumeral joint degenerative changes. You are unable to obtain magnetic resonance imaging (MRI) because of the patient's pacemaker. Does the patient have a rotator cuff tear?

LITERATURE REVIEW

Shoulder pain is a common chief complaint in the primary care setting and accounts for up to 10% of all physical therapy referrals.[1] The rotator cuff is the most common source of shoulder pain in these visits, with an estimated 4.5 million clinician visits annually for rotator cuff issues.[2,3] Risk factors for rotator cuff injuries include anatomic factors such as curved or hooked acromion (type II or type III acromion), acromial spurs, and os acromiale. Extrinsic factors such as increasing age, obesity, diabetes mellitus, smoking, and repetitive overhead activities also contribute to the risk of rotator cuff tears.[4]

Rotator cuff impingement syndrome is commonly comorbid with rotator cuff tears, and it can often be difficult to clinically differentiate shoulder pain from impingement syndrome without significant rotator cuff tear versus shoulder pain caused by rotator cuff tear without the aid of imaging. Shoulder arthroscopy remains the gold standard for diagnosis of rotator cuff tears; however, ultrasound and MRI are very effective at diagnosis of full-thickness tears (although both are slightly less effective for partial-thickness tears).

Ultrasound is widely available and can be used in the outpatient setting to diagnose rotator cuff tears. Multiple studies, including meta-analysis and systematic reviews, have shown that ultrasound and MRI have similar sensitivity and specificity for detecting full-thickness rotator cuff tears, and they have similar diagnostic performance for detecting partial-thickness tears.[5-13]

There are multiple advantages to using ultrasound instead of MRI for the diagnosis of rotator cuff tears in the primary care setting. They include lower cost, ability to perform a dynamic examination, ability to do examination under manipulation with immediate patient–clinician feedback, immediate side to side comparison, greater portability, decreased length of time for examination completion, and no contraindications to patients with metallic or electronic implanted devices such as a pacemaker or military shrapnel.[14,15]

MRI is the most considerable preoperative expense, and a cost savings in the United States of $6.9 billion could have been achieved if ultrasound were appropriately substituted for MRI diagnosis of shoulder pain between the years 2006 and 2020. In addition to cost savings, there are higher rates of patient satisfaction with shoulder ultrasonography over MRI.[16] There are no known contraindications to ultrasound examination as of the time of this writing.

The most significant disadvantages of ultrasound compared to MRI are the need for operator proficiency in obtaining and interpreting the images and the clinical patient time required to obtain the images. Multiple studies show that some degree of training and practice are necessary to be proficient in musculoskeletal ultrasound.[17,18]

There are many resources available, ranging from in-person and online courses to online didactics, some of which are free of cost. The American Medical Society for Sports Medicine (AMSSM) and the American Institute of Ultrasound in Medicine (AIUM) have online musculoskeletal ultrasound instructional videos that are free of charge and only require registration with the website.

Proficient in-office musculoskeletal ultrasonography not only increases patient satisfaction and decreases health care costs but is also potentially financially lucrative to the clinician. Medicare reimbursement for diagnostic musculoskeletal ultrasound studies has increased by 319% from 2000 to 2009.[19] Multiple guidelines for shoulder ultrasound have been published.[20-24] We condense these guidelines to be used by the primary care physician in evaluation of a rotator cuff tear in a way that can be used in the fast-paced outpatient office workflow present in most primary care giver's offices.

TABLE 36-1	Recommendations for Use of Point-of-Care Ultrasound in Clinical Practice		
Recommendation		**Rating**	**References**
Use of ultrasound as first-line imaging to diagnose full-thickness rotator cuff tears is as effective as magnetic resonance imaging.		A	5-13
The use of ultrasound as first-line imaging to diagnose rotator cuff tears is cost-effective.		A	16, 19, 25

A = consistent, good-quality patient-oriented evidence; B = inconsistent or limited-quality patient-oriented evidence; C = consensus, disease-oriented evidence, usual practice, expert opinion, or case series. For information about the SORT evidence rating system, go to http://www.aafp.org/afpsort.

PERFORMING THE SCAN

Before Starting Ultrasound Examination of the Rotator Cuff

We recommend using a high-frequency linear array probe for ultrasound of the rotator cuff as most structures are relatively superficial, and a higher frequency probe will give better detail to evaluate for defects in the rotator cuff. Diagnostic ultrasound of the rotator cuff has the highest yield for supraspinatus because it is the most commonly torn tendon of the rotator cuff, and it is easily visualized by ultrasound. In this chapter, we will primarily discuss ultrasound of the supraspinatus and then briefly discuss ultrasound of the remaining rotator cuff. The anatomy of the rotator cuff and upper arm is reviewed in **Figures 36-1 and 36-2.**

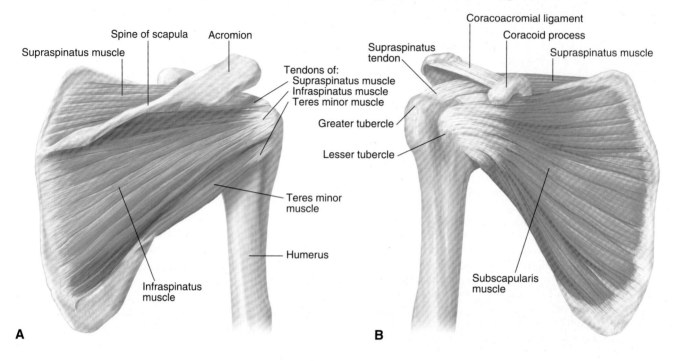

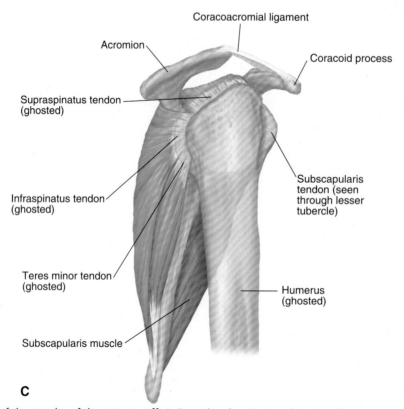

FIGURE 36-1. Anatomy of the muscles of the rotator cuff. A, Posterior view. B, Anterior view. C, Lateral view. Reprinted with permission from Gest TR. *Lippincott Atlas of Anatomy.* 2nd ed. Philadelphia, PA: Wolters Kluwer; 2020:50. Plate 2-16.

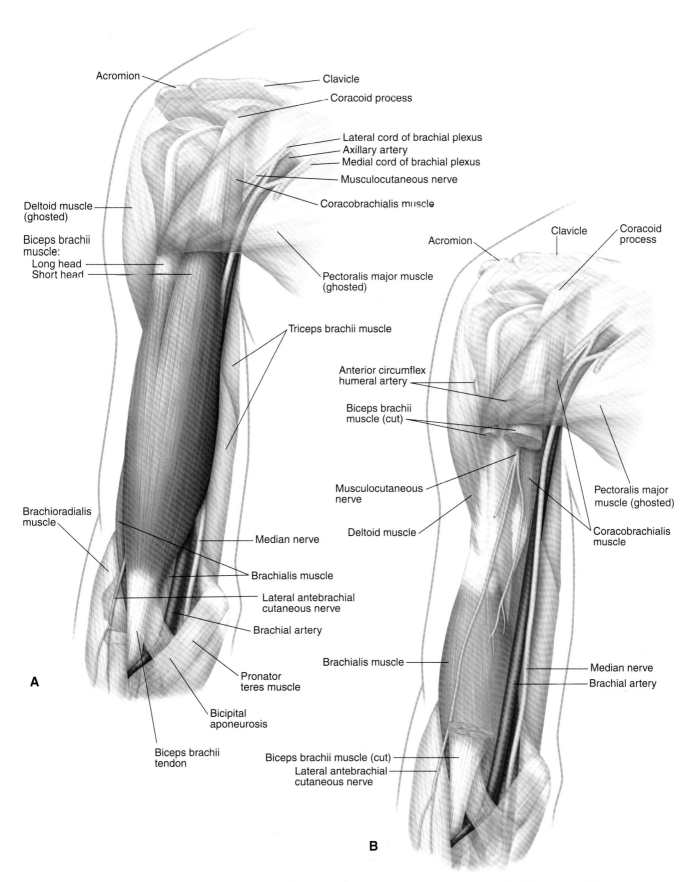

FIGURE 36-2. Anatomy of the muscles of the anterior arm. A, Superficial view. B, Deep view. Reprinted with permission from Gest TR. *Lippincott Atlas of Anatomy*. 2nd ed. Philadelphia, PA: Wolters Kluwer; 2020:51. Plate 2-17.

Supraspinatus

The supraspinatus is the most injured rotator cuff muscle. This makes the ability to diagnose a supraspinatus tear of great importance to the primary care physician.

Patient Positioning

We recommend placing the patient in the modified Crass position (**Figure 36-3**) as this will allow you to assess the supraspinatus as well as the rotator interval (the intra-articular portion of biceps tendon that indicates the most anterior aspect of the supraspinatus tendon). To do this, position the patient sitting upright with the affected shoulder next to the sonographer. The patient should place the palm of their hand on the posterior aspect of their iliac wing. This will flex the elbow, which should be pointing posteriorly, and place the shoulder in extension, abduction, and internal rotation, giving a good window to visualize the supraspinatus.

If the patient is unable to be positioned in the modified Crass position, the Crass position (**Figure 36-4**) can allow improved visualization of the supraspinatus compared to the neutral position and may be easier for a patient with a painful shoulder to maintain for the examination.

Ultrasound Examination

Landmarks help in ultrasound visualization of desired structures. The AC joint is a good starting landmark for the anterior shoulder and rotator cuff. First, you will place your ultrasound probe in an

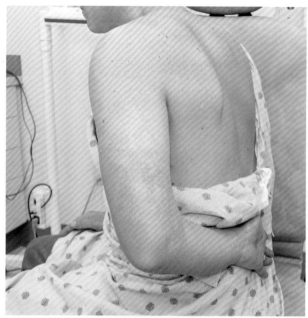

FIGURE 36-4. Crass position is another position that can be used to evaluate the supraspinatus; however, it does not allow visualization of the rotator interval nor distal tendon insertion because of the degree of internal rotation. It can be used in addition to the modified Crass position if you need an additional view of potential pathology or if the patient is unable to place their shoulder in the modified Crass position.

oblique coronal position along the clavicle in which you will visualize the AC joint in the long axis (**Figure 36-5**). You will then follow the acromion laterally toward the humeral head. **Figures 36-6 and 36-7** show probe positioning in the long- and short-axis evaluation of the supraspinatus. You will see the acromion is very superficial, and when you track to the edge, you will see an increase in depth to the humeral head (**Figure 36-8**). Sitting on top of the humeral head, you will see the supraspinatus. As you scan in the long axis along the supraspinatus, you will notice it has a "bird beak" appearance as the tendon tapers to its insertion on the greater tuberosity of the humerus, as is seen in **Figures 36-9 and 36-10**. The supraspinatus

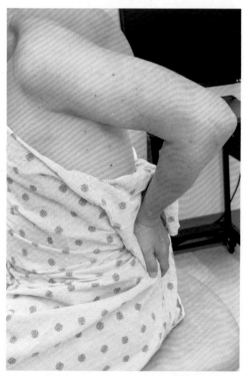

FIGURE 36-3. Modified Crass position. This is our recommended positioning of the patient when doing the ultrasound examination of the supraspinatus. Note that the elbow is pointed posteriorly, which gives a greater degree of external rotation than the Crass position does. The modified Crass position gives a better visualization of the supraspinatus insertion at the greater tubercle as well as better visualization of the rotator interval, both of which are common locations of pathology and should be evaluated in ultrasound examination.

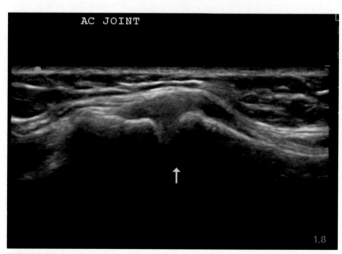

FIGURE 36-5. Long-axis view of the acromioclavicular (AC) joint. The depth of the AC joint is quite superficial. This patient also has degenerative changes and fluid within the joint. The AC joint (arrow) is a landmark that can be used for finding the acromion and supraspinatus.

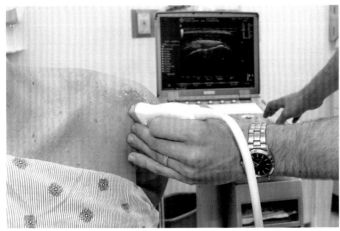

FIGURE 36-6. Probe positioning for the long-axis view of supraspinatus with a patient in the modified Crass position. The anterior aspect of the supraspinatus near the rotator interval is better visualized with the modified Crass positioning when compared to the Crass position or neutral positioning.

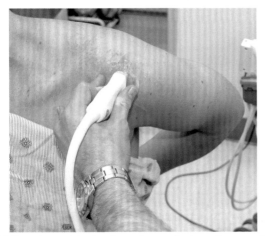

FIGURE 36-7. Probe positioning for a short-axis view of supraspinatus with a patient in the modified Crass position. Note that the patient's elbow is pointing posteriorly to allow a degree of external rotation to allow better visualization of the supraspinatus.

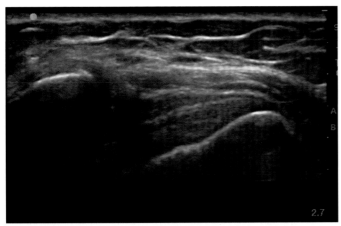

FIGURE 36-8. Step off from the acromion (very hyperechoic structure on the left-hand side) to the supraspinatus tendon that lies along the humeral head and is seen inserting into the greater tuberosity of the humerus. The acromion is a good landmark for finding the supraspinatus. Additionally, this view is used in dynamic impingement testing. It can be noted that this tendon is bunching as it passes deep to the acromion and this is evidence of potential chronic tendinosis.

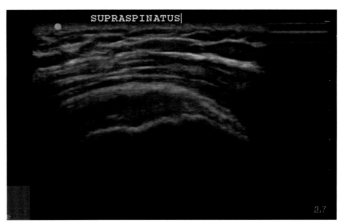

FIGURE 36-9. Normal appearance of supraspinatus in long axis. Note the "bird's beak appearance" of the tendon as it inserts onto the greater tuberosity. Also, note the hyperechoic tight fibrillar pattern that is linear and generally undisrupted. The hypoechoic portion on the far left and right hand of the screen is due to anisotropy and resolves with heel toeing the probe. Anisotropy is ubiquitous when imaging the rotator cuff because of the spherical geometry and curved nature of the rotator cuff tendon around the humeral head. Anisotropy should be ruled out as the etiology of any visualized potential pathology.

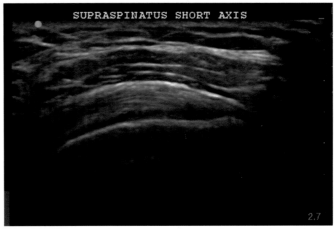

FIGURE 36-10. Normal appearance of supraspinatus in short axis. See Figure 40-7 for long-axis view of the same injury.

should have a uniform hyperechoic and fibrillar appearance along its length. Look along the entire length for any defects in this fibular pattern or hypoechoic regions, which could indicate a tear in the muscle or tendon. Possible defects should be evaluated in at least two planes to confirm pathology and to rule out anisotropy as a cause of the hypoechogenicity. **Figures 36-11 to 36-15** show different types of tears in the supraspinatus including partial-thickness tear, full-thickness tear with retraction, and full-thickness tear with glenohumeral effusion extending through the rotator cuff tear to the subdeltoid subacromial space. After you have scanned laterally to the insertion of the tendon of the supraspinatus, you can scan medially back to the origin along the spine of the scapula.

Dynamic Examination for Supraspinatus Impingement

Once you have scanned the supraspinatus and determined there is no tear or rupture, you can test for impingement of the supraspinatus at the acromion (► **Videos 36-1 and 36-2**).

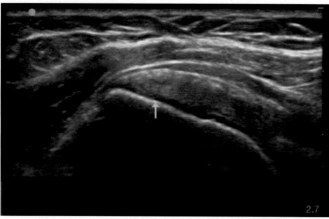

FIGURE 36-11. Long-axis view of a partial-thickness tear in the supraspinatus (arrow). It can be difficult to distinguish between partial-thickness tears and anisotropy, so multiple views from different angles should be utilized to confirm the diagnosis of tear versus anisotropy. See Figure 40-10 for short-axis view of the same injury.

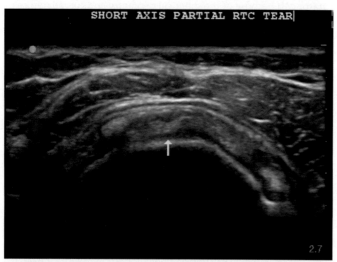

FIGURE 36-12. Short-axis view of a partial-thickness tear in the supraspinatus (arrow). See Figure 40-9 for the long-axis view of the same injury.

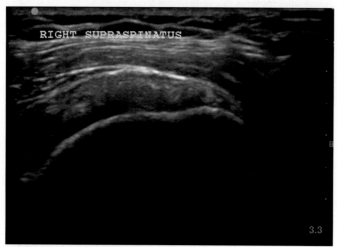

FIGURE 36-13. Long-axis visualization of supraspinatus with chronic tendinosis. Notice the thickening and disorganization of the tendon compared to a normal-appearing tendon such as in Figure 40-8. The normal hyperechoic fibrillar structure is disorganized and is not compact, tight, and linear as is seen in a normal tendon. Chronic tendinosis often accompanies impingement syndrome, and partial-thickness or full-thickness tears may be noted with tendinosis.

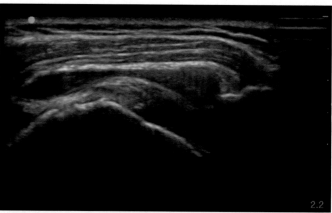

FIGURE 36-14. Full-thickness tear of the supraspinatus tendon with significant hypoechoic fluid seen around the hyperechoic tendon. This fluid is from a glenohumeral joint effusion and the full-thickness tear allows the fluid to leak from the joint capsule to the subdeltoid subacromial space.

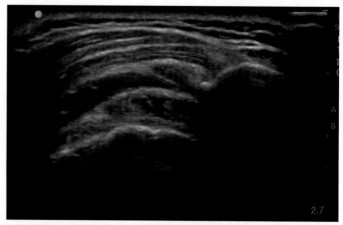

FIGURE 36-15. Short-axis view of full-thickness tear of supraspinatus with retraction from its insertion on the greater tuberosity.

Patient Positioning and Ultrasound Examination for Dynamic Impingement

Have the patient place their shoulder in 0° of abduction, neutral flexion, and neutral rotation with their elbow flexed at 90° as is seen in **Figure 36-16**. Once again start in the long axis at the AC joint and scan laterally along the acromion until you see the supraspinatus

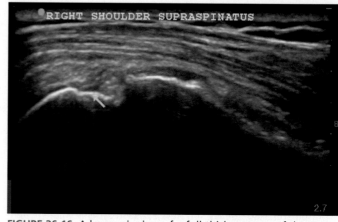

FIGURE 36-16. A long-axis view of a full-thickness tear of the supraspinatus with retraction from its insertion on the greater tuberosity. Note lack of "bird beak appearance" (arrow) and the bunched and disorganized appearance of the tendon because of retraction.

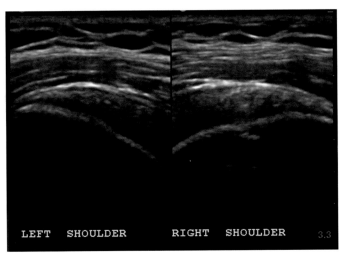

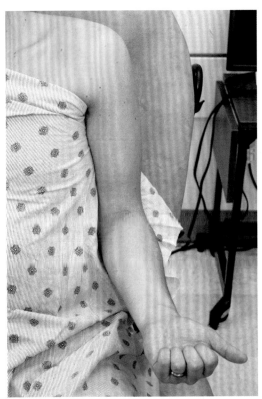

LEFT SHOULDER   RIGHT SHOULDER   3.3

FIGURE 36-17. Side-by-side comparison of a normal-appearing supraspinatus in long axis on the left and supraspinatus with chronic tendinosis on the right, which displays thickening and disorganization of the normally tight fibrillar pattern. This patient is a right-hand-throwing baseball player, which could account for the chronic tendinosis changes of his rotator cuff.

lying over the humeral head. The supraspinatus should be seen in the long axis. Be sure that the acromion, the humeral head, and the supraspinatus are in view at this time. Next, have the patient SLOWLY abduct their shoulder. You will need to keep the probe steady on the shoulder as the shoulder abducts so you can observe the supraspinatus. You will be able to see the supraspinatus contract and cause the humerus to abduct. This causes the supraspinatus to pass deep to the acromion. Look for catching, pinching, or bunching of the supraspinatus muscle as it passes deep to the acromion, which would be indicative of dynamic impingement. Figure 36-13 shows an example of supraspinatus with chronic tendinosis changes related to chronic shoulder impingement. **Figure 36-17** shows a side-by-side comparison of normal supraspinatus compared to chronic tendinosis often seen with chronic shoulder impingement. Remember that rotator cuff tears, tendinosis, and impingement are not mutually exclusive; rather, they are comorbid, and impingement is commonly a contributing factor to rotator cuff tears.

Infraspinatus and Teres Minor

Infraspinatus and teres minor are the primary external rotators of the shoulder and are less commonly injured than the supraspinatus; however, they can still be assessed by ultrasound for injury or rupture. If the patient presents with pain and/or weakness with external rotation, infraspinatus and teres minor may be evaluated by ultrasound.

Patient Positioning

Position the patient sitting upright with the affected shoulder next to the sonographer. Allow the patient's shoulder to sit with the elbow flexed at 90°, hand supinated, and the shoulder at neutral flexion, 0° of abduction, and in internal rotation (**Figure 36-18**).

Ultrasound Examination

Place the ultrasound probe in the axial position over the posterior fossa and visualize the glenohumeral joint. **Figures 36-19 and 36-20** show appropriate probe positioning. **Figures 36-21 and 36-22** show supraspinatus tendon and the posterior glenohumeral

FIGURE 36-18. Neutral positioning of the shoulder for evaluating long head of the biceps tendon, subscapularis, infraspinatus, teres minor, and dynamic impingement examination. It is not possible to visualize the entire supraspinatus in this position because of shadowing from the acromion, and the modified Crass position or Crass position is recommended for evaluation of the supraspinatus.

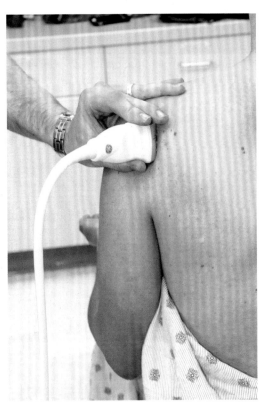

FIGURE 36-19. Probe positioning for the short-axis view of the infraspinatus and teres minor. Note that you can scan to the spine of the scapula to ensure that you are in the inferior fossa.

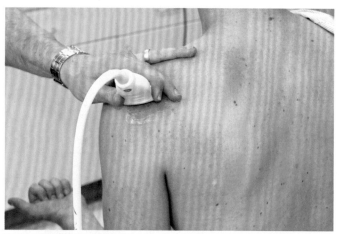

FIGURE 36-20. Probe positioning for a long-axis view of the infraspinatus and teres minor. Note that when positioning the patient, you can have the patient externally rotate for a dynamic examination (pictured) or internally rotate and have the patient place their hand on the opposite shoulder to better visualize the entire length of the muscle and tendon.

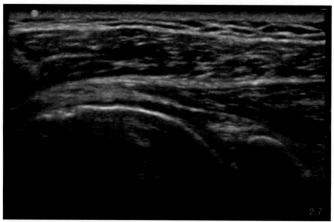

FIGURE 36-21. Tendon of infraspinatus in long axis inserting onto the greater tuberosity.

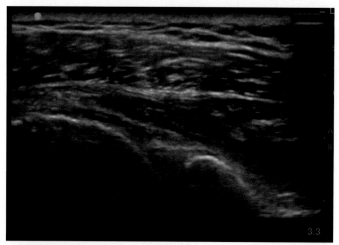

FIGURE 36-22. Glenohumeral joint with infraspinatus visualized in long axis. The outermost portion of the labrum can be visualized as a hyperechoic triangular structure between the humeral head and the glenoid. The majority of the labrum is intra-articular and it has a significant anisotropic property of the visualized portion. The labrum is generally not well visualized by ultrasound.

joint. Scan medially to the spine of the scapula to determine the supraspinatus fossa versus the infraspinatus fossa. You will see that the infraspinatus and teres minor are visualized in the long axis. Scan along the entire length of the infraspinatus and teres minor to their tendinous insertion on the greater tuberosity first in long axis and then in short axis, assessing for any defects or hypoechoic regions. Infraspinatus and teres minor will be deeper and more posterior than the supraspinatus, but will not be shadowed by the acromion as much of the supraspinatus is in the neutral position. Evaluate abnormalities by imaging them in at least two planes to confirm the pathology.

Long Head of Biceps Tendon

The importance of locating and scanning the long head of biceps tendon in evaluating the rotator cuff is 2-fold. The first is that the biceps tendon in the bicipital groove will act as a reference point when scanning the subscapularis and the anterior shoulder. When you are in doubt as to the anatomy in the anterior shoulder, relocate the biceps tendon and rescan to the previous location to reorient yourself in regard to anatomy. The second reason is that the long head of the biceps tendon runs in the bicipital groove and attaches at the labrum. This can be a source of pain in patients with impingement symptoms. There is also a correlation of fluid in the biceps tendon sheath with rotator cuff rupture,[1] so this can be used as additional evidence of a rotator cuff tear.

Patient Positioning

Have the patient sitting with hand supinated, elbow flexed and 90°, and shoulder in slight external rotation with the elbow abducted to the patient's side and in neutral flexion (Figure 36-18).

Visualizing the Biceps Tendon

Place the ultrasound probe axially on the anterior arm near the humeral neck and locate the biceps tendon in the short axis (**Figures 36-23 and 36-24**). This is the easiest way to visualize and

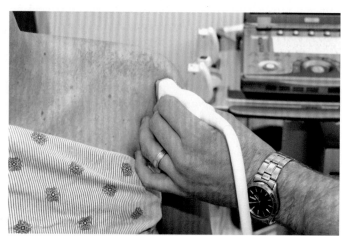

FIGURE 36-23. Probe placement for a long-axis view of the tendon of the long head of biceps brachii. The tendon will be seen in the bicipital groove. If you translate the probe medially, you will image the subscapularis in the short axis. Remember that as you scan inferior, you will scan pectoralis instead of the subscapularis, so confirming anatomy with a dynamic examination by internally rotating the shoulder and visualizing the subscapularis and its insertion at the lesser tubercle of the head of the humerus can help to differentiate these structures.

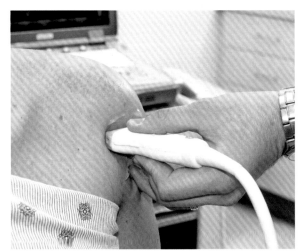

FIGURE 36-24. Probe placement for a short-axis view of the tendon of the long head of biceps brachii. You will see the tendon in the bicipital groove. Anisotropy can make tendon visualization difficult, so be sure to heel–toe and reposition the probe to minimize anisotropy.

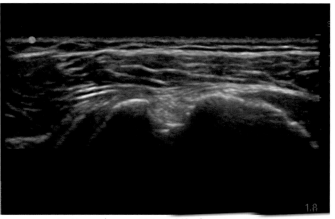

FIGURE 36-26. Normal appearance of the long head of biceps brachii tendon situated in the bicipital groove visualized in short axis.

to follow the biceps tendon from its musculotendinous junction through the bicipital groove of the humeral head superior to the origin at the glenoid.

Once the biceps tendon has been adequately assessed, scan to the more superior portion as the tendon enters the tendon sheath. It continues in the bicipital groove with the insertion of the subscapularis on the lesser tubercle medial to the biceps tendon. As the tendon continues superiorly, it then passes deep to the distal-most aspect of the supraspinatus tendon as it inserts on the greater tubercle of the humeral head. **Figures 36-25 and 36-26** show the normal appearance of the tendon of the long head of biceps brachii. As you scan, note any change in the hyperechoic and fibrillar pattern of the tendon or hypoechoic fluid seen in the tendon sheath. Any of these could indicate pathology in the biceps tendon. **Figures 36-27 to 36-30** show pathologic biceps tendons with fluid in the tendon sheath. Fluid in the biceps tendon sheath is also correlated with rotator cuff tear.[25] Next, scan the length of the tendon in the long axis. Defects or abnormalities should be visualized in the short and long axis to confirm pathology and rule out anisotropy.

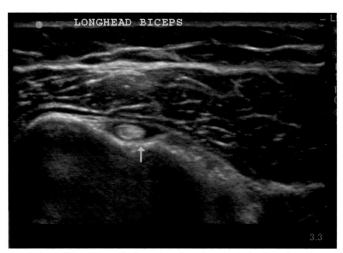

FIGURE 36-27. Short-axis view showing the tendon of the long head of biceps brachii situated in the bicipital groove with hypoechoic fluid surrounding it in the tendon sheath (arrow). This is commonly seen in the long head of biceps tendinitis and rotator cuff tears.

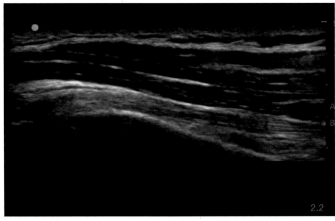

FIGURE 36-25. Normal appearance of the long head of biceps brachii tendon situated in the bicipital groove visualized in long axis.

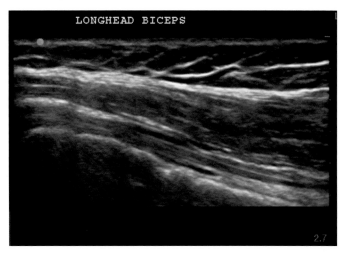

FIGURE 36-28. Long-axis view of the same patient as Figure 36-27 showing hypoechoic fluid in the tendon sheath of the long head of biceps brachii. This is commonly seen in the long head of biceps tendinitis and rotator cuff tears.

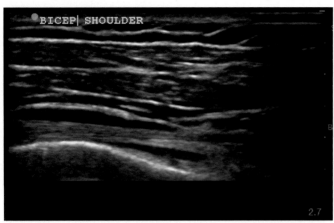

FIGURE 36-29. Long-axis view of the long head of biceps tendon with a prominent hypoechoic fluid present. This can be seen in the long head of biceps brachii tendinitis and frequently is seen with rotator cuff tears.

Sometimes non–rotator cuff pathology will be noted such as complete rupture of the long head of the biceps. **Figures 36-31 and 36-32** show complete rupture of the tendon of the long head of biceps brachii. The patient will usually present with a history of a traumatic pop, swelling, ecchymoses, and a "Popeye deformity" with distal retraction of the muscle body. If the patient is a surgical candidate and desires surgery, they should be referred to orthopedic surgery for consideration of repair. However, many patients, especially older patients, do quite well without surgical intervention. The Popeye deformity, however, will be permanent without surgical intervention even after strength and pain improve.

Subscapularis

The subscapularis is the major internal rotator of the shoulder. It is rare to have an isolated subscapularis tear; however, if your patient presents with a significant decrease in strength of internal rotation or significant pain with internal rotation, then ultrasound evaluation of subscapularis would be warranted. It is best viewed from the anterior of the shoulder.

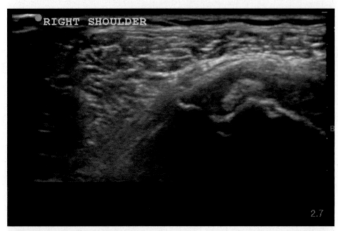

FIGURE 36-30. Biceps tendon subluxed in the bicipital groove. This is commonly accompanied by chronic tendinosis and can be an etiology of anterior shoulder pain. A dynamic examination may note the tendon subluxing and reducing with rotation of the shoulder and supination and pronation of the forearm.

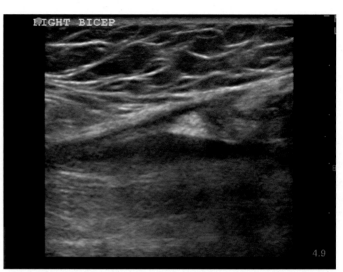

FIGURE 36-31. Long axis of the distal portion of complete rupture of tendon of the long head of biceps brachii with retraction. Note hypoechoic hematoma present around the hyperechoic ruptured and retracted tendon. The patient will usually have a "Popeye deformity" on physical examination with the long head of biceps muscle pronounced distally.

Patient Positioning

Have the patient sitting comfortably with hand supinated, elbow flexed to 90°, and shoulder in slight external rotation with the elbow abducted to the patient's side and in neutral flexion (**Figure 36-33**).

Ultrasound Examination

You will locate the biceps tendon in the short axis as described previously and scan superiorly until the subscapularis comes into view at the level of the humeral head (**Figure 36-34**). You will see the subscapularis insertion on the lesser tubercle medial to the biceps tendon (**Figure 36-35**). Your ultrasound probe will be directed axially, which will place the subscapularis in the long axis and the

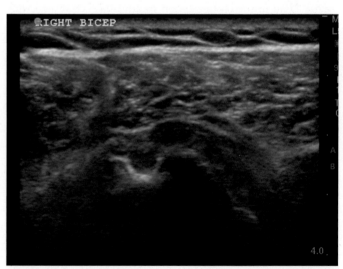

FIGURE 36-32. Bicipital groove in short axis showing complete rupture of the tendon of biceps brachii with retraction. Note there is no tendon seen in the bicipital groove. Be sure to heel-toe the probe to rule out anisotropy. Retracted tendon and muscle should be able to be visualized distally (see Figure 36-31). Often significant hematoma is present if the rupture is acute.

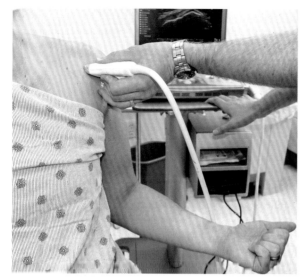

FIGURE 36-33. Probe placement for a long-axis view of the subscapularis. Note that the patient is placed in external rotation to better view the entire length of the subscapularis muscle body and tendon. The patient can undergo internal rotation for a dynamic examination. In this view, the subscapularis will be in the long axis, and the long head of biceps brachii tendon can be seen in the short axis.

biceps tendon in the short axis. Next, have the patient externally rotate their shoulder. This will better expose the musculotendinous junction and muscle body of the subscapularis. Scan the subscapularis medially in the long axis and then in short axis. Look for hyperechoic changes in muscle or tendon, a fibular pattern which could represent fluid or disruption in the muscle. **Figure 36-36** shows the corresponding MRI correlating the subscapularis tear, and **Figures 36-37 and 36-38** show a partial-thickness tear of the subscapularis. You can have the patient internally rotate the shoulder to observe the subscapularis in a dynamic examination. This is best seen in the long axis. This also confirms that you are looking at the subscapularis

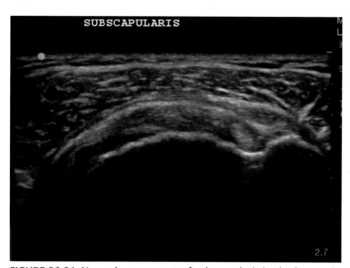

FIGURE 36-34. Normal appearance of subscapularis in the long axis. Note that the subscapularis and the long head of biceps are perpendicular to each other, so a long-axis view of the subscapularis visualizes the long head of biceps tendon in its short axis. The tendon of the subscapularis is seen inserting into the lesser tuberosity. The long head of biceps brachii is seen in the bicipital groove in its short-axis orientation.

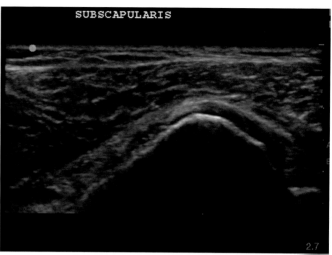

FIGURE 36-35. Normal appearance of subscapularis in the short axis. Note that the short axis (perpendicular) to subscapularis puts the long head of biceps tendon into its longitudinal axis if you scan all the way to the bicipital groove.

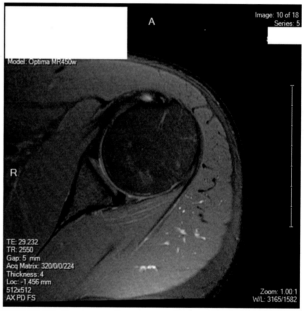

FIGURE 36-36. Corresponding magnetic resonance imaging to the ultrasound correlating subscapularis tear.

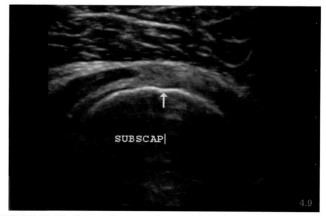

FIGURE 36-37. Short-axis view of a partial-thickness tear of the subscapularis (arrow). Subscapularis tears are much less common and often harder to visualize compared to those in supraspinatus.

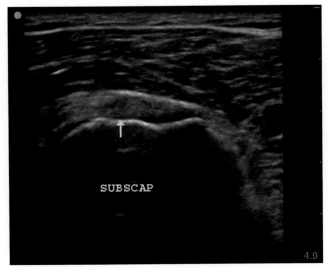

FIGURE 36-38. Long-axis view of partial-thickness tear (arrow) of the subscapularis. Subscapularis tears are much less common and often harder to visualize compared to those in supraspinatus.

versus other structures such as pectoralis, which inserts on the lateral lip of the distal bicipital groove of the humerus more distal than subscapularis but could be easily confused for subscapularis

on ultrasound examination. **Figure 36-39** shows a side-by-side comparison of insertion of pectoralis versus subscapularis.

PATIENT MANAGEMENT

Management of patients with full-thickness or retracted rotator cuff tears may differ from those with partial-thickness tears or impingement alone. In the patient with impingement syndrome, first-line treatment will include rotator cuff strengthening, range of motion, physical therapy, anti-inflammatory medications, acetaminophen, activity modification, and corticosteroid injection of subacromial space/subdeltoid bursa. If they continue to fail conservative therapy and are a surgical candidate, orthopedic referral for arthroscopic surgical intervention such as shoulder arthroscopy with subacromial decompression, distal clavicular excision, or long head of biceps tenodesis or tenolysis may provide relief of symptoms. If the patient is not a good surgical candidate, referral to primary care sports medicine may also be considered. If the patient has confirmed rotator cuff tear and is a surgical candidate, surgical referral should be considered earlier in the treatment course, especially for a full-thickness or retracted rotator cuff tears because surgical repair has better outcomes in the acute setting than in the chronic setting. **Figure 36-40** is a flowsheet that can be considered for the patient with shoulder pain with suspected rotator cuff impingement versus rotator cuff tear.

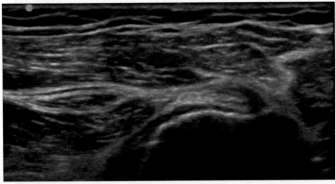

Pectoralis

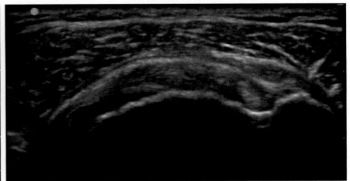

Subscapularis

FIGURE 36-39. Side-by-side comparison of pectoralis insertion on the distal portion of the lateral lip of the bicipital groove versus the subscapularis inserting more proximally at the lesser tuberosity. Note the long head of biceps tendon seen in the bicipital groove at the insertion of the subscapularis. Also note the larger muscle mass of the pectoralis. A dynamic examination can also aid in differentiating between these two structures.

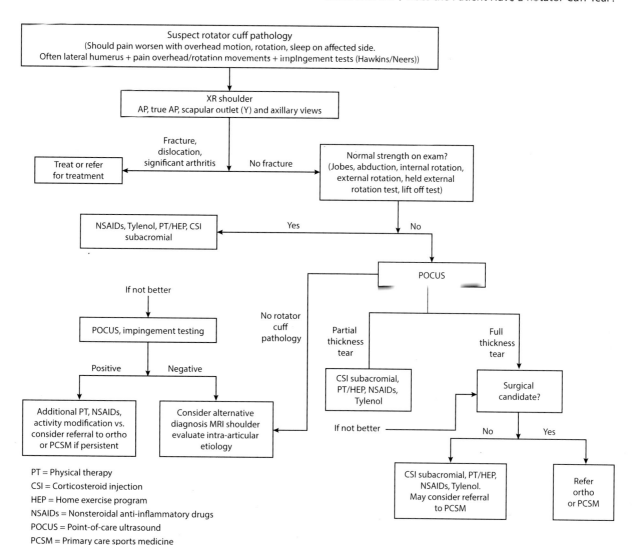

FIGURE 36-40. Flowsheet for the use of point-of-care ultrasound and treatment of the patient with shoulder pain and suspected rotator cuff tear. Although surgical intervention can greatly improve the quality of life of many who are good surgical candidates (especially those who are active), surgical treatment is not indicated for all patients with rotator cuff pathology. Many patients, even with full-thickness or retracted tears, can have good functional outcomes without surgery, especially if they are poor surgical or poor postoperative rehab candidates. Older patients who have multiple comorbidities or are unwilling or unable to undergo surgical intervention or postsurgical rehab may not benefit from surgical intervention. Postsurgical rehab may be quite extensive after rotator cuff repair. Rotator cuff repair often requires >6 to 12 months of rehab and recovery process to return to normal activity. AP, anteroposterior; MRI, magnetic resonance imaging.

PEARLS AND PITFALLS

Pearls

- The supraspinatus has the highest rate of injury and will have the highest sensitivity and specificity for ultrasound diagnosis of pathology.
- If unsure if your image shows pathology, you can try the following tricks:
  - Scan in multiple planes
  - Heel-toe the ultrasound probe to evaluate for anisotropy
  - Scan the unaffected side to have a normal comparison
- A dynamic examination can be used to:
  - Confirm anatomy
  - Better expose and visualize different parts of the muscle or tendon
  - Diagnose pathology
  - Distinguish pathology versus anisotropy

- When scanning the rotator cuff in the long and short axis, your probe will often be oblique compared to traditional axial, coronal, and sagittal planes.

Pitfalls

- Anisotropy can be mistaken for pathology. The spherical nature of the humeral head and natural curve of supraspinatus accentuate anisotropy.
- Small and partial-thickness tears can be difficult to visualize on ultrasound.
- Glenoid labrum and deeper intra-articular structures are poorly visualized with ultrasound.
- The humeral head is curved, and with it the rotator cuff; this magnifies anisotropy.

BILLING

CPT Code	Description	Global Payment	Professional Component	Technical Component
76881	Ultrasound, extremity, nonvascular, real time with image documentation; complete	$116.06	$31.87	$84.14
76882	Ultrasound, extremity, nonvascular, real time with image documentation; limited, anatomic specific	$36.52	$11.46	$25.06

CPT codes and average national reimbursement for Medicare in 2016. Payment data are from https://www.cms.gov/apps/physician-fee-schedule/search/search-criteria.aspx. See Chapter 2 for details on ultrasound billing.

References

1. Brar T. *Ferri's Clinical Advisor*. Philadelphia, PA: Elsevier; 2017:1118.e2-1118.e7.
2. McFarland EG. Examination of the shoulder. In Kim TK, Park HB, Rassi GE, et al., eds. *The Complete Guide*. New York, NY: Thieme Medical Publishers; 2006:142.
3. Oh LS, Wolf BR, Hall MP, et al. Indications for rotator cuff repair: a systematic review. *Clin Orthop Relat Res*. 2007;455:52.
4. Oliva F, Osti L, Padulo J, Maffulli N. Epidemiology of the rotator cuff tears: a new incidence related to thyroid disease. *Muscles Ligaments Tendons J*. 2014;4(3):309-314.
5. de Jesus JO, Parker L, Frangos AJ, Nazarian LN. Accuracy of MRI, MR arthrography, and ultrasound in the diagnosis of rotator cuff tears: a meta-analysis. *AJR Am J Roentgenol*. 2009;192:1701-1707.
6. Smith TO, Back T, Toms AP, Hing CB. Diagnostic accuracy of ultrasound for rotator cuff tears in adults: a systematic review and meta-analysis. *Clin Radiol*. 2011;66:1036-1048.
7. Lenza M, Buchbinder R, Takwoingi Y, Johnston RV, Hanchard NC, Faloppa F. Magnetic resonance imaging, magnetic resonance arthrography and ultrasonography for assessing rotator cuff tears in people with shoulder pain for whom surgery is being considered. *Cochrane Database Syst Rev*. 2013;(9):CD009020.
8. Teefey SA, Rubin DA, Middleton WD, et al. Detection and quantification of rotator cuff tears. Comparison of ultrasonographic, magnetic resonance imaging, and arthroscopic findings in seventy-one consecutive cases. *J Bone Joint Surg Am*. 2004;86-A:708.
9. Iannotti JP, Ciccone J, Buss DD, et al. Accuracy of office-based ultrasonography of the shoulder for the diagnosis of rotator cuff tears. *J Bone Joint Surg Am*. 2005;87:1305.
10. Teefey SA, Middleton WD, Payne WT, Yamaguchi K. Detection and measurement of rotator cuff tears with sonography: analysis of diagnostic errors. *AJR Am J Roentgenol*. 2005;184:1768.
11. Schibany N, Zehetgruber H, Kainberger F, et al. Rotator cuff tears in asymptomatic individuals: a clinical and ultrasonographic screening study. *Eur J Radiol*. 2004;51:263.
12. Ottenheijm RP, Jansen MJ, Staal JB, et al. Accuracy of diagnostic ultrasound in patients with suspected subacromial disorders: a systematic review and meta-analysis. *Arch Phys Med Rehabil*. 2010;91:1616.
13. Roy J-S, Braën C, Leblond J, et al. Diagnostic accuracy of ultrasonography, MRI and MR arthrography in the characterisation of rotator cuff disorders: a systematic review and meta-analysis. *Br J Sports Med*. 2015;49:1316-1328.
14. Smith J, Finnoff JT. Diagnostic and interventional musculoskeletal ultrasound: part 1. Fundamentals. *PM R*. 2009;1:64.
15. Hirahara AM, Panero AJ. A guide to ultrasound of the shoulder, part 1: coding and reimbursement. *Am J Orthop (Belle Mead NJ)*. 2016;45(3):176-182.
16. Middleton WD, Payne WT, Teefey SA, et al. Sonography and MRI of the shoulder: comparison of patient satisfaction. *AJR Am J Roentgenol*. 2004;183:1449.
17. Cole B, Twibill K, Lam P, Hackett L, Murrell GA. Not all ultrasounds are created equal: general sonography versus musculoskeletal sonography in the detection of rotator cuff tears. *Shoulder Elbow*. 2016;8(4):250-257. doi:10.1177/1758573216658800.
18. Day M, Phil M, McCormack RA, Nayyar S, Jazrawi L. Physician training ultrasound and accuracy of diagnosis in rotator cuff tears. *Bull Hosp Jt Dis (2013)*. 2016;74(3):207-211.
19. Sharpe R, Nazarian L, Parker L, Rao V, Levin D. Dramatically increased musculoskeletal ultrasound utilization from 2000 to 2009, especially by podiatrists in private offices. Department of Radiology Faculty Papers. Paper 16. http://jdc.jefferson.edu/radiologyfp/16. Accessed January 7, 2016.
20. Lee MH, Sheehan SE, Orwin JF, Lee KS. Comprehensive shoulder US examination: a standardized approach with multimodality correlation for common shoulder disease. *Radiographics*. 2016;36(6):1606-1627.
21. Amoo-Achampong K, Nwachukwu BU, McCormick F. An orthopedist's guide to shoulder ultrasound: a systematic review of examination protocols. *Phys Sportsmed*. 2016;44:1-10.
22. European Society of Musculo skeletal Radiology. Musculoskeletal ultrasound technical guidelines I. Shoulder. https://essr.org/content-essr/uploads/2016/10/shoulder.pdf. Accessed November 12, 2016.
23. AIUM practice parameter for the performance of a musculoskeletal ultrasound examination. http://www.aium.org/resources/guidelines/musculoskeletal.pdf. Accessed November 12, 2016.
24. Jacobson JA. Shoulder ultrasound. In *Fundamentals of Musculoskeletal Ultrasound*. 2nd ed. Philadelphia, PA: Saunders/Elsevier; 2007:3.e4-71.e4.
25. Hanusch BC, Makaram N, Utrillas-Compaired A, Lawson-Smith MJ, Rangan A. Biceps sheath fluid on shoulder ultrasound as a predictor of rotator cuff tear: analysis of a consecutive cohort. *J Shoulder Elbow Surg*. 2016;25(10):1661-1667.

CHAPTER 37

Does the Patient Have an Ankle Sprain or Fracture?

Tenley E. Murphy, MD, FAAFP, CAQSM and Patrick F. Jenkins, III, MD, CAQSM

● Clinical Vignette

A 28-year-old male presents with left lateral ankle pain. He was running on a trail and rolled his ankle. He described severe pain and was unable to finish his run. He had ankle sprains in the past but never had pain of this severity. He limps into the examination room. He has noticeable swelling throughout his ankle joint and tenderness to palpation over the distal lateral malleolus. Does the patient have an ankle sprain or fracture?

LITERATURE REVIEW

The ankle is the most frequently injured joint.[1] Acute ankle injuries account for more than 2 million injuries yearly, making it a common chief complaint in primary care offices.[2] The most common mechanism of injury is forced inversion of the plantarflexed foot, leading to a lateral ankle sprain. Ankle sprains are most common in sports that involve running and jumping including basketball, football, soccer, and cross country running.[1,3] It is the most common reason for missed athletic participation.[4]

Three bones, the distal tibia, distal fibula, and talus, form the ankle joint. The tibia and fibula are bound together by an interosseous membrane and the anterior and posterior tibiofibular ligaments distally.[5] The most distal portions of the tibia and fibula as well as the posterior tibiofibular ligament form a mortise.[1] This surface articulates with the trochlea of the talus.[6] Ligaments and tendons maintain the joint. The lateral ankle has three ligamentous structures that stabilize it. The anterior talofibular ligament attaches to the lateral malleolus proximally and neck of the talus distally. It is a weak band that is the most commonly injured ligament.[2] The posterior talofibular ligament is a much stronger ligament and extends from the lateral malleolus to the lateral tubercle of the talus.[1] The calcaneofibular ligament runs from the distal tip of the lateral malleolus.[1] The lateral joint capsule is also reinforced with peroneus brevis and longus.[2] Medially, the deltoid ligament adds stability to the joint. It begins at the medial malleolus and fans out to attach on the navicular, calcaneus, and anterior and posterior talus.[1] The capsule is also supported by the tibialis anterior and posterior, flexor digitorum longus, flexor hallucis longus, and extensor hallucis longus[2] (**Figure 37-1**).

The ankle is a hinge joint that acts to maintain balance and absorb impact as the total body weight is transferred to the foot.[7] Movement at the ankle is largely in the vertical plane—dorsiflexion and plantarflexion. Because the talus narrows in between the malleoli anteriorly, there is a small amount of eversion and inversion in the ankle joint.[1] Most, however, occurs in the talofibular joint. Because this is a stronger joint, inversion injuries typically occur at the ankle.[2] Most ankle injuries occur in the plantarflexed position with forced inversion, such as stepping on another player's shoe or off a curb. Although a lateral ankle sprain is most common in this

scenario, a fracture involving the lateral malleolus, distal fibula, or base of the fifth metatarsal is also a possibility. Injuries to the medial side are much less common, occurring in only 15% of ankle sprains.[2] This occurs when the foot is in the lateral position with forced eversion, such as a player falling on the lateral surface of the lower leg. Because of the strength of the deltoid ligament, an avulsion fracture of the medial malleolus is often seen, as well as a concurrent fibula fracture.[1]

Fractures occur in less than 15% of patients presenting with mechanisms consistent with an ankle sprain.[8] This led to the development of the Ottawa foot and ankle rules (OFAR) in 1992. Its purpose was and is to accurately rule out fracture in patients without radiography if the likelihood is low. These rules are given in **Table 37-1**.

The OFAR has a sensitivity of nearly 100% if applied within 48 hours of the injury and a specificity of 25% to 40%. When applying this, foot and ankle radiography is reduced by 30% to 40%.[10] The specificity, however, leaves room for improvement.

Ultrasound evaluation has the potential to be used as an adjunct to the physical examination.[11,12]

Although bony structures cannot be fully evaluated, the cortex can be visualized. Disruption of this cortex represents fractures.[13] Because of this, there have been multiple studies adding sonographic evaluation to the OFAR to improve the sensitivity and reduce unnecessary radiography. In these studies, the sonographer had received training on musculoskeletal ultrasound and had the opportunity to see normal anatomy and pathology before beginning. An ultrasound was done if a patient was positive on the OFAR. The patient had ultrasound evaluation of the injured leg. The result was interpreted and recorded at the time of evaluation before the X-rays were completed. The results showed a sensitivity of 87% to 100% and a specificity of 90% to 99%[14-17] in patients 16 years and older. By using the ultrasound to augment the OFAR, X-rays could be further decreased by almost two-thirds.[16] It is worth noting that only one study had navicular fractures. Because of the difficulty in visualizing the navicular, the sensitivity for detecting a fracture was 40%.[14] This is a possible limitation in adding sonographic evaluation to the OFAR. If the patient is tender over this point, X-rays should be considered regardless if ultrasound imaging shows a cortical disruption.

It is important to note that the OFAR were developed and validated in the emergency department setting. In that setting, fractures are said to occur in about 15% of patients presenting with acute ankle pain.[8] It has been argued that this prevalence is lower in the primary care setting as the velocity of injury is lower.[5] Being able to apply these rules in the primary care setting can be very useful. Although X-ray is readily available in the emergency department, that is not the case in most primary care offices.

Thus, ultrasound may be especially beneficial for ankle sprain management in primary care by preventing the need for a patient to travel to another location for X-rays and allowing for clinical decisions to be made more quickly for less cost.

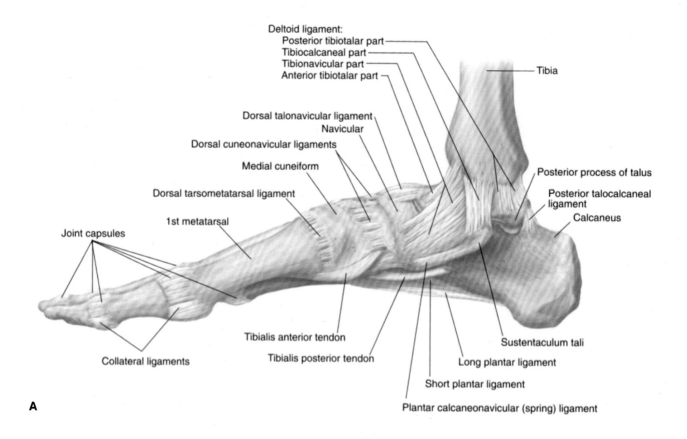

A

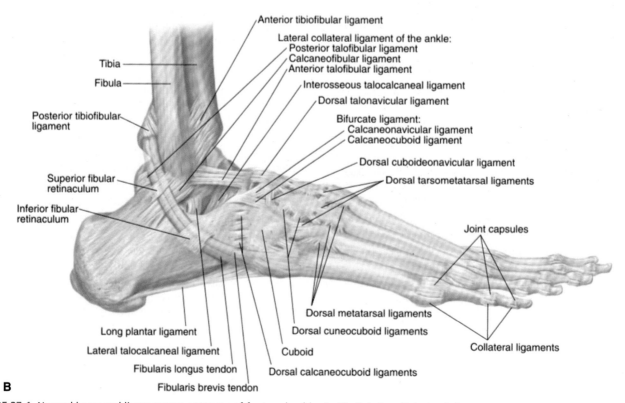

B

FIGURE 37-1. Normal bony and ligamentous anatomy of foot and ankle. A, Medial view. B, Lateral view.

| TABLE 37-1 | **Ottawa Foot and Ankle Rules** |

An ankle X-ray series is only required if there is pain in the malleolar zone (Figure 37-2) and any of these findings:

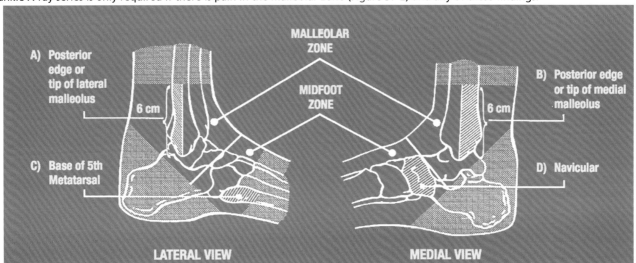

FIGURE 37-2. Areas of concern under Ottawa foot and ankle rules. From Stiell IG, McKnight RD, Greenberg GH, et al. Ottawa ankle rules for ankle injury radiography. http://www.ohri.ca/emerg/cdr/docs/cdr_ankle_poster.pdf. Copyright © 1992 and 2013, Ottawa Hospital Research Institute.

1. Bone tenderness over the posterior edge of the distal 6 cm of the fibula or tip of the lateral malleolus,

OR

2. bone tenderness over the posterior edge of the distal 6 cm of the tibia or tip of the medial malleolus,

OR

3. inability to take four complete steps both immediately and while seeking care.

A foot X-ray series is only required if there is pain in the midfoot zone (Figure 37-2) and any of these findings:

1. Bone tenderness at the base of the fifth metatarsal,

OR

2. bone tenderness over the navicular,

OR

3. inability to take for complete steps both immediately and while seeking care.[9]

Stiell IG, McKnight RD, Greenberg GH, et al. Ottawa ankle rules for ankle injury radiography. http://www.ohri.ca/emerg/cdr/docs/cdr_ankle_poster.pdf.

| TABLE 37-2 | **Recommendations for Use of Point-of-Care Ultrasound in Clinical Practice** |

Recommendation	Rating	References
The Ottawa foot and ankle rules (OFAR) effectively rule out fracture if negative and decrease X-rays.	A	8-10, 16
Adding sonographic evaluation to the OFAR can further reduce the number of X-rays needed without underdiagnosing fractures.	A	14-17
If the patient is tender over the navicular bone, ultrasonography may not be effective.	B	16

A = consistent, good-quality patient-oriented evidence; B = inconsistent or limited-quality patient-oriented evidence; C = consensus, disease-oriented evidence, usual practice, expert opinion, or case series. For information about the SORT evidence rating system, go to http://www.aafp.org/afpsort.

PERFORMING THE SCAN

1. **Preparation.** Position the patient sitting or supine, whichever is most comfortable for him/her. Position the affected leg in a way that exposes the area of concern. If the medial structures are causing the concern and the patient is sitting, a "frog-legged" position should be assumed. If the patient is lying supine and the concern is for the medial structures, externally rotate the leg and place a pillow or towel underneath the lateral side to better expose the surface (**Figure 37-3A**). If the concern is for the lateral structures and the patient is sitting, the knee should be flexed at 45° with the foot flat on the examination table.

If the patient is lying supine and the concern is for the lateral structures, the leg should be internally rotated to best display the lateral surface and a pillow or towel placed underneath the medial side to better expose the surface and put stress on the joint (**Figure 37-3B**). This will help level any contour the ankle has in its natural position.[18] Position the ultrasound machine so that it can be easily viewed while sonographically examining the patient. A linear array probe with a high frequency should be selected. The setting should be in a musculoskeletal or ankle setting and a shallow depth should be chosen.

2. **Reexamine the patient.** Confirm the area of maximal tenderness by gently palpating the ankle.

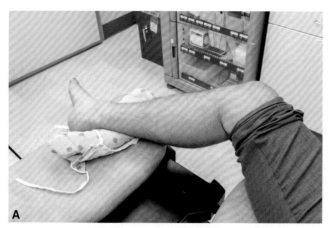
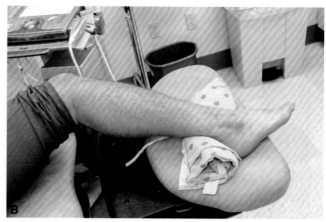

FIGURE 37-3. A, Supine positioning for sonographic evaluation of medial structures and supine positioning for sonographic evaluation of lateral structures (B).

3. **Evaluate the area of concern.** Place the transducer with the probe in the long axis over the area of maximal tenderness. Angle the probe perpendicular to the bony surface (**Figure 37-4**). Be sure to scan above and below the area of concern. If the tenderness is over the tibia or fibula, continue to scan distally to the tip of the malleolus. The surface of the bone should be smooth without any defects (**Figure 37-5**). Any area of cortical defect is likely to represent a fracture (**Figure 37-6**). Be sure to scan over the entire surface of the bone so as not to miss a fracture.

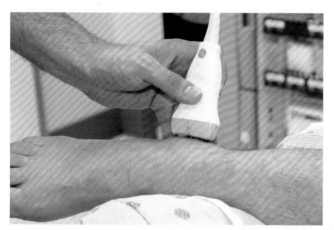

FIGURE 37-4. Angle the transducer so that it is perpendicular to the area of concern.

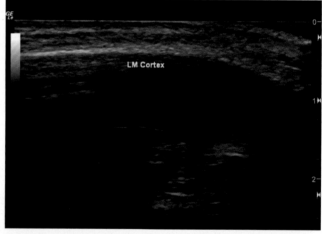

FIGURE 37-5. Normal cortex of lateral malleolus.

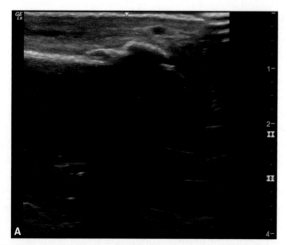
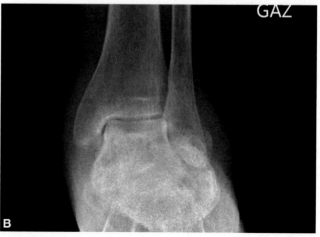

FIGURE 37-6. A, Cortical disruption of lateral malleolus on sonographic evaluation and corresponding X-ray demonstrating fracture of lateral malleolus (B).

PATIENT MANAGEMENT

If a patient's history and physical examination are concerning for an ankle sprain, the OFAR should be applied. If the OFAR are negative, no radiographic evaluation is needed and the patient can be treated for an ankle sprain. This includes early mobilization, anti-inflammatory medications, rest, ice, bracing, and rehabilitation exercises once the patient is able to tolerate them.[19]

If the rules are positive secondary to tenderness over the navicular, then a foot X-ray series should be ordered. There is inadequate evidence that navicular fractures can be ruled out with sonographic evaluation.[14] If the X-ray series is negative, typical ankle sprain treatment should be implemented. If the X-ray series shows a fracture, proper fracture management should begin and

necessary referrals made. If the OFAR are positive secondary to tenderness over the distal 6 cm of the posterior fibula or tibia, medial or lateral malleolus, or base of the fifth metatarsal, sonographic evaluation should be performed as detailed previously. There is consistent evidence that this can be used to rule out fracture.[14-17] If there is no cortical abnormality, a fracture can be ruled out and typical ankle sprain management should be started. If there is a cortical defect noted on ultrasonography, the appropriate X-ray series should be ordered to further evaluate the leg or the foot. If the fracture is not visible on X-ray, then it is likely a small, subclinical fracture and may be treated the same as typical ankle sprain. If the X-rays are positive for fracture, proper fracture care should be implemented and necessary referrals made (**Figure 37-7**).

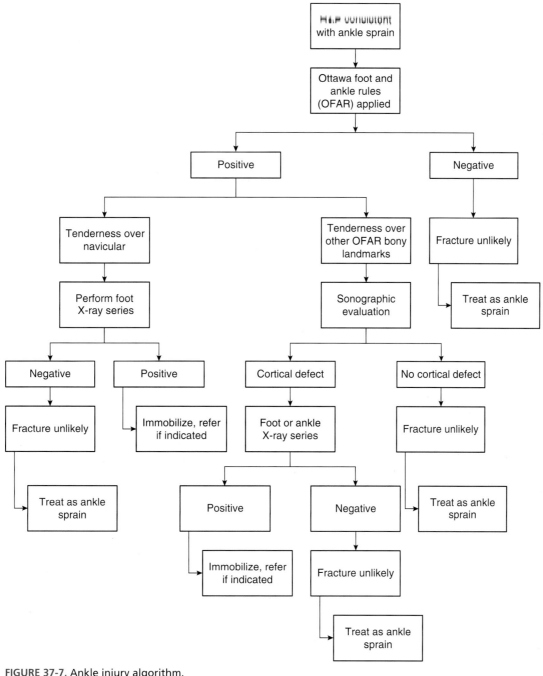

FIGURE 37-7. Ankle injury algorithm.

PEARLS AND PITFALLS

Pearls

- Use a towel or pillow underneath the side of the leg not being evaluated. This takes extra stress off the ligaments, flattens the contour of the surface anatomy, and opens up the joint space, allowing for better visualization of the internal structures.
- Because the ankle is a very bony joint, there is a lot of contour to it. This can make sonographic evaluation difficult because the linear array probe is not curved. Do not be afraid to use copious amounts of gel. It fills in the convexities, which will allow for better evaluation while also preventing the sonographer

from feeling the need to increase the pressure with which the probe is applied, which will cause discomfort to the patient.

Pitfalls

- Although the OFAR only include the distal 6 cm of the tibia or the fibula, fractures can occur above this. If a patient says there is pain elsewhere or palpation reveals tenderness elsewhere, do not be afraid to ultrasound other tender areas if needed.
- Sensitivity of ultrasound for navicular fracture may be low, and if there is concern for this, an X-ray should be obtained.

BILLING

CPT Code	Description	Global Payment	Professional Component	Technical Component
76882	Ultrasound, extremity, nonvascular, real time with image documentation; limited, anatomic specific	$36.52	$11.46	$25.06
76881	Ultrasound, extremity, nonvascular, real time with image documentation; complete	$116.01	$31.87	$84.14

CPT codes and average national reimbursement for Medicare in 2016. Payment data are from https://www.cms.gov/apps/physician-fee-schedule/search/search-criteria.aspx. See Chapter 2 for details on ultrasound billing.

References

1. Moore KL, Dalley AF, Agur AMR, eds. Lower limb. *Clinically Oriented Anatomy.* 6th ed. Philadelphia, PA: Lippincott Williams & Wilkins; 2010:508-669.
2. Ivins D. Acute ankle sprain: an update. *Am Fam Physician.* 2006;74(10)1714-1720.
3. Wexler RK. The injured ankle. *Am Fam Physician.* 1998;57(3):474-480.
4. Badylak J. Low ankle sprain. *Orthobullets.* http://www.orthobullets.com/foot-and-ankle/7028/low-ankle-sprain
5. Abbott C, Barry HC. Ankle and knee pain. In Sloane PD, Slatt LM, Ebell MH, Smith MA, Power D, Viera AJ, eds. *Essentials of Family Medicine.* 6th ed. Philadelphia, PA: Lippincott Williams & Wilkins; 2012:409-420.
6. Netter FH. Ankle and foot. In Netter FH, ed. *Atlas of Human Anatomy.* 5th ed. Philadelphia, PA: Elsevier; 2011:511-515.
7. Bickley LS, ed. *The Musculoskeletal System. Bates' Guide to Physical Examination and History Taking.* 10th ed. Philadelphia, PA: Lippincott Williams & Wilkins; 2009:571-641.
8. Bachmann LM, Kolb E, Koller MT, Steurer J, Riet GT. Accuracy of Ottawa ankle rules to exclude fractures of the ankle and mid-foot: systematic review. *BMJ.* 2003;326(7386):417-423.
9. Stiell IG, McKnight RD, Greenberg GH, et al. Ottawa ankle rules for ankle injury radiography. http://www.ohri.ca/emerg/cdr/docs/cdr_ankle_poster.pdf.
10. Stiell IG, Greenberg GH, McKnight RD, et al. A study to develop clinical decision rules for the use of radiography in acute ankle injuries. *Ann Emerg Med.* 1992;21(4):384-390.
11. McNally EG. Ankle joint and forefoot: anatomy and techniques. In McNally EG, ed. *Practical Musculoskeletal Ultrasound.* 2nd ed. Philadelphia, PA: Elsevier; 2014:253-268.
12. McNally EG. Disorders of the ankle and foot: medial. In McNally EG, ed. *Practical Musculoskeletal Ultrasound.* 2nd ed. Philadelphia, PA: Elsevier; 2014:301-314.
13. Court-Payen M. Disorders of the ankle and foot: lateral. In McNally EG, ed. *Practical Musculoskeletal Ultrasound.* 2nd ed. Philadelphia, PA: Elsevier; 2014:295-300.
14. Atilla OD, Yesilaras M, Kilic TY, et al. The accuracy of bedside ultrasonography as a diagnostic tool for fractures in the ankle and foot. *Acad Emerg Med.* 2014;21(9):1058-1061.
15. Canagasabey MD, Callaghan MJ, Carley S. The sonographic Ottawa foot and ankle rules study (the SOFAR study). *Emerg Med J.* 2011;28(11):838-840.
16. Tollefson B, Nichols J, Fromang S, Summer RL. Validation of the sonographic Ottawa foot and ankle rules (SOFAR) study in a large urban trauma center. *J Miss State Med Assoc.* 2016;57(2):35-38.
17. Ekinci S, Polat O, Günalp M, et al. The accuracy of ultrasound evaluation in foot and ankle trauma. *Am J Emerg Med.* 2013;31(11):1551-1555.
18. Beggs I, Bianchi S, Beuno A, et al. Musculoskeletal ultrasound technical guidelines, VI. Ankle. *European Society of Musculoskeletal Radiology.* https://essr.org/content-essr/uploads/2016/10/ankle.pdf
19. Tiemstra JD. Update on acute ankle sprains. *Am Fam Physician.* 2012;85(12):1170-1176.

Does the Patient Have Tendinopathy?

Michael Marchetti, DO

Clinical Vignette

A 55-year-old otherwise healthy female presents to clinic with anterior left knee pain. Six months ago, she began a new squat-heavy workout routine involving weekly gradual increases in weight. She progressed well for the first 3 months but then developed pain in her left knee, only when squatting. Her pain improved after resting for several days, so she resumed her workout regimen. After a few more months of increasing her squatting weight, her anterior knee pain slowly increased as well. This time, however, a few days' rest has not resolved the pain. She has not tried any medications. A knee sleeve offered no relief. Although she has no pain during her daily activities, she would like to continue working out and is wondering what is wrong and what can help. She is currently uninsured and cannot afford to pay out of pocket for an MRI. Does the patient have tendinopathy?

LITERATURE REVIEW

It has been reported that tendon injuries account for approximately 7% of all physician visits in the United States and up to 50% of them are sports related.[1-3] Traditionally, the diagnosis of acute or chronic tendinitis has been on clinical examination alone or with the help of MRI. This modality, however, is frequently overused and can also be associated with a significant financial cost to the patient and medical system. Most of the major tendons that are affected by injury are rather superficial; therefore, visualization under ultrasound is relatively simple. The substitution of ultrasound for MRI, when appropriate, would lead to savings of more than $6.9 billion over a 14-year period.[4]

Tendons are primarily composed of linear fibrils of type 1 collagen but are also composed of elastin, proteoglycans, and lipids all encased in a sheath called the epitenon. Tendons connect bone to muscle. The fibrils of the tendon are oriented along the direction of force of the muscle contraction. Contraction of the muscle causes the tendon to shorten and lengthen within its physiologic range.[5] Overuse is a common injury to tendons and is significantly more prevalent than complete ruptures.

It is common to label injuries to the tendon as a "tendinitis." This nomenclature may be incorrect, in that there are several studies that demonstrate little or no inflammation in the actual tendon.[6] The more acceptable term to describe this condition in and around an overused tendon is "tendinopathy." Looking at the histopathologic changes that occur in an overused tendon, there is little to no inflammation, but there is evidence of increased cellularity, disorganization of collagen fibers, and degeneration and thickening of the tendon.[7] It is generally believed that as a whole, a tendon has very limited blood supply. Most of the vascular structures of tendons are located in the epitenon and are concentrated near the

insertion into bone.[8] There is also a characteristic ultrasonographic appearance of a normal healthy tendon that changes when injured, which will be demonstrated later.

It should be noted that in certain areas, the tendon has direct communication with the joint space, making it necessary to rule out a joint effusion before characterizing something as a tenosynovitis. It is hypothesized that because the blood supply is scarce in a tendon, it leaves it vulnerable to injury, with relative difficulty of healing compared to a more vascular structure.[8] This also means that too much pressure with the probe can compress the tendon and possibly remove evidence of neovascularization, a common ultrasonographic characteristic of a tendinopathy.

Neovascularization is increase in blood flow around the tendon and is best viewed with the power Doppler mode on an ultrasound. The clinical significance is not fully understood, but it is known that normal tendons do not have this characteristic. It is believed by some that the higher levels of neovascularization correlates with pain, but that is not well proven.[9]

Anisotropy is an artifact resulting from an angulated transducer. Sometimes this will mimic hypoechoic changes in a tendon. It is necessary to make small adjustments with the transducer angle over a tendon, as anisotropy will disappear, whereas true pathologic findings will not.[10] It has been described that as little as 2° off of a perpendicular evaluation of a study can create this false positive.[11]

TABLE 38-1	Recommendations for Use of Point-of-Care Ultrasound in Clinical Practice		
Recommendation		**Rating**	**References**
Use ultrasound as the first-line imaging modality for the diagnosis of acute and chronic tendinopathy.		B	4, 9, 10, 11

A = consistent, good-quality patient-oriented evidence; B = inconsistent or limited-quality patient-oriented evidence; C = consensus, disease-oriented evidence, usual practice, expert opinion, or case series. For information about the SORT evidence rating system, go to http://www.aafp.org/afpsort.

PERFORMING THE SCAN

There are many anatomic locations in the body prone to tendinopathy but perhaps the two most common are the patella and the Achilles. Because of this, how to properly perform their scans will be demonstrated below.

Patella

1. The patella is best evaluated with the patient lying supine with hips and knees flexed with the foot flat. The tendon is tensed and straight in this position, which allows for best ultrasonographic evaluation.
2. The most effective way of visualizing a tendon with the goal of evaluating a tendinopathy is with a high-frequency linear transducer

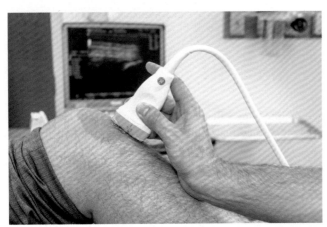

FIGURE 38-1. The probe is in long axis over a cushion of gel and light pressure. The examination of the patella tendon will take place at both the proximal and distal poles near the origin and insertion of the tendon as these are more likely to be the areas of greatest visual change.

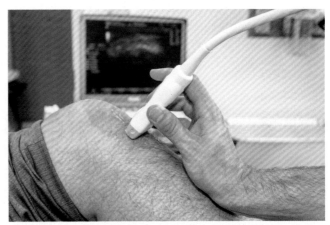

FIGURE 38-2. The probe is in short axis, which will better show neovascularization. Again, it is important to focus the examination on the distal and proximal poles of the patella tendon.

and a thick layer of gel and light pressure (**Figures 38-1 and 38-2**). The tendon will be evaluated in both the long and short axis looking for swelling, neovascularization, and disorganization of the collagen fibrils. **Figure 38-3** shows the difference between a normal and abnormal tendon.

3. It is important to note that the bony origin and insertion of the tendon should be evaluated as this can be common site for characteristic ultrasound findings for tendinopathy.

4. Once abnormal characteristics are identified or the probe is over an area of pain, the tendon should be evaluated with the Doppler to evaluate neovascularization. Neovascularization can be seen in **Figure 38-4**.

Achilles

1. The best position to scan the Achilles is with the patient prone and both feet hanging off the edge of the bed. This provides easy access to the Achilles but also allows for a dynamic examination

of the tendon. Again, the tendon should be evaluated in both the long and short axes (**Figures 38-5 and 38-6**).

2. The Achilles tendon gets its blood supply from three main areas: the musculotendinous and osteotendinous junctions and the paratenon, with the posterior tibial artery providing the major contribution.[12] Because of the unusual biomechanics and the decreased blood supply, there is an area of tendon about 4 to 6 cm above the calcaneus that is more prone to injury and tearing.[13]

3. The Achilles tendon connects the plantaris, gastrocnemius, and the soleus to the calcaneus. Because it has three attachments, it moves in more than one direction. Because of the three separate muscles, the tendon twists medially as it contracts, which leads to a concentration of forces as the muscles flex and relax.[14] Because of this the Achilles tendon needs to be evaluated in its length as the concentration of forces in this area makes it another area prone to injury. **Figure 38-7** shows a normal and abnormal tendon.

4. Once areas of abnormality or pain are identified, the power Doppler should be used to examine the tendon as well. This is demonstrated in **Figure 38-8** and Table 38-2.

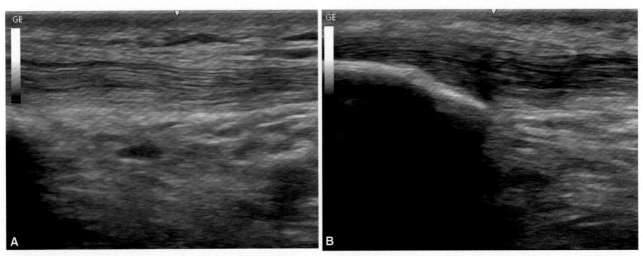

FIGURE 38-3. Image (A) shows a normal patella. This shows good linear-appearing fibrils with no fluid and hypoechoic texture. Image (B) shows an abnormal tendon, and the difference is subtle. There is increased fluid between the fibrils. This is identified as the dark areas between the white fibrils and increased heterogeneity.

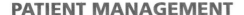
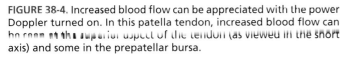

FIGURE 38-4. Increased blood flow can be appreciated with the power Doppler turned on. In this patella tendon, increased blood flow can be seen at the superior aspect of the tendon (as viewed in the short axis) and some in the prepatellar bursa.

PATIENT MANAGEMENT

There are many different options for treatment of tendinopathy, but it is important to know which are evidence based and most likely to lead to optimal patient outcomes.

The first-line treatment for most overuse injuries is nonsteroidal anti-inflammatory drugs (NSAIDs). There is good evidence to suggest that NSAID use within the first 4 weeks of injury can be beneficial, but there is little evidence to suggest that there is any benefit for chronic tendinopathy.[15] Neovascularization on ultrasound may be a marker of active inflammation and could suggest patients more likely to benefit from anti-inflammatory medications; however, this is speculative.

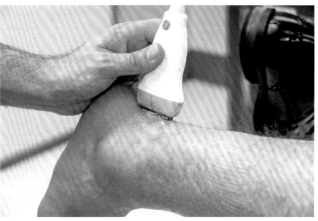

FIGURE 38-5. The probe is placed in long axis over a cushion of gel with very little pressure. The probe is supported with the examiner's hand resting on the posterior heel.

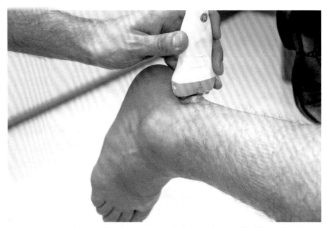

FIGURE 38-6. The probe is in short axis, which will allow for better visualization of the neovascularization seen in tendinopathy. Again, there is a good cushion of gel and light pressure.

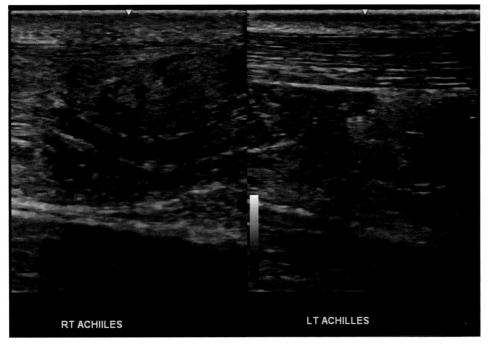

RT ACHIILES   LT ACHILLES

FIGURE 38-7. A normal (right) and an abnormal (left) Achilles. In the abnormal Achilles on the right, there is disorganized fibrils and edema within the tendon. This results in increased tendon thickness and heterogeneity. The tendon also appears more hypoechoic.

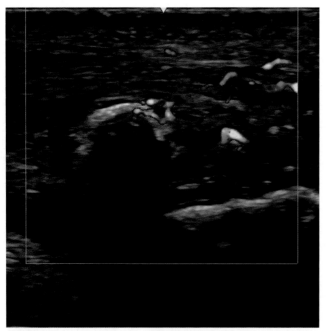

FIGURE 38-8. This Achilles tendon has calcifications, which can be seen as hyperechoic areas within the tendon. There is also increased signal with the power Doppler.

TABLE 38-2	Ultrasound Findings in Chronic Tendinopathy Hypoechoic Fluid Surrounding the Tendon or in the Tendon Sheath

1. Increased heterogeneity secondary to disorganization of the normal fibril pattern.
2. Decreased echogenicity of the tendon.
3. Thickening of the tendon diameter compared to normal or the unaffected contralateral side.
4. Hyperechoic calcifications with shadowing.
5. Increased Doppler flow because of neovascularization.

Nitroglycerin topical patches have been studied in a variety of tendinopathies and have shown good evidence to improve day and night pain, function, and outcomes of patients with Achilles tendinopathy.[16]

There is fairly strong evidence to suggest that a corticosteroid injection is beneficial for acute injuries (less than 6 weeks old), but there is little evidence to suggest benefit for chronic issues. There is also the established concern with the Achilles that it increases the risk of tendon rupture, but there have been studies that show that the use of imaging to guide the injection into the sheath has decreased this risk.[17]

There is some evidence for physical therapy. Eccentric strengthening exercises have shown an improvement in pain, function, and patient satisfaction in comparison to concentric exercises, stretching, and splinting. However, the level of evidence for this is low.[18] There is currently little evidence available to support the use of most physical therapy modalities including low-level laser therapy, iontophoresis, phonophoresis, therapeutic ultrasound, or deep friction massage.[15]

There are still too few studies showing high levels of evidence to support the use of growth factors and stem cells or platelet-rich plasma injections.[15] These forms of treatment are considered experimental by most health insurers and are largely not covered.

Surgery should be considered as a last resort but has generally had positive outcomes. It does, however, carry a substantial failure rate of 20% to 30% and is also associated with a much greater risk than the other forms of treatment (**Figure 38-9**).[15]

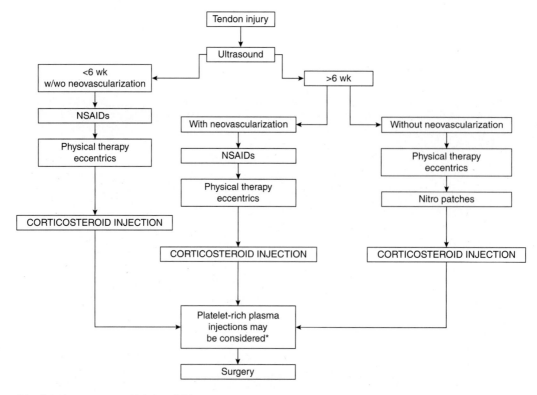

*Very little data to suggest this is beneficial
SORT evidence C.

FIGURE 38-9. Algorithm for suspected tendon injury. NSAID, nonsteroidal anti-inflammatory drug.

PEARLS AND PITFALLS

Pearls

- Chronic tendinosis is often unilateral so the contralateral side can often be referred to as a normal control.
- Ask the patient to put the probe directly over the area of pain for quick localization of abnormalities.
- Pressure from the probe can be used for sonopalpation. An abnormal tendon will often be tender to probe pressure.

Pitfalls

- Anisotropy can give false positives. Be sure to adjust the scan angle of the ultrasound beam to confirm a perpendicular orientation and rule out anisotropy.
- Too much pressure can give false negatives especially for Doppler, as small neovascular vessels may be occluded by the force.

BILLING

CPT Code	Description	Global Payment	Professional Component	Technical Component
76881	Ultrasound, extremity, nonvascular, real time with image documentations; complete	$116.01	$31.87	$84.14
76882	Ultrasound, extremity, nonvascular, real time with image documentations; limited, anatomic specific	$36.52	$25.06	$11.46

CPT codes and average national reimbursement for Medicare in 2016. Payment data are from https://www.cms.gov/apps/physician-fee-schedule/search/search-criteria.aspx. See Chapter 2 for details on ultrasound billing.

References

1. Kannus P, Natri A. Etiology and pathophysiology of tendon ruptures in sports. *Scand J Med Sci Sports*. 1997;7:107-112.
2. Kannus P. Etiology and pathophysiology of chronic tendon disorders in sports. *Scand J Med Sci Sports*. 1997;7:78-85.
3. Sharma P, Maffulli N. Tendon injury and tendinopathy: healing and repair. *J Bone Joint Surg Am*. 2005;87:187-202.
4. Parker L, Nazarian LN, Carrino JA, et al. Musculoskeletal imaging: Medicare use, costs, and potential for cost substitution. *J Am Coll Radiol*. 2008;5:182-188.
5. Teitz CC, Garrett WE Jr, Miniaci A, Lee MH, Mann RA. Tendon problems in athletic individuals. *Instr Course Lect*. 1997;46:569-582.
6. Khan KM, Cook JL, Bonar F, Harcourt P, Astrom M. Histopathology of common tendinopathies. Update and implications for clinical management. *Sports Med*. 1999;27:393-408.
7. Soslowsky LJ, Thomopoulos S, Tun S, et al. Neer Award 1999: Overuse activity injures the supraspinatus tendon in an animal model: a histologic and biomechanical study. *J Shoulder Elbow Surg*. 2000;9:79-84.
8. Carr AJ, Norris SH. The blood supply of the calcaneal tendon. *J Bone Joint Surg Br*. 1989;71:100-101.
9. Zanetti M, Metzdorf A, Kundert HP, et al. Achilles tendons: clinical relevance of neovascularization diagnosed with power doppler US. *Radiology*. 2003;227:556-560.
10. Van Holsbeeck M, Introcasco J. *Musculoskeletal Ultrasound*. 2nd ed. St Louis, MO: Mosby; 2001.
11. Crass JR, van de Vegte GL, Harkavy LA. Tendon echogenicity: ex vivo study. *Radiology*. 1988;167:499-501.
12. Ahmed IM, Lagopoulos M, McConnell P, Soames RW, Sefton GK. Blood supply of the achilles tendon. *J Orthop Res*. 1998;16:591-596.
13. Scheller AD, Kasser JR, Quigley TB. Tendon injuries about the ankle. *Orthop Clin North Am*. 1980;11:801-811.
14. Robinson P, White LM. The biomechanics and imaging of soccer injuries. *Semin Musculoskelet Radiol*. 2005;9:397-420.
15. Andres BM, Murrell GAC. Treatment of tendinopathy: what works, what does not, and what is on the horizon. *Clin Orthop Relat Res*. 2008;466(7):1539-1554. doi:10.1007/s11999-008-0260-1.
16. Paoloni JA, Appleyard RC, Nelson J, Murrell GA. Topical glyceryl trinitrate treatment of chronic noninsertional Achilles tendinopathy. A randomized, double-blind, placebo-controlled trial. *J Bone Joint Surg Am*. 2004;86-A:916-922.
17. Gill SS, Gelbke MK, Mattson SL, Anderson MW, Hurwitz SR. Fluoroscopically guided low-volume peritendinous corticosteroid injection for Achilles tendinopathy. A safety study. *J Bone Joint Surg Am*. 2004;86-A:802-806.
18. Woodley BL, Newsham-West RJ, Baxter GD. Chronic tendinopathy: effectiveness of eccentric exercise. *Br J Sports Med*. 2007;41:188-198; discussion 199.

PART 2

Is the Patient's Arthritis From Crystal Disease?

Mark H. Greenberg, MD, FACR, RMSK, RhMSUS

● Clinical Vignette

A 69-year-old woman presented with joint pain. She described several years of recurrent right knee and left first metatarsophalangeal (MTP) joint pain. Uric acid was elevated to more than 10 mg/dL in the past. Prednisone aborted each episode. No joint aspiration was done. The episodes in each joint occurred several times yearly and could occur simultaneously or separately. In between episodes, each joint was asymptomatic. Severe swelling, pain, erythema, and tenderness accompanied the inflammatory episodes. She could not walk when the joints flared up. Even gentle touch to the toe was unbearable. It always resolved within 14 days even without treatment. Joint x-rays showed only degenerative change commensurate with her age with the exception of calcium deposits in the medial and lateral menisci. Institution of colchicine and allopurinol stopped the inflammatory episodes. When colchicine was withdrawn, episodic swelling and pain in her right knee resumed. Uric acid level was found to be 5.4. Rheumatoid factor and anti-cyclic citrullinated peptide antibody were negative. There was no history or evidence of psoriasis. Her physician was uncertain as to why she continued to flare despite having a low uric acid. Is the patient's arthritis from crystal disease?

LITERATURE REVIEW

The major crystal diseases are gout and calcium pyrophosphate dihydrate (CPPD) crystal deposition disease. Gout is caused by the precipitation of monosodium urate (MSU), also known as uric acid crystals in joints and tendons. CPPD disease, often called pseudogout, is caused by the precipitation of CPPD crystals in joints and tendons. MSU crystals exhibit negative birefringence under polarized light. These crystals are needle-like in appearance and are yellow when parallel to polarized light. CPPD crystals are blue when parallel to polarized light, which is termed positive birefringence. CPPD crystals are shorter than MSU crystals and may be rhomboidal in shape.

Both conditions may occur in the same person and even in the same joint. Furthermore, crystal disease may occur concurrently with other joint problems, including joint infection, osteoarthritis, and rheumatoid arthritis.

Both diseases have a number of general similarities (see Table 39-1).

The diseases have similar and different joint predilections (see Table 39-2). Note that both often occur in the knee. Also note that inflammation of the first MTP joint is called podagra irrespective of the cause.

Risk factors for gout[1] include aging, elevated uric acid level, male gender, obesity,[2] alcohol use, hypertension, chronic kidney disease, high animal purine diet, and medication affecting uric acid level and/ or interfering with urate-lowering medications.[3,4] The prevalence rate for gout likely exceeds 3% of adults.[2] Pseudogout risk factors are aging and the "four H's": hypophosphatasia, hemochromatosis, hypomagnesemia, and hyperparathyroidism.[5] The prevalence of CPPD disease is not clearly known but is estimated to be between 4% and 7%.[5,6]

Diagnosis of crystal disease may be challenging. For both gout and pseudogout, the most accurate diagnosis is made when one can observe white blood cells in synovial fluid phagocytizing crystals. Classification criteria for both crystal diseases have been proposed and address the circumstance in which synovial fluid is not obtainable (the patient declines aspiration or there is no fluid to be aspirated) and during intercritical periods.[7-9] These criteria depend on other supporting evidence, including the clinical picture (including the pattern of joint involvement), laboratory tests, radiographs, and now ultrasound. These criteria are less specific for the diagnosis than when crystals are seen in synovial fluid. However, for gout, patients may be classified as having the condition even without the demonstration of crystals on synovial fluid analysis.[7,8]

For gout classification criteria, see Table 39-3.

For *pseudogout* proposed diagnostic criteria, see Table 39-4.

For an individual patient, the criteria for pseudogout are often circumstantial and, if definitive synovial fluid crystals are not present, we label the patient as having possible or probable pseudogout.

TABLE 39-1 Similarities Between Gout and Calcium Pyrophosphate Dihydrate

May mimic nearly any other form of arthritis and occur in any joint, including small joints
May have three phases: acute (severe inflammation), intercritical (clinically quiescent), and subacute (chronic)
May have crystal deposits in joints and soft tissue that are not causing any problem
Tend to be monoarticular (involving one joint at a time), less often oligoarticular (involving two to four joints), and occasionally polyarticular (involving five or more joints)
Absolute diagnosis is based on joint aspiration and rapid examination of synovial fluid using polarized microscopy.
Ultrasound may demonstrate distinct patterns that may support the diagnosis.

TABLE 39-2 Gout and Pseudogout Joint Predilection

Gout: first metatarsophalangeal joint, ankle, foot dorsum, and knee
Pseudogout: knee and wrist

TABLE 39-3 **Gout Classification Criteria**[7-9]

Clinical picture of a monoarticular or oligoarticular pattern of involvement of joints, including the first metatarsophalangeal joint (first MTP), ankle, and midfoot
Synovial fluid with white blood cells phagocytizing strongly negative birefringent needle-shaped crystals
Tophi on physical examination
Serum uric acid elevation (note that during an acute gout attack, uric acid levels may be high, low, or normal[10,11])
Radiographic evidence of gout-related bony erosion with overhanging edge[7,12]
Ultrasound finding of double contour sign

TABLE 39-4 **Pseudogout Proposed Diagnostic Criteria**[5,9,13,14]

Clinical picture of monoarticular or oligoarticular pattern of involvement of joints typically involving the wrists and knees
Synovial fluid with white blood cells phagocytizing weakly positive birefringent rhomboid-shaped crystals
Laboratory evidence for hypercalcemia or hyperparathyroidism, hypophosphatemia, or hemochromatosis may be corroborative
Radiographic finding of chondrocalcinosis involving the symphysis pubis, knee, wrist, tendons, spinal disks, and fascia (eg, Achilles tendon, plantar fascia, quadriceps, rotator cuff, triceps tendon) is corroborative. Other supporting radiographic findings include accelerated osteoarthritis-like picture, particularly in joints not typically affected by osteoarthritis (eg, wrists, metacarpophalangeal joints, elbows, and shoulders), intervertebral and sacroiliac vacuum phenomenon, subchondral cysts, hook-like osteophytes, particularly at the metacarpal heads, and joint space narrowing at the radiocarpal or patellofemoral joints.
Ultrasound finding of calcium pyrophosphate dihydrate crystal aggregates

It reminds us to consider this possibility and not conclusively label a patient with a different arthropathy.

A less common but diagnostically confounding manifestation of CPPD disease is the Crowned Dens Syndrome in which CPPD crystals deposit around the odontoid process, causing severe neck pain, fever, and elevated inflammatory markers.[5,15] This condition may imitate infection, tumor, and other inflammatory processes.

It is challenging to make the diagnosis of crystal disease in an intercritical period without the advantage of synovial fluid analysis. However, it is important to make the correct diagnosis because treatment targeting a different disease may be ineffective and expose patients to potentially toxic medications. Crystal disease in its quiescent (intercritical) or chronic phase needs to be considered when evaluating patients for the spectrum of polyarthropathies. Even more bewildering is the understanding that crystal disease may be only part of the picture or that the presence of crystals in radiographs or ultrasound may merely indicate the presence of crystals that are not clinically significant. Ultrasound can add important evidence in this regard.

Ultrasound is rapidly evolving into a useful tool for gout and pseudogout diagnosis and care.[16,17] When joint aspiration is not feasible, ultrasound may noninvasively support the diagnosis of crystal disease by detecting crystal aggregates. Ultrasound also locates and directs aspiration of tiny fluid collections.[18] Furthermore, ultrasound can monitor tophi dissolution in gout.[18,19] Ultrasound is highly specific in the detection of crystal aggregates[18,20,21] and does not require an actively inflamed joint. Although not as specific as observing active phagocytosis of MSU or CPPD crystal on microscopic evaluation of synovial fluid, ultrasound findings can be highly suggestive of the diagnosis.

Ultrasonic finding for crystal arthropathy have generated new terms: double contour sign (DCS), uratic sand, intracartilaginous deposits, intratendinous crystal clouds, and multiple shining dots.[18,20-22]

Ultrasound and gout. Findings on ultrasound examination can support the diagnosis of gout and may be useful in the early detection and monitoring of therapy.[19,23] The two classic US signs of gout are the **DCS** and **tophaceous deposits.**[22]

The DCS is a thick hyperechoic coating of urate (uric acid) crystals on the superficial aspect of joint cartilage. It is as thick as the underlying bony cortex but may vary in being intermittent or continuous, regular or irregular. It is not dependent on the angle of the ultrasound beam (insonation). In one study, the DCS specificity was 64%.[24] However, the occurrence of DCS along with Power Doppler evidence for hyperemia and elevated serum uric acid levels raised specificity to more than 90%.[24] The DCS is now included in the newest gout classification criteria.[7,8]

The description of tophaceous deposits varies widely, but in general, these deposits are visualized sonographically as hypoechoic to hyperechoic heterogeneous cloudy circumscribed areas that may be surrounded by a hypoechoic border or rim ("halo").[25] These aggregates of MSU crystals are sometimes described as hyperechoic cloudy areas.[26]

Interestingly, patients with hyperuricemia *without* acute gout symptoms may demonstrate DCS and tophi.[26] Despite what appears to be a dormant stage, tophi may aggregate and cause dactylitis, bone erosion, and chronic gouty arthropathy. Osteomyelitis may be mimicked by tophaceous bone destruction.[27] During an acute gouty attack, ultrasound may demonstrate increased fluid, joint recess widening, soft-tissue swelling, and enhanced Power Doppler signal.[22]

At the opposite end of the gouty spectrum, it has been demonstrated that in patients with asymptomatic hyperuricemia, a DCS may be seen at the first MTP.[28] Furthermore, patients with gout in an intercritical phase may have first MTP chronic synovitis and bone erosion demonstrated on ultrasound, implying an ongoing subclinical chronic process.[28] This may suggest that ultrasound scans be performed in all patients with hyperuricemia and a history of gout to differentiate subclinical gout activity from asymptomatic hyperuricemia.[28]

MSU patterns that may be sonographically visualized are as follows: intra-articular tophi (urate iceberg), DCS, MSU crystal aggregates, shining dots (crystal microaggregates or microtophi, also called uratic sand), soft tophaceous aggregates (urate clouds), and dense (hard) tophi. In addition, abnormal Power Doppler signal within and surrounding the joint may be detected. In tendons, there may be intratendinous urate deposits disrupting the normal fibrillary echotexture (can be hyperechoic linear lines, hyperechoic dots, clouds, frank tophi).[22] In addition to the foregoing ultrasound signs of uric acid deposition, bone erosions may be detected in disease of longer duration.[22]

Ultrasound is changing the way we think about the diagnosis and treatment of gout. Tophi are part of the clinical diagnostic criteria, yet we can identify them on ultrasound as microaggregates long before they become large nodular deposits that are clinically detectable. Ultrasonic imaging of the first MTP in asymptomatic hyperuricemic patients in search of uric acid crystals may potentially change the gout treatment paradigm in the future.

It is too early to determine the value of using ultrasound to monitor the efficacy of urate-lowering medication with respect to the resolution of tophi[19] and DCS.[29,30]

Ultrasound and pseudogout. CPPD crystal aggregates are seen as hyperechoic deposits of varied sizes, with or without acoustic shadowing. Typical locations are cartilage, tendons, and entheses. An enthesis is where tendons, ligaments, or fascia connect to bone. Knee meniscal and femoral condyle fibrocartilage are common areas in which CPPD crystal deposition is found. Knee meniscal calcification is found in most patients with CPPD deposition.[31] CPPD crystals differ from MSU crystals in that the latter reside on the superficial cartilage surface, whereas CPPD crystals are typically embedded in the cartilage itself. X-rays may or may not show calcium deposits in CPPD deposition disease. The distribution of CPPD crystals is often patchy. If enough CPPD crystals are present, you may see a "pseudo-double contour sign" which is composed of hyperechoic foci *within* the cartilage. Occasionally, with CPPD, calcium deposits on the surface of cartilage, the province of MSU crystals. However, with CPPD, this is often thin, patchy, and changes ultrasonic appearance with the angle of insonation. In contrast, MSU crystals have a steadfast appearance independent of the angle of insonation.

The presence of CPPD crystal deposition in cartilage or tendon does not establish clinical relevance. Corroborating evidence in favor of clinical relevance includes synovial fluid collection, synovial hypertrophy, and Power Doppler signal changes. There is consensus that ultrasound is more sensitive than conventional radiographs in detecting CPPD crystals.[32-34] CPPD crystals may be visualized on ultrasound in many asymptomatic joints and soft tissue, including the elbows, metacarpal phalangeal joints, shoulders, knees, wrists, feet, plantar fascia, and Achilles tendons.[34-36] Ultrasonic detection of hyperechoic calcium deposits at either the triangular fibrocartilage complex of the wrist or menisci of the knee may be considered to be evidence for CPPD crystal deposition disease and should raise suspicion for the disease.[37]

TABLE 39-5	Recommendations for Use of Point-of-Care Ultrasound in Clinical Practice		
Recommendation		**Rating**	**References**
Use of ultrasonography for assessing symptomatic joints by comparing the predictions based on ultrasonography signs with the identification of synovial fluid MSU crystals or with a combination of a validated clinical algorithm and MSU crystals.		A	24, 60-63
Using ultrasound for diagnosis of calcium pyrophosphate deposition disease, with microscopic crystal detection as a gold standard.		B	17, 18, 21, 31, 32, 34, 36, 38

Abbreviation: MSU, monosodium urate.

A = consistent, good-quality patient-oriented evidence; B = inconsistent or limited-quality patient-oriented evidence; C = consensus, disease-oriented evidence, usual practice, expert opinion, or case series. For information about the SORT evidence rating system, go to http://www.aafp.org/afpsort.

PERFORMING THE SCAN

A. **First MTP joint**—three views: dorsal longitudinal, medial longitudinal, and plantar longitudinal.

1. **Preparation.** The patient should be positioned sitting semiupright. The affected foot should have the hip partially flexed and the posterior heel in contact with the examination table. The distal foot should be hanging off the table (**Figure 39-1**). Alternatively, the patient may be supine with the leg extended and a cushion beneath the ankle for comfort. The first toe would be upright.

Position the ultrasound equipment appropriately, and select a high-frequency linear probe with a superficial high-frequency preset.

2. **Evaluate the dorsal longitudinal first MTP joint.** Place a transducer with the probe in a longitudinal position in the midline of the dorsum of the first toe over the MTP joint (**Figure 39-2**). Examine the distal metatarsal head and the

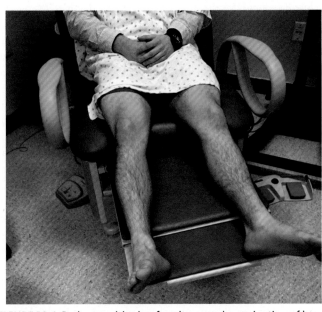

FIGURE 39-1. Patient positioning for ultrasound examination of lower extremity.

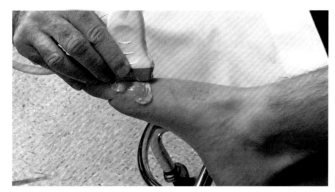

FIGURE 39-2. Probe position for dorsal first metatarsophalangeal joint ultrasound examination.

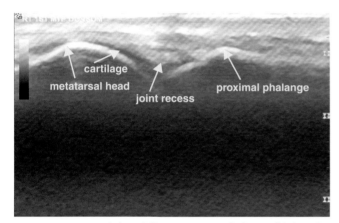

FIGURE 39-3. Normal dorsal first metatarsophalangeal joint ultrasound image.

proximal phalanx (**Figure 39-3**). Look at the dark cartilage overlying the metatarsal head, and observe for any abnormality within the cartilage or hyperechogenicity on the surface of the cartilage that might indicate a DCS or a cartilage interface sign (CIS). The CIS is due to synovial fluid in the dorsal recess produced by a change in impedance when the sound waves enter the cartilage. The CIS is hyperechoic but not nearly as thick as the DCS. The hyperechoic CIS will change dramatically with the angle of insonation, in contrast to the DCS, which will remain fairly constant with changes in probe angle. Look at the dorsal joint recess and examine it for distention and for crystal aggregates (**Figure 39-4**). Look at the bone of the metatarsal neck, the metatarsal head, and proximal phalanx for possible erosion. Turn on the Power Doppler, and set the pulse repetition frequency to a point where the baseline Power Doppler signal is slightly active for bone, and observe for any Power Doppler activity within the surrounding soft tissue of the joint.

3. **Evaluate the medial longitudinal first MTP joint.** Turn the Power Doppler off. Ask the patient to externally rotate the flexed knee into a "frog leg" position. Then rotate the probe gently in a medial slide but still in a longitudinal axis to the first toe (**Figure 39-5**). Examine the medial aspect of the metatarsal phalangeal joint. Interrogate the joint completely, including the soft tissues (**Figure 39-6**). Once again turn on the Power Doppler.

4. **Evaluate the plantar longitudinal first MTP joint.** Once you have completed the medial first MTP joint evaluation, turn the Power Doppler off and rotate the probe still in a longitudinal orientation to the inferior aspect of the first MTP joint (**Figures 39-7 and 39-8**). After evaluation of the joint, turn the Power Doppler back on to evaluate for inflammation.

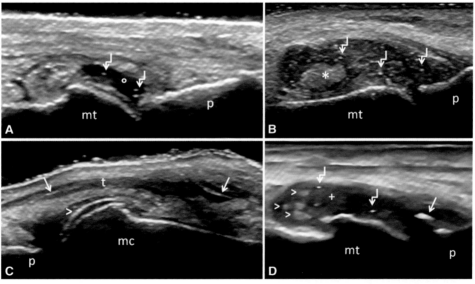

FIGURE 39-4. Gout. A and B, Longitudinal dorsal scan. Metatarsophalangeal joint. Broken arrows indicate hyperechoic spots within the synovial fluid (o). The asterisk indicates an intra-articular tophaceous deposit (urate iceberg) not generating acoustic shadow. C, Double contour sign (arrowhead) shown on longitudinal dorsal scan of a metacarpophalangeal joint. Intratendinous urate deposits appear as subtle hyperechoic bands not generating acoustic shadows (arrows). D, Monosodium urate crystal aggregates different in size, shape, and reflectivity. The broken arrows point shining dots representing dense crystal microaggregates. The arrowheads indicate soft tophaceous aggregates (urate clouds) and the arrow points a dense highly echogenic tophus (hard tophus) floating in the urate sand (+). mc, metacarpal bone; mt, metatarsal bone; p, proximal phalanx; t, finger extensor tendon. Reprinted with permission from Grassi W, Okano T, Filippucci E. Use of ultrasound for diagnosis and monitoring of outcomes in crystal arthropathies. *Curr Opin Rheumatol.* 2015;27(2):148. Figure 1.

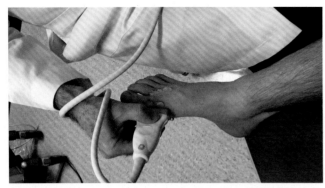

FIGURE 39-5. Position for medial first metatarsophalangeal joint ultrasound examination.

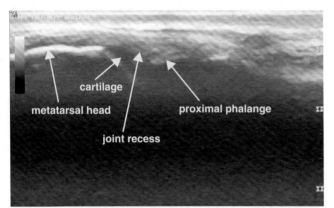

FIGURE 39-6. Normal medial first metatarsophalangeal joint ultrasound image.

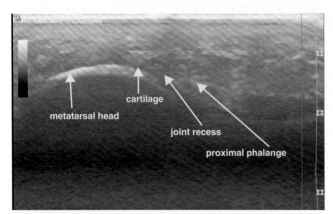

FIGURE 39-7. Position for plantar first metatarsophalangeal joint ultrasound examination.

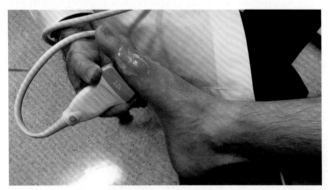

FIGURE 39-8. Normal plantar first metatarsophalangeal joint ultrasound image.

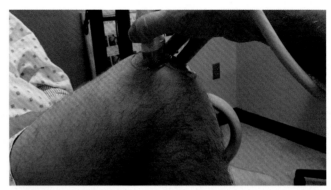

FIGURE 39-9. Probe position for evaluation of the anterior superior distal femoral cartilage.

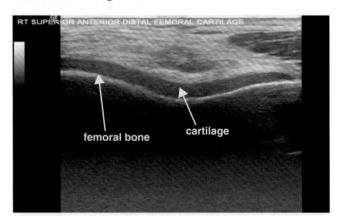

FIGURE 39-10. Ultrasound picture of normal distal anterior femoral cartilage.

B. **Knee**—three views: flexed suprapatellar transverse (femoral notch), medial meniscus longitudinal, and lateral meniscus longitudinal
   1. **Preparation.** The patient should be positioned sitting semiupright or supine. The knee should be maximally flexed. Use a linear probe with a mid-depth setting.
   2. **Evaluate the knee in a flexed suprapatellar transverse position (femoral notch).** Place the probe transverse to the limb at the superior portion of the patella. The probe should be perpendicular to the table (**Figure 39-9**). Move the probe slightly proximally until a hypoechoic "V-shaped" structure appears (**Figure 39-10**). This is the femoral notch. Toggle the probe up and down, and move it slightly medially and then slightly laterally to sharply define the cartilage covering the distal femur. Note that this is **not** the joint space itself but simply the articular cartilage covering the superior one-third of the femur. Look at the cartilage in terms of its depth and clarity as well as the cartilage surface. Look for calcifications within the cartilage and also for a DCS on the surface of the cartilage (**Figure 39-11**).
   3. **Evaluate the medial meniscus in longitudinal view.** Have the patient extend the knee, and place a bolster or pillow beneath the knee so that the knee is bent approximately 30°. Rotate the probe 90° (to a longitudinal position with respect to the limb) and place it just medial to the distal half of the patella (**Figure 39-12**). Slowly move the probe posteriorly until the joint space emerges, and then center the joint space in the field of view (Figure 39-12). Toggle the probe back and forth to clarify the picture of the medial meniscus, which is normally hyperechoic and triangular in shape ([**Figure 39-13**];

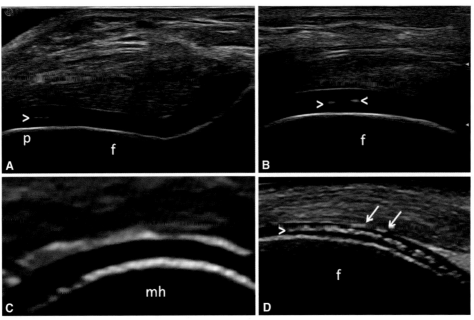

FIGURE 39-11. Calcium pyrophosphate dihydrate crystal deposition disease. Knee. Suprapatellar anterior transverse (A) and longitudinal (B) scans showing hyperechoic linear spots not generating acoustic shadowing, located within the hyaline cartilage the lateral femoral condyle (arrowheads). C, Gout. Double contour sign at metacarpal head (mh) level. D, Calcium pyrophosphate dihydrate (CPPD) crystal deposition disease. Hyperechoic deposits in the midzone generating a double contour that can be easily differentiated from that of gout because of the "sandwich" appearance (crystal in-between two layers of cartilage). Arrows indicate CPPD deposits at the outer profile of the hyaline cartilage. f, femur. Reprinted with permission from Grassi W, Okano T, Filippucci E. Use of ultrasound for diagnosis and monitoring of outcomes in crystal arthropathies. *Curr Opin Rheumatol.* 2015;27(2):151. Figure 4.

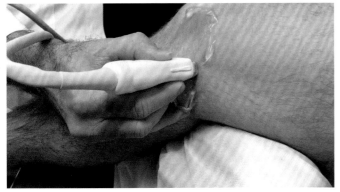

FIGURE 39-12. Probe position for evaluation of the medial meniscus.

note that the transducer fin is proximal, correlating with the left side of the figure). Another tip is to keep the proximal end of the probe stable and slightly rotate ("fan") the distal portion in either direction and then toggle the probe again. This will ensure that you will have a high-quality picture of the medial meniscus. Look for calcium deposits within the medial meniscus and the medial collateral ligament.

Continue to slide the probe posteriorly keeping the meniscus in focus to evaluate the posterior portion of the medial meniscus for calcium deposits.

4. **Evaluate the lateral meniscus in longitudinal view.** In the same knee position as the medial meniscal evaluation, take the linear probe, still in a longitudinal orientation, and place the probe just lateral to the distal half of the patella. Slowly slide the probe posteriorly still in longitudinal position until the joint space is noted (**Figure 39-14**). Center the joint

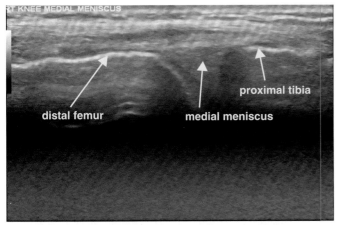

FIGURE 39-13. Normal medial meniscus ultrasound image.

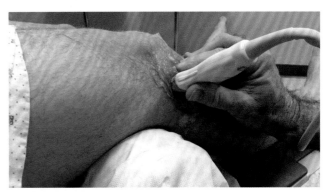

FIGURE 39-14. Probe position for evaluation of the lateral meniscus.

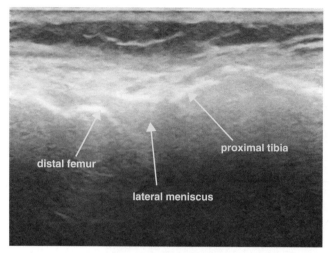

FIGURE 39-15. Normal lateral meniscus ultrasound image.

space in the field of view, and then toggle the probe back and forth to identify and sharpen the picture of the lateral meniscus. This should also be hyperechoic and triangular (**Figure 39-15**). You can fix the proximal portion of the probe and "fan" the probe slightly in either direction and then toggle the probe until you optimize the image. Look for calcifications within the meniscus and the lateral collateral ligament (**Figure 39-16**). Continue with the probe in the same position posteriorly to look at the posterior meniscus, toggling and fanning it along the way as needed.

PATIENT MANAGEMENT

In evaluating acute monoarthritis, ultrasound may give strong supporting diagnostic evidence for gout or CPPD deposition disease (**Figure 39-17**; Tables 39-6 and 39-7).

After establishing a diagnosis of acute gout or pseudogout, the first step is to abort the episode.[38,39] Anti-inflammatory medication such as nonsteroidal anti-inflammatory drugs (NSAIDs), glucocorticoids (intra-articular or oral), and colchicine is effective for both gout and pseudogout. Treatment duration should be 10 to 14 days or at least 3 days after the episode has completely subsided. Consider treatment for a longer period with a slower taper when

using oral steroids to avoid a rebound flare. Consideration of the choice of anti-inflammatory medication should be made in light of the patient's age, concurrent medications, renal/liver/cardiac status, and risk of gastrointestinal complications. Intra-articular steroids are particularly helpful but require certainty that there is no concomitant joint infection. We do not use intravenous colchicine because of safety concerns, and oral colchicine use is often limited by the side effect of diarrhea or other gastrointestinal symptoms. Other treatment modalities such as icing the affected joint and the use of analgesics might also be of help.[40]

Next, a search to determine modifiable risk/associated factors needs to be done and such factors mitigated if at all possible. For gout these would include medication or the dietary causes of hyperuricemia, obesity, hypertension, alcohol use, and hyperlipidemia.[41-44] Rarely, lead ingestion might be a cause. For pseudogout, a search for hemochromatosis, hypomagnesemia, and hyperparathyroidism should be undertaken. Hypothyroidism may or may not be associated with pseudogout.[45,46] Note that in contrast to some cases of gout, modifications of risk factors/associated conditions will not reduce recurrent episodes of acute CPPD deposition arthritis.[47]

For gout, if there are no modifiable risk/associated factors or if modifications are insufficient to halt acute attacks, then a decision will need to be made regarding chronic treatment. The occurrence of more than two episodes per year (fewer if the episodes are disabling) would be reason to chronically treat. Other reasons to treat gout on a chronic basis would be bone or joint destruction, the presence of tophi, gout associated with renal insufficiency, or recurrent uric acid kidney stones.

For chronic treatment of gout, the goal is to lower uric acid below 6.0 mg/dL.[38,39,48] If tophi are present, it has been suggested that the goal be to lower serum uric acid level to below 5.0 mg/dL. However, the suggested target serum uric acid levels are not data-driven values, and further research is needed to determine ideal targets.[49] Lowering serum uric acid level is done under prophylactic cover of an anti-inflammatory agent such as colchicine or a nonsteroidal anti-inflammatory agent. A urate-lowering agent such as allopurinol is added after the patient has been on an anti-inflammatory agent (eg, colchicine or NSAID) for 3 to 4 weeks, and then uric acid is slowly lowered. If an anti-inflammatory agent is not used prophylactically, then there is a risk of a seemingly paradoxical gouty flare,

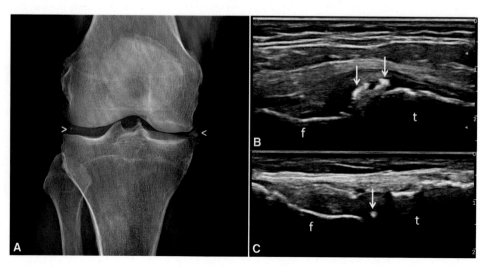

FIGURE 39-16. Calcium pyrophosphate dihydrate crystal deposition disease. A, Conventional radiography showing meniscal calcifications (arrowheads). B and C, Meniscal calcification appear as homogeneous hyperechoic aggregates not generating acoustic shadowing (arrows) on both medial (B) and lateral (C) longitudinal scan. f, femur; t, tibia. Reprinted with permission from Grassi W, Okano T, Filippucci E. Use of ultrasound for diagnosis and monitoring of outcomes in crystal arthropathies. *Curr Opin Rheumatol.* 2015;27(2):151. Figure 3.

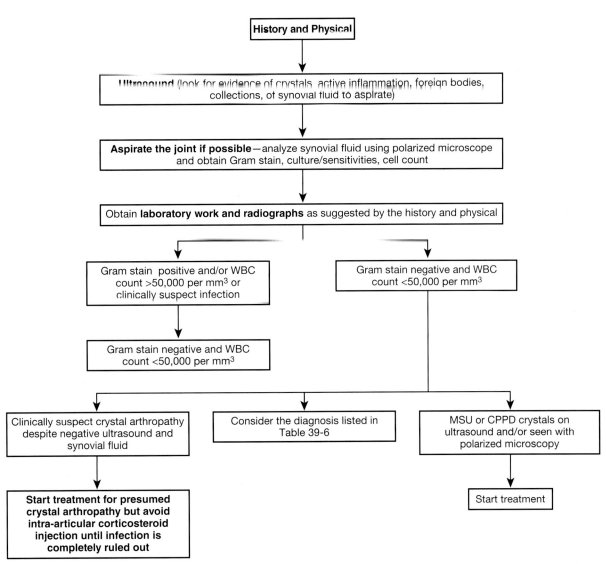

FIGURE 39-17. Acute monoarthritis algorithm. CPPD, calcium pyrophosphate dihydrate; MSU, monosodium urate; WBC, white blood cells.

that is, a flare that occurs when the uric acid is being lowered. Begin the urate-lowering medication at low dose, and increase the dose slowly every 2 to 4 weeks.[38] Once the goal of lower uric acid level is achieved, the anti-inflammatory agent can be withdrawn. It should be withdrawn 3 months after the goal of lower serum uric acid levels

is achieved if no tophi are present and 6 months after achieving the goal of lower uric acid level if tophi had been detected on clinical examination.[39] Continued laboratory monitoring for side effects and efficacy of the urate-lowering medication is extremely important.

For pseudogout, the reason to treat chronically would be multiple disabling episodes per year and possibly accelerated and severe destruction of joints. For recurrent or chronic pseudogout, chronic nonsteroidal anti-inflammatory agents might be useful if coupled with a proton pump inhibitor (PPI) to prevent gastrointestinal side effects, weighing the risk of potential gastrointestinal bleeding against the unknown risks of long-term PPI use. Again, comorbid conditions and concurrent medications will help determine the best agent to use. NSAIDs or low-dose colchicine might be effective. There have been only a few reports of the efficacy of chronic hydroxychloroquine[50] and methotrexate[51-55] to diminish flares of pseudogout. Reports for methotrexate efficacy are conflicting.[51-55]

Beyond diagnostic value, information from the ultrasound examination may help guide treatment in the proper clinical setting. For gout, it may show tophi that are undetectable on physical examination. It may also demonstrate bone erosions and

TABLE 39-6 **Monoarthritis Causes**

Gout
Calcium pyrophosphate dihydrate crystal deposition disease
Infection: bacterial, fungal, mycobacterium, viral, Lyme disease
Osteoarthritis
Internal derangement of joint
Sarcoidosis
Spondyloarthropathies
Aseptic necrosis of bone
Osteomyelitis
Foreign body synovitis
Other crystal diseases
Hemarthrosis
Intra-articular loose body
Atypical presentation of a polyarthropathy

TABLE 39-7   **Gout Versus Pseudogout Summary**

Disease	Clinical	Laboratory Tests	Radiograph, CT, MRI Findings	US Findings
Gout	Attacks typically start in the large toe, ankle, and foot dorsum and ascend over time to involve the knee, elbow, hand, and any joint. **Risk factors:** male gender, obesity, alcohol, diabetes, hypertension, diuretics, diet. See references 7 and 8 for classification criteria or access web-based calculator at http://goutclassificationcalculator.auckland.ac.nz or download the app RheumaHelper	**Serum uric acid, polarized microscopy** of synovial fluid or tophaceous material reveals strongly negative birefringent needle-shaped crystals	Bone or joint erosions with overhanging bony edges	**Double contour sign, deposits of urate crystals** forming tophi or aggregates, bony erosion, positive Power Doppler if active synovitis
Calcium pyrophosphate dihydrate deposition disease (CPPD disease), also known as **pseudogout**	Favors knee and wrist but can affect any joint. **Associated conditions:** age, osteoarthritis, hyperparathyroidism, hemochromatosis, hypomagnesemia, hypophosphatemia, hypothyroidism. See reference 59 (**Table 13-2** Revised Diagnostic Criteria for Calcium Pyrophosphate Dihydrate Crystal Deposition Disease)	**Polarized microscopy** of synovial fluid. See positive birefringent short needle-shaped or rhomboid crystals. Serum calcium, parathyroid hormone, ferritin, iron saturation, phosphate level, magnesium level, thyroid functions.	Calcific densities in cartilage most commonly in the knee, hip labrum, wrist triangular fibrocartilage, intervertebral disks, symphysis pubis. **Screen with radiographs: AP bilateral knees, AP pelvis/hips, bilateral PA hands.**	**Hyperechoic deposits** of varied sizes with or without acoustic shadowing present in cartilage, tendon, and enthesis.

Abbreviations: AP, anteroposterior; CT, computed tomography; MRI, magnetic resonance imaging; PA, posteroanterior; US, ultrasound.

Adapted from Helfgott RH. Overview of monoarthritis in adults. Post TW, ed. *UpToDate*. Waltham, MA: UpToDate Inc. http://www.uptodate.com. Accessed November 25, 2016.

PEARLS AND PITFALLS

Pearls

- Gout and pseudogout crystal arthropathy can imitate many other types of arthritis and may also occur together and concurrently with different types of arthritis in the same joint or patient.
- Aspiration of synovial fluid from an affected joint or bursa and examination under polarized microscopy is the single best diagnostic tool.
- Ultrasound improves detection of small amounts of synovial fluid and directly assists in accurate aspiration.
- Diagnostically, ultrasound provides strongly suggestive signs of gout and CPPD crystal deposition.
- The classic and most significant ultrasound sign of gout is the DCS. The DCS is included in validated gout classification criteria and may aid in identifying patients with gout in the absence of positive synovial fluid crystal analysis.
- The most significant ultrasound sign of CPPD deposition disease is hyperechoic calcium deposits within cartilage.
- Location of crystal diseases may overlap, but the first toe MTP is the domain for MSU crystals, and the knee is the realm for CPPD crystals. These two joints should be examined under ultrasound when crystal deposition arthropathy is suspected.
- Knee and wrist joints are frequently involved both in gout and in CPPD crystal deposition disease, but almost any joint may be affected by either disease.
- When gout is the clear diagnosis, ultrasound follow-up of MSU deposits can be used to help determine the efficacy of urate-lowering therapy.

Pitfalls

- Do not fail to look for the underlying causes of crystal arthropathy.
- Single and multiple joints may be involved in the same patient by different processes.
- Do not inject a joint with corticosteroids without making sure that it is not infected, even if you see crystals on microscopy.
- The medications we use to treat gout arthropathy have potential toxicities. Choose the patient and the medication carefully.
- Discovery of crystal deposition on a radiograph or ultrasound does not necessarily mean that the joint is subject to active or chronic arthropathy and may not necessitate treatment.
- Crystal arthropathy can imitate rheumatoid arthritis and psoriatic arthritis. In such cases, treatment targeting rheumatoid arthritis or psoriatic arthritis is ineffective and potentially toxic.
- It may take time and patience to search for crystal findings on ultrasound and under the polarizing microscope.
- Never lose the opportunity to aspirate inflamed joints even if it seems to be due to a crystal arthropathy because concomitant joint infection has been known to occur with crystal-induced arthritis.
- Do not fail to think of and rule out infection which may occur concurrently with crystal disease.
- Do not confuse a CIS with the DCS of gout.

the presence of subclinical inflammation. Ultrasound may also help monitor treatment efficacy such as the resolution of tophi. For CPPD deposition disease, ultrasound may prove useful in detecting subclinical chronic inflammation requiring treatment. For both diseases, it can aid in detecting minute fluid collections for aspiration and guide in the aspiration. With the exception of

the known utility of ultrasound-guided joint aspiration[56-58] and the DCS in gout, we await better studies to support evidence-based recommendations at this time.

The possible avenues of applying point-of-care ultrasound in clinical practice are listed and rated in Table 39-5. Coding for billing is described in the table "Billing for Limited Joint or Tendon Ultrasound Exam."

BILLING

CPT Code	Description	Global Payment	Professional Component	Technical Component
76882	Ultrasound of extremity—nonvascular limited	$36.52	$25.06	$11.46

CPT codes and average national reimbursement for Medicare in 2016. Payment data are from https://www.cms.gov/apps/physician-fee-schedule/search/search-criteria.aspx. See Chapter 2 for details on ultrasound billing.

References

1. Roddy E, Choi HK. Epidemiology of gout. *Rheum Dis Clin North Am.* 2014;40:155.
2. Juraschek SP, Miller ER III, Gelber AC. Body mass index, obesity, and prevalent gout in the United States in 1988-1994 and 2007-2010. *Arthritis Care Res (Hoboken).* 2013;65(1):127-132.
3. Lin HY, Rocher LL, McQuillan MA, Schmaltz S, Palella TD, Fox IH. Cyclosporine-induced hyperuricemia and gout. *N Engl J Med.* 1989;321:287.
4. Choi HK, Soriano LC, Zhang Y, Garcia Rodriquez LA. Antihypertensive drugs and risk of incident gout among patients with hypertension: population based case-control study. *BMJ.* 2012;344:d8190.
5. Rosenthal AK, Ryan LM. Calcium pyrophosphate deposition disease. *N Engl J Med.* 2016;374:2575-2584.
6. Neame RL, Carr AJ, Muir K, Doherty M. UK community prevalence of knee chondrocalcinosis: evidence that correlation with osteoarthritis is through a shared association with osteophyte. *Ann Rheum Dis.* 2003;62:513-518.
7. Neogi T, Jansen TL, Dalbeth N, et al. 2015 Gout classification criteria: an American College of Rheumatology/European League against rheumatism collaborative initiative. *Arthritis Rheumatol.* 2015;67:2557.
8. Neogi T, Jansen TL, Dalbeth N, et al. 2015 Gout classification criteria: an American College of Rheumatology/European League against rheumatism collaborative initiative. *Ann Rheum Dis.* 2015;74:1789.
9. McCarty D. Calcium pyrophosphate crystal deposition disease; pseudogout; articular chondrocalcinosis. In: McCarty D, ed. *Arthritis and Allied Conditions: A Textbook of Rheumatology.*11th ed. Philadelphia, PA: Lea & Febiger; 1989:1714-1715.
10. Logan JA, Morrison E, McGill PE. Serum uric acid in acute gout. *Ann Rheum Dis.* 1997;56:696.
11. Schlesinger N, Baker DG, Schumacher HR Jr. Serum urate during bouts of acute gouty arthritis. *J Rheumatol.* 1997;24:2265.
12. McQueen FM, Doyle A, Dalbeth N. Imaging in the crystal arthropathies. *Rheum Dis Clin North Am.* 2014;40:231.
13. Rosenthal AK, Ryan LM, McCarty DJ. Calcium pyrophosphate crystal deposition disease, pseudogout, and articular chondrocalcinosis. In: Koopman WJ, Moreland LW, eds. *Arthritis and Allied Conditions.* 15th ed. Philadelphia, PA: Lippincott Williams & Wilkins; 2005:2373.
14. Rosenthal AK. Pseudogout: presentation, natural history, and associated conditions. In: Wortmann RL, Schumacher HR Jr, Becker MA, Ryan LM, eds. *Crystal-Induced Arthropathies: Gout, Pseudogout, and Apatite-Associated Syndromes.* New York, NY: Taylor and Francis Group; 2006:99.
15. Lee GS, Kim RS, Park HK, Chang JC. Crowned dens syndrome: a case report and review of the literature. *Korean J Spine.* 2014;11(1):15-17.
16. Sivera F, Andrés M, Carmona L, et al. Multinational evidence-based recommendations for the diagnosis and management of gout: integrating systematic literature review and expert opinion of a broad panel of rheumatologists in the 3e initiative. *Ann Rheum Dis.* 2014;73:328-335.
17. Zhang W, Doherty M, Bardin T, et al. European League against rheumatism recommendations for calcium pyrophosphate deposition. Part I: Terminology and diagnosis. *Ann Rheum Dis.* 2011;70:563-570.
18. Grassi W, Meenagh G, Pascual E, Filippucci E. "Crystal clear"—sonographic assessment of gout and calcium pyrophosphate deposition disease. *Semin Arthritis Rheum.* 2006;36:197-202.
19. Perez-Ruiz F, Martin I, Canteli B. Ultrasonic measurement of tophi as an outcome measure for chronic gout. *J Rheumatol.* 2007;34:1888-1893.
20. Thiele RG, Schlesinger N. Diagnosis of gout by ultrasound. *Rheumatology.* 2007;46:1116-1121.
21. Frediani B, Filippou G, Falsetti P, et al. Diagnosis of calcium pyrophosphate dihydrate crystal deposition disease: ultrasonographic criteria proposed. *Ann Rheum Dis.* 2005;64:638-640.
22. Grassi W, Okano T, Filippucci E. Use of ultrasound for diagnosis and monitoring of outcomes in crystal arthropathies. *Curr Opin Rheumatol.* 2015;27(2):147-155.
23. Girish G, Glazebrook KN, Jacobson JA. Advanced imaging in gout. *AJR Am J Roentgenol.* 2013;201:515-525.
24. Löffler C, Sattler H, Peters L, Löffler U, Uppenkamp M, Bergner R. Distinguishing gouty arthritis from calcium pyrophosphate disease and other arthritides. *J Rheumatol.* 2015;42:513-520.
25. Chowalloor PV, Keen HI. A systematic review of ultrasonography in gout and asymptomatic hyperuricaemia. *Ann Rheum Dis.* 2013;72:638-645.
26. De Miguel E, Puig JG, Castillo C, Peiteado D, Torres RJ, Martín-Mola E. Diagnosis of gout in patients with asymptomatic hyperuricaemia: a pilot ultrasound study. *Ann Rheum Dis.* 2012;71:157.
27. Rousseau I, Cardinal É, Raymond-Tremblay D, Beauregard CG, Braunstein EM, Saint-Pierre A. Gout: radiographic findings mimicking infection. *Skeletal Radiol.* 2001;30:565.
28. Stewart S, Dalbeth N, Vandal AC, Allen B, Miranda R, Rome K. Ultrasound features of the first metatarsophalangeal joint in gout and asymptomatic hyperuricaemia: comparison with normouricaemic individuals. *Arthritis Care Res (Hoboken).* 2017;69(6):875-883.
29. Thiele RG, Schlesinger N. Ultrasonography shows disappearance of monosodium urate crystal deposition on hyaline cartilage after sustained normouricemia is achieved. *Rheumatol Int.* 2010;30:495-503.
30. Peiteado D, Villalba A, de Miguel E, Ordonez MC, MartinMola E. Longitudinal study of ultrasonography sensibility to change in patients with gout after one year of treatment. *Ann Rheum Dis.* 2010;69(suppl 3):713.
31. Filippou G, Filippucci E, Tardella M, et al. Extent and distribution of CPP deposits in patients affected by calcium pyrophosphate dihydrate deposition disease: an ultrasonographic study. *Ann Rheum Dis.* 2013;72:1836-1839.
32. Filippucci E, Scirè CA, Delle Sedie A, et al. Ultrasound imaging for the rheumatologist. XXV. Sonographic assessment of the knee with gout and calcium pyrophosphate deposition disease. *Clin Exp Rheumatol.* 2010;28:2-5.
33. Ellabban AS, Kamel SR, Omar HA, El-Sherif AM, Abdel-Magied RA. Ultrasonographic diagnosis of articular chondrocalcinosis. *Rheumatol Int.* 2012;32:3863-3868.
34. Gamon E, Combe B, Barnetche T, Mouterde G. Diagnostic value of ultrasound in calcium pyrophosphate deposition disease: a systemic review and meta-analysis. *RMD Open.* 2015;1:e000118.
35. Di Geso L, Tardella M, Gutierrez M, Filippucci E, Grassi W. Crystal deposition at elbow hyaline cartilage: the sonographic perspective. *J Clin Rheumatol.* 2011;17:344-345.

36. Ellabban AS, Kamel SR, Abo Omar HA, El-Sherif AM, Abdel-Magied RA. Ultrasonographic findings of Achilles tendon and plantar fascia in patients with calcium pyrophosphate deposition disease. *Clin Rheumatol.* 2012;31:697-704.

37. Naredo E, Uson J, Jimenez-Palop M, et al. Ultrasound-detected musculoskeletal urate crystal deposition: which joints and what findings should be assessed for diagnosing gout? *Ann Rheum Dis.* 2014;73:1522-1528.

38. Zhang W, Doherty M, Bardin T, et al; EULAR Standing Committee for International Clinical Studies including therapeutics. EULAR evidence based recommendations for gout. Part II: Management. Report of a task force of the EULAR Standing Committee for International Clinical Studies Including Therapeutics (ESCISIT). *Ann Rheum Dis.* 2006;65:1312.

39. Khanna D, Fitzgerald JD, Khanna PP, et al. 2012 American College of Rheumatology guidelines for management of gout. Part 1: Systematic nonpharmacologic and pharmacologic therapeutic approaches to hyperuricemia. *Arthritis Care Res (Hoboken).* 2012;64:1431.

40. Schlesinger N, Detry MA, Holland BK, et al. Local ice therapy during bouts of acute gouty arthritis. *J Rheumatol.* 2002;29:331.

41. Choi HK, Atkinson K, Karlson EW, Willett W, Curhan G. Alcohol intake and risk of incident gout in men: a prospective study. *Lancet.* 2004;363:1277.

42. Choi HK, Liu S, Curhan G. Intake of purine-rich foods, protein, and dairy products and relationship to serum levels of uric acid: the Third National Health and Nutrition Examination Survey. *Arthritis Rheum.* 2005; 52:283.

43. Choi HK, Atkinson K, Karlson EW, Willett W, Curhan G. Purine-rich foods, dairy and protein intake, and the risk of gout in men. *N Engl J Med.* 2004;350:1093.

44. Becker MA, Jolly M. Hyperuricemia and associated diseases. *Rheum Dis Clin North Am.* 2006;32:275.

45. Alexander GM, Dieppe PA, Doherty M, Scott DG. Pyrophosphate arthropathy: a study of metabolic associations and laboratory data. *Ann Rheum Dis.* 1982;41:377-381.

46. Ellman MH, Brown NL, Porat AP. Laboratory investigations in pseudogout patients and controls. *J Rheumatol.* 1980;7:77-81.

47. MacMullan P, McCarthy G. Treatment and management of pseudogout: insights for the clinician. *Ther Adv Musculoskelet Dis.* 2012;4(2):121-131.

48. Neogi T. Clinical practice. Gout. *N Engl J Med.* 2011;364:443.

49. Kiltz U, Smolen J, Bardin T, et al. Treat-to-target (T2T) recommendations for gout. *Ann Rheum Dis.* 2017;76:632-638.

50. Rothschild BM, Yakubov LE. Prospective six month, double-blind trial of hydroxychloroquine treatment of calcium pyrophosphate deposition disease. *Contemp Ther.* 1997;23:327-331.

51. Pascual E, Andrés M, Sivera F. Methotrexate: should it still be considered for chronic calcium pyrophosphate crystal disease? *Arthritis Res Ther.* 2015;17:89.

52. Andres M, Sivera F, Pascual E. Methotrexate is an option for patients with refractory calcium pyrophosphate crystal arthritis. *J Clin Rheumatol.* 2012;18:234.

53. Chollet-Janin A, Finckh A, Dudler J, Guerne PA. Methotrexate as an alternative therapy for chronic calcium pyrophosphate deposition disease: an exploratory analysis. *Arthritis Rheum.* 2007;56:688.

54. Doan TH, Chevalier X, Leparc JM, Richette P, Bardin T, Forestier R; French Society for Rheumatology Osteoarthritis Section. Premature enthusiasm for the use of methotrexate for refractory chondrocalcinosis: comment on the article by Chollet-Janin et al. *Arthritis Rheum.* 2008; 58:2210.

55. Finckh A, Mc Carthy GM, Madigan A, et al. Methotrexate in chronic-recurrent calcium pyrophosphate deposition disease: no significant effect in a randomized crossover trial. *Arthritis Res Ther.* 2014;16:458.

56. Raza K, Lee CY, Pilling D, et al. Ultrasound guidance allows accurate needle placement and aspiration from small joints in patients with early inflammatory arthritis. *Rheumatology.* 2003;42:976-979.

57. Koski JM, Hammer HB. Ultrasound-guided procedures: techniques and usefulness in controlling inflammation and disease progression. *Rheumatology.* 2012;51:vii31-vii35.

58. Cunnington J, Marshall N, Hide G, et al. A randomized double-blind, controlled study of ultrasound-guided corticosteroid injection into the joint of patients with inflammatory arthritis. *Arthritis Rheum.* 2010;62(7):1862-1869.

59. Klippel JH, Stone JH, Crofford LJ, White PH, eds. *Primer on the Rheumatic Diseases.* 13th ed. New York, NY: Springer; 2008:266, Table 13-2.

60. Lamers-Karnebeek FB, Van Riel PL, Jansen TL. Additive value for ultrasonographic signal in a screening algorithm for patients presenting with acute mono-/oligoarthritis in whom gout is suspected. *Clin Rheumatol.* 2014;33:555-559.

61. Lai KL, Chiu YM. Role of ultrasonography in diagnosing gouty arthritis. *J Med Ultrasound.* 2011;19:7-13.

62. Zufferey P, Valcov R, Fabreguet I, Dumusc A, Omoumi P, So A. A prospective evaluation of ultrasound as a diagnostic tool in acute microcrystalline arthritis. *Arthritis Res Ther.* 2015;17:188.

63. Newberry SJ, FitzGerald JD, Motala A, et al. Diagnosis of gout: a systematic review in support of an American College of Physicians clinical practice guideline. *Ann Intern Med.* 2017;166:27-36.

CHAPTER 40

Does the Patient Have Carpal Tunnel Syndrome?

Paul Bornemann, MD, RMSK, RPVI and Mohamed Gad, MD, MPH(c)

● Clinical Vignette

A 54-year-old female comes to the clinic complaining of weakness, numbness, and a painful tingling sensation in her right hand. It radiates to all of her fingers and up to her proximal forearm. It started 6 months ago and has been getting worse. She tells you that she now must take breaks from typing and that this is interfering with her job as a secretary. She has mild rheumatoid arthritis for which she takes methotrexate and takes levothyroxine for hypothyroidism. On physical examination, tapping the wrist elicited paresthesia. She also reported numbness in the thumb and first two fingers on wrist flexion. You suspect median nerve entrapment, but the patient has some atypical features. Does the patient have carpal tunnel syndrome?

LITERATURE REVIEW

Carpal tunnel syndrome (CTS) affects approximately 4% of adults, making it a common complaint encountered in the primary care setting.[1] Females are four times more likely to be affected than males especially between the ages of 50 and 60 years.[2] The end cause of CTS is entrapment of the median nerve in the carpal tunnel between the flexor retinaculum and the carpal bones.[3] However, the underlying pathophysiology that leads to this is complex and caused by an interplay between a multitude of factors. Increasing pressure inside the carpal tunnel leads to compression and traction of the median nerve, which in turn leads to obstruction of the venous outflow resulting in edema, ischemia, and nerve injury.[4] Additionally, inflammation of the surrounding synovial membranes and microcirculation can play a substantial role in the development of the disease (**Figure 40-1**).[5,6]

Factors increasing the risk for CTS can be from intrinsic damage to the nerve fibers, extrinsic compression of the nerve, or other idiopathic factors. Intrinsic risk factors lead to damage of median nerve fibers and include diabetes, alcoholism, vitamin deficiencies, and toxins.[7] Extrinsic factors cause compression on the median nerve from the outside and are often secondary to coexisting medical conditions such as hypothyroidism, pregnancy, menopause, obesity, chronic kidney failure, and connective tissue diseases.[8] Repetitive overuse injuries to the wrist and hand because of occupation, such as typing, have also been widely implicated as a risk factor for CTS.[9] Idiopathic factors, including female gender, older age, and genetic factors, have also been implicated in the development of CTS.[10]

Commonly, patients with CTS present to the clinic with a complaint of pain and paresthesias. The paresthesias usually affect the sensory distribution of the median nerve, which includes the thumb, index, and middle fingers. Atypical presentations can occur when the pain and paresthesias affect the entire hand and palm or radiate proximally up the arm. This can create a diagnostic challenge as these symptoms overlap with other common conditions such as epicondylitis and cervical radiculitis. With symptom progression, patients may complain of increased frequency of dropping items, difficulty using doorknobs, and opening jars because of a weakening grip. They may also complain of nighttime pain and discomfort that can be alleviated by shaking the wrists, which are known as the flick sign.

A full neurologic, dermatologic, and musculoskeletal examination of the upper extremities should be performed. Patients usually exhibit weakness of opposition and thumb abduction. Atrophy of the thenar eminence can also be a sign noticed in more severe cases. A number of provocative maneuvers can be done to elicit the symptoms of the patient. These include the Tinel sign that is positive if light tapping over the median nerve in the wrist reproduces the symptoms and the Phalen sign that is considered positive when forced wrist flexion for 30 seconds reproduces the symptoms. It's important to know that the physical examination signs in CTS are neither sensitive nor specific and a thorough history and physical should be obtained to exclude other conditions (**Figure 40-2**).[11,12]

The clinical assessment of CTS can be combined with diagnostic testing to confirm the diagnosis. Fowler et al. examined the use of ultrasound, nerve conduction studies, as well as the CTS-6 questionnaire and concluded that all three tests have comparable sensitivity and specificity and can accurately diagnose CTS.[13] Nerve conduction studies showing impaired median nerve conduction across the carpal tunnel but normal conduction along the proximal course of the median nerve are highly sensitive and specific for the diagnosis. Other neurologic conditions such as C6/C7 cervical radiculopathy, cervical spondylotic myelopathy, brachial plexopathy, and median neuropathy can be diagnosed using electrophysiologic testing, which also determines the location of the lesion, the severity of the injury, and the need for surgical intervention.[14]

Imaging studies can be used in CTS to detect structural abnormalities in the nerves, tendons, bones, and vasculature. CT and MRI scan can be used to visualize the surrounding structures and exclude masses and deformities; however, the diagnostic sensitivity and specificity are uncertain.[15] Ultrasonography, on the other hand, is known to be highly sensitive and specific for the diagnosis of CTS. Although the results of ultrasonography are operator dependent, there is evidence that novices can perform the examination at the level of experts after only 5 minutes of training.[16]

High-frequency ultrasonography can easily assess the median nerve at the inlet of the carpal tunnel because of its superficial position. The median nerve appears to be a rounded or oval structure with heterogeneous hypoechoic and hyperechoic areas, giving it a vesicular appearance. The use of ultrasonography is associated with multiple advantages in the outpatient setting. The patient is comfortable, the test is noninvasive and fast with a duration of

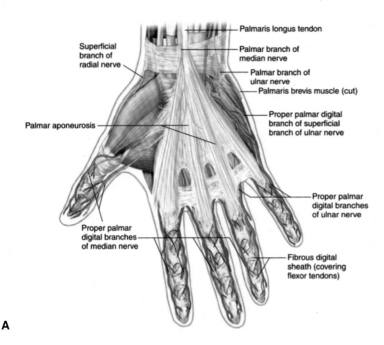

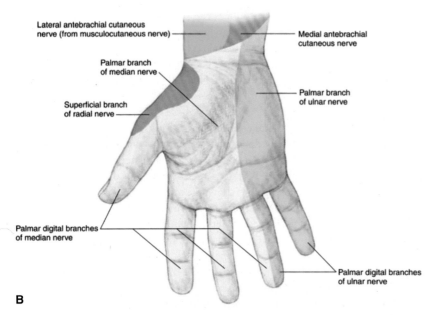

FIGURE 40-1. The sensory distribution of the median nerve. The median nerve innervates the radial two-thirds of the palm, thumb, index, middle, and half of the ring fingers. Note that sensory innervation of the palm is not affected in carpal tunnel syndrome as the palmar cutaneous nerve passes superficial to the flexor retinaculum. A, Dissection. B, Nerve territories. From Tank PW, Gest TR. *Lippincott's Atlas of Anatomy.* 2nd ed. Philadelphia, PA: Lippincott Williams & Wilkins; 2020.

fewer than 5 minutes per wrist. Additionally, it possesses the ability to assess local causes of nerve compression like mass lesions and tenosynovitis.[17] Ultrasonography can also be used to guide local corticosteroid injections into carpal tunnel space and may be more effective than blind injections.[18]

According to the 2016 Medicare national average, limited ultrasound of the median nerve is significantly less expensive than limited electrophysiologic testing. In addition to the increased cost, electrophysiologic testing is uncomfortable and can't assess the anatomy of the median nerve. When a correlation was made

TABLE 40-1 Recommendations for Use of Point-of-Care Ultrasound in Clinical Practice		
Recommendation	**Rating**	**References**
Use ultrasound of the median nerve cross-sectional area as an accurate carpal tunnel syndrome (CTS) diagnostic tool.	Level B	20
Assess the wrist with ultrasound even in patients with confirmed CTS to rule out reversible structural abnormalities.	Level C	20

A = consistent, good-quality patient-oriented evidence; B = inconsistent or limited-quality patient-oriented evidence; C = consensus, disease-oriented evidence, usual practice, expert opinion, or case series. For information about the SORT evidence rating system, go to http://www.aafp.org/afpsort.

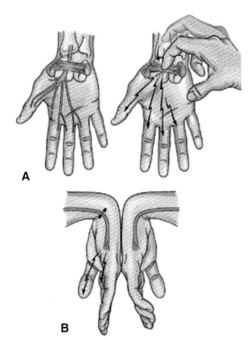

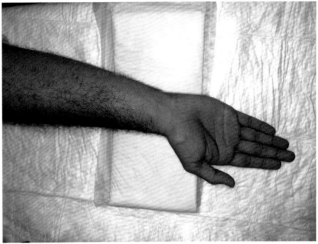

FIGURE 40-3. The correct wrist positioning for wrist ultrasound examination. The wrist is supported, placed in a supine position, and slightly extended (around 20°).

FIGURE 40-2. Illustration of Tinel and Phalen signs. In Tinel sign (A), light tapping over the median nerve in the wrist reproduces the sensory symptoms. In Phalen sign (B), forced wrist flexion for 30 seconds reproduces the symptoms. Reprinted with permission from Timby BK, Smith NE. *Introductory Medical-Surgical Nursing*. 12th ed. Philadelphia, PA: Wolters Kluwer; 2017. Figure 62.1.

between ultrasonography findings and electrophysiologic testing, it was found that an increased cross-sectional area is associated with a decreased nerve conduction velocity, making ultrasonography highly predictive of CTS.[19]

PERFORMING THE SCAN

1. **Preparation**. Position the patient sitting and facing the examiner. Position the forearm comfortably with the wrist supine, slightly extended (around 20°), and supported with a towel underneath the wrist. Position the ultrasound equipment appropriately and use a high-frequency, linear array ultrasound transducer. Use the MSK examination preset in the software settings (**Figures 40-3 and 40-4**).

2. **Evaluate the median nerve at the volar surface of the wrist by transverse axis ultrasound**. Use the distal palmar crease as a landmark and place the transducer there oriented transversally. This location is just proximal to the carpal tunnel. The carpal tunnel is enclosed by the flexor retinaculum superficially and extends from the pisiform to the scaphoid bones. The median nerve appears round or oval. It has a honeycomb appearance because of heterogenicity of the nerve fibers that appear hypoechoic compared to the supporting connective tissue. The surrounding tendons appear homogeneous and hyperechoic. The flexor carpi radialis (FCR) has a relatively constant position and may be used to identify the median nerve medial to FCR. After identifying the median nerve, freeze the image and calculate the cross-sectional area of the median nerve using circumferential trace mode. Normal median nerve should be uniform with a cross-sectional area less than 10 mm^2.[20] An

uneven, hypoechoic nerve or a cross-sectional area of more than 10 mm^2 is highly suggestive of median nerve edema and CTS. The swelling can be seen most proximal to the flexor retinaculum, which is a thin hyperechoic band (**Figures 40-5 through 40-9**).

3. **Evaluate the median nerve at the volar surface of the wrist by longitudinal axis ultrasound**. Assess the longitudinal axis by turning the transducer probe 90°. The median nerve should be identified as the striated structure that is slightly hypoechoic compared to normal tendons. The radius, lunate, and capitate bones should be identified as well as the hyperechoic deep tendons. Physiologically, the median nerve should have a uniform diameter

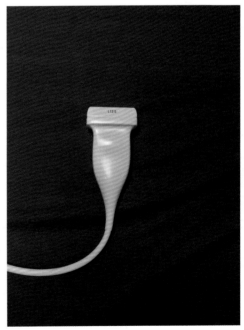

FIGURE 40-4. The linear array ultrasound transducer used in musculoskeletal examination.

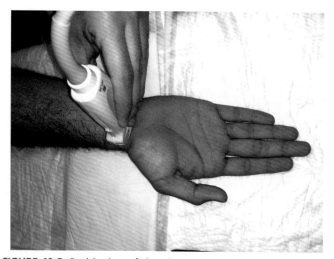

FIGURE 40-5. Positioning of the ultrasound probe. Using the distal palmar crease as a landmark, the transducer is placed transversally just proximal to the carpal tunnel.

and move with index finger movement. Findings suggestive of CTS include hypoechoic changes, enlargement of the median nerve with loss of the uniform diameter, and loss of the median nerve movements with the index finger (**Figures 40-10 and 40-11**).

4. **Evaluate the median nerve at the distal forearm by transverse axis ultrasound.** Move the transducer proximally and place it transversally over the pronator quadratus muscle. The pronator quadratus is the first muscle noted deep in the forearm with fibers running transversely. Other muscles in the area have fibers that run in the long access of the forearm. The median nerve can be identified between the flexor pollicis longus (FPL) and the flexor digitorum superficialis (FDS) tendons. Obtain the cross-sectional surface area of the median nerve for comparison to the previously obtained distal measurement in Step 2. In patients with CTS, the distal cross-sectional area is enlarged compared to the proximal area, usually at a ratio of 1.4:1 or greater. This can be particularly helpful when examining a patient with a bifid median nerve (**Figures 40-12 and 40-13**).

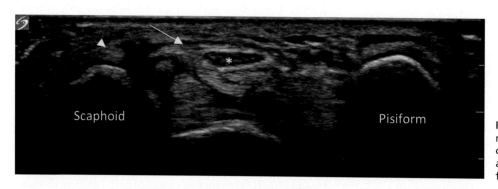

FIGURE 40-6. Cross-sectional image of a normal median nerve at the level of the carpal tunnel. Asterisk, median nerve; arrowhead, flexor carpi radialis; arrow, flexor retinaculum.

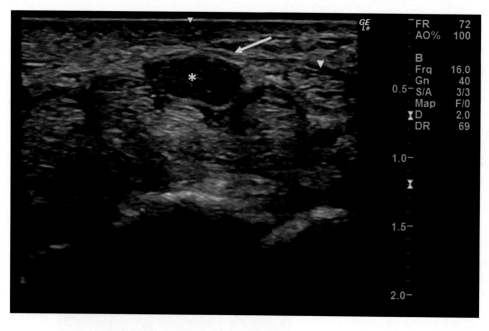

FIGURE 40-7. Cross-sectional image of an abnormal median nerve at the level of the carpal tunnel. Note the subjectively enlarged diameter, uneven appearance, and hypoechoic appearance. Asterisk, median nerve; arrowhead, flexor carpi radialis; arrow, flexor retinaculum.

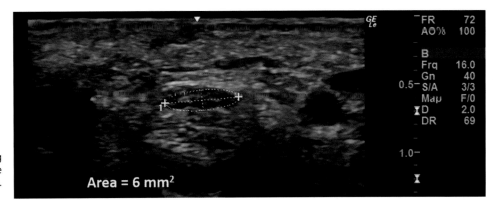

FIGURE 40-8. Cross-sectional image detailing the area of a normal median nerve at the level of the carpal tunnel in a healthy person. Note the cross-sectional area of 6 mm².

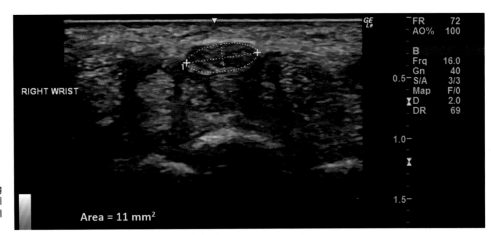

FIGURE 40-9. Cross-sectional image showing the area of median nerve in a case of carpal tunnel syndrome. Note the cross-sectional area of 11 mm².

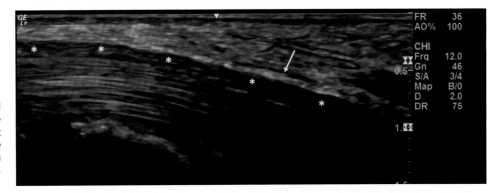

FIGURE 40-10. Longitudinal ultrasound view in a normal healthy individual. The nerve runs distal to proximal from the left to right side of the image. Please notice the uniform diameter of the median nerve. Asterisk, median nerve; arrow, flexor retinaculum.

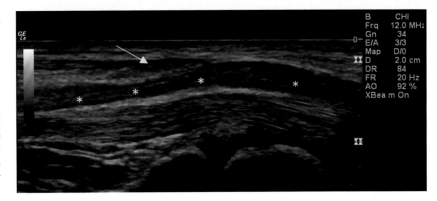

FIGURE 40-11. Longitudinal view of the median nerve in a patient with carpal tunnel syndrome. The nerve runs proximal to distal from the left to right side of the image. Note how the nerve becomes larger and more hypoechoic distal to the flexor retinaculum to do compression. Asterisk, median nerve; arrow, flexor retinaculum.

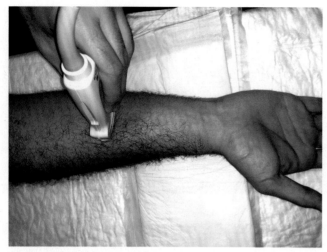

FIGURE 40-12. Positioning of the ultrasound probe in the distal forearm to visualize median nerve and assess its diameter.

PATIENT MANAGEMENT

When a patient presents with suspected CTS, a thorough history and physical examination are required. When the patient exhibits the typical features of CTS, pain, and paresthesia affecting the classic distribution of the median nerve (thumb, index, and middle finger), the diagnosis can be made clinically without further testing. However, when the patient exhibits atypical features such as symptoms including the entire wrist, palm, or radiating proximally to the forearm, the diagnosis is best confirmed with ultrasound imaging. A cross-sectional area of the median nerve greater than 10 mm² is positive for CTS. Patients diagnosed with CTS should be treated with conservative therapy if they suffer from mild to moderate disease.[21] The options available for conservative management include nocturnal wrist splinting, corticosteroid injections, systemic oral corticosteroids, as well as physical therapy.

Wrist splinting is used as a first-line therapy for mild to moderate CTS.[19] Wrist splinting can be used either all day long or only during sleep (nocturnal), with similar success rate. The splint works by stabilizing the wrist in a neutral position, helping reduce the overuse injury from flexion and extension to the median nerve. Nocturnal wrist splint has been demonstrated to be effective for short-term alleviation of symptoms.[22]

In addition to wrist splinting, medications can be used for relief of short-term symptoms. Studies have demonstrated that nonsteroidal anti-inflammatory drugs (NSAIDs) are not effective and should not be used.[23] Corticosteroids, on the other hand, can be used as a therapy, resulting in short-term relief of the symptoms. Even though CTS is usually not associated with an inflammatory reaction in the median nerve, their use has been associated with better outcomes compared to placebo.[24] Local corticosteroid injections are used first before trying systematic corticosteroids to decrease the risk of side effects associated with systematic use. Local injections are, however, not without their risks. The risk includes worsening of the median nerve compression because of an injection in the carpal tunnel, inadvertent injury to the median or the ulnar nerves because of intraneuronal injection, and rupture of the flexor tendons. Use of ultrasound to guide the corticosteroid injection can significantly lower the risk of complications.[25] Oral prednisolone is also very effective in short-term control of CTS symptoms.[26] Some studies suggest that local corticosteroid injections might be more effective than systematic use and should be put into consideration while determining the next step for the management of your patient.[27] It's noteworthy that a combination of wrist splinting and local corticosteroid injection is more effective than monotherapy with either.[27]

Indications for surgical intervention include symptoms that don't improve with conservative management, symptoms that are acute and progressive, mass lesions, or a systemic disease that's unlikely to improve. Surgical treatment of CTS involves decompression of the carpal tunnel and is usually very effective in ameliorating the symptoms and improving the prognosis and satisfaction of patients.[23] Failure of surgery may be attributed to poor surgical technique because of incomplete release of the transverse ligament or to a reaction fibrosis surrounding the median nerve. In cases of no improvement after the initial surgical intervention, a revision surgery is needed. Below is an algorithm that illustrates how to manage patients with CTS (**Figure 40-14**).

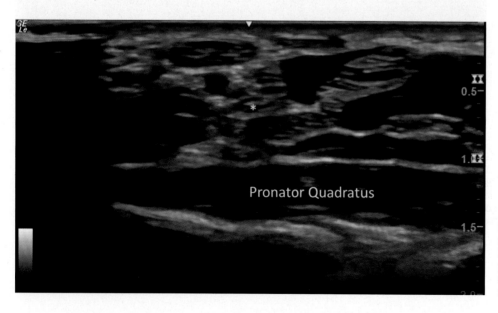

Pronator Quadratus

FIGURE 40-13. Distal forearm view in a normal individual. The median nerve is best identified by following it from a proximal location. Note the pronator quadratus running from left to right. Asterisk, median nerve.

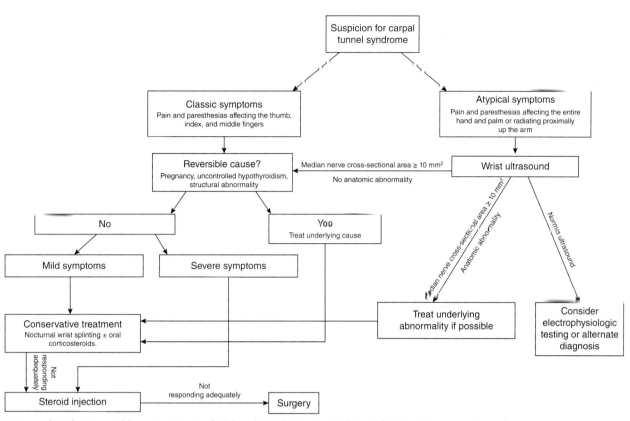

FIGURE 40-14. Flowchart to guide management decisions in patients presenting with symptoms suggestive of carpal tunnel syndrome.

PEARLS AND PITFALLS

Pearls

- Confirm the structure identified is the median nerve and not a nearby tendon by following it proximally in the forearm. The median nerve will dive deeper, whereas the tendons maintain the same depth. See ▶ **Video 40-1**.
- A bifid median nerve is a common normal variant. In these instances, it is more accurate to use the ratio of the total cross-sectional area of the two branches of the distal median nerve compared to the cross-sectional area of the proximal median nerve. A ratio of greater than 1.4 is positive.

Pitfalls

- Approximately 60% of individuals will have a palmaris longus tendon that is typically located immediately superficial to the median nerve above the flexor retinaculum. It is frequently mistaken for the median nerve by novices.
- If the ultrasound beam is not maintained perpendicular to the tendons and nerves of the wrist, it may lead to anisotropy in which the hyperechoic tendons are abnormally hypoechoic.

BILLING

CPT Code	Description	Global Payment	Professional Component	Technical Component
76882	Limited ultrasound, extremity, nonvascular, real time with image documentation	$36.52	$25.06	$11.46
76942	Ultrasonic guidance for needle placement (e.g., biopsy, aspiration, injection, localization device), imaging supervision, and interpretation	$61.58	$34.01	$27.57

CPT codes and average national reimbursement for Medicare in 2016. Payment data are from https://www.cms.gov/apps/physician-fee-schedule/search/search-criteria.aspx. See Chapter 2 for details on ultrasound billing.

PART 2

References

1. Atroshi I, Gummesson C, Johnsson R, Ornstein E, Ranstam J, Rosén I. Prevalence of carpal tunnel syndrome in a general population. *JAMA*. 1999;282(2):153-158.

2. Mondelli M, Giannini F, Giacchi M. Carpal tunnel syndrome incidence in a general population. *Neurology*. 2002;58(2):289-294.

3. Alfonso C, Jann S, Massa R, Torreggiani A. Diagnosis, treatment and follow-up of the carpal tunnel syndrome: a review. *Neurol Sci*. 2010;31(3):243-252.

4. Mackinnon SE, Dellon AL, Hudson AR, Hunter DA. Chronic nerve compression—an experimental model in the rat. *Ann Plast Surg*. 1984;13(2):112-120.

5. Ozkul Y, Sabuncu T, Kocabey Y, Nazligul Y. Outcomes of carpal tunnel release in diabetic and non-diabetic patients. *Acta Neurol Scand*. 2002;106(3):168-172.

6. Samii A, Unger J, Lange W. Vascular endothelial growth factor expression in peripheral nerves and dorsal root ganglia in diabetic neuropathy in rats. *Neurosci Lett*. 1999;262(3):159-162.

7. Taser F, Deger AN, Deger H. Comparative histopathological evaluation of patients with diabetes, hypothyroidism and idiopathic carpal tunnel syndrome. *Turk Neurosurg*. 2017;27(6):991-997.

8. Roshanzamir S, Mortazavi S, Dabbaghmanesh A. Does hypothyroidism affect post-operative outcome of patients undergoing carpal tunnel release? *Electron Phys*. 2016;8(9):2977-2981.

9. de Krom MC, Kester AD, Knipschild PG, Spaans F. Risk factors for carpal tunnel syndrome. *Am J Epidemiol*. 1990;132(6):1102-1110.

10. Aroori S, Spence RA. Carpal tunnel syndrome. *Ulster Med J*. 2008;77(1):6-17.

11. Pryse-Phillips WE. Validation of a diagnostic sign in carpal tunnel syndrome. *J Neurol Neurosurg Psychiatry*. 1984;47(8):870-872.

12. MacDermid JC, Wessel J. Clinical diagnosis of carpal tunnel syndrome: a systematic review. *J Hand Ther*. 2004;17(2):309-319.

13. Fowler JR, Cipolli W, Hanson T. A comparison of three diagnostic tests for carpal tunnel syndrome using latent class analysis. *J Bone Joint Surg Am*. 2015;97(23):1958-1961.

14. Jablecki CK, Andary MT, Floeter MK, et al. Practice parameter: electrodiagnostic studies in carpal tunnel syndrome. Report of the American Association of Electrodiagnostic Medicine, American Academy of Neurology, and the American Academy of Physical Medicine and Rehabilitation. *Neurology*. 2002;58(11):1589-1592.

15. Jarvik JG, Yuen E, Haynor DR, et al. MR nerve imaging in a prospective cohort of patients with suspected carpal tunnel syndrome. *Neurology*. 2002;58(11):1597-1602.

16. Crasto JA, Scott ME, Fowler JR. Ultrasound measurement of the cross-sectional area of the median nerve: the effect of teaching on measurement accuracy. *Hand (N Y)*. 2017;14(2):155-162. doi:1558944717731857.

17. Martinoli C, Bianchi S, Gandolfo N, Valle M, Simonetti S, Derchi LE. US of nerve entrapments in osteofibrous tunnels of the upper and lower limbs. *Radiographics*. 2000;20 Spec No:S199-S213; discussion S-7.

18. Babaei-Ghazani A, Roomizadeh P, Forogh B, et al. Ultrasound-guided versus landmark-guided local corticosteroid injection for carpal tunnel syndrome: a systematic review and meta-analysis of randomized controlled trials. *Arch Phys Med Rehabil*. 2018;99(4):766-775.

19. Mhoon JT, Juel VC, Hobson-Webb LD. Median nerve ultrasound as a screening tool in carpal tunnel syndrome: correlation of cross-sectional area measures with electrodiagnostic abnormality. *Muscle Nerve*. 2012;46(6):871-878.

20. Cartwright MS, Hobson-Webb LD, Boon AJ, et al. Evidence-based guideline: neuromuscular ultrasound for the diagnosis of carpal tunnel syndrome. *Muscle Nerve*. 2012;46(2):287-293.

21. McClure P. Evidence-based practice: an example related to the use of splinting in a patient with carpal tunnel syndrome. *J Hand Ther*. 2003;16(3):256-263.

22. Page MJ, Massy-Westropp N, O'Connor D, Pitt V. Splinting for carpal tunnel syndrome. *Cochrane Database Syst Rev*. 2012;(7):CD010003. doi:10.1002/14651858.CD010003.

23. O'Connor D, Marshall S, Massy-Westropp N. Non-surgical treatment (other than steroid injection) for carpal tunnel syndrome. *Cochrane Database Syst Rev*. 2003;(1):CD003219. doi:10.1002/14651858.CD003219.

24. Marshall S, Tardif G, Ashworth N. Local corticosteroid injection for carpal tunnel syndrome. *Cochrane Database Syst Rev*. 2007;(2):CD001554. doi:10.1002/14651858.CD001554.pub2.

25. Gottlieb NL, Riskin WG. Complications of local corticosteroid injections. *JAMA*. 1980;243(15):1547-1548.

26. Herskovitz S, Berger AR, Lipton RB. Low-dose, short-term oral prednisone in the treatment of carpal tunnel syndrome. *Neurology*. 1995;45(10):1923-1925.

27. Wong SM, Hui AC, Tang A, et al. Local vs systemic corticosteroids in the treatment of carpal tunnel syndrome. *Neurology*. 2001;56(11):1565-1567.

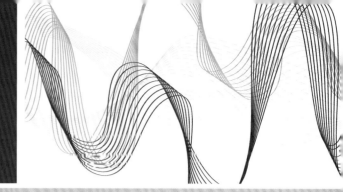

SECTION

2

SKIN AND SOFT TISSUE

CHAPTER

41

Does the Patient Have Cellulitis or an Abscess?

Casey Parker, MBBS, DCH, FRACGP and Matthew Fitzpatrick, MBBS

Clinical Vignette

A 7-year-old boy presents with fever, tachycardia, and a hot, painful swelling on the back of his leg. He reports a history of an insect bite a few days earlier. There is an area of erythema over most of his calf, and a small amount of pus is expressed from a central lesion, but you are unsure if there is an underlying collection that needs to be drained. You consider exploration under procedural sedation, but the patient's mother is anxious about proceeding unless it is absolutely necessary. You are concerned that he may not improve unless any collection is drained. Does the patient have cellulitis or an abscess?

LITERATURE REVIEW

Cellulitis is frequently encountered in emergency departments and general practice. The presence of an underlying abscess is important to identify, because this will require a drainage procedure rather than antibiotics alone.[1-5] Although superficial abscesses are often readily identified, deeper collections can be missed. The tissue edema and induration associated with cellulitis can also obscure the diagnosis.[6-8] When studied, the sensitivity of clinical examination alone is as low as 79%, with variable interobserver reliability.[8-10]

Ultrasound can be used to enhance management of skin and soft-tissue infections by augmenting the accuracy of the clinical examination.[10-13] In one study of adults presenting to an emergency department, the use of bedside ultrasound changed management in 56% of patients.[11,13] This included drainage of collections that had not been clinically apparent as well as a change to antibiotics alone rather than the performance of an unnecessary drainage procedure.[11] Similar results have been shown in children and adults.[10,13-15] Importantly, ultrasound has been shown to be useful in this setting even in the hands of novice ultrasonographers who have received only brief training.[13,14] Bedside ultrasound has also been shown to be at least as sensitive as computed tomography for locating superficial abscesses; however, it has not been as specific.[16]

The fact that ultrasound has been shown to alter clinical management is probably a better indicator of utility than specific sensitivity and specificity data. This is because there is wide variation within the literature and no readily available gold standard with which to compare results. Sensitivity data range from 77% to as high as 98%,[10-16] whereas specificity ranges from 62% to 88%.[10-16] This is in part a result of the heterogeneity of inclusion criteria, with some studies enrolling all patients with skin and soft-tissue infections and others obtaining images in only those patients who are considered high risk clinically. In addition, in most studies, the gold standard test of incision and drainage is not applied to all patients, which is understandable because it is quite invasive. Instead, surrogate markers are used to determine false-negative results, for example, patient deterioration despite antibiotics. It is important to note that, in general, the specificity is low, indicating the presence of false-positive results. Lymph nodes, serosanguineous collections, and vascular structures can all be confused with infective collections.[16-19]

Despite these limitations, it is clear that bedside ultrasonography can be a useful adjunct to the clinical history and examination. It is a cheap and simple test that can be readily performed following only brief training and can be used to make meaningful changes to patient management.

TABLE 41-1 Recommendations for Use of Point-of-Care Ultrasound in Clinical Practice

Recommendations	Rating	References
In skin and soft tissue infections, point-of-care ultrasound should be used to augment the clinical examination to increase the rate of identification of underlying collections.	A	8-15
Point-of-care ultrasound should be used in place of CT scanning as the first-line investigation.	B	16
Point-of-care ultrasound for evaluation of skin and soft-tissue infections can be performed at the point of care effectively by practitioners with only brief training.	A	13, 14

Abbreviation: CT, computed tomography.

A = consistent, good-quality patient-oriented evidence; B = inconsistent or limited-quality patient-oriented evidence; C = consensus, disease-oriented evidence, usual practice, expert opinion, or case series. For information about the SORT evidence rating system, go to http://www.aafp.org/afpsort.

PERFORMING THE SCAN

1. Use the high-frequency linear transducer. Using plenty of gel, scan the area of interest from above to below. It works best if you make a number of passes over the area, scanning from one side to the other systematically. Repeat the scanning in the horizontal plane (**Figure 41-1**).
2. Differentiate cellulitis from an abscess. Cellulitis classically has a cobblestone appearance because of increased subcutaneous fluid (**Figure 41-2**). Early findings show thickening and increased echogenicity of the subcutaneous tissue. Note that this appearance is due to inflammatory edema, and it is difficult to differentiate cellulitis from noninfective edema using ultrasound alone. It is also sometimes difficult to differentiate gross edema from pus that has not coalesced into an abscess. The presence of hyperemia seen on color Doppler mode makes infection more likely (**Figure 41-3**). Needle aspiration may be required to clarify the diagnosis.

3. An abscess will usually appear as a discrete area of hypoechoic fluid (**Figure 41-4**). They may have a sharp edge or an enhancing ring; however, they may merge with the surrounding cellulitis (**Figure 41-5**). There may be posterior acoustic enhancement (**Figure 41-6**). If you find an abscess, try and estimate the size, extent, and the exact location. Determine whether it pierces the fascial layer or whether there is involvement of underlying joints or muscles.

PATIENT MANAGEMENT

The management of simple cellulitis consists of treatment with appropriate antibiotics. These should have cover against both staphylococci and streptococci. The Infectious Diseases Society of America recommends empirical treatment with oral antibiotics for a total of 5 days unless there are signs of a systemic inflammatory

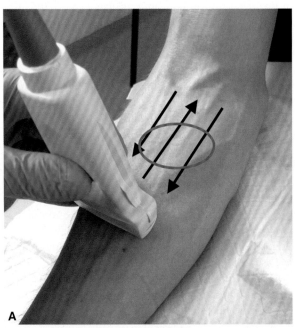
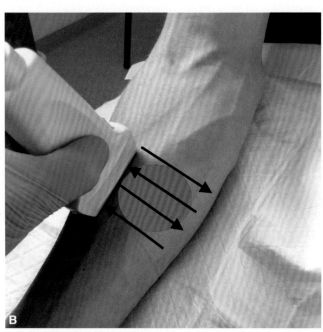

FIGURE 41-1. Scan in both the vertical (A) and horizontal (B) planes over the affected area.

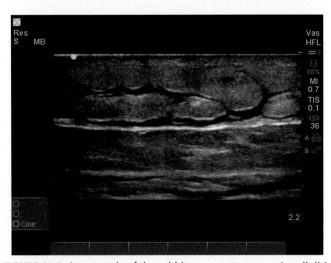

FIGURE 41-2. An example of the cobblestone pattern seen in cellulitis or edema.

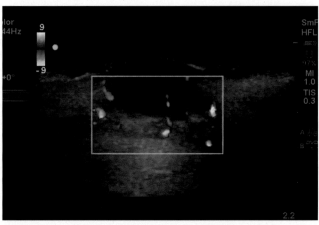

FIGURE 41-3. An example of hyperemia caused by cellulitis.

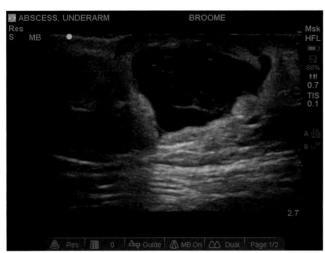

FIGURE 41-4. An abscess in the axilla illustrating the presence of heterogeneous material within the cavity.

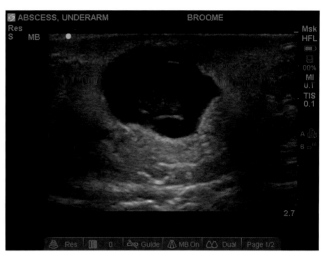

FIGURE 41-6. This figure demonstrates the effect of posterior acoustic enhancement. Note that the tissue directly behind the abscess is brighter than the tissue to either side.

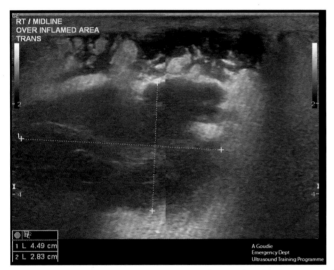

FIGURE 41-5. This abscess does not have a distinct border but instead has merged with the surrounding tissue.

response, in which case intravenous antibiotics are recommended. Cultures of blood, aspirate, or swabs are not recommended in simple cellulitis in immunocompetent patients. An antibiotic active against methicillin-resistant *Staphylococcus aureus* is recommended

for patients with purulent infections who have failed initial antibiotic treatment or have markedly impaired host defenses. They are also recommended in patients with severe infection as indicated by the presence of systemic inflammatory response syndrome plus hypotension.[20]

If an abscess is found within a soft-tissue infection, it is recommended that this collection be drained. Drainage techniques vary and may include incision and drainage or fine-needle aspiration. Either may be appropriate; however, there are some data that suggest superior outcomes from initial incision and drainage, particularly in loculated collections.[4]

There is evidence that small abscesses may be conservatively managed with antibiotics alone; however, ultrasound-guided fine-needle aspiration could also be considered.[12] It can be useful to rescan the area after or during needle aspiration in order to ensure that as much purulent fluid as possible has been drained, thus leaving the cavity empty.

Traditionally, abscess cavities have been left to heal by secondary intention, often with the addition of packing material. A systematic review has shown that primary closure of abscess cavities is associated with faster healing and a similar rate of abscess recurrence, whereas abscess packing has been shown to be more painful without improving outcomes[21,22] (Table 41-2 and **Figure 41-7**).

TABLE 41-2 Modified Treatment Recommendations for SSTI From the IDSA Guidelines, 2014

Disease Entity	Drug	Adult Dose	Pediatric Dose
Simple SSTI	Dicloxacillin—PO	500 mg QID	25-50 mg/kg QID
	Cephalexin—PO	500 mg QID	25-50 mg/kg QID
SSTI with SIRS	Nafcillin or Oxacillin—IV	1-2 g every 4 h	100-150 mg/kg daily in four divided doses
	Cefazolin—IV	1 g 8 hourly	50 mg/kg daily in three divided doses
MRSA SSTI[a]	Vancomycin—IV	30 mg/kg daily in two divided doses	40 mg/kg daily in four divided doses
	Linezolid	600 mg BID	10 mg/kg BID
	Clindamycin—IV or PO	450 mg QID	25-40 mg/kg daily in three divided doses
	Trimethoprim and Sulfamethoxazole—PO	One double-strength tablet BID	8 mg/kg BID (based on Trimethoprim)

[a]IDSA Guidelines recommend empiric treatment for MRSA in patients with severe infection or purulent infections after initial antibiotics have failed.

Abbreviations: BID, twice daily; IDSA, Infectious Diseases Society of America; IV, intravenous; MRSA, methicillin-resistant *Staphylococcus aureus*; PO, orally; QID, four times per day; SIRS, systemic inflammatory response syndrome; SSTI, skin and soft-tissue infection.

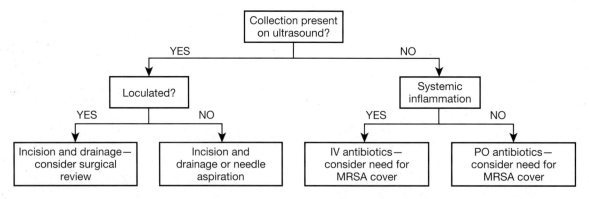

FIGURE 41-7. Proposed algorithm for the integration of ultrasound into skin infection clinical management. MRSA, methicillin-resistant Staphylococcus aureus

PEARLS AND PITFALLS

Pearls

- Ensure you are scanning with an adequate depth. Collections can reside deeper than expected. Important structures such as vessels and nerves may be just beneath the infected tissue—it is important to localize these to allow safe surgical management (**Figure 41-8**).
- Always scan a wide area of skin to ensure there are no collections outside of the area of cellulitis. This will enhance the sensitivity of your technique.
- Look for the presence of loculations within the abscess. If present, these can make needle aspiration less effective, because all of the pockets of infection may not be cleared. Sometimes increasing the gain can make these clearer (**Figure 41-9**).
- It can be difficult to obtain accurate images when assessing the fingers or feet. The use of a water bath instead of a gel will improve image quality in these situations (**Figures 41-10 and 41-11**).

Pitfalls

- Lymph nodes can also masquerade as abscesses. They will usually have a hyperechoic center and will demonstrate color flow when Doppler is applied. A healthy lymph node will display branching vascular architecture. An avascular area within a lymph node may indicate an abscess within the node (**Figure 41-12**).
- Some abscesses are isoechoic to the surrounding tissue. Compress the area and look for swirling of the material within the collection (▶ **Video 41-1**).
- Ultrasound can be used to identify necrotizing fasciitis, it has poor negative predictive value and should not be used to rule out the condition. Typically, findings include thickened, edematous soft-tissue overlying fluid in the deep fascial layer. Gas-forming organisms within this layer can create microscopic bubbles that interfere with the penetration of the ultrasound beam. This gas causes an air–fluid interface that gives the underlying tissue a "dirty gray" appearance. This sign can be

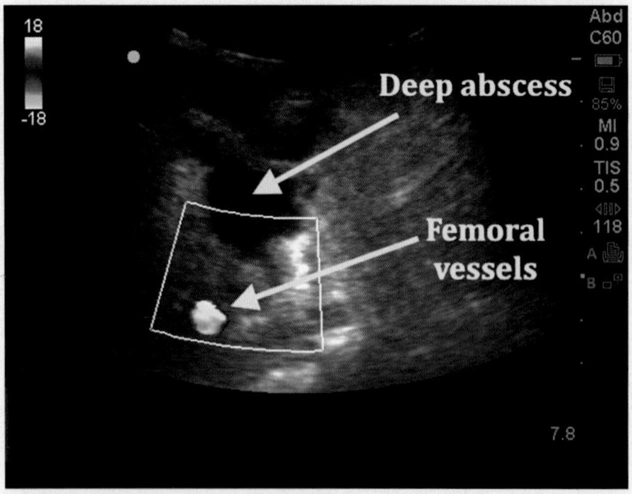

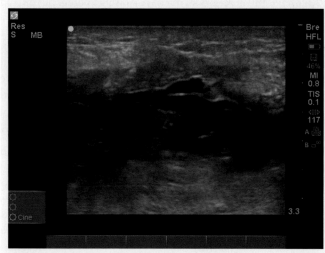

FIGURE 41-8. This image shows an abscess overlying the femoral neurovascular bundle.

FIGURE 41-9. This is an example of a loculated abscess that may not be adequately aspirated with only a needle.

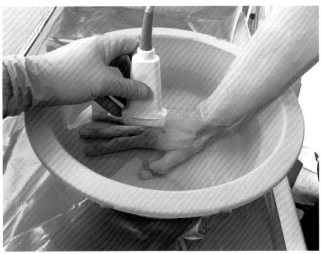

FIGURE 41-10. This demonstrates the technique for using a water bath to obtain more accurate images when examining the extremities.

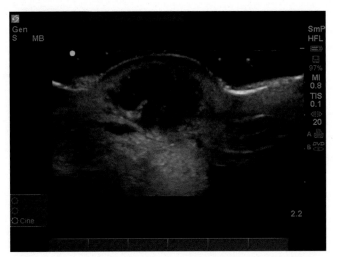

FIGURE 41-11. This is an abscess on the finger that has been taken using a finger bath as illustrated in Figure 41-9.

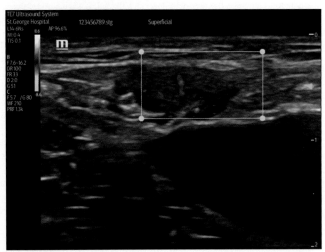

FIGURE 41-12. This is an example of a normal lymph node with an organized internal structure and a typical vascular pattern.

subtle but is a marker of a potentially severe infection that requires prompt surgical management and potentially broader spectrum antibiotic cover (**Figures 41-13 and 41-14** and ▶ **Video 41-2**).

- It is always good practice to scan the tissue overlying any collection you are about to incise so as not to cut other important structures. Assess your predicted track with color Doppler to ensure that there are no overlying superficial vessels prior to the procedure.
- Occasionally, an abscess will exhibit similar echogenicity as the surrounding tissue, making it very difficult to identify. Gentle compression will cause the fluid in the abscess to swirl around, differentiating it from the surrounding tissue. This should be performed every 1 to 2 cm throughout the area of cellulitis.
- It's generally better to be sure that a collection is not actually a vascular structure prior to incision. Press down on the collection to see if it is pulsatile. Arteries will expand with each heartbeat. Color Doppler mode should always be used to assess for flow within a structure prior to incision (**Figure 41-15**).

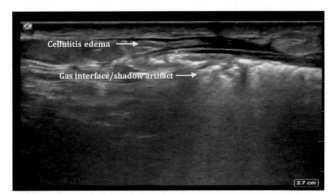

FIGURE 41-13. This is an example of necrotizing fasciitis showing an area of cellulitis overlying fluid in the deep fascial layer as well as a gas interface in the infected tissue. Courtesy of Christopher Partyka, MD.

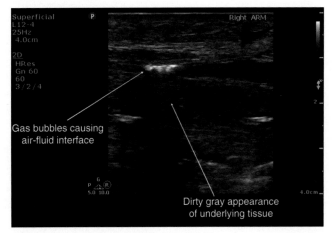

FIGURE 41-14. An image of the air–fluid interface caused by gas particles in the deep fascia in a patient with necrotizing fasciitis. (Courtesy of Dr Adrian Goudie.)

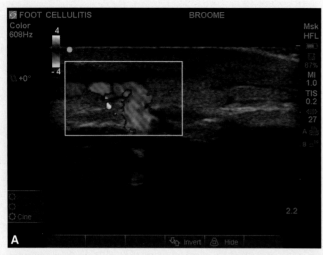 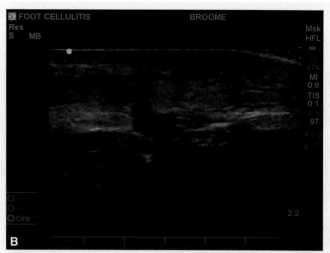

FIGURE 41-15. These images demonstrate the importance of using color Doppler mode (A) to look for the presence of vessels prior to incision. What looks like an abscess (B) is actually a vessel.

BILLING

There are no specific codes for evaluation of the skin and soft tissue. Instead, the area of the body examined is used to determine the code.

CPT Code	Description	Global Payment	Professional Component	Technical Component
76882	Ultrasound, extremity, nonvascular, real time with image documentation; limited	$36.52	$25.06	$11.46
76775	Ultrasound, abdominal, real time with image documentation; limited	$58.72	$29.36	$29.36
76604	Ultrasound, chest, real time with image documentation	$89.15	$27.57	$61.58

CPT codes and average national reimbursement for Medicare in 2016. Payment data are from https://www.cms.gov/apps/physician-fee-schedule/search/search-criteria.aspx. See Chapter 2 for details on ultrasound billing.

References

1. Lee MC, Rios AM, Aten MF, et al. Management and outcome of children with skin and soft tissue abscesses caused by community-acquired methicillin-resistant *Staphylococcus aureus. Pediatr Infect Dis J.* 2004;23:123-127.
2. Llera JL, Levy RC. Treatment of cutaneous abscess: a double-blind clinical study. *Ann Emerg Med.* 1985;14:15-19.
3. McCaig LF, McDonald LC, Mandal S, Jernigan DB. *Staphylococcus aureus*-associated skin and soft tissue infections in ambulatory care. *Emerg Infect Dis.* 2006;12:1715-1723.
4. Liu C, Bayer A, Cosgrove SE, et al. Clinical practice guidelines by the Infectious Diseases Society of America for the treatment of methicillin-resistant *Staphylococcus aureus* infections in adults and children. *Clin Infect Dis.* 2011;52:e18-e55.
5. Singer AJ, Taira BR, Chale S, Bhat R, Kennedy D, Schmitz G. Primary versus secondary closure of cutaneous abscesses in the emergency department: a randomized controlled trial. *Acad Emerg Med.* 2013;20:27-32.
6. Stevens DL, Bisno AL, Chambers HF, et al; Infectious Diseases Society of America. Practice guidelines for the diagnosis and management of skin and soft-tissue infections. *Clin Infect Dis.* 2005;41:1373-1406.
7. Swartz MN. Clinical practice. Cellulitis. *N Engl J Med.* 2004;350:904-912.
8. Giovanni JE, Dowd MD, Kennedy C, Michael JG. Interexaminer agreement in physical examination for children with suspected soft tissue abscesses. *Paediatr Emerg Care.* 2011;27(6):475-478.
9. Marin J, Bilker W, Lautenbach E, Alpern ER. Reliability of clinical examinations for pediatric skin and soft-tissue infections. *Pediatrics.* 2010;126(5):925-930.
10. Iverson K, Haritos D, Thomas R, Kannikeswaran N. The effect of bedside ultrasound on diagnosis and management of soft tissue infections in a pediatric ED. *Am J Emerg Med.* 2012;30:1347-1351.
11. Tayal V, Nael Hasan N, Norton HJ, Tomaszewski CA. The effect of soft-tissue ultrasound on the management of cellulitis in the emergency department. *Acad Emerg Med.* 2006;13:384-388.

12. Marin J, Dean AJ, Bilker WB, Panebianco NL, Brown NJ, Alpern ER. Emergency ultrasound-assisted examination of skin and soft tissue infections in the pediatric emergency department. *Acad Emerg Med.* 2013;20(6):545-553.
13. Squire BT, Fox JC, Anderson C. ABSCESS: applied bedside sonography for convenient evaluation of superficial soft tissue infections. *Acad Emerg Med.* 2005;12(7):601-606.
14. Berger T, Garrido F, Green J, Lema PC, Gupta J. Bedside ultrasound performed by novices for the detection of abscess in ED patients with soft tissue infections. *Am J Emerg Med.* 2012;30:1569-1573.
15. Sivitz AB, Lam SHF, Ramirez-Schrempp D, Valente JH, Nagdev AD. Effect of bedside ultrasound on management of pediatric soft-tissue infection. *J Emerg Med.* 2010;39(5):637-643.
16. Gaspari R, Dayno M, Briones J, Blehar D. Comparison of computerized tomography and ultrasound for diagnosing soft tissue abscesses. *Crit Ultrasound J.* 2012;4:5.
17. Chau CL, Griffith JF. Musculoskeletal infections: ultrasound appearances. *Clin Radiol.* 2005;60:149-159.
18. Loyer EM, Kaur H, David CL, DuBrow R, Eftekhari FM. Importance of dynamic assessment of the soft tissues in the sonographic diagnosis of echogenic superficial abscesses. *J Ultrasound Med.* 1995;14(9):669-671.
19. Loyer EM, DuBrow RA, David CL, Coan JD, Eftekhari F. Imaging of superficial soft-tissue infections: sonographic findings in cases of cellulitis and abscess. *AJR Am J Roentgenol.* 1996;166:149-152. doi:10.2214/ajr.166.1.8571865.
20. Stevens DL, Bisno AL, Chambers HF, et al; Infectious Diseases Society of America. Practice guidelines for the diagnosis and management of skin and soft tissue infections: 2014 update from the Infectious Diseases Society of America. *Clin Infect Dis.* 2014;59(2):e10-e52.
21. Singer AJ, Thode HC, Chale S, Taira BR, Lee C. Primary closure of cutaneous abscesses: a systematic review. *Am J Emerg Med.* 2011;29(4):361-366. doi:10.1016/j.ajem.2009.10.004.
22. O'Malley GF, Dominici P, Giraldo P, et al. Routine packing of simple cutaneous abscesses is painful and probably unnecessary. *Acad Emerg Med.* 2009;16(5):470-473. doi:10.1111/j.1553-2712.2009.00409.x.

Is a Foreign Body Present?

Jennifer S. Lee, DO, MPH and Joshua R. Pfent, MD

Clinical Vignette

A 56-year-old woman presents to the clinic with a chief complaint of pain on the bottom of her foot. Eight weeks ago, she stepped on a sewing needle while barefoot, and since then, she has been having pain in her foot. The needle had been standing straight up in the carpet, and she immediately withdrew her foot after feeling pain. Only a broken portion of the needle was found on the floor. She says she can feel a painful bump on the bottom of her foot. Is a foreign body present?

LITERATURE REVIEW

A foreign body is defined as any object or material that becomes embedded or placed inside the body that does not naturally arise from it. Foreign bodies in the skin and other external soft tissues are commonly treated in the office or emergency department, and up to 70% are able to be removed in those settings.[1] Ultrasound can be a helpful diagnostic tool for the detection of a foreign body and is recommended for use in the outpatient setting. Risk factors that can increase exposure to foreign bodies include trauma, age, physical and mental disability, and occupation.[2]

There are many different types of foreign bodies that can be acquired. Ninety-five percent of foreign bodies are from wood, glass, or metal. Splinters refer to trauma from wood, plants, metal, or plastic. Vegetative foreign bodies have a higher risk of inflammation and infection and should be removed promptly. Less than 15% of wooden foreign bodies, which are radiolucent, are detectable with radiographs.[1] Glass embedment typically occurs from trauma with broken and shattered glass, which can leave small, retained pieces within the wound. The high spatial resolution of ultrasound allows identification of foreign bodies smaller than a millimeter.[3] Fishhooks, bullets, pencil lead, gravel, and teeth are some other unique objects that can become embedded in patients.

If left untreated, foreign bodies may cause pain and increase the risk of infection and scarring from the retained material. Early identification of the foreign body aids in removal and is ideally done within 24 hours due to wound healing. Delayed presentation may have obvious inflammation, infection, scarring, induration, and pigmentation defects of the overlying tissue. Deterioration of organic material may lead to variations in foreign body appearance itself.

The presence of a foreign body has historically been identified using radiographs as the modality of choice. Although radiographs can identify radiopaque substances such as metal or stone, this often leaves the need for other modalities to identify radiolucent materials. In a study by Anderson et al. (1982), only 15% of radiolucent foreign bodies could be seen radiographically.[4] The use of ultrasound to locate foreign bodies was first described in 1978 and has since been found to be an accurate modality in locating foreign bodies, both radiopaque and radiolucent.[5] Studies have mainly consisted of either a series of human case reports in vitro that cannot control for foreign body size and location or nonhuman in vivo studies using cubes of beef or chicken thighs that are implanted with foreign bodies of various materials.[6] An in vivo study by Tahmasebi et al. (2014) found a 97.9% sensitivity for the identification of a radiolucent foreign body, similar to a study by Gilbert et al. (1990) that found a sensitivity of 95.4%.[7,8] One study found that for the evaluation of foreign bodies in the hand by ultrasonography, the specificity was 99% (confidence interval [CI], 96%-100%).[6]

Even with the aid of ultrasonography, a combination of other factors can increase the difficulty of locating a foreign body. If the foreign body is very small or is not superficially located, it may be more difficult to see. A thorough history, such as one of penetrating trauma, may define the mechanism of injury to help determine possible depth. If the foreign body is superficial, it may be identified by external visualization and palpation alone. Air at the removal site can mimic a foreign body and the introduction of air may occur when flushing to cleanse the wound. Scar tissue that distorts normal anatomic structures or the presence of calcifications may result in difficult identification or false-positive scans.[1] Furthermore, the foreign body may elude sonographic detection if it is oriented in a way that makes it difficult to detect. Obtaining adequate visualization of the foreign body underscores the importance of optimal positioning of the patient and the potential need for axial, sagittal, and coronal ultrasound scans or additional modalities.

It has been well established that ultrasonography is an accurate method for the diagnosis of foreign body.[6,9,10] Evidence supports that if the clinical history and sonographic findings are positive for a foreign body, no further imaging workup is necessary.[9] Ultrasonography is a useful aid in foreign body removal and can provide reassurance to the patient and clinician that all foreign body material has been extracted.

TABLE 42-1	Recommendations for Use of Point-of-Care Ultrasound in Clinical Practice		
Recommendation		Rating	References
Foreign bodies are effectively located using ultrasonography in the outpatient setting		B	1, 3, 5-9

A = consistent, good-quality patient-oriented evidence; B = inconsistent or limited-quality patient-oriented evidence; C = consensus, disease-oriented evidence, usual practice, expert opinion, or case series. For information about the SORT evidence rating system, go to http://www.aafp.org/afpsort.

PERFORMING THE SCAN

1. **Preparation**. Position the patient such that they can remain still and comfortable for an extended period of time. The body part that is affected should be at a comfortable height to scan, as upright as possible, and easily accessible. Position the

ultrasound equipment appropriately and select a high-frequency linear probe with a soft tissue preset. Adjust the focal point to the appropriate depth once you identify the object to enhance resolution (**Figures 42-1 and 42-2**).

2. **Use gel or water bath to allow visualization**. A generous amount of gel should be used on the surface of the skin to aid in visualization. With surfaces that are painful or uneven, using a water bath may be helpful. Hold the probe just above the surface of the skin while underwater (**Figures 42-3 and 42-4**).

3. **Localize the foreign body using ultrasound**. Using a slow and gentle rolling technique, search for the foreign body. Thoroughly assess the entire area, as objects may be oriented such that they elude detection. Note that visualizing the foreign body perpendicular to the transducer minimizes potential for errors. Once identified, orient the probe to measure the length, width, and depth. Proper orientation aids in the removal process and helps confirm that the entire foreign body has been removed. Take note of important anatomic structures nearby. These structures may be injured, may dictate removal technique, or may contraindicate removal of the foreign body depending on the medical setting (**Figures 42-5 and 42-6**).

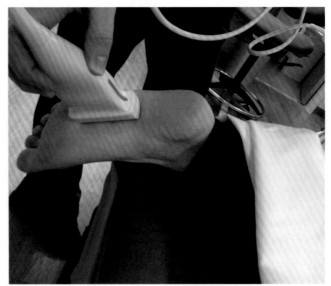

FIGURE 42-2. Patient positioning and linear probe placement for evaluation of foreign body in foot.

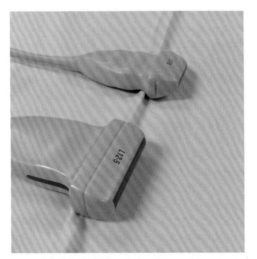

FIGURE 42-1. High-frequency linear probes.

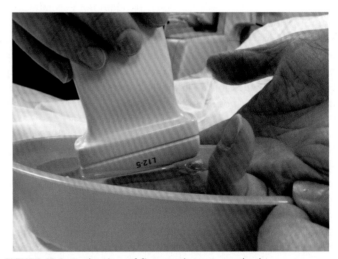

FIGURE 42-3. Evaluation of finger using a water bath.

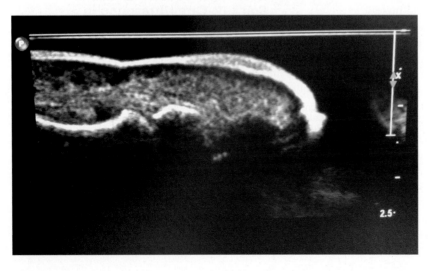

FIGURE 42-4. Image from evaluation of finger using water bath; no foreign body present.

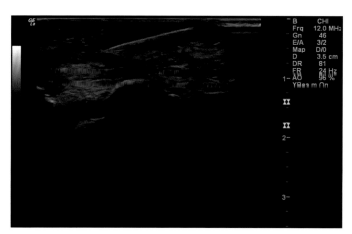

FIGURE 42-5. Needle visualized in the subcutaneous tissue of the plantar aspect of the foot.

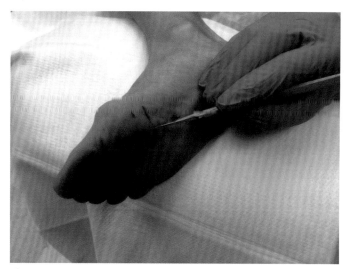

FIGURE 42-8. Incision at the point of intersecting lines.

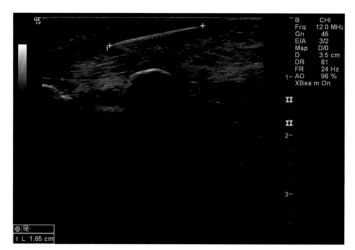

FIGURE 42-6. Measurement of the foreign body.

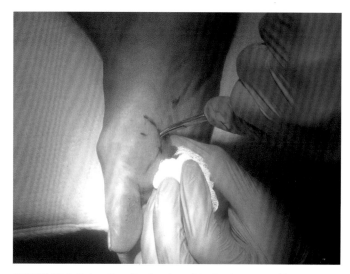

FIGURE 42-9. Extracting the foreign object using curved hemostat.

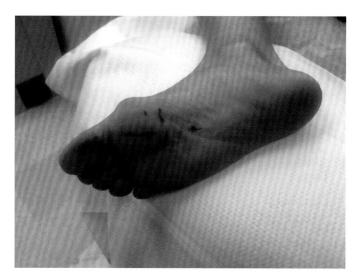

FIGURE 42-7. Lines drawn to indicate dimensions and point of entry.

4. **Mark the skin, noting the length and width of the foreign object**. With the foreign body visualized on ultrasound, use a sterile marker on the skin to make longitudinal and horizontal locations on all four sides of the probe. These markings should mark both the dimensions of the foreign body and the desired point of entry. This technique will aid in minimizing the incision size necessary to remove the foreign body (**Figures 42-7 and 42-8**).

5. **Remove the foreign body**. After incising the skin, use the appropriate instrument to dissect down to the level of the foreign body. This entire retrieval process can be done under continuous ultrasound guidance, or it can be used as an adjunct if the foreign body is still difficult to retrieve (**Figures 42-9 and 42-10**).

6. **Confirm that the entire foreign body has been removed**. Measure the dimensions of the foreign body that has been removed. Compare these with the measurements taken during your initial assessment to confirm that the entire foreign body was removed. Additionally, complete removal may be confirmed by reimaging with ultrasound (**Figure 42-11**).

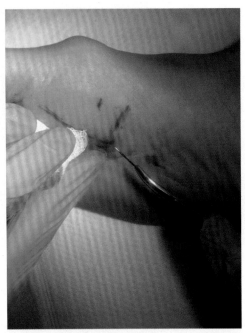

FIGURE 42-10. Removal of foreign body.

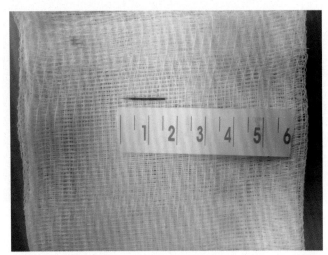

FIGURE 42-11. Measurement of foreign body after removal matched the initial assessment.

PATIENT MANAGEMENT

Management of the wound after removal of a foreign body includes debridement and irrigation with generous amounts of normal saline. If there are no signs of infection at the sight of penetration, prophylactic antibiotics are generally not indicated. Certain wounds such as animal and human bites and contaminated penetrating objects are the exception and should be treated accordingly. If there are

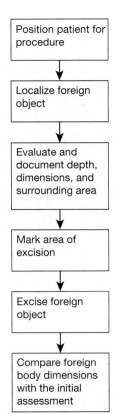

FIGURE 42-12. Treatment algorithm for evaluation of foreign body.

signs of an infection, treat with the appropriate antibiotic regimen. Any penetrating wound warrants evaluation for history of tetanus vaccination. Identify if the patient is up to date on their tetanus vaccination and then treat according to **Figure 42-12**.

PEARLS AND PITFALLS

Pearls

- Note surrounding anatomic structures for safety.
- Obtain optimal position for scanning and patient comfort.
- Apply generous amount of gel to ultrasound site to aid visualization.
- Adjust settings appropriately for depth.

Pitfalls

- Inadequate patient positioning to obtain image
- Failure to document with image
- Failure to measure the object
- Failure to remove entire foreign body

BILLING

CPT Code	Description	Global Payment	Professional Component	Technical Component
76882	Ultrasound, **extremity**, nonvascular, real time with image documentation, limited	$36.54	$25.08	$11.46
10120	Incision and removal of foreign body simple	$153.06	n/a	n/a

CPT codes and average national reimbursement for Medicare in 2016. Payment data are from https://www.cms.gov/apps/physician-fee-schedule/search/search-criteria.aspx. See Chapter 2 for details on ultrasound billing..

References

1. Gibbs T. The use of sonography in the identification, localization, and removal of soft tissue foreign bodies. *J Diagn Med Sonography*. 2006;22:5-21.
2. Halaas G. Management of foreign bodies in the skin. *Am Fam Phys*. 2007;76(5):683-690.
3. Ng SY, Songra AK, Bradley PF. A new approach using intraoperative ultrasound imaging for the localization and removal of multiple foreign bodies in the neck. *Int J Oral Maxillofacial Surg*. 2003;32(4):433-436.
4. Anderson MA, Newmeyer WL, Kilgore ES. Diagnosis and treatment of retained foreign bodies in the hand. *Am J Surg*. 1982;144(1):63-67.
5. Hassani SN, Bard RL. Real time ophthalmic ultrasonography. *Radiology*. 1978;127:213-219.
6. Bray PW, Mahoney JL, Campbell JP. Sensitivity and specificity of ultrasound in the diagnosis of foreign bodies in the hand. *J Hand Surg*. 1995;20(4):661-666.
7. Tahmasebi M, Zareizadeh H, Motamedfar A. Accuracy of ultrasonography in detecting radiolucent soft-tissue foreign bodies. *Indian J Radiol Imaging*. 2014;24(2):196-200.
8. Gilbert FJ, Campbell RS, Bayliss AP. The role of ultrasound in the detection of non-radiopaque foreign bodies. *Clin Radiol*. 1990;41(2):109-112.
9. Callegari L, Leonardi A, Bini A, et al. Ultrasound-guided removal of foreign bodies: personal experience. *Eur Radiol*. 2009;19(5):1273-1279.
10. Soudack M, Nachtigal A, Gaitini D. Clinically unsuspected foreign bodies: the importance of sonography. *J Ultrasound Med*. 2003;22(12):1381-1385.

PART 2

Is This Soft Tissue Mass Concerning?

Ximena Wortsman, MD

● Clinical Vignette

A 69-year-old man with a 3-month history of a slow-growing lump in the right dorsal region presents to the outpatient clinic. The patient has a history of diabetes type II and a melanoma surgery in the anterior aspect of the right leg 3 years ago. At that time, histologic examination demonstrated an in situ tumor with tumor-free margins, and the last positron-emission tomography–computed tomography (PET–CT) study, performed 1 year ago, showed no signs of metastases. On physical examination today, there is a 3 cm painless and skin-colored palpable mass in the right dorsal region. Is this soft tissue mass concerning?

LITERATURE REVIEW

Soft tissue lumps and bumps are common reasons for primary care consultations, and the underlying causes can range from benign to life-threatening lesions. Lumps can result from growths, called masses, that are discrete from the surrounding tissue, or from indiscrete entities, called pseudomasses, that can mimic masses on physical examination (ie, hematomas or abscesses). Additional concerns arise when the location is in cosmetically sensitive regions such as the face or in very active corporal segments such as the digits or the plantar foot surface.[1]

Recent developments in ultrasound technology allow for improved evaluation of superficial soft tissue masses and for assessment of many of their attributes. High-frequency ultrasound probes (≥15 MHz) can discriminate structures as small as 0.1 mm. This is a degree of resolution that is not possible with commercially available MRI or CT units.[2,3] Although high-frequency ultrasound can usually penetrate to depths of 6 to 8 cm, which is usually adequate to visualize most soft tissue masses, if deeper penetration is needed a lower-frequency probe should be used.[2] In addition to penetration, high-frequency ultrasound may have other limitations. These include the inability to visualize pigments such as melanin[3] and difficulty in detecting in situ skin cancers or other lesions measuring less than 0.1 mm.

Features of masses that can usually be assessed include dermatologic from nondermatologic origins, solid from cystic structure, or endogenous tissues from foreign bodies. The internal and external degree of vascularity in a mass or pseudomass can be evaluated along with the relation of the lesion to the neighboring structures. Assessment of these characteristics can be suggestive of benignancy versus malignancy, among other features.[2,4-6] If needed, ultrasound can guide percutaneous procedures such as a puncture, biopsy, or drainage. The recommendations and level of evidence for using point-of-care ultrasound in soft tissue masses are shown in Table 43-1.

Normal Sonographic Anatomy of the Superficial Layers

The layers of the skin from superficial to deep are the epidermis, dermis, and hypodermis (also called the subcutaneous tissue). The epidermis appears as a single hyperechoic line in the skin located throughout most of the body (nonglabrous skin). In contrast, in the skin of the palms and soles (glabrous skin), the epidermis appears as a bilaminar hyperechoic layer. The echogenicity of the epidermis is mainly due to the keratin content of the stratum corneum, which is increased in the palms and soles.

The dermis presents as a hyperechoic band less bright than the epidermis. In the areas of the body most exposed to sun such as the face and the dorsum of the forearms, a hypoechoic band located in the upper dermis can be detected. This is caused by a deposit of glycosaminoglycan and is called the subepidermal low echogenicity band (SLEB). The SLEB is a sign of photodamage or photoaging.

The hypodermis, also called subcutaneous tissue, is composed of hypoechoic fatty lobules and hyperechoic septa. Low-velocity vessels that include arteries with peak systolic ≤15 cm/s are usually detected in the hypodermis[2,7] (Figure 43-1).

Abnormal Sonographic Findings

Epidermal Cysts

Epidermal cysts are caused by epidermal remnants that become ectopically located in the dermis or hypodermis. Intact epidermal cysts are well-defined, round or oval-shaped structures located in the dermis or hypodermis. Typically, they are 2 cm or smaller in diameter, but occasionally, they can present as large structures that measure more than 5 cm. They appear anechoic or hypoechoic and produce the posterior acoustic enhancement artifact that is typically seen with fluid-filled structures. Sometimes, when these cysts present with an oval shape and hypoechoic appearance they resemble the sonographic features of testes. This has been called

TABLE 43-1	Recommendations for Use of Point-of-Care Ultrasound in Clinical Practice		
Recommendation		**Rating**	**References**
Point-of-care ultrasound should be used to determine the risk for malignancy of a soft tissue mass and help guide the decision on need for biopsy.		C	2-6, 8, 16, 18, 19, 22, 23, 26-28
Point-of-care ultrasound should be used to differentiate solid from cystic soft tissue masses.		C	1-21, 24-26

A = consistent, good-quality patient-oriented evidence; B = inconsistent or limited-quality patient-oriented evidence; C = consensus, disease-oriented evidence, usual practice, expert opinion, or case series. For information about the SORT evidence rating system, go to http://www.aafp.org/afpsort.

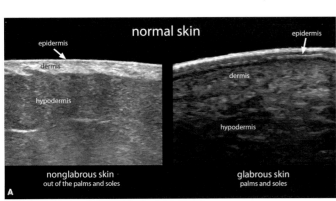

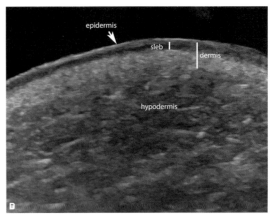

FIGURE 43-1. A, Ultrasonographic anatomy of the normal skin (gray scale). B, Subepidermal low echogenicity band (SLEB) in the dermis.

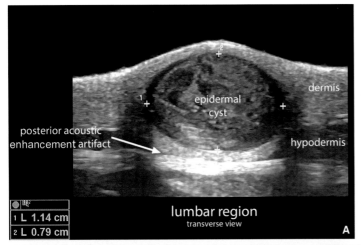

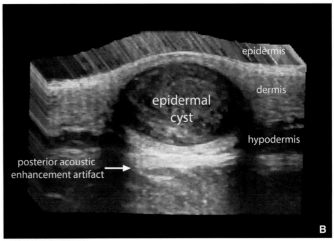

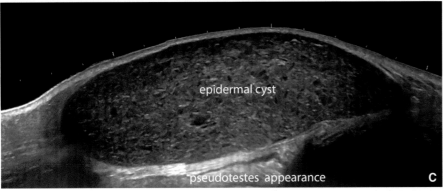

FIGURE 43-2. A-C, Intact epidermal cyst (lumbar region; A, gray scale; B, 3D reconstruction; C, panoramic view). A and B demonstrate a 1.1 cm (transverse) × 0.8 cm (thickness), well-defined, oval-shaped, hypoechoic dermal and hypodermal structure that produces posterior acoustic enhancement artifact. C shows the pseudotestes appearance of an intact epidermal cyst.

"pseudotestes appearance." In some cases, a connecting tract to the epidermis, called a punctum, can be detected. If the cyst ruptures, keratin is released, causing a foreign body–like reaction and inflammation. When inflamed, they can become enlarged with peripheral hypervascularity. Even when inflamed or ruptured, they tend to conserve the posterior acoustic enhancement artifact[8-11] (**Figures 43-2 and 43-3**).

Pilonidal Cysts

Pilonidal cysts are commonly located in the intergluteal region. Traditionally, it was thought that they were caused by the embedding of hair in the subcutaneous tissue, resulting in inflamed tracts.[12,13]

A more recent report with sonographic and histologic correlation suggests that they are, in fact, a localized form of hidradenitis suppurativa.[12] Pilonidal cysts seem to be generated from dysfunction of hair follicles secondary to inflammation of skin in regions with a high presence of terminal hair and apocrine glands. This can happen when skin is exposed to high levels of friction, humidity, and other unknown factors. Affected skin creates abnormally high amounts of keratin and new hair tracts that become retained in the dermis and hypodermis. This perpetuates the inflammatory process and generates hypoechoic saclike or bandlike dermal or hypodermal structures. These structures are usually connected to the base of dilated hair follicles and become filled with nests of hyperechoic

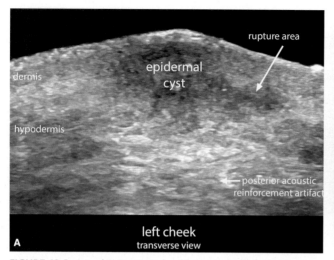

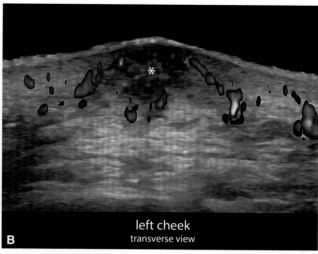

FIGURE 43-3. A and B, Ruptured epidermal cyst (left cheek; transverse views; A, gray scale; B, color Doppler). Ill-defined, hypoechoic dermal and hypodermal structure (asterisk) that produces posterior acoustic enhancement artifact. Notice the spread of the keratinous component in A (arrow) and the peripheral increase in vascularity on color Doppler (B).

linear structures that correspond to fragments of hair. When pilonidal cysts become inflamed, they can show prominent hypervascularity in their periphery with low-velocity arterial and venous vessels on color Doppler imaging[12-14] (**Figure 43-4**).

Superficial Fluid Collections

Dermal and hypodermal fluid collections are commonly caused by seromas, hematomas, and abscesses. Seromas appear as easily compressible anechoic fluid collections. They can be laminar or show a saclike morphology and may last for several months. Hematomas can vary in their ultrasound appearance according to their age. In early phases, the fresh blood may appear as hyperechoic deposits within an anechoic dermal or hypodermal fluid collection. Over days, the fluid becomes fully anechoic, although it may still contain some echogenic debris. At later stages, the content of the hematoma becomes hypoechoic because of the presence of fibrinous granulation and scar tissue (**Figure 43-5**).

If a fluid collection becomes infected, it may become an abscess. In this case, prominent internal echoes and increased peripheral vascularity are commonly detected. Additionally, abscesses can manifest as confluent lacunar areas with irregular borders and multiple internal echoes. Seromas, hematomas, and abscesses all tend to present a posterior acoustic enhancement artifact (**Figure 43-6**).[15,16] (See Chapter 41 for more details.)

Lipomas

Lipomas are the most common soft tissue masses. They can present with fibrous tissue components (fibrolipoma) or capillary vessels (angiolipoma). On ultrasound, they tend to manifest as a well-defined oval-shaped mass with hypoechoic (fibrolipoma) or hyperechoic (angiolipoma) echostructure. They tend to follow the axis of the skin layers and contain internal hyperechoic linear septa. They can present in hypodermal, subfascial, or intramuscular locations, and occasionally may show slightly lobulated margins. On color Doppler, they commonly appear as hypovascular masses, although some present a low level of internal vascularity with slow velocity (≤15 cm/s) arterial and/or venous vessels (**Figure 43-7**). Lipomas are commonly single tumors, but they can also present as multiple masses in the same or different body areas. Lipomas are benign masses, but it is important to differentiate them from other potentially malignant lesions such as liposarcomas.[3,8,15]

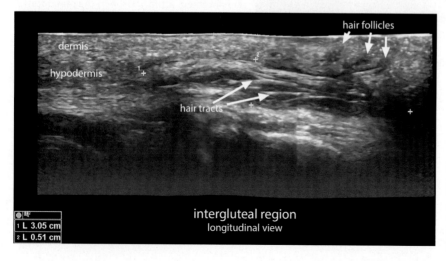

FIGURE 43-4. Pilonidal cyst (intergluteal region; longitudinal view; gray scale). 3.0 cm (long) × 0.5 cm (thickness) hypoechoic, dermal and hypodermal, saclike structure that contains multiple fragments of hair tracts (some of them marked with arrows pointing up) and connected to the dilated base of the regional hair follicles (arrows pointing down).

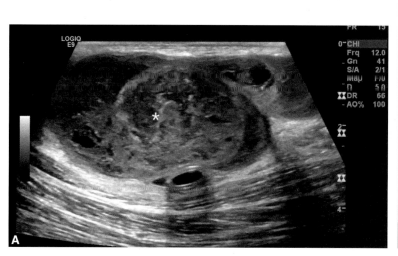

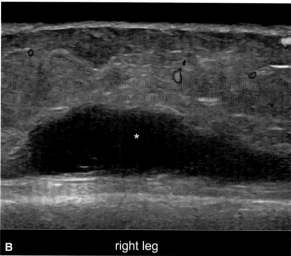

FIGURE 43-5. A and B, Hematoma. A, An acute hematoma of the thigh shows heterogeneous hyperechoic material (asterisk). B, A chronic hematoma (anterior aspect of the right leg; longitudinal view; color Doppler ultrasound) shows anechoic deep hypodermal fluid collection (asterisk).

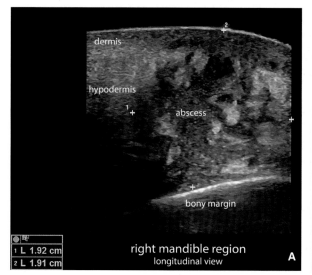

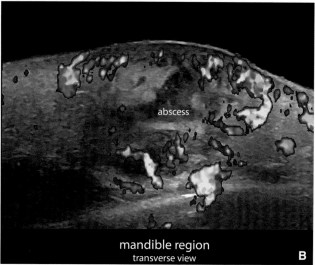

FIGURE 43-6. A and B, Abscess (right mandible region). A (gray scale, longitudinal view) and B (color Doppler, transverse view) demonstrate a 1.9 cm (long) × 1.9 cm (thickness) hypoechoic dermal and hypodermal fluid collection that presents multiple echoes and irregular margins.

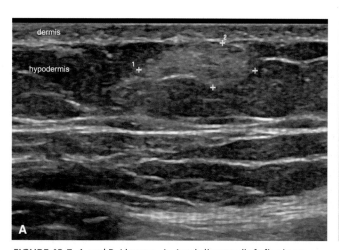

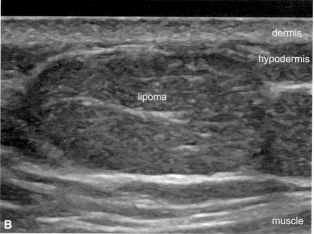

FIGURE 43-7. A and B, Lipoma. A, Angiolipoma (left flank; transverse view) gray scale ultrasound image demonstrates a well-defined, oval-shaped, hyperechoic hypodermal structure. B, Fibrolipoma (left lumbar region; transverse view) gray scale ultrasound shows a well-defined, oval-shaped, hypoechoic structure that follows the axis of the skin and presents hyperechoic fibrous septa.

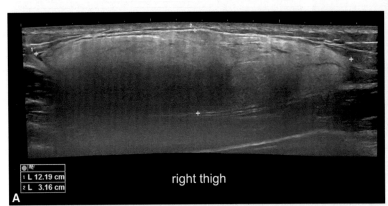

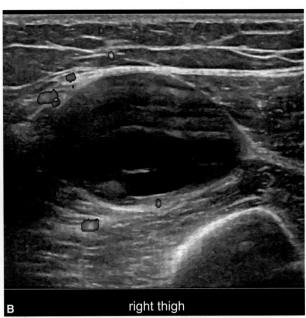

FIGURE 43-8. A and B, Liposarcoma. A, Angioliposarcoma (gray scale; longitudinal view; anterior aspect of the right thigh) presents a 12.19-cm-long oval-shaped hyperechoic hypodermal mass with heterogeneous areas mainly in the lower part (right side of the image). B, Myxoid liposarcoma (color Doppler; anterior aspect of the right thigh; transverse view) shows a well-defined, mixed echogenicity mass in the anterior muscular compartment. The mass presents hypoechoic and anechoic areas with some septa, and a slight increase in vascularity in the periphery.

Liposarcoma

There are several histologic subtypes of liposarcomas, including well-differentiated, ill-differentiated, and myxoid (cystic) variants. Their appearance on ultrasound may change according to the subtypes. Among the ultrasound signs suggestive of liposarcomas are the presence of intratumoral nodules, thick septa (more than 2 mm of thickness), large size (measuring more than 5 cm), normal fat echogenicity in less than 25% of the mass, intralesional cystic areas, heterogeneous echogenicity, ill-defined or irregular margins, fascial attachment, increased echogenicity of the adjacent hypodermis, and focal or diffuse intralesional hypervascularity (**Figure 43-8**).[17,18]

Lymphadenopathy

Lymph nodes are located in the anatomic sites of drainage of the lymphatic fluid. Benign lymph nodes tend to conserve their oval shape (long axis more than twice the short axis) and echostructure (hypoechoic thin and regular cortex and hyperechoic medulla).

The size is ≤1 cm in transverse axis, and the vascularity is centripetal with a vascular hilum entering in one of the borders (**Figure 43-9**).

Malignant lymph nodes tend to have a round shape, diffuse hypoechoic structure with loss of the medulla echogenicity, size ≥1 cm (transverse view), and cortical vascularity (**Figure 43-10**). Other ultrasonographic signs of malignancy are the presence of hypoechoic nodules within the lymph node[15,19] (see Chapter 6 for more details).

Thrombosed Venous Vascular Malformation

Vascular malformations are caused by errors in morphogenesis of the vascular system. They can be classified as high flow (arterial or arteriovenous) and low flow (venous, lymphatic or capillary). Vascular malformations are commonly congenital; however, in some cases, they can be acquired secondary to trauma or occur without a recognizable trigger. Venous vascular malformations are the most likely to thrombose. When this occurs, patients commonly complain of a sudden growth or pain at the site of the lesion. On ultrasound,

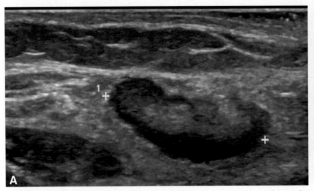

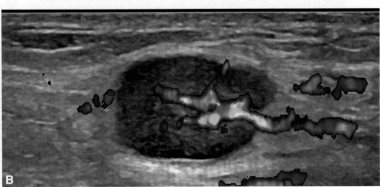

FIGURE 43-9. A and B, Benign lymph nodes A, Gray scale and B, Color Doppler show oval-shaped hypodermal nodules with a hypoechoic rim (cortex) and hyperechoic center (medulla). Notice the vascular hilum (colors) at the right border in (B) with a centripetal distribution of flow within the lymph node.

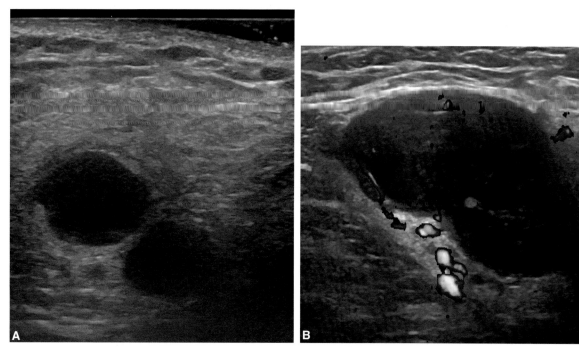

FIGURE 43-10. A and B, Malignant lymph nodes. A, Gray scale (transverse view) shows two round, fully hypoechoic hypodermal nodules in the supraclavicular fossa. B, Power Doppler demonstrates an oval-shaped mainly hypoechoic axillary lymph node with loss of the medulla echogenicity pattern and prominent cortical vascularity.

nonthrombosed venous vascular malformations usually appear as a dermal or hypodermal network of tubules or lacunar areas that are anechoic and easily compressible with the probe. On the spectral curve analysis, there is a monophasic venous flow. However, in the presence of thrombosis, there is dilation and hypoechoic material within the thrombosed parts of the vessels and/or lacunar areas

(**Figure 43-11**). Additionally, the affected vessels are noncompressible or partially compressible with the probe, and the monophasic flow is decreased or not detected.[1,2,20,21]

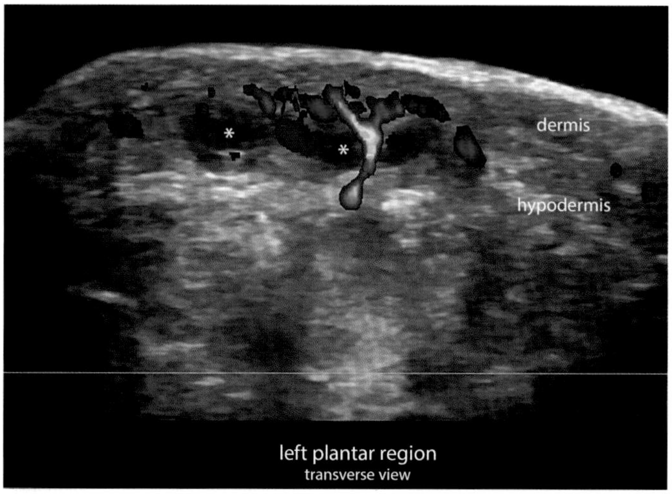

Soft Tissue Metastases

According to their distance from the primary tumor, metastases can be classified as

- satellites: <2 cm from the primary tumor
- in-transit: ≥2 cm from the primary tumor
- nodal: at the regional lymph nodes

Soft tissue metastases are usually located in the hypodermis and present as hypoechoic masses with ill-defined, irregular, polylobulated, or spiculated margins. Vascularity is variable and can frequently vary from slightly vascular to hypervascular. Occasionally, several metastatic hypoechoic nodules that follow the lymphatic drainage paths are detected (**Figure 43-12**).[15,19,22,23]

PERFORMING THE SCAN

Step 1: Choose the correct probe. When scanning superficial soft tissue masses, use machines working with high-frequency linear probes, usually ≥12 MHz and with availability of color Doppler. If the mass is located in the muscle or subcutaneous tissue, lower-frequency linear probes (12-14 MHz) may be preferred.[24,25] However, for studying cutaneous lesions, linear or compact linear probes with a frequency ≥15 MHz are needed. The high frequency makes it possible to focus the field of view in the superficial layers, and the color Doppler application supports the assessment of the vascularity patterns at the periphery and within the mass (**Figure 43-13**).

Step 2: Position the patient. Position the patient with the lesion facing the operator and close to the machine location (**Figure 43-14**). Visually inspect and palpate the mass.

dermis

hypodermis

left plantar region
transverse view

FIGURE 43-11. Thrombosed venous vascular malformation (left plantar region, color Doppler, transverse view) shows hypoechoic lacunar areas (asterisk) in the border between dermis and hypodermis that present a dilated lumen without detectable flow. These lacunar areas were noncompressible in the examination. In the periphery of the lacunar areas, there is increased vascularity, which corresponded to low-velocity arterial vessels secondary to inflammation. Decreased echogenicity and thickening of the dermis, as well as increased echogenicity of the underlying hypodermis, are also detected due to regional inflammation. Additionally, the increased blood flow in the periphery of the lesion generates a posterior acoustic enhancement artifact.

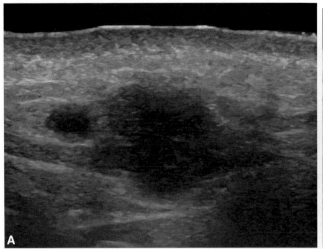
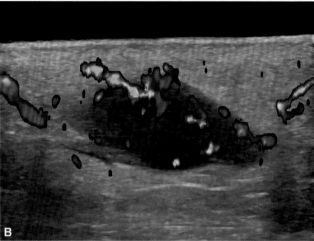

FIGURE 43-12. A and B, Soft tissue metastases. A, Squamous cell carcinoma metastasis. Gray scale (left side of the neck; transverse view) shows an ill-defined hypodermal mass attached to the fascial layer with lobulated and spiculated margins. B, Melanoma metastasis. Color Doppler (lateral aspect of the right leg; longitudinal view) presents an ill-defined, oval-shaped hypodermal mass with hypervascularity and increased echogenicity of the adjacent hypodermis due to edema.

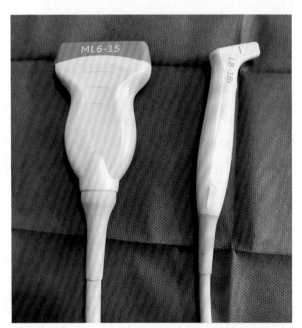

FIGURE 43-13. Examples of linear and compact linear probes used in soft tissue examinations.

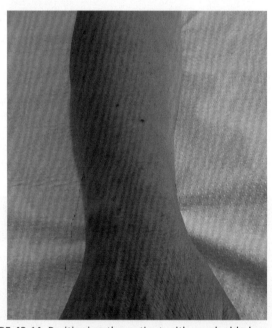

FIGURE 43-14. Positioning the patient with a palpable lump in the right forearm facing the operator.

Step 3: Scan the area of concern. Apply a copious amount of gel if the lesion is located in the superficial skin to allow the probe to stand off the skin while scanning. For deeper masses, use a thin layer of gel (**Figure 43-15**) and apply the probe directly to the skin. A gray scale sweep in at least two perpendicular axes is performed for assessing the nature of the lesion (mass or pseudomass; solid and/or cystic). In some cases, compression of the lesion may support the assessment of components (eg, dense fluid versus scarring). Color Doppler is applied in at least two perpendicular axes for viewing the pattern of vascularity of the lesion (avascular, hypovascular, hypervascular, center, and/or periphery). A scanning of the lesion using different frequency probes may provide a better observation of the lesion and surrounding structures at variable depth (**Figure 43-16**).

PATIENT MANAGEMENT

The management of the patients with soft tissue masses varies according to the sonographic signs presented by the mass such as nature (solid or cystic), the presence of vascularity, and the definition of the borders, among other factors. Sonographic signs concerning for malignancy are listed in **Table 43-2**.[26-28] Patients with fluid collections such as abscesses or solid masses might benefit from an ultrasound-guided drainage or biopsy procedure, respectively[19,29] (see Chapter 58 on FNA and core needle biopsy).

A proposal for managing soft tissue masses according to their main ultrasound features is presented in **Figure 43-17**.

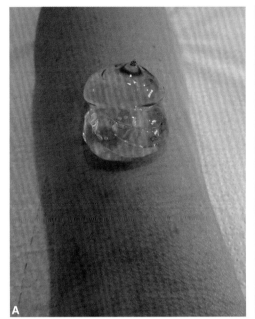
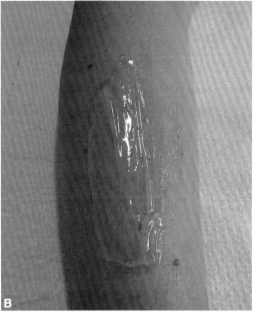

FIGURE 43-15. A and B, Application of a different amount of gel to adjust the focal area of observation. A, A copious amount of gel if the lesion is located in the skin or dermis. B, A thin layer of gel if the lesion is located in the hypodermis or deeper soft tissue structures.

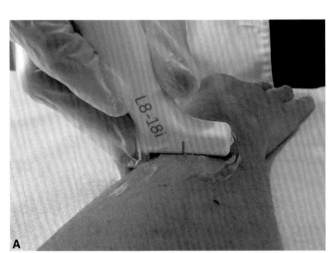
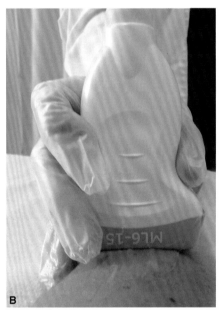

FIGURE 43-16. A and B, Scanning the lesion using different frequency probes for a better observation of the lesion and surrounding structures.

TABLE 43-2	**Malignant Sonographic Features of Soft Tissue Masses**

Rapid growth

Size greater than 5 cm (Figure 43-8A)

Ill-defined masses with heterogeneous echogenicity (Figure 43-12A)

Irregular, polylobulated, or spiculated margins (Figure 43-12A)

Medium to high intralesional vascularity (Figure 43-12B)

Perilesional edema (Figure 43-12B)

Infiltration of deeper and/or adjacent structures

Severe pain

History of malignancy

From DiDomenico P, Middleton W. Sonographic evaluation of palpable superficial masses. *Radiol Clin North Am.* 2014;52(6):1295-1305. doi:10.1016/j.rcl.2014.07.011; Hung EH, Griffith JF, Ng AW, Lee RK, Lau DT, Leung JC. Ultrasound of musculoskeletal soft-tissue tumors superficial to the investing fascia. *AJR Am J Roentgenol.* 2014;202(6):W532-W540. doi:10.2214/AJR.13.11457; Prativadi R, Dahiya N, Kamaya A, Bhatt S. Chapter 5 Ultrasound characteristics of benign vs malignant cervical lymph nodes. *Semin Ultrasound CT MR.* 2017;38(5):506-515. doi:10.1053/j.sult.2017.05.005.

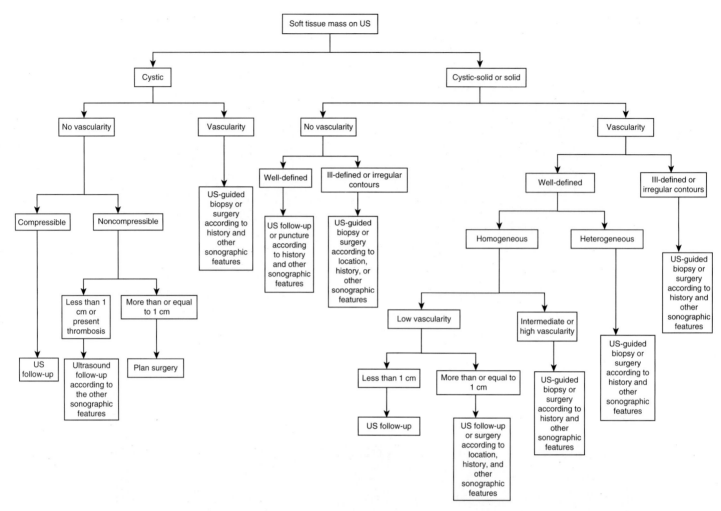

FIGURE 43-17. Algorithm for managing soft tissue masses according to main point-of-care ultrasound (POCUS) features.

PEARLS AND PITFALLS

Pearls

- The discrimination of benign features versus those concerning for malignancy in a soft tissue mass should not rely only on a single sonographic feature. It is recommended to use two or more.
- Compression with the probe can support the diagnosis of a fluid collection because seromas or hematomas are usually compressible.
- Besides a real-time percutaneous-guided ultrasound drainage or biopsy procedure, a cutaneous marking of a mass can be performed.[19,22,23,29] Whatever method is used, the usage of sonography can increase the precision and safety of the procedure.
- Spectral curve analysis is suggested for supporting the type of flow (arterial or venous) and may help to make the diagnosis of a vascular malformation. Remember that the colors of the box in color Doppler do not imply the type of flow but are just directions of the flow (toward and away from the probe).

- Panoramic views can be helpful for viewing large size lesions.
- Optional gray scale and power Doppler 3D reconstructions can be added to the examination in order to improve the clinical understanding of the images.

Pitfalls

- Occasionally, metastatic lymph nodes can present pseudo-cystic anechoic areas. This appearance has been reported for lymphomas and melanomas and is not related to necrosis. It is believed that the presence of compact hypercellular tumoral nests in these cases allows the passage of the sound waves and mimic cystic areas. The usage of power or color Doppler can support these cases because they can show vascularity within the pseudocystic regions.[19,29]
- Although large size of a mass is a risk factor for malignancy, the specificity of this finding is low, and many large masses are benign.

BILLING

CPT Code	Description	Global Payment	Professional Component	Technical Component
76882	Ultrasound, extremity, nonvascular, real time with image documentation; limited	$36.52	$25.06	$11.46
76775	"Ultrasound, abdominal, real time with image documentation; limited"	$58.72	$29.36	$29.36
76604	"Ultrasound, chest, real time with image documentation"	$89.15	$27.57	$61.58

CPT codes and average national reimbursement for Medicare in 2016. Payment data are from https://www.cms.gov/apps/physician-fee-schedule/search/search-criteria.aspx. See Chapter 2 for details on ultrasound billing.

References

1. Wortsman X. Sonography of dermatologic emergencies. *J Ultrasound Med.* 2017;36(9):1905-1914.
2. Wortsman X. Common applications of dermatologic sonography. *J Ultrasound Med.* 2012;31:97-111.
3. Wortsman X, Wortsman J, Clinical usefulness of variable frequency ultrasound in localized lesions of the skin. *J Am Acad Dermatol.* 2010;62:247-256.
4. Barcaui Ede O, Carvalho AC, Lopes FP, Piñeiro-Maceira J, Barcaui CB. High frequency ultrasound with color Doppler in dermatology. *An Bras Dermatol.* 2016;91(3):262-273.
5. Alfageme Roldán F. Ultrasound skin imaging. *Actas Dermosifiliogr.* 2014;105(10):891-899.
6. Mandava A, Ravuri PR, Konathan R. High-resolution ultrasound imaging of cutaneous lesions. *Indian J Radiol Imaging.* 2013;23(3):269-277.
7. Wortsman X, Wortsman J, Carreño L, Morales C, Sazunic I, Jemec GBE. Sonographic anatomy of the skin, appendages and adjacent structures. In Wortsman X, Jemec GBE, eds. *Dermatologic Ultrasound with Clinical and Histologic Correlations.* 1st ed. New York, NY: Springer; 2013:15-35.
8. Wortsman X, Bouer M. Common benign non-vascular skin tumors. In Wortsman X, Jemec GBE, eds. *Dermatologic ultrasound with clinical and histologic correlations.* 1st ed. New York, NY: Springer; 2013:119-175.
9. Huang CC, Ko SF, Huang HY, et al. Epidermal cysts in the superficial soft tissue: sonographic features with an emphasis on the pseudotestis pattern. *J Ultrasound Med.* 2011;30:11-17.
10. Yuan WH, Hsu HC, Lai YC, Chou YH, Li AF. Differences in sonographic features of ruptured and unruptured epidermal cysts. *J Ultrasound Med.* 2012;31:265-272.
11. Jin W, Ryu KN, Kim GY, Kim HC, Lee JH, Park JS. Sonographic findings of ruptured epidermal inclusion cysts in superficial soft tissue: emphasis on shapes, pericystic changes, and pericystic vascularity. *J Ultrasound Med.* 2008;27:171-176.
12. Wortsman X, Castro A, Morales C, Franco C, Figueroa A. Sonographic comparison of morphologic characteristics between pilonidal cysts and hidradenitis suppurativa. *J Ultrasound Med.* 2017;36:2403-2418.
13. Solivetti FM, Elia F, Panetta C, Teoli M, Bucher S, Di Carlo A. Preoperative advantages of HF sonography of pilonidal sinus. *G Ital Dermatol Venereol.* 2012;147:407-411.
14. Mentes O, Oysul A, Harlak A, Zeybek N, Kozak O, Tufan T. Ultrasonography accurately evaluates the dimension and shape of the pilonidal sinus. *Clinics (Sao Paulo).* 2009;64:189-192.
15. Wortsman X, Azocar P, Bouffard JA. Conditions that can mimic dermatologic diseases. In Wortsman X, Jemec GBE, eds. *Dermatologic Ultrasound with Clinical and Histologic Correlations.* 1st ed. New York, NY: Springer; 2013:505-569.
16. Subramaniam S, Bober J, Chao J, Zehtabchi S. Point of care ultrasound for diagnosis of abscess in skin and soft tissue infections. *Acad Emerg Med.* 2016;23(11):1298-1306. doi: 10.1111/acem.13049.
17. Murphey MD, Arcara LK, Fanburg-Smith J. From the archives of the AFIP: imaging of musculoskeletal liposarcoma with radiologic-pathologic correlation. *Radiographics.* 2005;25(5):1371-1395.
18. Le CK, Harvey G, McLean L, Fischer J. Point-of-care ultrasound use to differentiate hematoma and sarcoma of the thigh in the pediatric emergency department. *Pediatr Emerg Care.* 2017;33(2):135-136.
19. Wortsman X. Skin cancer. In Wortsman X, ed. *Atlas of Dermatologic Ultrasound.* New York, NY: Springer; 2018.
20. Peer S, Wortsman X. Hemangiomas and vascular malformations. In Wortsman X, Jemec GBE, eds. *Dermatologic Ultrasound with Clinical and Histologic Correlations.* 1st ed. New York, NY: Springer; 2013:183-248.
21. White CL, Olivieri B, Restrepo R, McKeon B, Karakas SP, Lee EY. Low-flow vascular malformation pitfalls: from clinical examination to practical imaging evaluation—part 1, lymphatic malformation mimickers. *AJR Am J Roentgenol.* 2016;206(5):940-951.
22. Nazarian LN, Alexander AA, Kurtz AB, et al. Superficial melanoma metastases: appearances on gray-scale and color Doppler sonography. *AJR Am J Roentgenol.* 1998;170(2):459-463.
23. Catalano O, Voit C, Sandomenico F, et al. Previously reported sonographic appearances of regional melanoma metastases are not likely due to necrosis. *J Ultrasound Med.* 2011;30(8):1041-1049.
24. Wortsman X. Technical considerations and guidelines for the dermatologic ultrasound examination. In Wortsman X, ed. *Atlas of Dermatologic Ultrasound.* New York, NY: Springer; 2018.
25. Wortsman X, Alfageme F, Roustan G, et al. Guidelines for performing dermatologic ultrasound examinations by the DERMUS group. *J Ultrasound Med.* 2016;35(3):577-580.
26. DiDomenico P, Middleton W. Sonographic evaluation of palpable superficial masses. *Radiol Clin North Am.* 2014;52(6):1295-1305. doi:10.1016/j.rcl.2014.07.011.
27. Hung EH, Griffith JF, Ng AW, Lee RK, Lau DT, Leung JC. Ultrasound of musculoskeletal soft-tissue tumors superficial to the investing fascia. *AJR Am J Roentgenol.* 2014;202(6):W532-W540. doi:10.2214/AJR.13.11457.
28. Prativadi R, Dahiya N, Kamaya A, Bhatt S. Chapter 5 Ultrasound characteristics of benign vs malignant cervical lymph nodes. *Semin Ultrasound CT MR.* 2017;38(5):506-515. doi:10.1053/j.sult.2017.05.005.
29. Gaspari RJ, Sanseverino A. Ultrasound-guided drainage for pediatric soft tissue abscesses decreases clinical failure rates compared to drainage without ultrasound: a retrospective study. *J Ultrasound Med.* 2018;37(1):131-136. doi:10.1002/jum.14318.

Does the Patient Have a Hernia?

John Rocco MacMillan Rodney, MD, FAAFP, RDMS and William MacMillan Rodney, MD, FAAFP, FACEP

● Clinical Vignette

A 2-month-old male presents for a well-child visit with a scrotal bulge that his mother noticed has worsened since birth. She states that the bulge is bilateral but enlarges on the right side when the infant cries. On examination, the infant is well appearing but there are palpable masses in the scrotum bilaterally that enlarge with deep palpation of the abdomen. Does the patient have a hernia?

LITERATURE REVIEW

Abdominal hernias are projections of omental fat, intestines, and occasionally other organs through defects in the abdominal fascia, diaphragm, or mesentery. Abdominal hernias are divided into internal and external hernias. In this chapter, we will be referring to external or abdominal wall hernias.

Hernias encompass a significant burden of disease throughout the world. In 2009, hernias were the fifth most common diagnosis leading to an outpatient visit in the United States.[1] This results in approximately 3.6 million outpatient visits, 380,000 hospitalizations, and 1300 deaths in the United States per year.[2] Direct and indirect costs for hernias in 2004 were estimated at 6 billion dollars per year in the United States.[3] True incidence, however, is difficult to assess because many hernias are asymptomatic and may not be detected or repaired. Historically, the estimated incidence in the United States has been projected at 5% to 6%.[4] Prevalence is bimodal, with peaks in infants because of congenital hernias and then again later in life as the incidence of groin hernias increases with age. Men are at a higher risk of having a hernia compared to women with a ratio of 8:1.

Inguinal, femoral, and ventral hernias are the most common hernia types. Inguinal hernias are located in the groin, with abdominal contents entering the inguinal canal and at times extending into the scrotum in men. Inguinal hernias can be further subdivided into direct and indirect types. Direct inguinal hernias originate from a fascial defect in Hesselbach's triangle. Hesselbach's triangle's borders are the inferior epigastric artery laterally, the lateral margin of the rectus sheath medially, and the inguinal ligament inferiorly. Indirect hernias originate from openings in the deep inguinal ring. Femoral hernias occur inferior to the inguinal ligament and medial to the common femoral vein. Inguinal hernias are the most common hernias in both sexes, but femoral hernias occur more commonly in women.[7] Ventral hernias typically occur in the midline between the rectus abdominis muscles. Frequently, they occur secondary to fascial defects from prior surgeries. Although they may occur near the umbilicus, they are not true umbilical hernias. True umbilical hernias are most common in children and will usually close spontaneously by 2 years of age. Spigelian hernias are rare and occur at the lateral border of the lower rectus abdominis muscles. Most hernias are obvious on physical examination, but occult hernias can also occur. Occult hernias are more likely to be small and spontaneously reducing, especially in the supine position. In these cases, ultrasound can be helpful. Point-of-care ultrasound has the unique versatility to examine patients in supine, standing, and other positions, which cause the patient pain. One meta-analysis showed ultrasound for inguinal hernia sensitivity was 96.6% and specificity was 84.8%.[8,9] False positives were less likely to occur when the patient presented with complaints of pain at the site of suspected hernia.[10] Possible false positives include lipoma of the spermatic cord or round ligament, varicoceles, or lymphadenopathy. Ultrasound can also detect inflammation causing osteitis pubis, tendinopathies, or other hip pathology that are in the differential of groin pain.[10]

When assessing the groin for hernias, there are specific anatomic landmarks that assist in identifying and classifying hernias. These are the inguinal ligament, inferior epigastric vessels, femoral canal, spermatic cord or round ligament if present, and the superficial and deep inguinal rings. Familiarity with the anatomic relationships of these structures is important (**Figure 44-1**).[11-15]

Many hernias will spontaneously reduce, and therefore, all symptomatic locations should be examined in the supine position while relaxed and with the Valsalva maneuver. If a hernia is not easily visualized in the supine position, the examination should be repeated with the patient standing and in any other position that reproduces the symptoms.

It is also helpful to know the appearance of other structures commonly visualized while assessing for hernias.[11,12] Herniated bowel will have alternating echogenic and hypoechoic layers from lumen to serosa and may have hyperechoic air with shadow visible inside (**Figure 44-2**). Normal bowel will also be seen peristalsing (▶ **Video 44-1**). Herniated fat is homogeneous and isoechoic to hyperechoic with hyperechoic septations (**Figure 44-3**).

Incarcerated hernias are hernias that are not reducible spontaneously or with manual maneuvers. The morbidity and mortality associated with hernias is primarily because of incarceration and the increased risk of associated emergent repair (standardized mortality risk 1.4 compared to average), which is increased 20 times when bowel is resected.[5] Strangulation occurs when incarcerated hernias develop complications secondary to ischemia. Strangulation can be difficult to assess until permanent damage occurs.

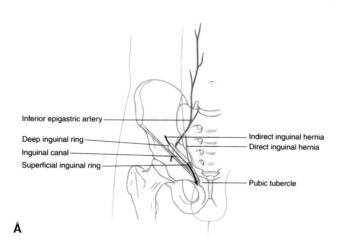

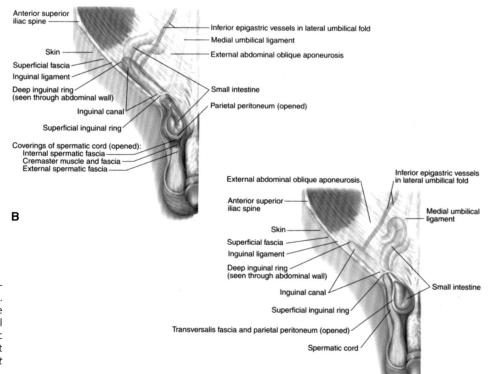

FIGURE 44-1. A, Anatomic landmarks distinguishing direct hernias from indirect hernias. B, The indirect inguinal hernia entering the deep inguinal ring. C, The direct inguinal hernia coursing medial to the epigastric vessels. Reprinted with permission from Gest TR. The abdomen. In: Gest TR, ed. *Lippincott Atlas of Anatomy*. 2nd ed. Philadelphia, PA: Wolters Kluwer; 2020:243. Plate 5-11.

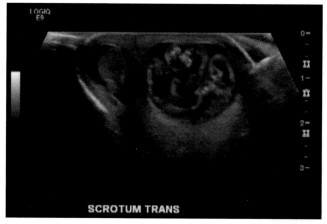

FIGURE 44-2. Herniated bowel in a short-axis view of the scrotum. Bowel is on the right side of the image. Note the alternating hyperechoic and anechoic layers. A testicle can be seen on the left side of the image.

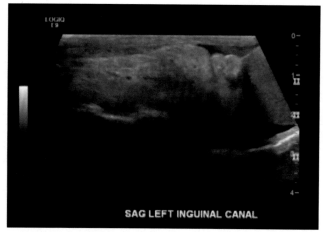

FIGURE 44-3. Herniated fat in a longitudinal view of the inguinal canal. Note the homogeneous, isoechoic appearance with hyperechoic septations. The testicle is seen on the right of the image.

TABLE 44-1	Recommendations for Use of Point-of-Care Ultrasound in Clinical Practice		
Recommendation		**Rating**	**References**
Ultrasound is recommended for initial assessment when clinical diagnosis is uncertain.		B	7-9, 20
Signs of strangulation are unpredictable, but abdominal wall thickness can indicate bowel wall pathology.		B	6
Ultrasound has good sensitivity and specificity for detection of groin hernias.		B	7-9, 13, 20
In females with a groin hernia, they should be assessed for a femoral hernia because of increased risk of recurrence if not repaired.		D	7
Symptomatic, large, recurrent (including nonstrangulated incarcerated) hernias should be referred for repair within 1 month.		C	20

A = consistent, good-quality patient-oriented evidence; B = inconsistent or limited-quality patient-oriented evidence; C = consensus, disease-oriented evidence, usual practice, expert opinion, or case series. For information about the SORT evidence rating system, go to http://www.aafp.org/afpsort.

PERFORMING THE SCAN

Step 1: Prepare for the examination. Preface ultrasound assessment with a thorough history and palpation of the areas in question with and without Valsalva maneuvers. Hernias should generally be

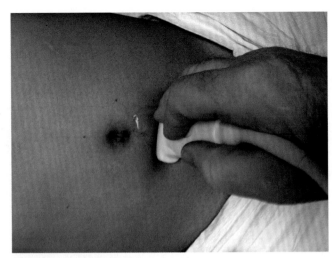

FIGURE 44-4. Probe positioning for transverse imaging of the linea alba to assess for fascial defects.

assessed using a high-frequency linear transducer 7 to 18 MHz. For the deep inguinal ring or deeper ventral hernias, it may be beneficial to change to a 5 MHz curvilinear transducer. Start the examination with the patient in the supine position.

Step 2: Assess for ventral hernias. In transverse position with light probe pressure, examine the midline from subxiphoid to pubis (**Figure 44-4**). Visualize a thickened linear white midline structure tenting upward. This is the linea alba and should be continuous as you travel from superior to inferior (**Figure 44-5**). This will detect

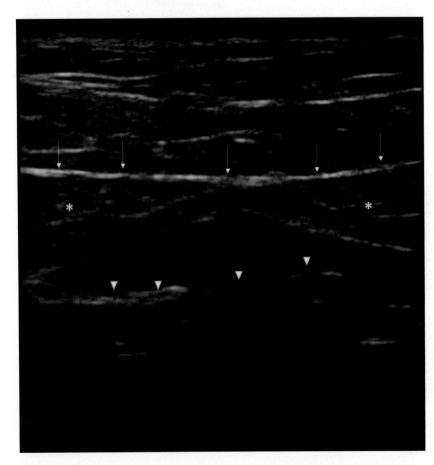

FIGURE 44-5. Ultrasound of normal linea alba. The top layer of tissue is the dermis and subdermal fat. The rectus sheath fascial layer is seen below (long arrows). The two rectus abdominus muscles are below (asterisk). The area of meeting of the recuts sheath and two rectus abdominus muscles is the linea alba (center long arrow). The parietal peritoneum is below (arrowheads).

ventral and umbilical hernias. Repeat this movement just lateral to the rectus bilaterally if a spigelian hernia is suspected.

Step 3: Assess for inguinal hernias. In males, start by placing the probe in the transverse position on the testicle (**Figure 44-6**). In females, position similarly but over the mons pubis. Testicles will have a characteristic oval homogeneous ground glass appearance (**Figure 44-7**).

Next find the spermatic cord (or in females the round ligament). The spermatic cord is most easily recognized by visualizing the pampiniform venous plexus, which appears as multiple small anechoic circular structures that can be highlighted with color Doppler.

Follow it proximally to the superficial ring, just superior to the inguinal ligament and lateral to the pubic bone. Continue to follow it laterally along the inguinal canal. The spermatic cord and associated structures will disappear through the deep inguinal ring. Scan it in both short and long axis. Next repeat the scan in the long axis of the inguinal canal and spermatic cord. Protrusion of hypoechoic fat or bowel from below the peritoneum is diagnostic for an inguinal

hernia. Trace the hernia to its origin. If it is located lateral to the inferior epigastric artery, it is an indirect hernia. If not, it is a direct hernia (**Figures 44-8 to 44-11** and ▶ **Video 44-2**).

Step 4: Assess for femoral hernias. In short axis, trace the external iliac artery inferiorly as it crosses the inguinal ligament and becomes the common femoral artery. The common femoral artery will be a minimally compressible anechoic structure lateral to the easily compressed common femoral vein. Color Doppler can be used to aid identification of the vessels (**Figure 44-12**). A femoral hernia will appear medial to the vein as a bulge of fat or intestine just distal to the inguinal ligament.

Step 5: Perform dynamic maneuvers. If no hernia is visualized, repeat all the above steps with and without Valsalva. If no hernia is visualized in the supine position with Valsalva, then the patient should be reimaged standing.

Step 6: Assess for incarceration or strangulation. If a hernia is identified, then it should immediately be assessed for reducibility. This can be done with gentle, constant pressure toward

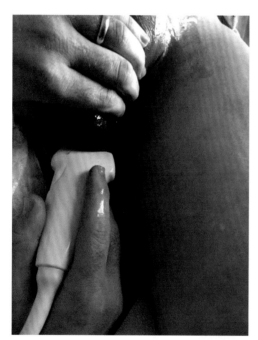

FIGURE 44-6. Probe positioning for a transverse view of the testicle.

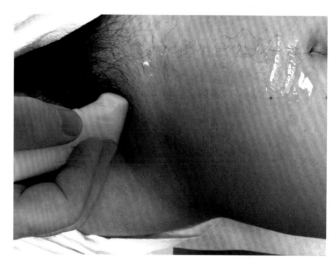

FIGURE 44-8. Probe seen in position tracing spermatic cord in short axis up to the inguinal ligament.

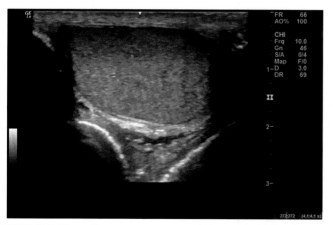

FIGURE 44-7. Normal homogeneous, ground glass testicular appearance.

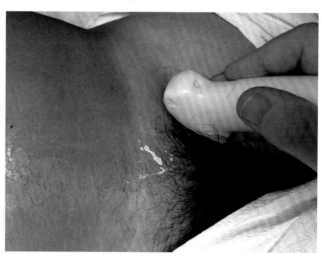

FIGURE 44-9. Probe position sagittal and just superior to the inguinal ligament midway between the anterior iliac spine and the pubis. This is where the deep inguinal ring can be found.

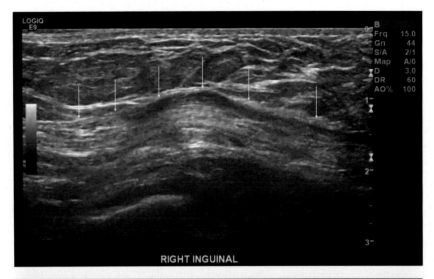

FIGURE 44-10. Normal spermatic cord (arrows) in inguinal canal. The pampiniform plexus is visible evidenced by multiple small hypoechoic structures.

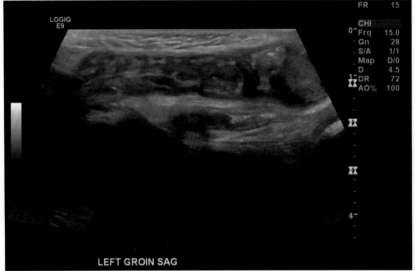

FIGURE 44-11. Longitudinal herniated bowel. Note the fascial defect visible on the left side of the image. A testicle is seen on the right side of the image.

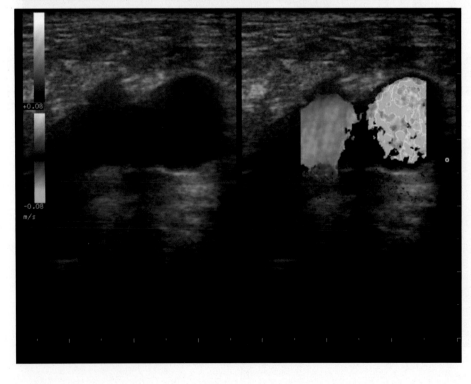

FIGURE 44-12. Femoral canal with and without color Doppler. The vein is on the left (medial) and the artery is on the right. A femoral hernia would be seen just medial (left on this image) to the larger, but compressible femoral vein.

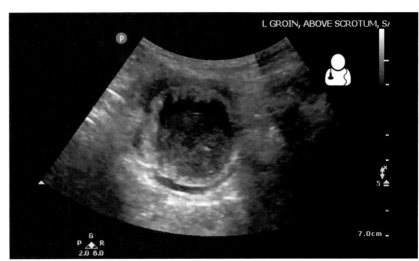

FIGURE 44-13. Short-axis image of strangulated bowel in a hernia. Note the thickened bowel wall, anechoic fluid around the bowel wall, and lack of blood flow on power Doppler. Courtesy of Ben Smith, https://www.ultrasoundoftheweek.com.

the fascial defect with the ultrasound probe or an examiner's digit. If a hernia is not able to be reduced easily, then it is incarcerated, and signs of strangulation should be ruled out. Signs of strangulation include free fluid in the hernia sac, thickened bowel wall (>5 mm) in the hernia, and fluid in the herniated bowel loop. Less helpful signs include loss of peristalsis, which is nonspecific, and failure to visualize Doppler flow, which is a late sign[6] (**Figure 44-13**).

PATIENT MANAGEMENT

Current recommendations for hernia management depend on the presence or risk of strangulation, the presence of symptoms, and the patient's ability to tolerate surgery. Initially, it is most important to determine if a hernia is strangulated or incarcerated. If there are signs of acute abdomen on physical examination or if imaging findings are suggestive, strangulation should be considered. Strangulated hernias are surgically repaired emergently. Incarcerated inguinal and umbilical and all femoral hernias should be repaired urgently because of their risk of subsequent strangulation and the difficulty in diagnosing early compromised blood flow.

The next branch of decision making is to determine if the hernia is symptomatic or asymptomatic. Symptomatic, healthy patients without signs of incarceration or strangulation should be repaired electively. The European Hernia Association guidelines suggest watchful waiting for patients with nonincarcerated asymptomatic hernias.[7]

The recommended method for hernia repairs in general is tension-free repair with mesh. However, suture repairs without mesh remain a valid technique, especially in pediatric surgery. Recurrence rates are low with either method. Patients who are poor surgical candidates with a reducible hernia can use a truss to manually maintain hernia reduction. The European Hernia Society guidelines recommend considering watchful waiting for patients who are not significantly symptomatic and have easily reduced hernias.[7] Patients should be advised to return immediately if their hernias become incarcerated or they develop worsening abdominal pain or symptoms of abdominal obstruction associated with the hernia (**Figure 44-14**).

PEARLS AND PITFALLS

Pearls

- Use the unique capabilities of ultrasound to image the patient in Valsalva, standing, and position of pain when diagnosis is in question.
- It is important to assess bilateral groins if an inguinal hernia is found because it is common for inguinal hernias to be bilateral and this may influence treatment. It is also recommended to assess for femoral hernias in females with inguinal hernias because of increased rates of co-occurance.[7]

Pitfalls

- Fat in a suspected hernia may originate from herniated omental fat or a lipoma of the spermatic cord or round ligament. Therefore, it should be traced back to the abdominal wall defect to confirm that it is a true hernia.
- Signs of strangulation are often late; do not wait for loss of blood flow on Doppler, because need for bowel resection increases mortality.

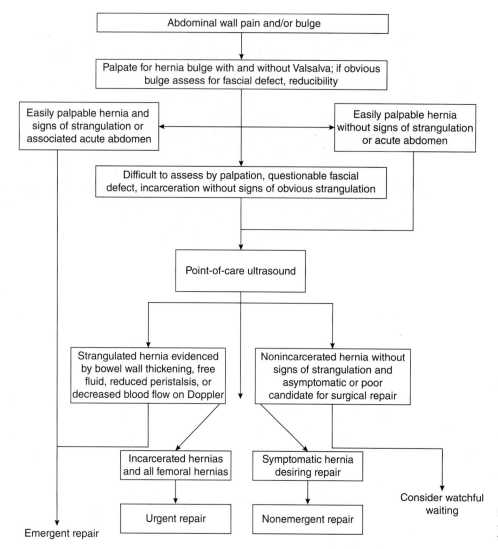

FIGURE 44-14. Algorithm showing recommended pathways for diagnosis and treatment of abdominal wall hernias.

BILLING

CPT Code	Description	Global Payment	Professional Component	Technical Component
76705	Limited abdominal ultrasound	$92.73	$30.08	$62.66

CPT codes and average national reimbursement for Medicare in 2016. Payment data are from https://www.cms.gov/apps/physician-fee-schedule/search/search-criteria.aspx. See Chapter 2 for details on ultrasound billing.

References

1. Peery AF, Dellon ES, Lund J, et al. Burden of gastrointestinal disease in the United States: 2012 update. *Gastroenterology.* 2012;143(5):1179.e3-1187.e3. doi:10.1053/j.gastro.2012.08.002.

2. Everhart JE. Abdominal wall hernia. In Everhart JE, ed. *The Burden of Digestive Diseases in the United States.* Washington, DC: US Government Printing Office, US Department of Health and Human Services, Public Health Service, National Institutes of Health, National Institute of Diabetes and Digestive and Kidney Diseases; 2008.

3. Everhart JE, Ruhl CE. Burden of digestive diseases in the United States part I: overall and upper gastrointestinal diseases. *Gastroenterology.* 2009;136(2):376-386. doi:10.1053/j.gastro.2008.12.015.

4. Lassandro F, Iasiello F, Pizza NL, et al. Abdominal hernias: radiological features. *World J Gastrointest Endosc.* 2011;3(6):110-117. doi:10.4253/wjge.v3.i6.110.

5. Nilsson H, Stylianidis G, Haapamäki M, Nilsson E, Nordin P. Mortality after groin hernia surgery. *Ann Surg.* 2007;245(4):656-660.

6. Rettenbacher T, Hollerweger A, Macheiner P, et al. Abdominal wall hernias: cross-sectional imaging signs of incarceration determined with sonography. *AJR Am J Roentgenol.* 2001;177(5):1061-1066.

7. Simons MP, Aufenacker T, Bay-Nielsen M, et al. European Hernia Society guidelines on the treatment of inguinal hernia in adult patients. *Hernia.* 2009;13(4):343-403. doi:10.1007/s10029-009-0529-7.

8. Alabraba E, Psarelli E, Meakin K, et al. The role of ultrasound in the management of patients with occult groin hernias. *Int J Surg.* 2014;12(9):918-922. doi:10.1016/j.ijsu.2014.07.266.

9. Robinson A, Light D, Nice C. Meta-analysis of sonography in the diagnosis of inguinal hernias. *J Ultrasound Med.* 2013;32(2):339-346.

10. McSweeney SE, Naraghi A, Salonen D, Theodoropoulos J, White LM. Hip and groin pain in the professional athlete. *Can Assoc Radiol J.* 2012;63(2):87-99. doi:10.1016/j.carj.2010.11.001.

11. Yoong P, Duffy S, Marshall TJ. The inguinal and femoral canals: a practical step-by-step approach to accurate sonographic assessment. *Indian J Radiol Imaging.* 2013;23(4):391-395. doi:10.4103/0971-3026 .125586.

12. Lee RK, Cho CC, Tong CS, Ng AW, Liu EK, Griffith JF. Ultrasound of the abdominal wall and groin. *Can Assoc Radiol J.* 2013;64(4):295-305. doi:10.1016/j.carj.2012.07.001.

13. Bradley M, Morgan D, Pentlow B, Roe A. The groin hernia—an ultrasound diagnosis? *Ann R Coll Surg Engl.* 2003;85(3):178-180.

14. Jamadar DA, Jacobson JA, Morag Y, et al. Sonography of inguinal region hernias. *AJR Am J Roentgenol.* 2006;187(1):185-190.

15. LeBlanc KE, LeBlanc LL, LeBlanc KA. Inguinal hernias: diagnosis and management. *Am Fam Physician.* 2013;87(12):844-848.

PART 2

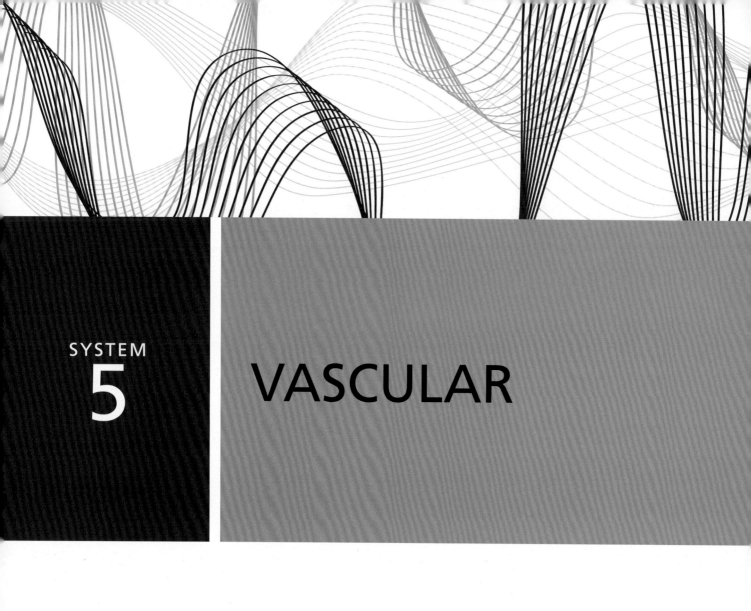

VASCULAR

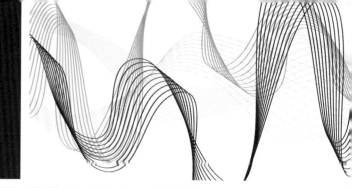

CHAPTER
45

Does the Patient Have a Lower Extremity Deep Venous Thrombosis?

Paul Bornemann, MD, RMSK, RPVI

Clinical Vignette

A 43-year-old male presents to the clinic with the complaint of acute onset of left lower extremity pain and swelling. It started the day before presentation after he returned from a 12-hour plane ride. He has no history of thrombosis, surgery, or malignancy. He does have a family history significant for multiple family members with thromboses. Does the patient have a lower extremity deep venous thrombosis?

LITERATURE REVIEW

Lower extremity DVTs occur at an annual rate of 1.92 per 1000 people. Major risk factors include increasing age, trauma, surgery, immobilization, and cancer; however, half of all DVTs are idiopathic. Up to 7.7% of initial DVTs recur within 2 years.[1] Patients who have had two prior DVTs are 1.73 times more likely to have a future DVT than those who have had only one in the past.[2] Up to 60% of proximal DVTs may embolize to the pulmonary vasculature, and the mortality rate is 9% within the first month after an initial DVT.[1]

DVTs can be classified by their location in the lower extremity. Proximal DVTs involve the deep veins of the thigh such as the common femoral vein, the deep femoral vein, the femoral vein, and the popliteal vein. The femoral vein, which is a true deep vein, had previously been known as the superficial femoral vein. The name, however, has been changed to avoid confusion with true superficial veins. Distal DVTs involve the deep veins of the calf and include the posterior tibial vein and the peroneal vein. Thrombosis almost never occurs in the anterior tibial vein, and it is usually not included in diagnostic evaluations.[3]

Thrombosis of the superficial veins is known as superficial thrombophlebitis. The superficial veins of the lower extremity coarse through the subcutaneous tissue, and unlike the deep veins, are not located with a paired artery. The two main superficial veins of the lower extremity are the greater saphenous and small saphenous veins. Superficial thrombophlebitis does not cause pulmonary embolization but can progress to thrombosis of a deep vein. This is more likely to happen if the affected area of the superficial vein

is within 5 cm of a deep vein or has a thrombosed segment greater than 5 cm in length[4] (**Figure 45-1**).

The preferred tests used to diagnose DVT have changed greatly over the past several decades. Prior to the 1980s, venography was the primary diagnostic tool. Venography was invasive, painful, and also carried a 10% risk of causing an iatrogenic DVT.[5] Because of these limitations, there was need for a less invasive diagnostic tool. In the 1980s, Talbot first described how ultrasound could be used to differentiate a thrombosed vein from a normal vein. He noted

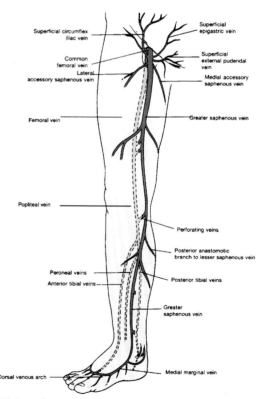

FIGURE 45-1. A schematic diagram demonstrates the veins of the lower extremity, which are divided into femoral, deep, and perforating veins. Reprinted with permission from Sussman C, Bates-Jensen BM. Wound care: a collaborative practice manual for health professionals. 4th ed. Philadelphia, PA: Wolters Kluwer Health/Lippincott Williams & Wilkins; 2011. Figure 11.4.

differences in B-Mode appearance, Pulsed Wave Doppler wave forms, and collapsibility with light compression from the transducer.[6] Raghavendra et al later confirmed that the accuracy of ultrasound was comparable to venography.[7]

Although ultrasound was effective and noninvasive, the examination required assessment of the entire lower extremity and was time-consuming. Research shifted toward finding ways to abbreviate the examination without reducing the accuracy. Raghavendra et al were able to show that collapsibility was the most important ultrasonographic finding and that Doppler studies were not a necessary component of the examination.[8]

It was known at the time that the vast majority of DVTs started in the calf veins and propagated proximally. The remaining few that did not start in the calves usually started in the pelvic or superficial veins, and isolated femoral vein DVTs were thought to be rare. Building on this theory, Lensing found that evaluating for collapsibility of only the common femoral vein and popliteal vein had a sensitivity of 100% and a specificity of 99% for proximal DVT.[9] This technique would later come to be known as the 2-point compression examination.

Although Lensing's 2-point evaluation was fast and accurate for the detection of proximal DVTs, the sensitivity for isolated calf vein thrombosis was only 36%.[9] However, the clinical significance of these distal DVTs was being called into question. A systematic review found that distal DVTs were unlikely to embolize, and that the most serious risk was a 20% chance of propagation to a proximal DVT in 1 to 2 weeks.[10] Therefore, initial 2-point ultrasound examinations that were negative would need to be followed up by repeat ultrasonography before DVT could be definitely ruled out. Birdwell et al[11] and Cogo et al[12] showed in separate studies that withholding anticoagulation in patients with negative ultrasonography was safe, pending follow-up scanning in 5 to 7 days.

Nonetheless, follow-up testing was cumbersome and patients were not always sure to return. There was a desire to find ways to use ultrasound to rule out DVT more efficiently. Wells et al showed that a low pretest probability of thrombosis in combination with a negative proximal leg ultrasound was able to sufficiently rule out DVT without the need for repeat scanning.[13] Fancher et al later showed that a negative D-Dimer assay along with low pretest probability was also sufficient to rule out a DVT.[14] Finally, it was shown that patients with a moderate or high pretest probability could forgo follow-up scanning if their initial ultrasound was done in conjunction with a negative D-dimer assay or if there was a negative ultrasound evaluation of the full leg including the calf veins.[15-17]

By this time, clinicians had shown that ultrasound could be effective and efficient at diagnosing DVTs. However, drawbacks remained, including the fact that ultrasonography required the availability of radiology suits or vascular labs with expensive equipment and highly trained personnel. Trottier et al were the first to demonstrate that DVT ultrasonography could be performed effectively at the bedside with inexpensive, portable ultrasound units and by ultrasonographers with limited training—only 35 prior training scans.[18] Blaivas et al later showed that emergency room physicians with only 5 hours of training were able to accurately perform 2-point ultrasonography with an average time of less than 4 minutes.[19] Not to be outdone, Jang et al gave a group of emergency medicine, internal medicine, and family medicine physicians only 10 minutes of initial training. After scanning 199 patients, 45 of whom had DVTs, they found that they had a sensitivity of 100% and a specificity of 99% compared with ultrasonography performed in the radiology suite.[20] Some experts have argued that 10 minutes of training is not adequate.[21] However, Jang's study does support that extensive training is not required to perform ultrasonography for DVT at the bedside.

Some controversy has arisen recently around whether 2-point compression ultrasound is truly an adequate examination of the proximal leg. The 2-point concept initially arose after early studies compared ultrasound with venography and showed that nearly all proximal leg DVTs involved the common femoral or popliteal vein and that isolated femoral vein DVTs were rare.[9,22] The controversy stems from several recent studies that have compared 2-point compression with full leg Duplex ultrasonography. These studies have found a higher-than-expected rate of isolated femoral vein DVTs, which in theory would have been missed by the 2-point compression technique.[23-27] However, in consideration of these findings, it is important to realize that these studies used full leg Duplex ultrasonography as the gold standard, an examination that can have false positives. Some studies have shown a false-positive rate as high as 14% for proximal DVTs when full leg Duplex is compared with venography, the true gold standard.[28] Additionally, 2-point compression combined with follow-up ultrasound or D-dimer testing has been shown to have equal outcomes to full leg Duplex in two large prospective trials.[12,16]

Given all of this, 2-point compression ultrasonography is a reasonable choice when used appropriately. Scanning of the femoral vein in addition to the 2-point compression scan can be considered optional until further data are available to make a definitive recommendation. In order to appropriately rule out DVT, all negative proximal scans (whether the femoral vein is included or not) must be combined with one of the three following: a low pretest probability of thrombosis, a negative D-dimer, or a follow-up ultrasound in 5 to 7 days (**Table 45-1**).

TABLE 45-1 **Recommendations for Use of Point-of-Care Ultrasound in Clinical Practice**		
Recommendation	**Rating**	**References**
Limited compression ultrasonography of the common femoral vein and popliteal vein along with pretest probability, D-dimer testing or follow-up ultrasonography can effectively rule in or rule out DVT.	A	4, 11-14
Point-of-care ultrasound for the evaluation of DVT can be performed at the point-of-care effectively by practitioners with only brief training.	A	18-20

A = consistent, good-quality patient-oriented evidence; B = inconsistent or limited-quality patient-oriented evidence; C = consensus, disease-oriented evidence, usual practice, expert opinion, or case series. For information about the SORT evidence rating system, go to http://www.aafp.org/afpsort.

Abbreviation: DVT, deep venous thrombosis.

PERFORMING THE SCAN

1. **Preparation.** The patient should be positioned sitting semi upright to allow for venous pooling in the lower extremities. The effected leg should be positioned with the hip partially flexed and externally rotated and with the knee partially flexed in a "frog leg" position. Position the ultrasound equipment appropriately and select a high-frequency, linear array probe with a vascular preset (**Figure 45-2**).

2. **Evaluate the common femoral vein for compressibility.** Place the transducer with the probe in the transverse position in the midline of the surface of the leg which is facing forward and just below the groin, with the probe marker pointing to the patient's right side. Find the common femoral vein and artery. The vein will be located medial to the artery (remember the

mnemonic NAVL; nerve, artery, vein, lymphatics). Scan proximally and distally until the junction of the common femoral vein and the greater saphenous vein is found. The greater saphenous vein will run in the subcutaneous tissue and then dive deeply to join the common femoral vein from above. Evaluate this location for compressibility. Press down with the transducer applying at least enough pressure to see the arterial walls begin to deform and increase in pulsation. In a normal vein, the walls should completely collapse, so that the vein is no longer visible. If the vein does not completely collapse, then a clot is present. Perform this maneuver every 1 cm as the probe is moved distally. Continue until the bifurcation of the common femoral vein into the femoral vein and deep femoral vein. This location, including both the femoral and deep femoral vein origins, should also be evaluated for compressibility (**Figures 45-3 through 45-6** and ▶ **Videos 45-1 and 45-2**).

3. **Evaluate the popliteal vein.** Place the transducer with probe in the transverse position in the midline of the posterior surface of the knee at the level of the most proximal popliteal crease, with the probe marker pointing to the patient's right. Angle the transducer toward the superior boarder of the patella on the opposite side of the leg. Find the popliteal vein and the artery; the vein should be superficial to the artery. The mnemonic "pop

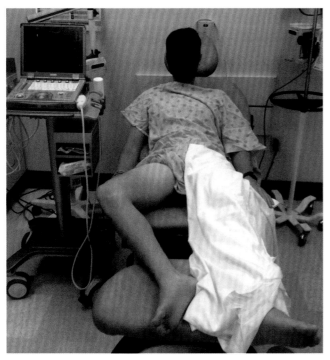

FIGURE 45-2. Patient positioning for the deep venous thrombosis examination.

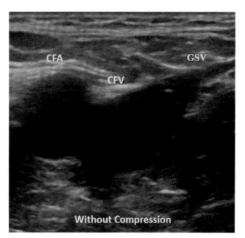

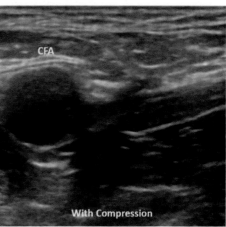

FIGURE 45-4. Compressed and noncompressed images of a normal common femoral vein at the junction of the greater saphenous vein. CFA, common femoral artery; CFV, common femoral vein; GSV, greater saphenous vein.

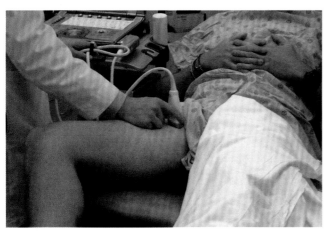

FIGURE 45-3. Probe placement for scanning of the common femoral vein.

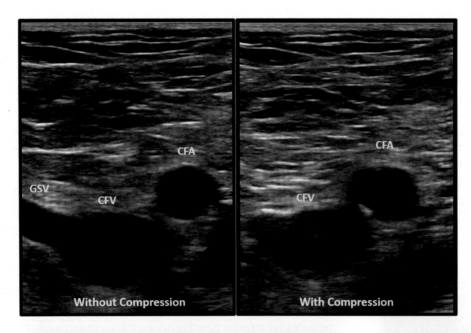

FIGURE 45-5. Compressed and noncompressed images of a common femoral vein thrombosis at the junction of the greater saphenous vein. CFA, common femoral artery; CFV, common femoral vein; GSV, greater saphenous vein.

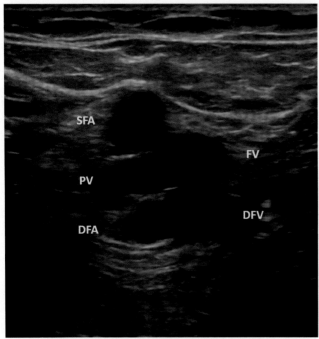

FIGURE 45-6. The bifurcation of the common femoral vein into the femoral and deep femoral veins. The evaluation for compressibility of the common femoral vein should start at the junction with the greater saphenous vein and continue at least to this point. DFA, deep femoral artery; DFV, deep femoral vein; FV, femoral vein; PV, perforating branch of the femoral vein; SFA, superficial femoral artery.

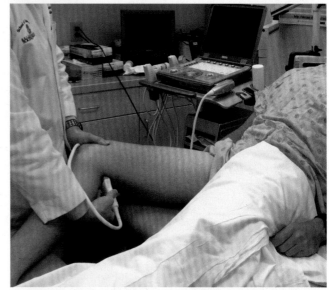

FIGURE 45-7. Probe placement for scanning of the popliteal vein.

on top" can be used to help remember this relationship. Evaluate the popliteal vein for compressibility at this location and then every 1 cm distally until the calf veins are seen branching from the popliteal vein. The calf veins are the anterior tibial, posterior tibial, and peroneal veins. They tend to split into two veins with a single-paired artery and run in the facial planes between the gastrocnemius and soleus muscles. However, variations are common and there may be a single vein or three veins with a paired artery (**Figures 45-7 through 45-10**).

4. **Complete a full leg venous evaluation (optional).** This step adds considerably to the amount of time required to complete the evaluation and is technically more challenging. However, there may be some instances where a full leg examination is desired. In order to complete a full leg evaluation, the full length of the femoral vein must be evaluated. After completing the evaluation of compressibility of the common femoral vein, the examination should continue. The femoral vein should be checked for compressibility every 1 cm distally until it becomes too deep to visualize, usually at the level of the adductor canal. The examination can be continued from below, starting at the level of the superior popliteal crease and checking for compressibility every 1 cm proximally until the vein can no longer be visualized. Finally, the posterior tibial and peroneal veins should be assessed for compressibility. Start at the bifurcation from the popliteal vein and continue to the level of the ankle. It can be helpful to move the transducer to a medial window through the calf muscles once

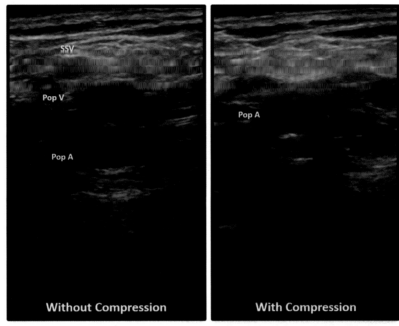

FIGURE 45-8. Compressed and noncompressed images of a normal popliteal vein. Pop A, popliteal artery; Pop V, popliteal vein; SSV, small saphenous vein.

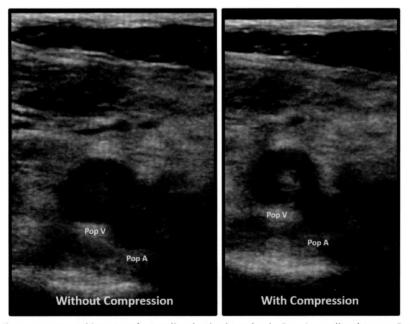

FIGURE 45-9. Compressed and noncompressed images of a popliteal vein thrombosis. Pop A, popliteal artery; Pop V, popliteal vein.

the calf veins become difficult to see. The anterior tibial artery does not need to be routinely assessed as an isolated thrombosis there is almost never seen[3] (**Figures 45-11 through 45-13**).

5. **Evaluate any location not already evaluated that is symptomatic.** Symptoms including pain and swelling can localize thrombi. Symptoms in the posterior thigh may come from the deep femoral vein. Symptoms along the greater saphenous vein or lesser saphenous vein should prompt evaluation of these vessels. Consider evaluation of the calf veins if symptoms localize to the calf. Calf symptoms localizing to the anterior lateral aspect should prompt a consideration of evaluation of the anterior tibial vein (**Figure 45-14**).

PATIENT MANAGEMENT

When planning patient management, the first step is to determine the pretest probability of DVT with a validated tool such as the Well's score. If a patient is low risk, he or she can be evaluated initially with a proximal leg ultrasound or a D-dimer. Given that a bedside proximal leg ultrasound can be completed in less than 4 minutes, often it will be the option of choice in primary care. Additionally, if the D-dimer is positive, the patient must then have a proximal leg ultrasound to further evaluate. However, if the D-dimer is negative, then a DVT is effectively ruled out. If the proximal leg ultrasound is negative, then a DVT is ruled out (**Table 45-2**).

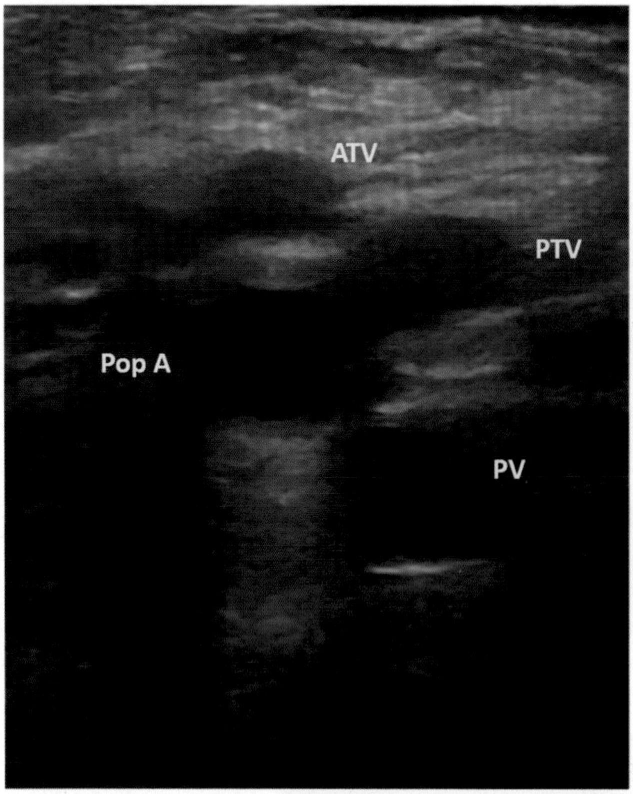

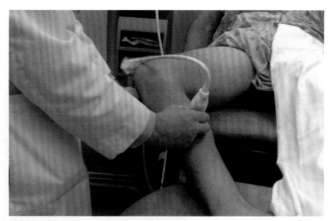

FIGURE 45-11. Probe placement for a medial window of the mid-calf veins.

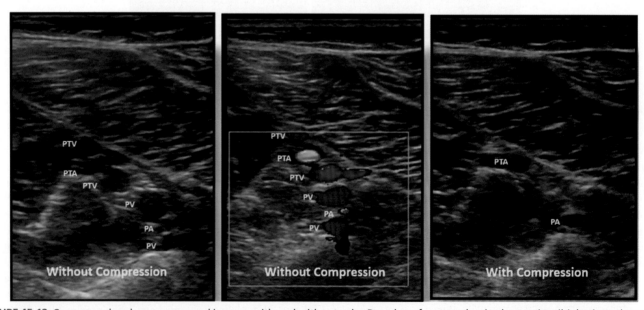

FIGURE 45-10. The trifurcation of the popliteal vein. The evaluation for compressibility of the popliteal vein should continue at least to this point. ATV, anterior tibial vein; Pop A, popliteal artery; PTV, posterior tibial vein; PV, peroneal vein.

If the patient is moderate or high risk, the initial step should be ultrasound. Usually, proximal ultrasound will be chosen over full leg ultrasound as it is faster and technically less challenging. If the proximal ultrasound is negative, a D-dimer can be obtained, and if also negative, then a DVT has been ruled out. If the D-dimer is positive or not available, the patient will need to have a repeat proximal leg ultrasound in 7 to 10 days. If the follow-up ultrasound is negative, then a DVT is ruled out. If there is concern that the patient will not follow-up in 7 to 10 days, initial compression ultrasonography involving the full leg can be considered. If full leg ultrasound is negative, then DVT is ruled out without the need for D-dimer testing or follow-up. However, a full leg ultrasound is considerably more time-consuming and technically more difficult to perform.

If at any point the ultrasound is positive, then DVT is ruled in and the patient should be treated. Treatment will be determined by the type of thrombosis that is diagnosed. Proximal DVTs should be treated with anticoagulation for at least 90 days. Indefinite anticoagulation should be given to patients with a history of prior proximal DVT or pulmonary embolism. It should also be considered for an initial unprovoked DVT when the patient is considered at low risk for bleeding complications from anticoagulation. Distal DVTs can be treated with 90 days

FIGURE 45-12. Compressed and noncompressed images, with and without color Doppler, of a normal-paired posterior tibial vein and a paired peroneal vein in the mid-calf. PA, peroneal artery; PTA, posterior tibial artery; PTV, posterior tibial vein; PV, peroneal vein.

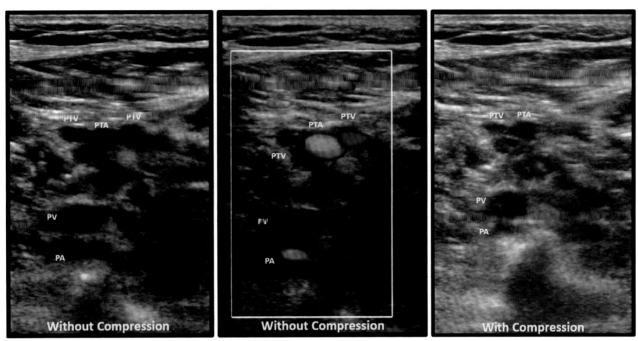

FIGURE 45-13. Compressed and noncompressed images, with and without color Doppler, of a paired posterior tibial vein and single peroneal vein in the mid-calf. The posterior tibial vein on the left of the artery in the image and the peroneal veins are thrombosed and noncompressible. They also have no flow demonstrated on color Doppler. PA, peroneal artery; PTA, posterior tibial artery; PTV, posterior tibial vein; PV, peroneal vein.

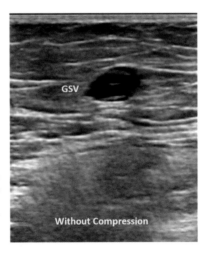
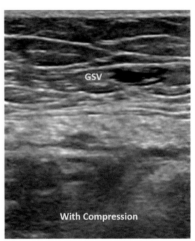

FIGURE 45-14. A thrombosed superficial vein, also known as superficial thrombophlebitis. Here, the greater saphenous vein can be seen with echogenic material in the lumen and to be noncompressible. Superficial veins usually run in the subcutaneous tissue and do not have paired arteries. GSV, greater saphenous vein.

TABLE 45-2 Pretest Probability of Deep Venous Thrombosis	
Finding	**Score**
Active cancer (patient receiving treatment for cancer within the previous 6 mo or currently receiving palliative treatment)	1
Paralysis, paresis, or recent plaster immobilization of the lower extremities	1
Recently bedridden for 3 d or more, or major surgery within the previous 12 wk requiring general or regional anesthesia	1
Localized tenderness along the distribution of the deep venous system	1
Entire leg swollen	1
Calf swelling at least 3 cm larger than that on the asymptomatic side (measured 10 cm below tibial tuberosity)	1
Pitting edema confined to the symptomatic leg	1
Collateral superficial veins (nonvaricose)	1
Previously documented deep-vein thrombosis	1
Alternative diagnosis at least as likely as deep-vein thrombosis	−2

A score of 2 or higher is considered high risk. A score of less than 2 is low risk.

From Wells PS, Anderson DR, Rodger M, et al. Evaluation of D-dimer in the diagnosis of suspected deep-vein thrombosis. *N Engl J Med.* 2003;349(13):1227-1235. Copyright © 2003 Massachusetts Medical Society. Reprinted with permission from Massachusetts Medical Society.

of anticoagulation if they are significantly symptomatic or if the patient is high risk for progression to a proximal DVT. Otherwise the patient can be followed with ultrasound every 1 to 2 weeks to rule out proximal progression. Superficial thrombophlebitis is treated with aspirin, unless it affects a segment of superficial vein longer than 5 cm or is within 5 cm of a junction with a deep vein, in which case it is treated with 30 days of anticoagulation (**Figure 45-15** and **Table 45-3**).

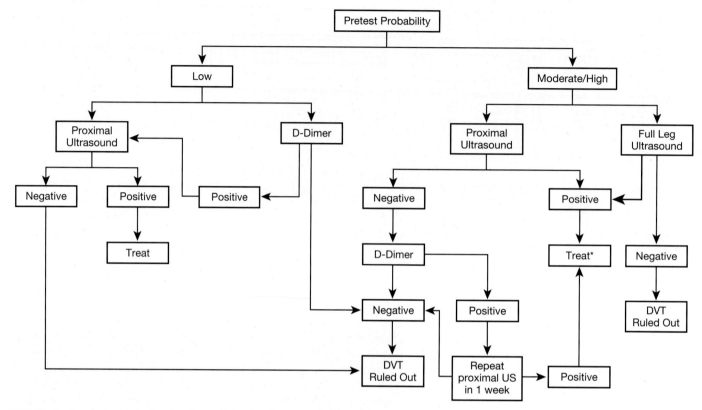

FIGURE 45-15. An algorithm for the diagnosis and treatment of deep venous thrombosis.

TABLE 45-3	Recommendations for Treatment of Thromboses
Type of Thrombosis	**Treatment**
Proximal DVT	Anticoagulation for 90 d or long term if high risk for recurrence or prior thrombosis
Distal DVT	Generally, not treated. Consider 90 d of anticoagulation if they are significantly symptomatic or if the patient is at a high risk for progression to a proximal DVT
Superficial thrombophlebitis	Aspirin, unless it affects a segment of superficial vein longer than 5 cm or is within 5 cm of a junction with a deep vent, in which case it is treated with 30 d of anticoagulation

Abbreviation: DVT, deep venous thrombosis.

Reprinted from Bates SM, Jaeschke R, Stevens SM, et al. Diagnosis of DVT: antithrombotic therapy and prevention of thrombosis, 9th ed: American College of Chest Physicians evidence-based clinical practice guidelines. *Chest.* 2012;141(2 suppl):e351S-e418S. Copyright © 2012 The American College of Chest Physicians. With permission.

PEARLS AND PITFALLS

Pearls

- Use Color Doppler to help visualize vessels and differentiate arteries from veins. Veins are normally low flow and it may be difficult to visualize color changes within them. Try augmenting flow by squeezing the patient's calf muscles or having the patient contract the calves by plantar-flexing the ankle.

- Deeper vessels can be difficult to visualize, especially in obese patients or those with large amounts of edema. In these instances, use a lower frequency, or switch to the curvilinear probe.
- If veins are small or difficult to visualize, have the patient place the lower extremities in a more dependent position by sitting more upright or hanging the feet over the edge of the examination table. This will increase venous pooling and enlarge the diameter of the veins.

Pearls and Pitfalls, Continued

- Chronic DVTs can sometimes be differentiated from acute DVTs by some of their ultrasonographic characteristics. Acute DVTs tend to cause the vein to enlarge, to be only loosely attached to the vein wall (or free floating) and to deform slightly with compression. Chronic DVTs tend to be small, to be well incorporated into the vein wall with wall thickening, to have irregular margins, and to have recanalized channels running through them.

Pitfalls

- The most common mistake made by novices is nonvisualization of the popliteal vein. Be sure not to mistake a lymph node or the tibial nerve for the vein. Color Doppler can be used to help differentiate as mentioned in the pearl section.
- There are several perforating veins branching from the popliteal vein in the popliteal fossa proximal to the trifurcation. These include the gastrocnemius deep veins and small saphenous veins superficial veins. Be sure to follow these proximally as they will be seen branching from the larger popliteal vein.

The popliteal vein will lie inferiorly and medially relative to the popliteal artery proximal to the branching of these perforating veins.

- Veins are normally easy to collapse. Be sure not to apply too much pressure when first searching for a vein or it will be collapsed and unable to be visualized.
- Be sure to compress veins from directly above with a perpendicular angle to the probe. Veins visualized from more acute or oblique angles will be difficult to compress and could result in false-positive results.
- Normal variations in the popliteal vein anatomy are relatively common. It can be duplicated or trifurcated proximal or distal to the popliteal fossae. It can also be located deep to the popliteal vein. Color Doppler can be used to differentiate the vein from the artery if there is doubt.
- A noncollapsible, thrombosed vein can be mistaken for an artery, and if enough pressure is applied, the normal artery can be collapsed and mistaken for the vein. Arteries are difficult to collapse and will begin to pulsate as they are compressed.

BILLING

CPT Code	Description	Global Payment	Professional Component	Technical Component
93970	Duplex scan of extremity veins including responses to compression and other maneuvers; complete bilateral study	$188.79	$35.82	$152.96
93971	Duplex scan of extremity veins including responses to compression and other maneuvers; unilateral or limited study	$114.63	$22.93	$91.71

CPT codes and average national reimbursement for Medicare in 2016. Payment data are from https://www.cms.gov/apps/physician-fee-schedule/search/search-criteria.aspx. See Chapter 2 for details on ultrasound billing.

References

1. Cushman M, Tsai AW, White RH, et al. Deep vein thrombosis and pulmonary embolism in two cohorts: the longitudinal investigation of thromboembolism etiology. *Am J Med.* 2004;117(1):19-25.
2. Schulman S, Wåhlander K, Lundström T, Clason SB, Eriksson H. Secondary prevention of venous thromboembolism with the oral direct thrombin inhibitor ximelagatran. *N Engl J Med.* 2003;349(18):1713-1721.
3. Mattos MA, Melendres G, Sumner DS, et al. Prevalence and distribution of calf vein thrombosis in patients with symptomatic deep venous thrombosis: a color-flow duplex study. *J Vasc Surg.* 1996;24(5):738-744.
4. Bates SM, Jaeschke R, Stevens SM, et al. Diagnosis of DVT: antithrombotic therapy and prevention of thrombosis, 9th ed: American College of Chest Physicians evidence-based clinical practice guidelines. *Chest.* 2012;141(2 suppl):e351S-e418S.
5. Cronan JJ. History of venous ultrasound. *J Ultrasound Med.* 2003;22(11):1143-1146.
6. Talbot S. Use of real-time imaging in identifying deep venous obstruction: a preliminary report. *Bruit.* 1982;(7):41-42.
7. Raghavendra BN, Rosen RJ, Lam S, Riles T, Horii SC. Deep venous thrombosis: detection by high-resolution real-time ultrasonography. *Radiology.* 1984;152(3):789-793.
8. Raghavendra BN, Horii SC, Hilton S, Subramanyam BR, Rosen RJ, Lam S. Deep venous thrombosis: detection by probe compression of veins. *J Ultrasound Med.* 1986;5(2):89-95.
9. Lensing AW, Prandoni P, Brandjes D, et al. Detection of deep-vein thrombosis by real-time B-mode ultrasonography. *N Engl J Med.* 1989;320(6):342-345.
10. Philbrick JT, Becker DM. Calf deep venous thrombosis. A wolf in sheep's clothing? *Arch Intern Med.* 1988;148:2131-2138.
11. Birdwell BG, Raskob GE, Whitsett TL, et al. The clinical validity of normal compression ultrasonography in outpatients suspected of having deep venous thrombosis. *Ann Intern Med.* 1998;128(1):1-7.
12. Cogo A, Lensing AW, Koopman MM, et al. Compression ultrasonography for diagnostic management of patients with clinically suspected deep vein thrombosis: prospective cohort study. *BMJ.* 1998;316(7124):17-20.
13. Wells PS, Anderson DR, Bormanis J, et al. Value of assessment of pretest probability of deep-vein thrombosis in clinical management. *Lancet.* 1997;350(9094):1795-1798.
14. Fancher TL, White RH, Kravitz RL. Combined use of rapid D-dimer testing and estimation of clinical probability in the diagnosis of deep vein thrombosis: systematic review. *BMJ.* 2004;329(7470):821.
15. Tick LW, Ton E, Van Voorthuizen T, et al. Practical diagnostic management of patients with clinically suspected deep vein thrombosis by clinical probability test, compression ultrasonography, and D-dimer test. *Am J Med.* 2002;113(8):630-635.
16. Bernardi E, Camporese G, Büller HR, et al; Erasmus Study Group. Serial 2-point ultrasonography plus D-dimer vs whole-leg color-coded Doppler ultrasonography for diagnosing suspected symptomatic deep vein thrombosis. *JAMA.* 2008;300(14):1653-1659.
17. Stevens SM, Woller SC, Graves KK, et al. Withholding anticoagulation following a single negative whole-leg ultrasound in patients at high pretest probability for deep vein thrombosis. *Clin Appl Thromb Hemost.* 2013;19(1):79-85.
18. Trottier SJ, Todi S, Veremakis C. Validation of an inexpensive B-mode ultrasound device for detection of deep vein thrombosis. *Chest.* 1996;110(6):1547-1550.
19. Blaivas M, Lambert MJ, Harwood RA, Wood JP, Konicki J. Lower-extremity Doppler for deep venous thrombosis—can emergency physicians be accurate and fast? *Acad Emerg Med.* 2000;7:120-126.

20. Crisp JG, Lovato LM, Jang TB. Compression ultrasonography of the lower extremity with portable vascular ultrasonography can accurately detect deep venous thrombosis in the emergency department. *Ann Emerg Med.* 2010;56(6):601-610.

21. Blaivas M. Point-of-care ultrasonographic deep venous thrombosis evaluation after just ten minutes' training: Is this offer too good to be true? *Ann Emerg Med.* 2010;56(6):611-613.

22. Cogo A, Lensing AW, Prandoni P, Hirsh J. Distribution of thrombosis in patients with symptomatic deep vein thrombosis. *Arch Intern Med.* 1993;153:2777-2780.

23. Frederick MG, Hertzberg BS, Kliewer MA, et al. Can the US examination for lower extremity deep venous thrombosis be abbreviated? A prospective study of 755 examinations. *Radiology.* 1996;199(1):45-47.

24. Maki DD, Kumar N, Nguyen B, et al. Distribution of thrombi in acute lower extremity deep venous thrombosis: implications for sonography and CT and MR venography. *AJR Am J Roentgenol.* 2000;175(5):1299-1301.

25. Caronia J, Sarzynski A, Tofighi B, et al. Resident performed two-point compression ultrasound is inadequate for diagnosis of deep vein thrombosis in the critically ill. *J Thromb Thrombolysis.* 2014;37(3):298-302.

26. Adhikari S, Zeger W, Thom C, Fields JM. Isolated deep venous thrombosis: implications for 2-point compression ultrasonography of the lower extremity. *Ann Emerg Med.* 2015;66:262-266.

27. Zitek T, Baydoun J, Yepez S, Forred W, Slattery DE, Budhram G. Mistakes and pitfalls associated with two-point compression ultrasound for deep vein thrombosis. *West J Emerg Med.* 2016;17(2):201-208.

28. Heijboer H, Cogo A, Büller HR, Prandoni P, Wouter ten Cate J. Detection of plethysmography and real-time compression ultrasonography in hospitalized patients. *Arch Intern Med.* 1992;9(152):1901-1903.

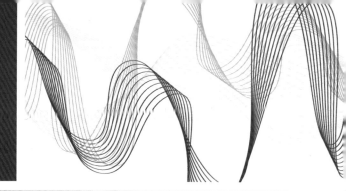

CHAPTER

46

What Is the Patient's Central Venous Pressure?

Matthew Fentress, MD

Clinical Vignette

A 63-year-old obese man with congestive heart failure (CHF) and chronic obstructive pulmonary disease (COPD) presents with shortness of breath and cough for 3 days. There is no history of fever or chills. His medications include a diuretic, β-blocker, angiotensin-converting enzyme inhibitor, and inhalers for his COPD. Blood pressure and pulse are normal, oxygen saturation is 96%, and weight is unchanged from the last known one 3 months prior. His body habitus makes it difficult for jugular venous pulse (JVP) to appreciate. Lung examination shows faint bilateral wheezes without crackles, and lower extremities show trace bilateral edema, all of which are relatively stable for this patient. You consider increasing his diuretic dose for a mild CHF exacerbation. What is the patient's central venous pressure?

LITERATURE REVIEW

Ultrasound-based inferior vena cava (IVC) measurements and their relationship to right atrial pressure (RAP) were first described in 1979.[1,2] Central venous pressure (CVP) is synonymous with RAP in the absence of vena cava obstruction,[1] and its measurement— either by physical examination, echocardiography, or central venous catheter—is often considered a critical tool for the accurate assessment of intravascular volume. Physical examination findings can be difficult to interpret, and accurate fluid assessment is often enhanced by a combination of history, physical examination, laboratory, and radiographic findings.[3-7] Although it does not provide a direct measure of circulating blood volume, CVP is frequently used in clinical practice as a surrogate for intravascular volume status, and historically has been used in critically ill hospitalized patients to guide fluid management.[8] CVP estimation via a central venous catheter is the gold standard for evaluating RAP,[1] but is not an option in the outpatient setting. Therefore, the estimation of CVP with point-of-care ultrasound of the IVC can add valuable information to the clinical volume assessment in an outpatient setting.

CVP may be estimated with ultrasound by combining two IVC measurements, (1) the maximum IVC diameter and (2) the respiratory variation, often expressed as the IVC collapsibility index

(IVCCI). The IVC collapsibility index, sometimes also called the caval index, is defined as the difference between the maximum and minimum IVC diameters divided by the maximum IVC diameter, often expressed as a percentage (**Figure 46-1**). The IVC is a highly compliant blood vessel whose size is easily altered by changes in CVP and intravascular volume. Inspiratory effort creates negative intrathoracic pressure, which, in turn, increases right ventricular diastolic filling, increases capacitance in the pulmonary vasculature, and effectively increases right ventricular cardiac output. The combined effect increases blood flow from the IVC to the right atrium, and the IVC, therefore, tends to collapse during inspiration.

The current body of evidence from the cardiology, emergency medicine, and critical care literature overall supports IVC ultrasound as a safe, accessible, noninvasive, and reliable tool for estimating CVP (**Table 46-1**). In general, a dilated IVC with minimal respiratory variation is associated with elevated CVP, whereas a narrow IVC with significant respiratory variation is associated with low CVP. A large systematic review by Ciozda et al in 2016, which included 21 studies with a total of 1430 combined patients, found consistent correlations between IVC measurements and CVP.[9] The authors concluded, "Sonographic measurement of IVC diameter and collapsibility is a valid method of estimating CVP and RAP. Given the ease, safety, and availability of this non-invasive technique, broader adoption and application of this method in clinical settings is warranted." A joint consensus statement in 2010 from the American Society of Echocardiography and the American College of Emergency Physicians (ASE and ACEP) also endorsed the use of focused bedside cardiac ultrasound for intravascular volume assessment, among other cardiac parameters.[10] IVCCI correlation to CVP is reportedly strongest at low (<20%) and high (>60%) values, suggesting that the closer IVCCI is to 0% or 100%, the more likely the patient is to be volume-overloaded or volume-depleted, respectively.[11] However, many studies have used an IVCCI threshold of 50% as a marker of low or high CVP. For instance, IVCCI greater than 50% has been

$$IVCCI = \frac{IVC\ Diameter\ Maximum - IVC\ Diameter\ Minimum}{IVC\ Diameter\ Maximum} \times 100$$

FIGURE 46-1. Calculation for IVCCI. IVC, inferior vena cava; IVCCI, IVC collapsibility index.

associated with CVP less than 10 mm Hg in one study, whereas IVCCI less than 50% was associated with CVP greater than 10 mm Hg.[12] Another study similarly found that IVCCI greater than 50% was a strong predictor of CVP less than 8 mm Hg, with an NPV of 96%.[13] Novices with less than 1 hour of training in this examination can achieve 90% accuracy after only 21 practice examinations.[14]

Despite good overall evidence supporting the utility of IVC to estimate CVP, and widespread clinical use, the optimal technique for IVC measurement has not been established.[15] Most studies measure the IVC in the longitudinal plane approximately 2 to 4 cm caudal to the right atrial junction. This is generally supported by the ASE guideline,[16] which recommends measuring the IVC in its long axis via the subcostal window, just caudal to the hepatic veins that lie approximately 0.5 to 3.0 cm caudal to the right atrial junction. However, there is scant high-quality evidence that demonstrates the superiority of one sampling location over another. One study found good correlation between IVC measurements taken 2 cm caudal from the hepatic vein and at the level of the left renal vein, but poor correlation of those taken at the IVC-atrial junction, concluding that the IVC should not be measured at the IVC-atrial junction.[17] Respirophasic variation of the IVC is usually measured during passive respiration, but some influential studies and guidelines have advocated use of a "sniff" maneuver in which the patient forcibly inhales,[16,18] and one study has shown that this maneuver improves accuracy.[19] In addition, the "eye-ball" estimation method may be as reliable as measuring with calipers.[20] Many studies use M-mode to measure IVC collapsibility, but it is possible that this practice introduces unintended variability. The IVC moves an average of 21.7 mm in a craniocaudal direction during respiration,[21] which means that measurements taken along a fixed M-mode line during respiration could actually be measuring two completely different sections of the IVC. In addition, it may also not always be possible to measure the true perpendicular diameter using the M-mode cursor, further contributing to inaccuracies. For these reasons, routine use of M-mode to obtain IVC measurements should generally be avoided, especially for novices.

There are several further limitations to the use of IVC to estimate CVP. Several patient factors can cause IVC enlargement in the absence of concomitantly increased CVP including large body surface area, athletic training, prominent Eustachian valve, narrowing of the IVC-RA junction, and web or tissue present in the IVC.[1] Furthermore, certain conditions may cause increased RAP, and therefore increased CVP, without necessarily increasing total intravascular volume, such as tachycardia and tricuspid regurgitation,[22] as well as cardiac tamponade and massive pulmonary embolism. The clinician should be aware of these potential limitations and alternative diagnoses.

IVC assessment with point-of-care ultrasound, as an adjunct to the clinical volume status examination, has been studied for the management of heart failure in the inpatient and outpatient settings.[18,20,23,24] One study of outpatients with heart failure identified discrepancies between ultrasound and physical examination volume assessment in nearly one-third of participants, and also found that novices with ultrasound were better able to predict hospital admission risk than experts with clinical assessment alone.[20] Furthermore, the presence of hypervolemia on both clinical examination and IVC ultrasound was more predictive of emergency room (ER) visit or hospital admission than either examination alone, suggesting that even experts

may be more accurate if they add IVC ultrasound to their clinical assessment. Another study that followed patients admitted into the hospital with heart failure exacerbations found that IVC size and collapsibility on discharge was a significant predictor of hospital readmission, even outperforming physical examination parameters and routine laboratory studies such as renal function.[25] Outpatient IVC measurements have also been used to assess dry weight and fluid status in dialysis patients,[22,26,27] and have demonstrated prognostic significance in heart failure patients.[28]

In recent years, there has been debate over several aspects of IVC ultrasound, ranging from basic questions about how to properly measure the IVC, to questions about the clinical utility of these measurements. For instance, some studies have questioned the ability of CVP to predict fluid responsiveness, and the relationship between CVP and blood volume.[29,30] The reliability of IVC measurements to predict CVP in critically ill patients has also been called into question by several studies.[31,32] For the outpatient clinician, it is worth noting that these studies were largely performed in hospitalized and perioperative patients, not in an outpatient population. Furthermore, the studies usually focused on the assessment of *fluid responsiveness* in critically ill patients and not on volume assessment for diuretic management in heart failure patients.

Overall, the literature suggests that point-of-care ultrasound of the IVC to estimate CVP and inform fluid management in the outpatient setting can be a very useful adjunct to the clinical assessment. However, robust data on the scale of a systematic review or meta-analysis is still lacking, and more research is still needed to clarify the optimal role for IVC ultrasound in the outpatient setting.

TABLE 46-1	Recommendations for Use of Point- of-Care Ultrasound in Clinical Practice		
Recommendation		**Rating**	**References**
Point-of-care ultrasound measurement of inferior vena cava diameter and respiratory variation may be used to estimate central venous pressure in the outpatient setting.		C	9, 11-13, 34

A = consistent, good-quality patient-oriented evidence; B = inconsistent or limited-quality patient-oriented evidence; C = consensus, disease-oriented evidence, usual practice, expert opinion, or case series. For information about the SORT evidence rating system, go to http://www.aafp.org/afpsort.

PERFORMING THE SCAN

1. **Preparation.** Place the patient in the supine position and arrange the ultrasound equipment to the right of the patient. Select a low-frequency (2.5-5 mHz) phased array or a curvilinear transducer. The examination may be completed in the "cardiac" or "abdomen" mode. Note that if it is performed in the Cardiac mode, the probe marker will appear on the right side of the screen and the image will be flipped right to left on the screen compared with the Abdomen mode. Images obtained in both modes are used in this chapter.

2. **Identify the IVC.** Obtain a subxiphoid view of the heart (see Chapters 8-11 for further details on cardiac imaging). Bring the right atrium into the center of the screen. Rotate the probe

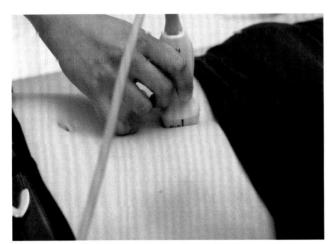

FIGURE 46-2. Patient position and probe placement for imaging the inferior vena cava.

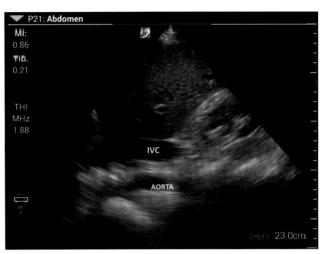

FIGURE 46-4. The inferior vena cava (IVC) visualized via the coronal transhepatic window. Notice that in this view the IVC and aorta are visualized together. The IVC is the vessel visualized closer to the top of the screen. In these images, the abdominal convention is being used—the probe marker is to the left which corresponds with the cranial end of the patient.

90° and point it toward the ground, so it is perpendicular to the patient's body, with the marker pointing toward the patient's head (**Figure 46-2**). Rock the probe toward the patient's head to obtain a longitudinal view of the IVC emptying into the right atrium (**Figure 46-3**). The IVC will be seen as a thin-walled, intrahepatic, tubular structure that connects directly with the right atrium. The hepatic vein will also be seen emptying into the IVC approximately 0.5 to 3 cm caudal to the right atrial junction. If the IVC is not immediately seen, fan the probe gradually from right to left until it comes into view. The aorta may easily be confused with the IVC. The aorta is thick-walled, pulsatile, lies to the left of the IVC, and does not connect directly to the right atrium. If the IVC is difficult to image clearly in the subxiphoid window, an alternate approach is to use the transhepatic coronal window. Start with the same approach used to view Morrison's pouch in the FAST examination (Chapter 50), then scan more anteriorly and cephalad to visualize the IVC coursing alongside the liver[33] (**Figure 46-4**).

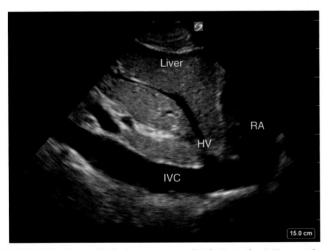

FIGURE 46-3. Normal inferior vena cava (IVC). Note the IVC emptying into the right atrium and the hepatic vein joining the IVC just caudal to the right atrium. In this image, the cardiac convention is being used—the probe marker is to the right which corresponds with the cranial end of the patient. HV, hepatic veins; RA right atrium.

3. **Measure maximum IVC diameter.** Measure the maximum IVC diameter at end-expiration approximately 2 to 3 cm caudal to the right atrial junction, or just caudal to the hepatic vein. This can be accomplished by obtaining a longitudinal image of the IVC emptying into the right atrium, as described earlier. Freeze the image and, if needed, use the cine function to identify the point in the respiratory cycle when the IVC is at its maximum diameter. Use calipers or the "eye ball" method to measure the IVC diameter (**Figure 46-5**). Be certain to measure along the true long-axis of the IVC when using calipers, because measurements obtained even a short distance off-axis can result in a falsely small diameter (**Figure 46-6**).

4. **Measure IVC respiratory variation.** Respiratory variation is evaluated by comparing the maximum (end-expiratory) IVC diameter with the minimum (end-inspiratory) IVC diameter. In clinical practice, many clinicians make a visual assessment of respiratory variation simply by watching the IVC throughout the respiratory cycle. A more precise method involves measuring both the maximum *and* minimum IVC diameters. Using the same longitudinal view of the IVC described earlier to measure the maximum diameter, identify the point in the respiratory cycle when the IVC is at its minimum diameter. Use calipers or the "eye ball" method to measure the minimum diameter of the IVC at approximately the same region where the maximum diameter was measured (**Figure 46-7** and ⏵ **Videos 46-1 and 46-2**). Once again, be certain to measure along the true long-axis of the vessel to maximize accuracy. Respiratory variation can be augmented by having the patient inhale forcibly, also known as the "sniff" maneuver.

5. **Calculate IVCCI.** The IVCCI is the difference between the maximum and minimum diameters divided by the maximum diameter and expressed as a percentage (Figure 46-1). For instance, if the maximum diameter is 1.5 cm, and the minimum diameter is 0.5 cm, the IVCCI is $(1.5 - 0.5)/1.5 = 0.67 = 67\%$. An IVC with nearly complete respiratory collapse will have an IVCCI near 100%, whereas the IVCCI will approach 0% when the IVC has minimal respiratory collapse.

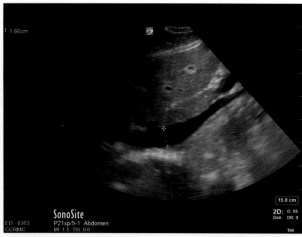 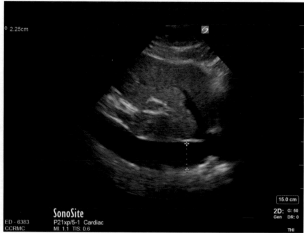

FIGURE 46-5. A, Normal inferior vena cava (IVC) at maximum diameter during end-expiration. The diameter is 1.66 cm. In this image, the abdominal convention is being used—the probe marker is to the left which corresponds with the cranial end of the patient. B, Plethoric IVC at maximum diameter during end-expiration. The diameter is 2.25 cm. In this image, the cardiac convention is being used—the probe marker is to the right which corresponds with the cranial end of the patient.

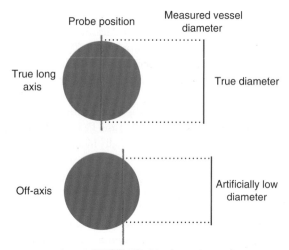

FIGURE 46-6. Effects of imaging off-axis. If a two-dimensional plane of the IVC is taken off the midline, then the diameter may appear falsely smaller.

PATIENT MANAGEMENT

Bedside ultrasound of the IVC may be performed as an adjunct to the physical examination in any outpatient whose fluid assessment remains uncertain after initial evaluation, and in whom accurate fluid assessment guides next steps in proper management. A common example is a patient with chronic heart failure in whom the physical examination is equivocal and whose care will be improved by appropriate diuretic titration. It should be viewed as one piece of diagnostic information among many and must always be incorporated with essential facets of the history, physical examination, and available labs or imaging to assess a patient's fluid status. A suggested patient management algorithm for using IVC ultrasound for CHF management can be found in **Figure 46-8**.

If the maximum IVC measures greater than 2.1 cm in diameter and has an IVCCI of less than 50%, this patient has a high estimated

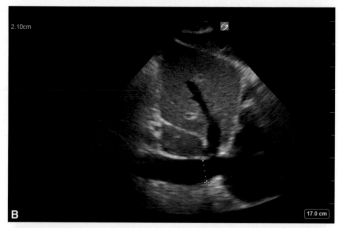

FIGURE 46-7. Respirophasic variation of a plethoric inferior vena cava (IVC). A, Here, the IVC is measured at end-expiration and is 2.82 cm. B, Here, the IVC is measured at inspiration and is 2.10 cm. This corresponds to an IVC collapsibility index >50%. In these images, the abdominal convention is being used—the probe marker is to the left which corresponds with the cranial end of the patient.

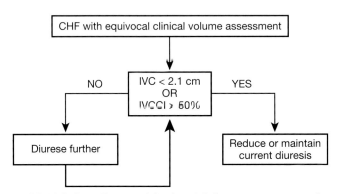

FIGURE 46-8. IVC ultrasound for heart failure management algorithm. CHF, congestive heart failure; IVC, inferior vena cava; IVCCI, IVC collapsibility index.

CVP of more than 10 mm Hg (Table 46-1). This patient is likely hypervolemic and may be further diuresed. There are multiple causes of increased right atrial pressure besides hypervolemia, including cardiac tamponade, massive pulmonary embolism, pulmonary hypertension, and mitral regurgitation, which could produce a similar IVC appearance.

If the IVC measures less than or equal to 2.1 cm in diameter and has an IVCCI of more than 50%, this patient is likely euvolemic or hypovolemic with a CVP in the low range of 0 to 5 mm Hg (**Table 46-2**). This patient is not likely to benefit from further diuresis, and depending on the clinical context, may require a reduction in diuretic dosing.

If the IVC findings are outside of these parameters—ie, diameter >2.1 cm with IVCCI greater than 50%, or diameter ≤2.1 cm with IVCCI less than 50%—the estimated CVP falls in the intermediate range of 5 to 10 mm Hg (Table 46-2). Echocardiographers can use secondary echocardiography signs of elevated RAP to more precisely estimate a patient's CVP when the IVC findings fall in this intermediate zone, but this is generally beyond the scope of point-of-care ultrasound clinicians.

As discussed earlier, there is some debate about the utility of point-of-care IVC ultrasound for CVP estimation and clinical decision-making. It is not a perfect test, and further research is still needed. Yet given its safety, evidence base, accessibility and ease of use, it may have a role as an extension of the physical examination for fluid status assessment and offers the potential to improve diagnosis and treatment in the outpatient setting.

PEARLS AND PITFALLS

Pearls

- Make sure to visualize the hepatic vein entering the IVC, and the IVC entering the right atrium, to avoid confusion with the aorta.
- If the IVC is difficult to visualize via the subcostal approach because of body habitus or overlying bowel gas, try to visualize it via a transhepatic coronal approach. Position your probe in the same position used to evaluate Morrison's Pouch during the FAST examination (Figure 46-4).
- Place one to two fingers from the hand, holding the ultrasound probe on the patient's body to help steady it. This will minimize out-of-plane movement during patient respiration, especially if the "sniff test" is used.

Pitfalls

- Do not mistake the aorta for the IVC. The aorta is thick-walled, pulsatile, does not connect to the right atrium, and lies to the left of the IVC. Color Doppler may be used to help distinguish IVC from aorta if in doubt.
- Avoid routine use of M-mode to measure IVC collapsibility, because the craniocaudal movement of the IVC during respiration could cause these measurements to be inaccurate.
- Beware that measurements obtained even a small distance off-axis can result in falsely low measurements (Figure 46-6).
- A dilated, noncollapsing IVC can occur in settings other than intravascular volume overload, such as cardiac tamponade, mitral regurgitation, and aortic sclerosis.

BILLING

Reimbursement for focused ultrasound of the IVC

CPT Code	Description	Global Payment	Professional Component	Technical Component
93979	Duplex scan of inferior vena cava, limited study	$178.66	$25.42	$153.24

CPT codes and average national reimbursement for Medicare in 2016. Payment data are from https://www.cms.gov/apps/physician-fee-schedule/search/search-criteria.aspx. See Chapter 2 for details on ultrasound billing.

TABLE 46-2	Estimation of CVP by IVC Diameter and Collapse	
	IVC Diameter <2.1 cm	IVC Diameter ≥2.1 cm
IVC collapse < 50%	Low normal (0-5 cm H$_2$O)	Normal (5-10 cm H$_2$O)
IVC collapse ≥ 50%	Normal (5-10 cm H$_2$O)	Elevated (>10 cm H$_2$O)

Abbreviations: CVP, central venous pressure; IVC, inferior vena cava.
Adapted from Rudski LG, Lai WW, Afilalo J, et al. Guidelines for the echocardiographic assessment of the right heart in adults: a report from the American Society of Echocardiography endorsed by the European Association of Echocardiography, a registered branch of the European Society of Cardiology, and the Canadian Society of Echocardiography. *J Am Soc Echocardiogr.* 2010;23(7):685-713. Copyright © 2010 by the American Society of Echocardiography. With permission.

References

1. Beigel R, Cercek B, Luo H, Siegel RJ. Noninvasive evaluation of right atrial pressure. *J Am Soc Echocardiogr.* 2013;26:1033-1042.

2. Natori H, Tamaki S, Kira S. Ultrasonographic evaluation of ventilatory effect on inferior vena caval configuration. *Am Rev Respir Dis.* 1979;120(2):421-427.

3. Wang CS, FitzGerald JM, Schulzer M, Mak E, Ayas NT. Does this dyspneic patient in the emergency department have congestive heart failure? *JAMA.* 2005;294(15):1944-1956.

4. Hanson J, Lam SW, Alam S, et al. The reliability of the physical examination to guide fluid therapy in adults with severe falciparum malaria: an observational study. *Malar J.* 2013;12:348.

5. Saugel B, Kirsche SV, Hapfelmeier A, et al. Prediction of fluid responsiveness in patients admitted to the medical intensive care unit. *J Crit Care.* 2013;28(4):537.e1-537.e9.

6. Demeria DD, MacDougall A, Spurek M, et al. Comparison of clinical measurement of jugular venous pressure versus measured central venous pressure. *Chest.* 2004;126:747S.

7. McGee S, Abernethy WB III, Simel DL. The rational clinical examination. Is this patient hypovolemic? *JAMA.* 1999;281(11):1022-1029.

8. Boldt J, Lenz M, Kumle B, Papsdorf M. Volume replacement strategies on intensive care units: results from a postal survey. *Intensive Care Med.* 1998;24:147-151.

9. Ciozda W, Kedan I, Kehl DW, Zimmer R, Khandwalla R, Kimchi A. The efficacy of sonographic measurement of inferior vena cava diameter as an estimate of central venous pressure. *Cardiovasc Ultrasound.* 2016;14:33.

10. Labovitz A, Noble VE, Bierig M, et al. Focused cardiac ultrasound in the emergent setting: a consensus statement of the American Society of Echocardiography and American College of Emergency Physicians. American Society of Echocardiography Consensus Statement. *J Am Soc Echocardiogr.* 2010;23(12):1225-1230. doi:10.1016/j.echo.2010.10.005.

11. Stawicki SP, Braslow BM, Panebianco NL, et al. Intensivist use of hand-carried ultrasonography to measure IVC collapsibility in estimating intravascular volume status: correlations with CVP. *J Am Coll Surg.* 2009;209(1):55-61.

12. Kircher BJ, Himelman RB, Schiller NB. Noninvasive estimation of right atrial pressure from the inspiratory collapse of the inferior vena cava. *Am J Cardiol.* 1990;66(4):493-496.

13. Nagdev AD, Merchant RC, Tirado-Gonzalez A, Sisson CA, Murphy MC. Emergency department bedside ultrasonographic measurement of the caval index for noninvasive determination of low central venous pressure. *Ann Emerg Med.* 2010;55(3):290-295.

14. Gómez Betancourt M, Moreno-Montoya J, Barragan-Gonzalez AM, Ovalle JC, Bustos Martinez YF. Learning process and improvement of point-of-care ultrasound technique for subxiphoid visualization of the inferior vena cava. *Crit Ultrasound J.* 2016;8:4.

15. Stone MB, Huang JV. Inferior vena cava assessment; correlation with CVP and plethora in tamponade. *Glob Heart.* 2013;8(4):323-327.

16. Rudski LG, Lai WW, Afilalo J, et al. Guidelines for the echocardiographic assessment of the right heart in adults: a report from the American Society of Echocardiography endorsed by the European Association of Echocardiography, a registered branch of the European Society of Cardiology, and the Canadian Society of Echocardiography. *J Am Soc Echocardiogr.* 2010;23(7):685-713. doi:10.1016/j.echo.2010.05.01.

17. Wallace DJ, Allison M, Stone MB. Inferior vena cava percentage collapse during respiration is affected by the sampling location: an ultrasound study in healthy volunteers. *Acad Emerg Med.* 2010;17:96-99.

18. Perera P, Mailhot T, Riley D, Mandavia D. The RUSH exam: Rapid Ultrasound in SHock in the evaluation of the critically ill. *Emerg Med Clin North Am.* 2010;28:29-56.

19. Brennan JM, Blair JE, Goonewardena S, et al. Reappraisal of the use of inferior vena cava for estimating right atrial pressure. *J Am Soc Echocardiogr.* 2007;20:857-861.

20. Saha NM, Barbat JJ, Fedson S, Anderson A, Rich JD, Spencer KT. Outpatient use of focused cardiac ultrasound to assess the inferior vena cava in patients with heart failure. *Am J Cardiol.* 2015;116(8):1224-1228.

21. Blehar DJ, Resop D, Chin B, Dayno M, Gaspari R. Inferior vena cava displacement during respirophasic ultrasound imaging. *Crit Ultrasound J.* 2012;4:18.

22. Mandelbaum A, Ritz E. Vena cava diameter measurement for estimation of dry weight in haemodialysis patients. *Nephrol Dial Transplant.* 1996;11(supp2):24-27.

23. Gundersen GH, Norekval TM, Haug HH, et al. Adding point of care ultrasound to assess volume status in heart failure patients in a nurse-led outpatient clinic. A randomised study. *Heart.* 2016;102:29-34.

24. Dalen H, Gundersen GH, Skjetne K, et al. Feasibility and reliability of pocket-size ultrasound examinations of the pleural cavities and vena cava inferior performed by nurses in an outpatient heart failure clinic. *Eur J Cardiovasc Nurs.* 2015;14(4):286-293.

25. Goonewardena SN, Gemignani A, Ronan A, et al. Comparison of hand-carried ultrasound assessment of the inferior vena cava and N-terminal pro-brain natriuretic peptide for predicting readmission after hospitalization for acute decompensated heart failure. *JACC Cardiovasc Imaging.* 2008;1(5):595-601.

26. Yanagiba S, Ando Y, Kusano E, Asano Y. Utility of the inferior vena cava diameter as a marker of dry weight in nonoliguric hemo- dialyzed patients. *ASAIO J.* 2001;47:528-532.

27. Brennan JM, Ronan A, Goonewardena S, et al. Hand carried ultrasound measurement of the inferior vena cava for assessment of intravascular volume status in the outpatient hemodialysis clinic. *Clin J Am Soc Nephrol.* 2006;1:749-753.

28. Pellicori P, Carubelli V, Zhang J, et al. IVC diameter in patients with chronic heart failure: relationships and prognosis. *JACC Cardiovasc Imaging.* 2013;6(1):16-28.

29. Marik PE, Baram M, Vahid B. Does central venous pressure predict fluid responsiveness? A systematic review of the literature and the tale of seven mares. *Chest.* 2008;134(1):172-178.

30. Marik PE, Cavallazzi R. Does the central venous pressure predict fluid responsiveness? An updated meta-analysis and a plea for some common sense. *Crit Care Med.* 2013;41:1774-1781.

31. Alavi-Moghaddam M, Kabir A, Shojaee M, Manouchehrifar M, Moghimi M. Ultrasonography of inferior vena cava to determine central venous pressure: a meta-analysis and meta-regression. *Acta Radiol.* 2016;58:537:541.

32. Ng L, Khine H, Taragin BH, Avner JR, Ushay M, Nunez D. Does bedside sonographic measurement of the inferior vena cava diameter correlate with central venous pressure in the assessment of intravascular volume in children? *Pediatr Emerg Care.* 2013;29(3):337-341.

33. Kulkarni AP, Janarthanan S, Harish MM, et al. Agreement between inferior vena cava diameter measurements by subxiphoid versus transhepatic views. *Indian J Crit Care Med.* 2015;19(12):719-722.

34. Dipti A, Soucy Z, Surana A, Chandra S. Role of inferior vena cava diameter in assessment of volume status: a meta-analysis. *Am J Emerg Med.* 2012;30(8):1414-1419.

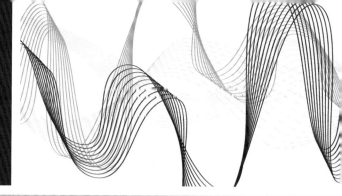

Does the Patient Have an Abdominal Aortic Aneurysm?

Neil Jayasekera, MD and Naman Shah, MD, PhD

Clinical Vignette

With the encouragement of family members, a 65-year-old man with a long-term smoking history and consequent chronic obstructive pulmonary disease (COPD) presents to clinic for a "checkup." He has not seen a doctor in 15 years. He feels tired but otherwise has no medical complaints and is in stable condition. Other than having findings consistent with COPD, his physical examination is unremarkable. A review of the US Preventive Services Task Force (USPSTF) guidelines recommends screening this patient for an abdominal aortic aneurysm (AAA). Does the patient have an abdominal aortic aneurysm?

LITERATURE REVIEW

About 10,000 to 15,000 people a year in the United States die from complications of an AAA.[1] AAAs are focal dilatations of the aorta at least 50% greater than the normal vessel size. Generally, a diameter of >3 cm is used as the cutoff for the diagnosis of AAA. Once present, AAAs will continue to expand, though the rate of expansion can vary greatly and is influenced by underlying risk factors. Risk factors for AAAs include age, male sex, smoking, hypertension, atherosclerosis, hyperlipidemia, family history, and connective tissue disorders such as Marfan and Ehlers-Danlos syndromes. The most important modifiable risk factor is smoking. Smokers are 3 to 5 times more likely to develop an AAA than nonsmokers.[2]

The most concerning complication of AAAs is rupture. When AAAs rupture, mortality rates are as high as 80% to 95%.[3] Rupture rates in asymptomatic patients with AAAs depend on the size, rate of expansion, and location of the aneurysm. The greatest risk factor in an asymptomatic patient is an AAA diameter that exceeds 5.0 cm.[3] At this size, the risk for rupture exceeds the risk of mortality from elective surgical repair. Elective surgical repair is associated with mortality rates of 5%. If an AAA becomes symptomatic, mortality rates for emergent surgical repair are as high as 50%.[3] Thus, finding AAAs by screening, while they are still asymptomatic, is critical.

The accuracy of physical examination in diagnosing AAAs is notoriously poor.[4] One meta-analysis showed the physical examination

to have a sensitivity ranging from 29% for AAAs of 3.0 to 3.9 cm, 50% for AAAs of 4.0 to 4.9 cm, and 76% for AAAs of 5.0 cm or greater.[5] Although the sensitivity of abdominal palpation increases with increasing aneurysmal size, it remains too low to be reliable at any size. In addition, the examination leads to many false positives.

Ultrasound examinations of the abdominal aorta, on the other hand, are highly accurate. They have been shown to have a high correlation with gold standards including computed tomography and intraoperative measurements of the abdominal aorta.[6,7] Additionally, ultrasound has the benefits of being rapid, cost-effective, noninvasive, and lacking radiation exposure.

Thus, ultrasound is the preferred screening method endorsed by the USPSTF. They recommend one-time AAA for all men 65 to 75 years of age who have ever smoked.[8] The number needed to screen to save one AAA-related death is 216. For context, 400 breast cancer screening examinations need to be performed to save one breast cancer–related death.

Despite these recommendations, screening rates remain low. One study showed that only 9.2% of eligible patients received appropriate screening in primary care practices. If screening recommendations were followed, it is estimated that mortality from complications of AAA could be cut in half.[9]

Primary care providers are well positioned to help increase screening of patients for AAA. There is good evidence that practitioners with focused training—typically several hours to a few days—can accurately perform point-of-care ultrasound (POCUS) screening for AAA. A systematic review of studies performed in the emergency department found a pooled sensitivity and specificity of 99% and 98%, respectively.[10] Multiple studies support primary care physicians performing POCUS AAA screening in clinic.[11-17] A 2012 prospective, observational study in Canada showed that office-based ultrasound screening examinations for AAA are reliable. The author—a rural family physician who had focused ultrasound training including 50 supervised aorta scans—compared the results of his office-based scans to hospital-performed scans in the same patients. The average discrepancy in aorta diameters between the two groups was only 2 mm and the office-based scans had a sensitivity and specificity of 100%. The average office-based scan in this study took only 212 seconds, which is helpful data for physicians that work in a busy clinic and feel they may not have time to do office-based ultrasound.[17]

TABLE 47-1	Recommendations for Use of Point-of-Care Ultrasound in Clinical Practice		
Recommendation		**Rating**	**References**
Point-of-care ultrasound has a higher sensitivity and specificity for the evaluation of abdominal aortic aneurysm (AAA) than physical examination findings.		A	4, 5
Point-of-care ultrasound can be utilized to screen patients for AAA in men, above the age of 65, who have a smoking history.		A	8
Point-of-care ultrasound for the evaluation of AAA can be performed by trained nonradiologists with similar sensitivity and specificity of hospital-performed, radiologist-reviewed ultrasounds.		A	12, 21

A = consistent, good-quality patient-oriented evidence; B = inconsistent or limited-quality patient-oriented evidence; C = consensus, disease-oriented evidence, usual practice, expert opinion, or case series. For information about the SORT evidence rating system, go to http://www.aafp.org/afpsort.

In addition to screening asymptomatic patients, ultrasound can be valuable in diagnosing patients presenting with symptomatic AAA. Despite the high mortality rate of a patient with an AAA with rupture, the classic triad of abdominal pain, hypotension, and a pulsatile mass is present in only 50% of patients on presentation.[18] Timely diagnosis of a ruptured AAA is important, as patients that make it to the operating room decrease their mortality in half.[19] Primary care doctors see many patients with acute back pain and undifferentiated abdominal pain where a ruptured AAA may be in the differential diagnosis. Performing a bedside aorta scan in these patients, in a setting where there is limited availability or a significant time delay in obtaining a formal study, can be potentially lifesaving.

PERFORMING THE SCAN

1. **Preparation.** Have the patient lie in the supine position. Position the ultrasound machine so you can easily view the images while scanning the patient. Use a phased array or a curvilinear, abdominal probe (3.5-5.0 MHz) to do the scan. Place the probe in a transverse plane, with the probe marker pointing to the right, just below the xiphoid process (**Figure 47-1**).

2. **Scan through the aorta in a transverse plane.** Find the vertebral body shadow. The only structure directly above the vertebral body is the aorta. Use the vertebral body as a landmark to find the aorta as attempting to look for the aorta on first glance can be difficult, and it is easy to misidentify the aorta as the inferior vena cava (IVC) or other large vessels branching off the aorta. Adjust the depth so the vertebral body shadow and aorta are in the middle of the screen (**Figure 47-2**). Scan down the aorta from the xiphoid process to the umbilicus in 1- to 2-cm intervals. Place

ultrasound gel along the path of the aorta so there is minimal disruption and removal of the probe from the abdomen. If you lose sight of the aorta by removing the probe or there is poor visualization, start the scan again. It is important to see the aorta in a continuous plane as you scan through it from the proximal to distal landmarks, described later.

3. **Visualize proximal landmarks.** As you progress down the aorta from the xiphoid to the umbilicus, you will first encounter the celiac artery. The celiac artery branches off the aorta and splits into the common hepatic artery and the splenic artery. This configuration has the appearance of a "seagull" (**Figure 47-3**). The superior mesenteric artery (SMA) branches anteriorly off the aorta approximately 1 cm distal to the celiac artery. It will run parallel and track from directly anterior, then to the right of the aorta. The renal arteries branch from the left and right sides of the aorta approximately 1 cm distal to the SMA. At this location, the SMA will appear as a smaller artery in cross section anterior to the aorta (**Figure 47-4**). The left renal vein can be seen branching from the IVC and running to the left kidney, coursing posterior to the SMA but anterior to the aorta. The portal vein will be seen running parallel to the left renal vein at this level but will be anterior to the SMA (**Figure 47-5**). Although you may not see the renal arteries, themselves, it is important to visualize the celiac artery, SMA, or renal vein to be sure you have scanned to a level proximal to the renal arteries as almost all AAAs are infrarenal in location.

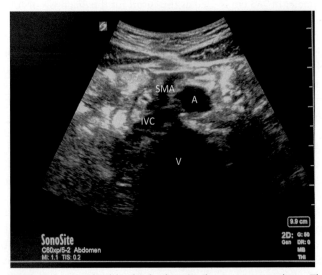

FIGURE 47-2. Vertebral body shadow in the transverse plane. The vertebral body can serve as a landmark that is easy to find and helps identify the aorta. The aorta lies superficial and to the left while the IVC lies superficial and to the right. A, aorta; IVC, inferior vena cava; SMA, superior mesenteric artery; V, vertebral body.

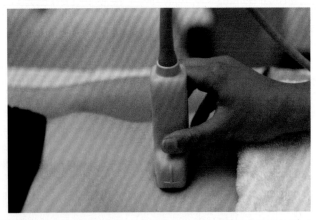

FIGURE 47-1. Patient and probe positioning. The patient is placed in the supine position. Note the use of the curvilinear probe, placed in the midline with the transverse orientation and with the probe marker toward the patient's right.

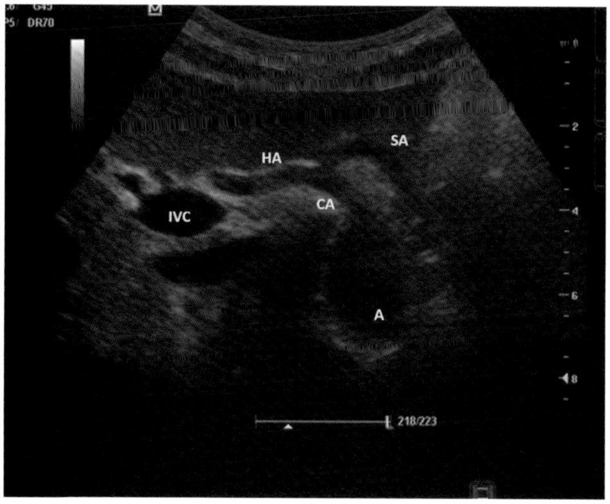

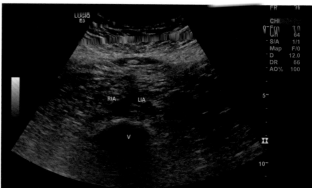

FIGURE 47-6. The iliac bifurcation at the level of the umbilicus. LIA, left common iliac artery; RIA, right common iliac artery; V, vertebral body.

aneurysm that is defined as greater than 1.5 cm in diameter. The iliac arteries dive down deep into the pelvis just below the umbilicus (**Figure 47-6** and ▶ **Video 47-1**).

5. **Scan through the aorta in a longitudinal plane.** Reposition the probe as in step 1. When the aorta is visualized in the transverse plane, slowly rotate the probe to a longitudinal plane maintaining visualization of the aorta the entire time. Repeat the scan with the probe in the longitudinal plane from the proximal landmarks to the distal landmarks. The celiac artery and SMA are the best proximal landmarks in the longitudinal plan as they will be visualized in the midline of the aorta with the celiac artery branching proximally and the SMA branching inferiorly. The renal arteries will not be visualized as they will be out of this plane of view. Similarly, the distal iliac artery bifurcation will only appear as a tapering of the aorta as the common iliacs branch laterally out of the plane of view (**Figure 47-7** and ▶ **Video 47-2**).

6. **Perform measurements.** Representative measurements at the proximal, mid-, and distal aorta can be obtained but are not always necessary. At a minimum, measure any area that appears to approach an abnormal diameter, defined as 3 cm or larger. Measurements should be obtained in both the transverse and

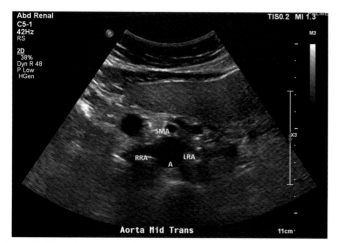

FIGURE 47-3. The aorta at the level of the celiac artery in transverse plane. The celiac artery branches into the common hepatic artery and splenic artery. A, aorta; CA, celiac artery; HA, common hepatic artery; IVC, inferior vena cava; SA, splenic artery.

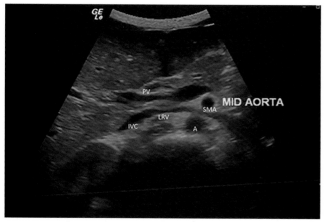

FIGURE 47-4. The aorta at the level of the renal arteries in transverse plane. A, aorta; LRA, left renal artery; RRA, right renal artery; SMA, superior mesenteric artery.

4. **Visualize distal landmarks.** With the probe just above the umbilicus, fan distally to visualize the aorta branch into the common iliac arteries. Assess the proximal iliac arteries for an

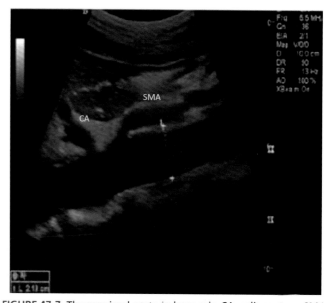

FIGURE 47-5. The aorta at the level of the left renal vein in transverse plane. A, aorta; IVC, inferior vena cava; LRV, left renal vein; PV, portal vein; SMA, superior mesenteric artery.

FIGURE 47-7. The proximal aorta in long axis. CA, celiac artery; SMA, superior mesenteric artery.

PART 2

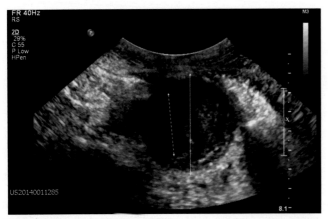

FIGURE 47-8. Ultrasound positive for a distal AAA in transverse plane. The correctly measured diameter from outer wall to outer wall was calculated as 3.8 cm (solid arrow). There is also a mural thrombus with a pseudo-lumen that measures smaller (hashed arrow). It is important to not mistake a pseudo-lumen for the aortic diameter.

longitudinal plane. Make sure each measurement is obtained with the probe at a 90° angle to the aorta. Do not scan at an oblique angle as it is possible you will overestimate the diameter. The diameter should be measured from the outer walls of the aorta, including the hyperechoic muscular wall. AAAs often contain mural thrombi that can create an area of canalization called a pseudo-lumen, which can lead to incorrect measurement if it is obtained only of the internal lumen without including the outer walls (**Figure 47-8**).

PATIENT MANAGEMENT

Asymptomatic patients with AAAs will need to have follow-up ultrasounds scheduled or be referred to a vascular surgeon depending on the size of the AAA. Patients with AAA of 3.0 to 3.9 cm should

be scheduled for follow-up ultrasound in 1 to 3 years. Patients with AAA of 4.0 to 4.9 cm should be scheduled for 12-month-interval aorta scans to assess for progression. Patients with an AAA of 5 to 5.5 cm should have repeat ultrasound in 6 months or be referred to a vascular surgeon for follow-up. We recommend referral at 5 cm as some patients at higher risk for rupture, such as women, may choose to have repair performed at 5 to 5.5 cm. Any AAA greater than 5.5 cm should be referred to a vascular surgeon for elective repair. If a repeat examination of a known AAA shows interval growth that is >0.5 cm/year, refer for vascular surgery regardless of aneurysm size because of increased risk for rupture.[20]

In patients with asymptomatic AAA, regardless of size, interventions of modifiable risk factors including smoking cessation, hypertension control, and management of hyperlipidemia should be initiated. AAA is also a coronary artery disease equivalent so all patients with known AAA should be started on a low-dose aspirin and a statin to decrease their risk of myocardial infarction in the future.

In any patient with risk factors for AAA presenting with symptoms that could be attributable to AAA including acute abdominal, back, or flank pain, emergent POCUS examination can be performed. Ultrasound has low sensitivity for confirming rupture so if AAA is present it should be assumed to be the source of symptoms until proven otherwise. Any patient with a possible symptomatic AAA should be immediately stabilized and referred for emergent evaluation. Computed tomography (CT) angiography is the preferred diagnostic test after ultrasound to confirm the size and evaluate for signs of rupture. Vascular surgery should be involved in the care as early as possible in any patient with potentially symptomatic AAA (**Figures 47-9 and 47-10**).

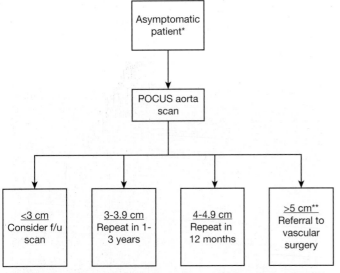

FIGURE 47-9. The asymptomatic patient. *US Preventive Services Task Force (USPSTF) screening criteria, other clinical concern, or asymptomatic abdominal mass found on physical examination. **We recommend a conservative 5-cm cutoff for referral to vascular surgery (some recommend 5.5 cm) to take into account the acceptable range of variation between measurements. If the rate of expansion is >0.5 cm/year on a repeat scan, refer patient to vascular surgery regardless of aorta diameter. POCUS, point-of-care ultrasound.

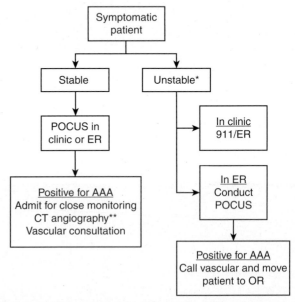

FIGURE 47-10. The symptomatic patient. *Unstable patients may have signs of hypotension or shock. Referral/diagnosis should occur while simultaneously stabilizing the patient (ie, monitored bed, large bore intravenous access, transfusion of blood). **A CT angiogram can assess if there is involvement of the renal arteries and dictate the type of surgery required in the stable patient. A negative POCUS for AAA evaluation should lead to a search for an alternative diagnosis. AAA, abdominal aortic aneurysm; CT, computed tomography; POCUS, point-of-care ultrasound.

PEARLS AND PITFALLS

Pearls

- Before screening patients, providers should check if the patient has already been screened incidentally through an alternative imaging modality (abdominal CT or magnetic resonance imaging [MRI]) ordered for another purpose.
- To minimize bowel gas that will prevent imaging of the aorta, have the patient be NPO at least 4 to 12 hours prior to a screening examination if possible. However, examination should not be delayed if patient has eaten in that time frame. In these instances, push down with the probe to move away bowel loops filled with air. Many times this maneuver will allow the vertebral column/shadow and aorta to come into view (▶ Video 47-3).
- Use shape, compressibility, and Doppler to discriminate the IVC (triangle shaped, compressible, monophasic waveform, venous sound) from the aorta (round, noncompressible, biphasic waveform, arterial sound).
- Distal AAAs (infrarenal) are common and proximal AAAs are rare. Proximal AAAs usually have distal involvement. Because of this reasoning, some authors start the aorta scan at the umbilicus and work upward, toward the xiphoid process.

Pitfalls

- Although the signs and symptoms of aortic dissection can mimic AAA, the pathophysiology and management between these two entities are different. Although an aortic dissection "flap" can be found with POCUS, the diagnostic test to assess for a dissection is a CT angiogram of the aorta. A thoracic and abdominal CT angiogram of the aorta should be ordered if there is concern for aortic dissection.
- If an AAA is found, be sure to take measurements that include the hyperechoic muscular walls. Measurement only including the lumen could be misleading if there is mural thrombus formation in an AAA, as commonly happens.
- The number one misdiagnosis for a ruptured AAA is ureteral colic. AAA that is rupturing can have the same presentation as patients passing a kidney stone with abdominal pain, flank pain, and hematuria. In an evaluation with a patient with flank pain, it is important to assess for AAA even if hydronephrosis is present. A large AAA with rupture can compress the neighboring ureter and cause hydronephrosis.

BILLING

CPT Code	Description	Global Payment	Professional Component	Technical Component
76775	Ultrasound, retroperitoneal (eg, renal, aorta, nodes), real time with image documentation, limited	$116.80	$29.38	$87.42

CPT codes and average national reimbursement for Medicare in 2016. Payment data are from https://www.cms.gov/apps/physician-fee-schedule/search/search-criteria.aspx. See Chapter 2 for details on ultrasound billing.

References

1. Underlying Cause of Death, 1999-2015 Request [Internet]. [cited 2016 Dec 9]. https://wonder.cdc.gov/ucd-icd10.html
2. Aggarwal S, Qamar A, Sharma V, Sharma A. Abdominal aortic aneurysm: a comprehensive review. *Exp Clin Cardiol.* 2011;16(1):11-15.
3. Metcalfe D, Holt PJ, Thompson MM. The management of abdominal aortic aneurysms. *BMJ.* 2011;342:d1384.
4. Lynch RM. Accuracy of abdominal examination in the diagnosis of non-ruptured abdominal aortic aneurysm. *Accid Emerg Nurs.* 2004;12(2):99-107.
5. Lederle FA, Simel DL. The rational clinical examination. Does this patient have abdominal aortic aneurysm? *JAMA.* 1999;281(1):77-82.
6. Leopold GR, Goldberger LE, Bernstein EF. Ultrasonic detection and evaluation of abdominal aortic aneurysms. *Surgery.* 1972;72(6):939-945.
7. Wanhainen A, Bergqvist D, Björck M. Measuring the abdominal aorta with ultrasonography and computed tomography—difference and variability. *Eur J Vasc Endovasc Surg.* 2002;24(5):428-434.
8. Fleming C, Whitlock EP, Beil TL, Lederle FA. Screening for abdominal aortic aneurysm: a best-evidence systematic review for the U.S. Preventive Services Task Force. *Ann Intern Med.* 2005;142(3):203-211.
9. Thompson SG, Ashton HA, Gao L, Buxton MJ, Scott RA; Multicentre Aneurysm Screening Study (MASS) Group. Final follow-up of the Multicentre Aneurysm Screening Study (MASS) randomized trial of abdominal aortic aneurysm screening. *Br J Surg.* 2012;99(12):1649-1656.
10. Rubano E, Mehta N, Caputo W, Paladino L, Sinert R. Systematic review: emergency department bedside ultrasonography for diagnosing suspected abdominal aortic aneurysm. *Acad Emerg Med.* 2013;20(2):128-138.

11. Abdominal Aortic Aneurysm—American Family Physician [Internet]. [cited 2016 Dec 9]. http://www.aafp.org/afp/2015/0415/p538.html
12. Ruff AL, Teng K, Hu B, Rothberg MB. Screening for abdominal aortic aneurysms in outpatient primary care clinics. *Am J Med.* 2015;128(3):283-288.
13. Sisó-Almirall A, Gilabert Solé R, Bru Saumell C, et al. Feasibility of hand-held-ultrasonography in the screening of abdominal aortic aneurysms and abdominal aortic atherosclerosis [in Spanish]. *Med Clínica.* 2013;141(10):417-422.
14. Oviedo-García AA, Algaba-Montes M, Segura-Grau A, Rodríguez-Lorenzo Á. Ultrasound of the large abdominal vessels [in Spanish]. *Semergen Soc Esp Med Rural Generalista.* 2016;42(5):315-319.
15. Steinmetz P, Oleskevich S. The benefits of doing ultrasound exams in your office. *J Fam Pract.* 2016;65(8):517-523.
16. Bonnafy T, Lacroix P, Desormais I, et al. Reliability of the measurement of the abdominal aortic diameter by novice operators using a pocket-sized ultrasound system. *Arch Cardiovasc Dis.* 2013;106(12):644-650.
17. Blois B. Office-based ultrasound screening for abdominal aortic aneurysm. *Can Fam Physician.* 2012;58(3):e172-e178.
18. Kiell CS, Ernst CB. Advances in management of abdominal aortic aneurysm. *Adv Surg.* 1993;26:73-98.
19. Hoffman M, Avellone JC, Plecha FR, et al. Operation for ruptured abdominal aortic aneurysms: a community-wide experience. *Surgery.* 1982;91(5):597-602.
20. Chaikof EL, Dalman RL, Eskandari MK, et al. The Society for Vascular Surgery practice guidelines on the care of patients with an abdominal aortic aneurysm. *J Vasc Surg.* 2018;67(1):2.e2-77.e2.
21. Costantino TG, Bruno EC, Handly N, Dean AJ. Accuracy of emergency medicine ultrasound in the evaluation of abdominal aortic aneurysm. *J Emerg Med.* 2005;29(4):455-460.

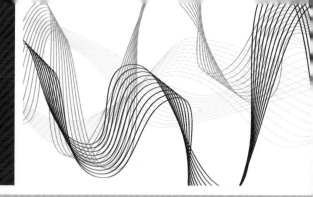

Does the Patient Have Carotid Stenosis?

Nicholas LeFevre, MD

Clinical Vignette

A 72-year-old man with hyperlipidemia, hypertension, and poorly controlled type II diabetes mellitus presents to the office of his primary care clinician for a walk-in visit. He describes an episode the night prior where the vision in his left eye became black "like a curtain coming down." His vision returned to normal within 5 minutes. You are concerned this may represent amaurosis fugax. Does the patient have carotid stenosis?

LITERATURE REVIEW

The prevalence of severe carotid stenosis in the general population has been variably reported between 0% and 3.1%.[1] The 2011 American Heart Association guidelines on the prevention of stroke indicate a prevalence of severe stenosis of less than 1% in those who are asymptomatic. In those identified with asymptomatic stenosis, there is a less than 1% annual attributable stroke risk.[2] Symptoms typical for carotid territory ischemia include weakness, paresthesia, or sensory deficits of the face, arm, or leg or transient ipsilateral blindness (amaurosis fugax). Syncope, vertigo, ataxia, dysarthria, and decreased level of consciousness are not causally related to carotid artery atherosclerotic disease.[3] Other groups with high (>20%) prevalence of severe carotid stenosis include smokers in whom coronary artery bypass graft (CABG) is planned and those with symptomatic peripheral artery disease.[3] Auscultation of a carotid bruit does not predict the presence of severe stenosis in asymptomatic patients and alone is not an indication for carotid artery ultrasound.[3,4]

After several major trials in the last two decades, it is widely recognized that intervention—either carotid endarterectomy (CEA) or carotid artery stenting (CAS)—for severe carotid stenosis in symptomatic patients carries benefit in decreasing the rate of future stroke. The North American Symptomatic Carotid Endarterectomy Trial (NASCET) established that threshold at 70% stenosis by its imaging criteria (which are now widely used).[5,6] The European Carotid Surgery Trial (ECST), using slightly different diagnostic criteria, reported an 80% stenosis threshold for meaningful intervention.[7] Unfortunately, patients meeting these criteria often have high surgical risk and both CEA and CAS carry with them significant perioperative morbidity and mortality. Thirty-day stroke or mortality rates of 2.4% to 3% are cited in high-volume centers, but rates as high as 6% are reported. Rates of myocardial infarction after CEA are high (2.2%).[8] Newer strategies like carotid stenting have lower myocardial infarction but higher perioperative stroke rates associated with them.[9] With the high rates of complications associated with these interventions, the consequences of overdiagnosis may be high. Thus, diagnostic testing should be limited to the groups most likely to benefit from treatment (Table 48-1). As such, many specialty societies now have strong recommendations against routine screening in asymptomatic patients including the U.S. Preventive Services Task Force, the American Heart Association, and the American College of Radiology.[2,4,10] Other countries have even gone on to recommend corroborative studies like magnetic resonance imaging (MRI) prior to intervention.[11]

The American Institute of Ultrasound in Medicine (AIUM) has published practice parameters for "Ultrasound Examination of the Extracranial Cerebrovascular System," which recommends imaging components for a complete study (Table 48-2.).[12] Ultrasound

TABLE 48-1 Indications for Carotid Stenosis Evaluation by Ultrasound

Screen or Consider Screening	Do Not Routinely Screen
1. Typical neurologic symptoms, ipsilateral amaurosis fugax, contralateral stroke or TIA including weakness, sensory loss, or paresthesia 2. High-risk patients >65 undergoing CABG 3. Symptomatic peripheral artery disease	1. Asymptomatic patients, regardless of age 2. Patients with abdominal aortic aneurysm 3. Patients with an asymptomatic auscultated carotid bruit 4. Patients with atypical neurologic symptoms including syncope or presyncope

Abbreviation: CABG, coronary artery bypass graft; TIA, transient ischemic attack.

Reprinted from Ricotta JJ, Aburahma A, Ascher E, et al. Updated Society for Vascular Surgery guidelines for management of extracranial carotid disease. *J Vasc Surg.* 2011;54(3):e1-31. Copyright © 2011 Society for Vascular Surgery. With permission.

TABLE 48-2	American Institute of Ultrasound in Medicine Practice Parameters for the Performance of an Ultrasound Examination of the Extracranial Cerebrovascular System

Required B-Mode/Gray-Scale Images	Required Color Doppler Images	Required Spectral Doppler Images with Peak Systolic Velocity
1. Long axis, common carotid 2. Long axis, carotid bifurcation 3. Long axis, internal carotid 4. Short axis, proximal internal carotid	1. Long axis, distal common carotid 2. Long axis, proximal and mid-internal carotid 3. Long axis, external carotid (showing branch) 4. Long axis, vertebral artery	1. Proximal common carotid 2. Middle or distal common carotid (2-3 cm below bifurcation). 3. Proximal internal carotid 4. Mid- to distal internal carotid 5. Proximal external carotid 6. Vertebral artery (in neck or near origin)

From American Institute of Ultrasound in Medicine, American College of Radiology, Society of Radiologists in Ultrasound. AIUM practice guideline for the performance of an ultrasound examination of the extracranial cerebrovascular system. *J Ultrasound Med.* 2012;31(1):145-54. Copyright © 2016 by the American Institute of Ultrasound in Medicine. Reprinted by permission of John Wiley & Sons, Inc.

examination of the carotid arteries requires more advanced knowledge and technical skill than the majority of point-of-care ultrasound (POCUS) studies and, as such, is not commonly performed by most POCUS providers. The most effective POCUS studies are generally those that answer focused clinical questions, improve patient care, are relatively fast to perform, and can be reliably performed by nonradiologists with limited training. For most providers, carotid Doppler imaging will fall outside of these parameters. A focused version of the complete examination may, however, have utility in certain practice settings, such as where resources are limited. Such a focused examination will be proposed here. As the highest incidence of clinically important pathology lies at the internal carotid artery (ICA), excluding the vertebral artery and external carotid artery (ECA) from a point-of-care study protocol would miss relatively little clinically important pathology.

Most laptop-sized point-of-care machines, when the appropriate linear high-frequency probe is installed, will have vascular calculations packages included. The ability to adjust Doppler angles may be limited when compared to machines more commonly found in radiology departments. Handheld units may lack pulsed-wave/spectral Doppler entirely. There have been few studies of carotid ultrasound by primary care providers. There are no validated limited protocols, including that proposed here. Investigating ways to make the study more accessible to point-of-care providers with limited training, Ray et al studied the accuracy of gray-scale plaque evaluation alone without Doppler. After a period of training, reviewers were able to identify all but one case of severe (>50%) stenosis by gray-scale imaging alone.[13] A study of European internists with 6 weeks of training showed a sensitivity and specificity for plaque detection alone (not including Doppler evaluation for stenosis severity) of 78.5% and 93.6%,

respectively.[14] All of the small-scale studies to date have evaluated the ability of providers to identify plaque on gray-scale imaging and none have included Doppler imaging.

With the power of showing patients their anatomy and pathology in real time, another argument for carotid ultrasound at the point of care would lie with its ability to induce behavior change in those with high cardiovascular risk. Across several trials, patients shown their carotid plaque on ultrasound have greater understanding of their cardiovascular risk. Despite better understanding, most trials have not shown a meaningful effect on behavior change (including smoking cessation rates).[15-18] One large European trial did show a reduction in Framingham risk at 1 year in patients shown their carotid plaque (or intima-media thickness) compared to controls who were not.[19] Key recommendations for use of carotid sonography at the point of care are discussed in **Table 48-3**.

PERFORMING THE SCAN

1. **Position the patient and select the examination**. A linear high-frequency probe should be used and the vascular/arterial examination settings selected. The ultrasound machine should face the sonographer and sit on the patient's right side. The patient should be supine with their head slightly tilted away from the side of the examination. Others prefer to sit at the head of the bed facing the patient's feet (**Figure 48-1**).
2. **Survey the carotid in gray-scale/B-mode imaging**. The study relies on complete visualization of the carotid from the clavicle to the angle of the mandible. The probe may be positioned to visualize the artery anteriorly or from a posterolateral view (**Figures 48-2 and 48-3**). Longitudinal images of the common carotid (**Figure 48-4**), carotid bifurcation (**Figure 48-5**), and

TABLE 48-3	Recommendations for Use of Point-of-Care Ultrasound in Clinical Practice		
Recommendation		**Rating**	**References**
Routine screening for carotid stenosis is recommended against several major specialty societies and the United States Preventive Services Task Force (USPSTF), this does not change in the point-of-care setting.		A	2, 4, 10
Point-of-care carotid ultrasound for identification of carotid plaque using gray-scale imaging alone may be reliable for triaging patients with a potential stenosis > 50%.		C	13, 14
Using point-of-care ultrasound plaque visualization as a teaching tool for patients at high cardiovascular risk may alter physician prescribing and lower Framingham risk, but does not improve rates of smoking cessation.		B	15, 16, 17, 18, 19

A = consistent, good-quality patient-oriented evidence; B = inconsistent or limited-quality patient-oriented evidence; C = consensus, disease-oriented evidence, usual practice, expert opinion, or case series. For information about the SORT evidence rating system, go to http://www.aafp.org/afpsort.

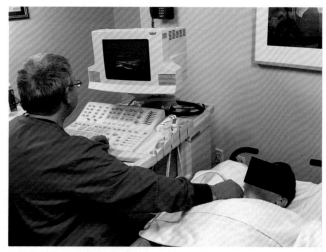

FIGURE 48-1. Ergonomics for performing the examination.

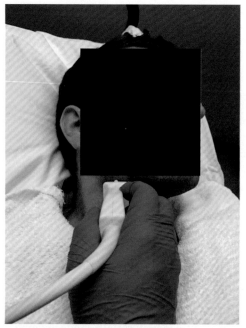

FIGURE 48-2. Anterior probe orientation.

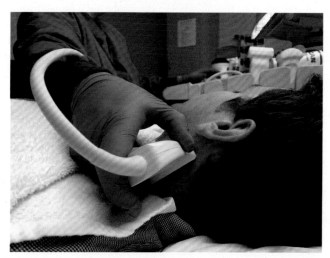

FIGURE 48-3. Posterolateral probe orientation.

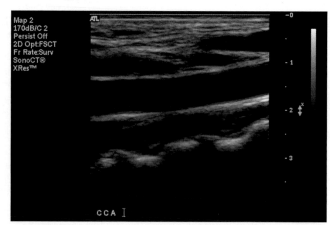

FIGURE 48-4. B-mode image of the common carotid artery (CCA).

ICA should be saved. A short axis image of the proximal internal carotid should be saved. The bifurcation of the common carotid into the internal and external carotid may be visualized at varied points from mid-cervical all the way to the angle of the mandible. The external carotid can be identified as the smaller of the two vessels at bifurcation and usually has branches, whereas the internal carotid does not (**Figure 48-6**).

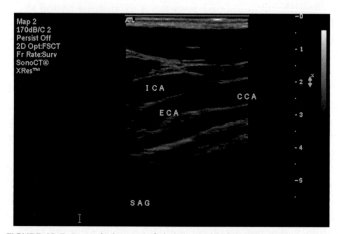

FIGURE 48-5. B-mode image of the carotid bifurcation.

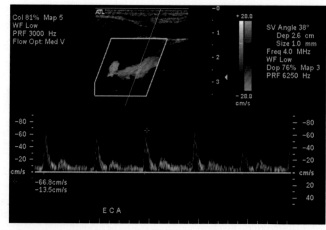

FIGURE 48-6. Doppler signature of the external carotid artery. Note the branch shown with color flow.

3. **Document any plaque seen in longitudinal and short axis**. If plaque is visualized it should be documented in both longitudinal and short axis and a visual estimation of percent stenosis by luminal diameter made. This is a visual estimation. Best images are obtained when the vessel is directly perpendicular to the ultrasound probe (**Figure 48-7**).

4. **Repeat the survey with color Doppler applied**. When transitioning to Doppler evaluation, it should be noted that the vessel can no longer be perpendicular to the ultrasound probe and must always be on an angle on the screen (such that the "angle of insonation" is always less than 60°). Heel-toe maneuver of the probe may be necessary (caudally angled toward the clavicle and cranially angled toward the mandible) to maintain these angles (**Figure 48-8**). Color images should be saved (**Figures 48-9** and **48-10**). In a focused point-of-care study, imaging of the vertebral arteries and ECA could be excluded as the ECA (which supplies the face) is not a source of embolic phenomena, and the vertebral artery is evaluated for different indications.

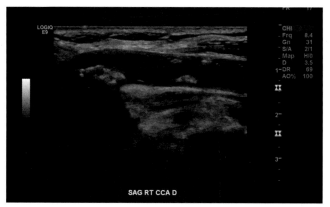

FIGURE 48-7. Note the presence of plaque (with posterior acoustic shadowing) in the distal CCA near the bifurcation.

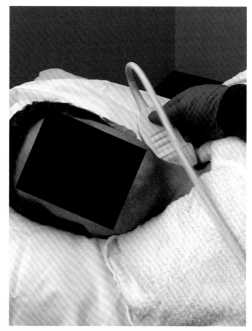

FIGURE 48-8. Exaggerated heel-toe maneuver.

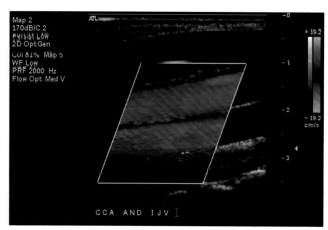

FIGURE 48-9. Color Doppler at the CCA. Note the thinner-walled internal jugular vein above. Red and blue represent flow toward or away from the probe, not arterial or venous.

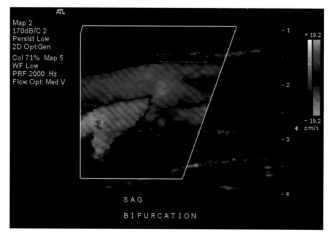

FIGURE 48-10. Color flow at the bifurcation.

5. **Apply pulsed-wave Doppler and measure peak systolic velocities**. Ensuring that the angle correction is kept to less than 60° (ideally 45°-60°), pulsed-wave Doppler tracings should be obtained at the proximal and mid-common carotid and at the proximal and mid-ICA. If an area of increased velocity is seen on color imaging, the pulsed-wave Doppler gate should be placed directly through the middle of it and this velocity measured (**Figures 48-11 to 48-13**). The peak systolic velocity (PSV) should be measured.

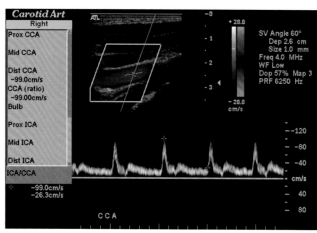

FIGURE 48-11. Peak systolic velocity of 99.0 cm/s in the common carotid.

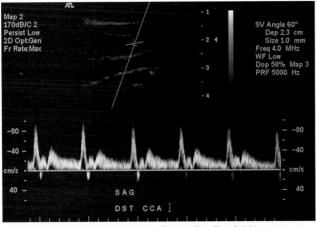

FIGURE 48-12. Pulsed-wave Doppler at the distal CCA.

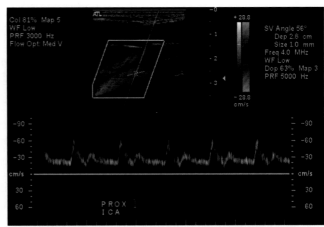

FIGURE 48-13. Pulsed-wave Doppler at the proximal internal carotid artery (ICA).

6. **Interpret the degree of stenosis present according to established criteria.** There are many described Doppler criteria for carotid stenosis. In the United States, the most common are based on the NASCET and were defined by the Society of Radiologists in Ultrasound.[20] Other criteria such as the modified NASCET index are described.[21] All rely upon plaque visualization, PSV, and the ratio of PSV in the ICA to the PSV in the CCA (**Table 48-4**).

PATIENT MANAGEMENT

Patients with symptomatic carotid atherosclerotic disease and reliable imaging suggesting a stenosis greater than 50% by any available criteria should be referred for comprehensive imaging at an accredited vascular imaging lab where available (**Figures 48-14 and 48-15**). Pending those results, vascular surgery consultation may be indicated. Medical management of carotid stenosis is beyond the scope of this review. There is variable evidence that showing a patient their atherosclerotic plaque in real time may aid in their understanding of cardiovascular risk.[15-18,22]

TABLE 48-4	Society of Radiologists in Ultrasound Criteria for Ultrasound Diagnosis of ICA Stenosis				
Stenosis Degree	ICA PSV (cm/s)	Plaque/Diameter	ICA/CCA PSV Ratio	ICA EDV (cm/s)
Normal	<125	None	<2.0	<40
<50%	<125	<50%	<2.0	<40
50%-69%	125-230	>50%	2.0-4.0	40-100
>70% to near occlusion	>230	>50%	>4.0	>100
Near Occlusion	High, low, or undetectable	Visible	Variable	Variable
Total Occlusion	Undetectable	Visible, no detectable lumen	N/A	N/A

Abbreviation: CCA, common carotid artery; EDV, end diastolic velocity; ICA, internal carotid artery; PSV, peak systolic velocity.

Reprinted with permission from Grant EG, Benson CB, Moneta GL. Carotid artery stenosis: gray-scale and Doppler US diagnosis—Society of Radiologists in Ultrasound Consensus Conference. *Radiology.* 2003;229(2):340-346.

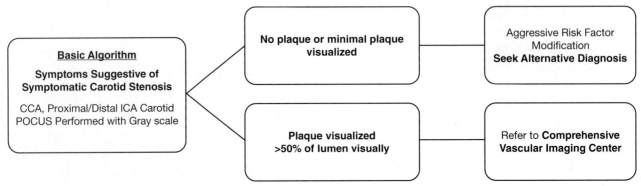

FIGURE 48-14. Ultrasound detection of plaque alone may be a more reliable basic skill to learn, as such it is presented as an optional basic protocol. POCUS, point-of-care ultrasound.

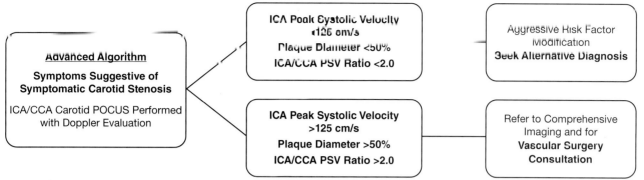

FIGURE 48-15. For providers skilled enough to accurately measure Doppler velocities, plaque that is greater than 50% obstructing by Doppler may not require advanced imaging. POCUS, point-of-care ultrasound.

PEARLS AND PITFALLS

Pearls

- The ECA is usually smaller than the ICA and runs anteriorly toward the face rather than posteriorly. It usually has branches, whereas the ICA will not. Tapping anterior to the ear on the preauricular branch of the temporal artery while observing a Doppler tracing ("temporal tap maneuver") will alter the ECA tracing but will minimally affect the ICA tracing.[19]
- B-mode/gray-scale imaging alone is sufficient for plaque detection, but Doppler imaging is required to determine the degree of stenosis. The presence of plaque alone in inexperienced hands should trigger comprehensive imaging when screening is indicated.
- Peak systolic velocity > 125 cm/s or ICA/CCA PSV ratio > 2.0 is associated with a significant stenosis of more than 50%.

Pitfalls

- The degree of stenosis can be dramatically underestimated when the Doppler gate angle or angle of insonation is incorrect (**Figure 48-16**).
- The pulsed-wave gate should always be directly in the middle of the vessel as turbulent flow is naturally seen at the margins[19] (**Figures 48-17 and 48-18**). Turbulent flow is seen as a "filling in" of the Doppler signal rather than "hollow" signals of laminar flow (broad vs narrow bandwidth).
- Anatomic variants are possible including vessel tortuosity, which may artificially raise velocities and make imaging more challenging. When encountered, these patients should be referred to more experienced sonographers.[19]

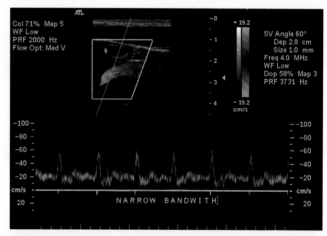

FIGURE 48-17. Sharp narrow bandwidth signal when the middle of the vessel is sampled.

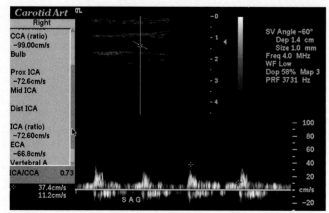

FIGURE 48-16. Spuriously low velocities are seen when the angle of insonation is 0° (vessel parallel).

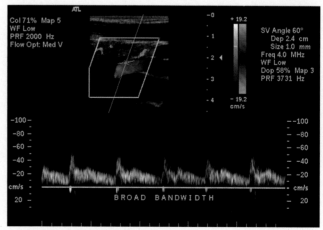

FIGURE 48-18. Distorted broad bandwidth signal when the vessel margin is sampled.

BILLING

CPT Code	Description	Global Payment	Professional Component	Technical Component
93880	Duplex scan of extracranial arteries; complete bilateral study	$206.63	$40.82	$165.42
93882	Duplex scan of extracranial arteries; unilateral or limited study	$131.76	$25.78	$105.98

CPT codes and average national reimbursement for Medicare in 2016. Payment data are from https://www.cms.gov/apps/physician-fee-schedule/search/search-criteria.aspx. See Chapter 2 for details on ultrasound billing.

References

1. de Weerd M, Greving JP, Hedblad B. Prevalence of asymptomatic carotid artery stenosis in the general population: an individual participant data meta-analysis. *Stroke*. 2010;41(6):1294-1297.

2. Goldstein LB, Bushnell CD, Adams RJ. Guidelines for the primary prevention of stroke: a guideline for healthcare professionals from the American Heart Association/American Stroke Association. *Stroke*. 2011;42(2):517-584.

3. Ricotta JJ, Aburahma A, Ascher E. Updated society for vascular surgery guidelines for management of extracranial carotid disease. *J Vascular Surg*. 2011;54(3):e1-e31.

4. LeFevre ML. Screening for asymptomatic carotid artery stenosis: U.S. Preventive Services Task Force recommendation statement. *Ann Internal Med*. 2014;161(5):356-362.

5. The North American Symptomatic Carotid Endarterectomy Trial Collaborators. Beneficial effect of carotid endarterectomy in symptomatic patients with high-grade carotid stenosis. *N Engl J Med*. 1991;325(7):445-453.

6. Ferguson GG, Eliasziw M, Barr HW. The North American Symptomatic Carotid Endarterectomy Trial: surgical results in 1415 patients. *Stroke*. 1999;30(9):1751-1758.

7. European Carotid Surgery Trialists' Group. Randomised trial of endarterectomy for recently symptomatic carotid stenosis: final results of the MRC European Carotid Surgery Trial (ECST). *Lancet* (London, England). 1998;351(9113):1379-1387.

8. Executive Committee for the Asymptomatic Carotid Atherosclerosis Study. Endarterectomy for asymptomatic carotid artery stenosis. *JAMA*. 1995;273(18):1421-1428.

9. Murad MH, Shahrour A, Shah ND, Montori VM, Ricotta JJ. A systematic review and meta-analysis of randomized trials of carotid endarterectomy vs stenting. *J Vascular Surg*. 2011;53(3):792-797.

10. Brott TG, Halperin JL, Abbara S. 2011 ASA/ACCF/AHA/AANN/AANS/ACR/ASNR/CNS/SAIP/SCAI/SIR/SNIS/SVM/SVS guideline on the management of patients with extracranial carotid and vertebral artery disease. *Stroke*. 2011;42(8):e464-e540.

11. Wardlaw JM, Chappell FM, Stevenson M. Accurate, practical and cost-effective assessment of carotid stenosis in the UK. *Health Technol Assess* (Winchester, England). 2006;10(30):iii-iv, ix-x, 1-182.

12. American Institute of Ultrasound in Medicine; American College of Radiology; Society of Radiologists in Ultrasound. AIUM practice guideline for the performance of an ultrasound examination of the extracranial cerebrovascular system. *J Ultrasound Med*. 2012;31(1):145-154.

13. Bhandari T, Socransky SJ. Is B-mode ultrasound alone a sufficient screening tool for carotid stenosis? A pilot study. *Crit Ultrasound J*. 2014;6(1):17. doi:10.1186/s13089-014-0017-x.

14. Ray A, Tamsma JT, Hovens MM, op 't Roodt J, Huisman MV. Accuracy of carotid plaque detection and intima-media thickness measurement with ultrasonography in routine clinical practice. *Eur J Int Med*. 2010;21(1):35-39.

15. Wyman RA, Gimelli G, McBride PE, Korcarz CE, Stein JH. Does detection of carotid plaque affect physician behavior or motivate patients? *Am Heart J*. 2007;154(6):1072-1077.

16. Rodondi N, Collet TH, Nanchen D. Impact of carotid plaque screening on smoking cessation and other cardiovascular risk factors: a randomized controlled trial. *Arch Int Med*. 2012;172(4):344-352.

17. Johnson HM, Turke TL, Grossklaus M. Effects of an office-based carotid ultrasound screening intervention. *J Am Soc Echocardiogr*. 2011;24(7):738-747.

18. Hollands GJ, Hankins M, Marteau TM. Visual feedback of individuals' medical imaging results for changing health behaviour. *Cochrane Database Syst Rev*. 2010. doi:10.1002/14651858.CD007434.pub2.

19. Näslund U, Ng N, Lundgren A, et al. Visualization of asymptomatic atherosclerotic disease for optimum cardiovascular prevention (VIPVIZA): a pragmatic, open-label, randomised controlled trial. *Lancet* (London, England). 2018;393(10167):133-142.

20. Grant EG, Benson CB, Moneta GL. Carotid artery stenosis: gray-scale and Doppler US diagnosis—Society of Radiologists in Ultrasound Consensus Conference. *Radiology*. 2003;229(2):340-346.

21. Hathout GM, Fink JR, El-Saden SM, Grant EG. Sonographic NASCET index: a new Doppler parameter for assessment of internal carotid artery stenosis. *Am J Neuroradiol*. 2005;26(1):68-75.

22. Pellerito JS, Polak JF. *Introduction to Vascular Ultrasonography: ExpertConsult*. 6th ed. Philadelphia, PA: Saunders/Elsevier; 2012.

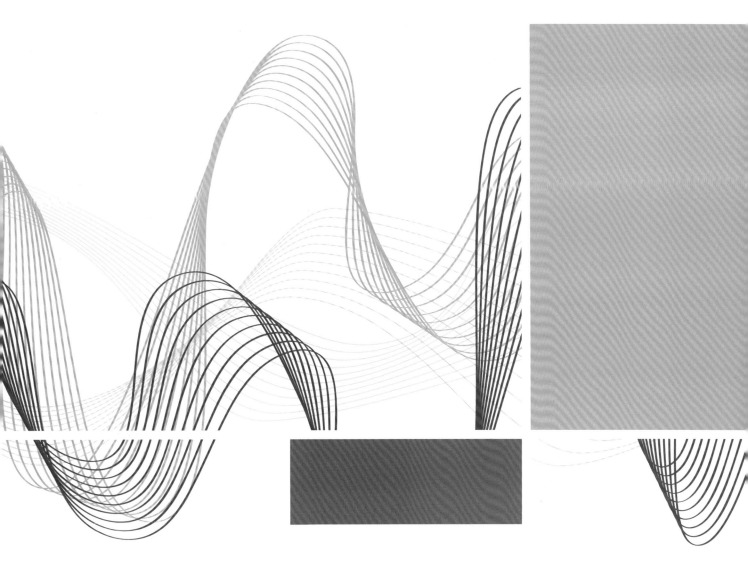

PART 3

COMBINING INTO PROTOCOLS

CHAPTER 49

Cardiopulmonary Limited Ultrasound Examination (CLUE)

Zachary B. Self, MD, FAAFP and T. Laura Bertani, MD

Clinical Vignette

A 54-year-old man presents to your medical clinic with the chief complaint of shortness of breath. He endorses a 3-day history of minimally productive cough, occasional wheeze, and dyspnea on exertion. He denies fevers, chills, and chest pain. His past medical history is significant for chronic obstructive pulmonary disease, diabetes, hypertension, and tobacco abuse.

LITERATURE REVIEW

With the increasing availability and portability of ultrasound, it has become more commonly used in physical examination, particularly in the setting of undifferentiated chest pain or shortness of breath. Quick-look cardiopulmonary ultrasound can assist in rapid patient evaluation and medical decision making when typical history and physical examination fail to yield a diagnosis. Protocols for such "quick-look" examinations have shown their worth in the inpatient, outpatient, emergency, critical care, and resource-limited settings[1-7] and the ability to train practitioners in these locations to utilize and interpret such protocols.[4,8-12] Focused cardiopulmonary ultrasound, being fast, increasingly more accessible, and free from known adverse effects to its performance other than possible misdiagnosis, provides significant advantages over more invasive, time-consuming, or radiating imaging counterparts. These advantages are ideal as part of the initial evaluation or in the setting of acute cardiopulmonary decompensation requiring rapid diagnosis and intervention.

Multiple cardiac ultrasound examinations, signs, and protocols have been developed and multiple names applied to this form of imaging, including focused cardiac ultrasound, bedside cardiovascular ultrasound examination, bedside echocardiography, hand-held cardiac ultrasound, ultrasound stethoscope, and quick-look cardiac ultrasound, all may apply to similar types of fast, bedside ultrasound examination meant to aid medical decision making in real time or for comparative monitoring throughout a patient's course. It is important to delineate these types of examinations from limited echocardiography, which also makes the interpreter responsible for any and all incidental findings that may be obtained in the views demonstrated on ultrasound, whereas bedside or focused ultrasound is meant to answer quick, yes or no questions regarding the patient's cardiopulmonary status.[12]

One of the most well-known and studied quick-look cardiopulmonary examinations is the cardiopulmonary limited ultrasound examination, or CLUE, published by Kimura et al. initially in 2011.[13] The examination allows for rapid evaluation of right and left heart function as well as pulmonary pathology in less than 5 minutes.[13] CLUE is meant to quickly augment physical examination findings to provide an initial evaluation or to follow a patient clinically throughout their course without the need for specific measurements and instead by simply classifying positive and negative findings. The

original protocol comprises four views and four signs: the parasternal long-axis view to evaluate for both left ventricular (LV) dysfunction and left atrial (LA) dilation, longitudinal apical views of both lung apices to evaluate for pulmonary edema, and the subcostal view of the longitudinal inferior vena cava (IVC) entering the right atrium to evaluate for increased central venous pressure.[13] The aforementioned views were selected for their ease of access for new users and ability to obtain in supine, intubated, or restrained patients, increasing their applicability to multiple scenarios.[1] In 2015, the protocol was expanded to include the evaluation of the right atrium in the subcostal view and bilateral views of the lung bases to evaluate for pleural effusion.

LV systolic dysfunction on the CLUE protocol is defined as an anterior leaflet of the mitral valve failing to approach the ventricular septum within 1 cm. This finding has previously been shown to have an approximate sensitivity of 65% and a specificity of 92% in comparison to formal echocardiogram and magnetic resonance imaging.[14,15] In the original CLUE study, this finding was shown to have a sensitivity and specificity of 69% and 91%, respectively, for an LV ejection fraction of less than 40%. The finding also had a positive correlation with in-hospital mortality.[13] Multiple evaluations have found that point-of-care assessment for decreased LV function is superior to physical examination findings alone but inferior to complete formal echocardiography.[1,13,16]

LA dilation is considered positive if the anterior–posterior view of the left atrium is larger than the overlying aorta during end-diastole. Even minimal LA dilation signals prolonged elevated LA pressure and diastolic dysfunction.[17-19] When studied by Kimura et al. in 2010, it was found to have a sensitivity and specificity of 59% and 79% for any LA enlargement, 80% and 74% for at least moderate LA enlargement, and 90% and 68% for severe enlargement.[18] In the 2011 initial CLUE protocol, the sensitivity and specificity were found to be 75% and 72% compared to formal echocardiography.[13] If LA enlargement is absent in the setting of other identified cardiac dysfunction, there is likely good cardiac compensation or adequate diuresis.[1]

The next windows in the protocol are the apical lung views for B-lines or ultrasound lung comets, sometimes referred to as "comet tail artifact." Comet tails are composed of linear reverberation, largely artifact, caused by interlobular septa thickened by fluid from inflammation or fibrosis.[20,21] A positive "comet tail sign" (particularly if focal B-lines are noted) in conjunction with a hyperdynamic LV and a negative "IVC plethora sign" should prompt consideration of an underlying infectious etiology and possible sepsis (see Table 49-1).[1,20,21] This sign has been noted to be an independent predictor of mortality greater than positive LV dysfunction.[13] Positive LA enlargement and B-lines suggest a cardiac cause, whereas comet tails alone could indicate isolated lung such as interstitial lung disease. Liteplo et al.[22] reported a specificity of 89% but a low sensitivity of 40% for congestive heart failure (CHF) with just two apical views. These can be improved by combining with the 85% to 90% sensitivity of N-terminal pro-brain natriuretic peptide or evaluation for basal lung effusions with ultrasound.[22,23]

TABLE 49-1 Diagnostic Patterns in CLUE

Disorder	C	L	U	E	S_R	S_I
LV systolic dysfunction, compensated	•	++/−				
Diastolic dysfunction, compensated		•				
Atrial fibrillation (paroxysmal or chronic)		•				
Severe mitral regurgitation/stenosis, compensated		•				
Severe multivessel CAD, compensated	+/−					
Symptomatic aortic valve disease, compensated		•				
CHF exacerbation, HFpEF		•	++/−	•		•
CHF exacerbation, HFrEF	•	•	++/−	•		•
Cardiogenic pulmonary edema		++/−	•	++/−		++/−
ARDS, noncardiogenic pulmonary edema			•	+/−−		+/−
Interstitial lung disease (acute or chronic)			++/−		+/−	
COPD with cor pulmonale			+/−−		•	•
Pneumonia or small pulmonary embolism			+/−−	+/−		
Submassive pulmonary embolism			+/−−	+/−	•	•
Cardiogenic shock	++/−	•	•	+/−		
Tamponade				•		•
RV myocardial infarction					•	•
Chronic right heart failure severe TR					•	•
Septic or hypovolemic shock						

Abbreviations: ARDS, adult respiratory distress syndrome; C, cardiac dysfunction; CAD, coronary artery disease; CHF, congestive heart failure; CLUE, cardiopulmonary limited ultrasound examination; COPD, chronic obstructive pulmonary disease; E, pleural (or pericardial) effusion sign; HFpEF, heart failure with preserved ejection fraction; HFrEF, heart failure with reduced ejection fraction; L, LA enlargement sign; LV, left ventricle; S_I, subcostal IVC plethora sign; S_R, subcostal right ventricular (RV) enlargement sign; TR, tricuspid regurgitation; U, ultrasound lung comet tail sign; •, present; ++/−, frequently present; +/−, commonly present; and +/− −, occasionally present.

From Kimura BJ, Shaw DJ, Amundson SA, et al. Cardiac Limited Ultrasound Examination Techniques to Augment the Bedside Cardiac Physical Examination. *J Ultrasound Med.* 2015;34(9):1683-1690. Copyright © 2016 by the American Institute of Ultrasound in Medicine. Reprinted by permission of John Wiley & Sons, Inc.

Ultrasound is far more sensitive than chest radiography for detecting pleural effusions in the costophrenic angle, detecting as few as 2 mL of pleural fluid compared to the 200 mL required to see pleural effusions on anterior posterior chest x-ray.[1,13,23] Findings combined with other positive cardiac findings could indicate CHF, whereas isolated findings could indicate interstitial lung disease, pulmonary embolism, or malignancy.[1] Studies have indicated poorer outcomes in patients with pleural effusions on ultrasound in the setting of CHF, pneumonia, and malignancy.[24-26]

The subcostal right ventricular view is new to the CLUE protocol as of the 2015 update by Kimura et al.[1] This sign is defined as a right ventricle approaching or equal to the LV, whereas a normal size is approximately two-thirds of the LV on this view. An enlarged right ventricle has been shown to be useful in identifying, when combined with other findings, cor pulmonale, pulmonary embolism, and right-sided myocardial infarction.[1,27-29]

The second subcostal view is the evaluation of the IVC for volume overload, which is defined as an anteroposterior diameter of the IVC nearly equal to the aorta and lacks a variation of greater than 50% with respirations.[1] A positive IVC plethora sign has been associated with increased in-hospital mortality,[13] and readmission to the hospital in patients with CHF.[30] Additionally, the IVC is always positive in the cases of tamponade and shock secondary to right heart failure.[1]

Overall, the CLUE protocol serves as a rapid evaluation of a patient to augment available history and physical examination in initial and ongoing medical decision making. Multiple studies have described the sensitivity and specificity of individual clue findings, which is significantly less than the gold standard of formal echocardiography.[1,4,5,10,13,16] However, CLUE is a quick and simple pathway for appropriately trained practitioners to evaluate the cardiac and pulmonary status of a patient in acute distress when formal echocardiography is not practical or available.[1,13,18] Although individual signs in the protocol have been assessed in terms of diagnostic accuracy and application to a variety of clinical settings, only further study can establish the utility of CLUE overall in terms of affecting patient outcomes.

TABLE 49-2 Recommendations for Use of Point-of-Care Ultrasound in Clinical Practice

Recommendation	Rating	References
Cardiopulmonary limited ultrasound examination (CLUE) can be used as a point-of-care modality to evaluate circulatory or respiratory distress	B	1-4, 6, 9, 10, 13, 17-19
CLUE can be performed with limited training when guided by an experienced provider or with training throughout a residency program	B	11, 12

A = consistent, good-quality patient-oriented evidence; B = inconsistent or limited-quality patient-oriented evidence; C = consensus, disease-oriented evidence, usual practice, expert opinion, or case series. For information about the SORT evidence rating system, go to http://www.aafp.org/afpsort.

PERFORMING THE SCAN[1]

1. **Preparation.** Bring ultrasound with a low-frequency transducer (typically 2-3 MHz) for cardiac imaging to the bedside. Place patient in the supine position. Explain the purpose of the examination to the patient. Apply gel to the locations where the probe will be placed during the examination.

2. **Evaluate for LV systolic dysfunction sign.** Place transducer to the left of the patient's sternum in the third or fourth intercostal space with probe marker directed to the patient's right shoulder (**Figure 49-1**). Obtain parasternal long-axis view of the heart. Visualize anterior leaflet of the mitral valve (**Figure 49-2**). If the anterior mitral valve leaflet does not encroach on the ventricular septum to a distance of less than 1 cm by subjective estimate,

then the "LV systolic dysfunction sign" is considered to be present[14] (**Figure 49-3** and ⏵ **Videos 49-1 and 49-2**)

3. **Evaluate for LA enlargement sign.** While interrogating the heart from the same parasternal long-axis view, as described previously (**Figure 49-1**), compare the anteroposterior diameter of the LA to that of the aorta (**Figure 49-4**). If the LA diameter is larger than the aorta during the entire cardiac cycle, then the "LA enlargement sign" is present[18] (**Figure 49-5** and ⏵ **Video 49-3**).

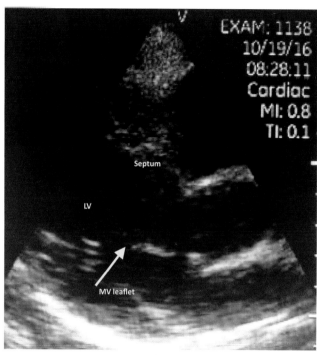

FIGURE 49-3. Parasternal long-axis view with "left ventricular systolic dysfunction sign" present. LV, left ventricle; MV, mitral valve.

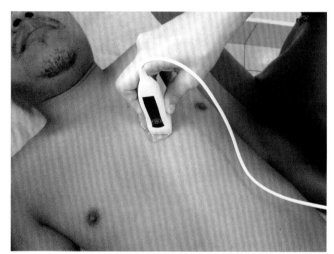

FIGURE 49-1. Probe placement to obtain parasternal long-axis view of heart.

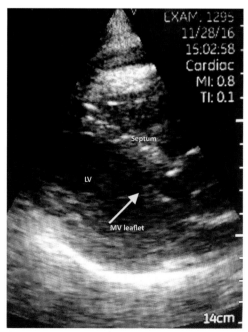

FIGURE 49-2. Parasternal long-axis view without "LV systolic dysfunction sign." LV, left ventricle; MV, mitral valve.

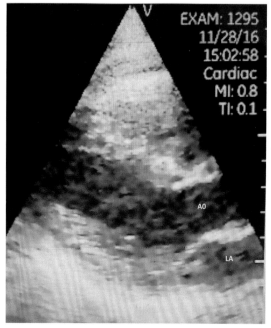

FIGURE 49-4. Parasternal long-axis view without "LA enlargement sign." AO, aorta; LA, left atrium.

PART 3

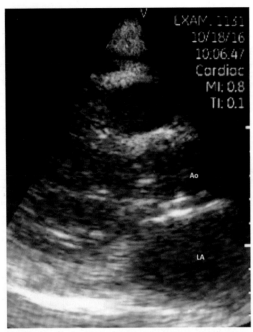

FIGURE 49-5. Parasternal long-axis view with "LA enlargement sign" present.

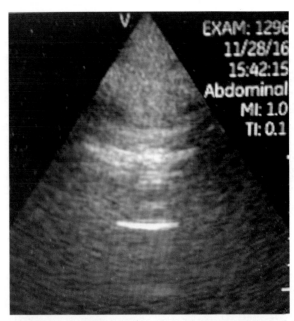

FIGURE 49-7. Lung ultrasound without "ultrasound lung comet tail sign."

4. **Evaluate for ultrasound lung comet tail sign.** Place the transducer in a sagittal position (probe marker toward head of patient) on the patient's anterior chest wall at the midclavicular line in the third intercostal space **(Figure 49-6)**. Perform the examination over the anteroapices of each lung. If at least three B-lines are noted in a single view, then "ultrasound lung comet tail sign" is present[21,31] **(Figures 49-7 and 49-8** and ▶ **Video 49-4)**.

5. **Evaluate for effusion (pleural) sign.** Place the transducer in the posterolateral axillary line at the costophrenic angle in a coronal position (marker toward patient's head). Obtain this view on each side of the patient **(Figure 49-9)**. An anechoic area between the lung and diaphragm is indicative of pleural

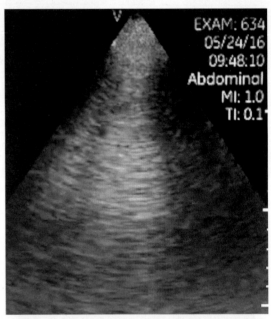

FIGURE 49-8. Lung ultrasound with "ultrasound lung comet tail sign" present.

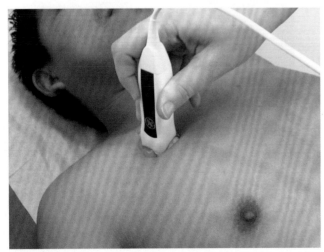

FIGURE 49-6. Probe placement to evaluate for "ultrasound lung comet tail sign."

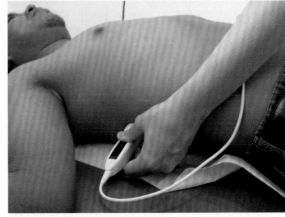

FIGURE 49-9. Probe placement to evaluate for "effusion (pleural) sign."

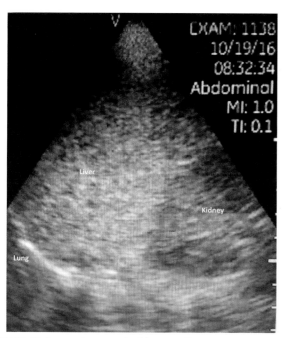

FIGURE 49-10. Lung ultrasound without "effusion (pleural) sign."

fluid and a positive "effusion (pleural) sign"[32] (**Figures 49-10 and 49-11** and ▶ **Videos 49-5 and 49-6**).

6. **Evaluate for right ventricular (RV) enlargement sign.** Place the transducer under the patient's xiphoid process and obtain a subcostal 4-chamber view of the heart (**Figure 49-12**). Consider the RV area in relation to the LV area (**Figure 49-13**). If the RV area is nearly equal to or equal to the LV area, then "RV enlargement sign" is present[33] (**Figure 49-14** and ▶ **Videos 49-7 and 49-8**).

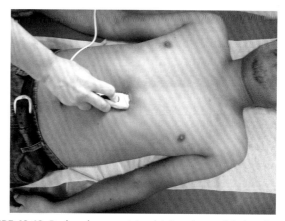

FIGURE 49-12. Probe placement to obtain subcostal 4-chamber view of heart.

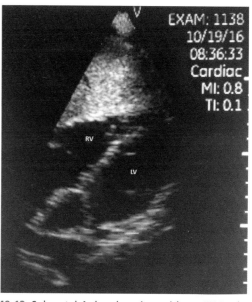

FIGURE 49-13. Subcostal 4-chamber view without "RV enlargement sign." LV, left ventricle; RV, right ventricle.

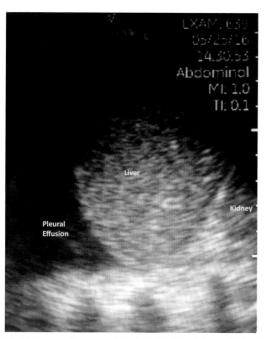

FIGURE 49-11. Lung ultrasound with "effusion (pleural) sign" present.

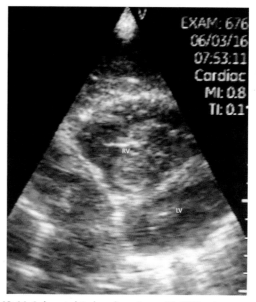

FIGURE 49-14. Subcostal 4-chamber view with "RV enlargement sign" present. LV, left ventricle; RV, right ventricle.

PART 3

7. **Evaluate for IVC plethora sign.** From the subcostal view, rotate the transducer from the 9 to the 12 o'clock position (probe marker toward patient's head) and visualize the intrahepatic IVC (**Figures 49-15 and 49-16**). The "IVC plethora sign" is present if the IVC diameter is dilated (ie, approaching the diameter of the adjacent aorta) and does not demonstrate respiratory variation of more than 50%[34] (**Figure 49-17** and ▶ **Videos 49-9 and 49-10**).

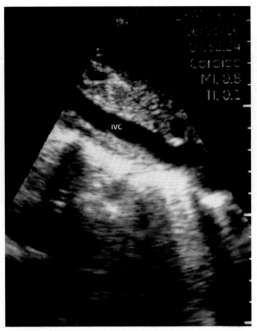

FIGURE 49-17. IVC ultrasound with "IVC plethora sign" present. IVC, inferior vena cava.

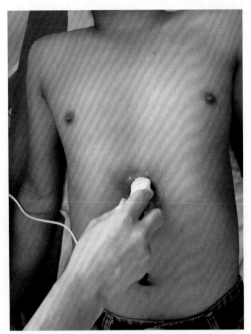

FIGURE 49-15. Probe placement to evaluate for "inferior vena cava (IVC) plethora sign."

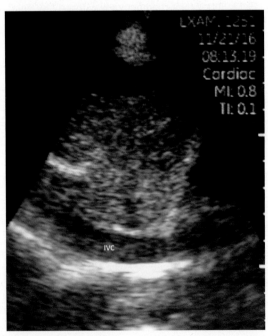

FIGURE 49-16. IVC ultrasound without "IVC plethora sign." IVC, inferior vena cava.

PATIENT MANAGEMENT

Utilizing point-of-care ultrasound within the organizational framework of the "CLUE protocol," it is possible to quickly narrow the differential diagnosis to the most likely etiology of the patient's presenting symptoms. The lengthy list of potential diagnoses for a patient presenting with undifferentiated dyspnea can efficiently and accurately be pared to a far more manageable list of probable pathologies.

A positive "LV systolic dysfunction sign" prompts one to consider systolic dysfunction (CHF exacerbation, heart failure with reduced ejection fraction [HFrEF]) as the etiology of the acute presenting symptoms.

However, if there is a negative "LV systolic dysfunction," but a positive "LA enlargement sign," one should consider the possibility of diastolic dysfunction (CHF exacerbation, heart failure with preserved ejection fraction [HFpEF]) as a potential cause of current symptomatology.

If—in the context of positive "LV systolic dysfunction sign" and/or positive "LA enlargement sign"—the examiner notes a positive "comet tail sign," this would further support decompensated heart failure as a likely cause of the patient's symptoms.

Conversely, a negative "LV systolic dysfunction sign" and a negative "LA enlargement sign" coupled with a positive "comet tail sign" should prompt consideration of noncardiogenic pulmonary edema (if B-lines are diffuse) or possibly infectious etiology (ie, pneumonia, if B-lines are focal).

A positive "effusion sign" may be produced by any number of underlying pathologic processes (cardiogenic, infectious, malignancy, etc.). Nevertheless, the effusion itself—particularly if large—may be a significant contributor to patient respiratory symptoms and, as such, should prompt further investigation and possibly intervention (ie, diagnostic/therapeutic thoracentesis).

A positive "RV enlargement sign"—particularly if believed to be new—should prompt strong consideration of pulmonary embolus

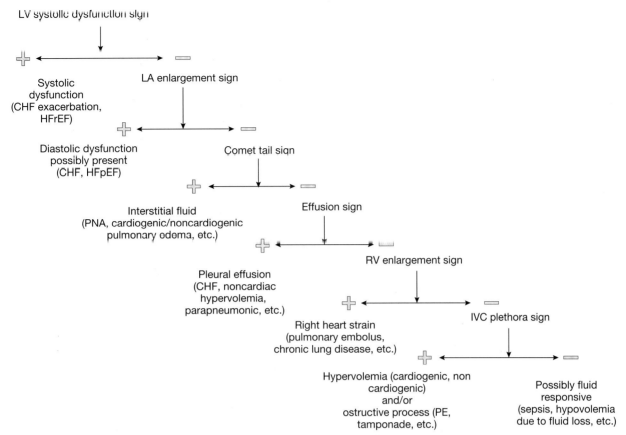

FIGURE 49-18. Clue protocol algorithm. CHF, congestive heart failure; HFpEF, heart failure with preserved ejection fraction; HFrEF, heart failure with reduced ejection fraction; IVC, inferior vena cava; LA, left atrium; LV, left ventricle; PE, pulmonary embolism; PNA, pneumonia; RV, right ventricle.

as a possibility. However, if evaluating a patient with known history of chronic lung disease, a positive "RV enlargement sign" may be due to the patient's chronic condition and may or may not be related to acute symptoms.

A positive "IVC plethora sign" encountered with positive "LV systolic dysfunction sign" and/or "LA enlargement sign" and positive "comet tail sign" lends further support to acute decompensated heart failure as the most likely cause of symptoms. If, in the absence of "LV systolic dysfunction sign" or "LA enlargement sign," one encounters an "IVC plethora sign" and "comet tail sign," noncardiac causes of hypervolemia should be strongly considered. A positive "IVC plethora sign" noted in addition to a positive "RV enlargement sign" should lend further support to the possibility of pulmonary embolus as potential diagnosis.

A positive "comet tail sign" (particularly if focal B-lines are noted) in conjunction with a hyperdynamic LV and a negative "IVC plethora sign" should prompt consideration of an underlying infectious etiology and possible sepsis.

As with any other investigative finding (physical examination, laboratories, etc.), no single portion of the CLUE protocol taken in isolation is 100% sensitive or 100% specific for ruling in or ruling out pathology. However, when taken into consideration in the context of clinical history and pertinent physical examination findings, the information derived from progressing through the CLUE protocol can be exceedingly helpful in allowing the clinician to rapidly narrow the differential diagnosis, arrive at the most likely suspected diagnosis, and guide timely and appropriate patient management (**Figure 49-18**).

PEARLS AND PITFALLS

Pearls

- "Work backward" in terms of blood flow. Start at LV function, then work backward to the left atrium, then to the lungs for comet tails and effusions, then evaluate the right heart and IVC.[12]
- When obtaining the parasternal long-axis view, adjust the probe until both the aortic and mitral valves are in view. The tricuspid valve should not be in this view.

- The parasternal window is generally between the third and fifth intercostal spaces; keep in mind that if a move to lower rib spaces is necessary to get a good image, the axis may be slightly off.
- If the apex of the LV is seen on the parasternal long-axis view, try rotating the probe clockwise a little to avoid foreshortening the view.

PART 3

Pearls and Pitfalls, Continued

- The interventricular septum should be almost horizontal on a parasternal long-axis view.
- In the apical views of bilateral lungs, keep in mind that some ultrasounds are designed to filter out artifact, which are needed in order to properly visualize B-lines or comet tails. Make sure any such filters are turned off, if possible, before viewing the lungs.
- When evaluating pleural effusions, note that blood or purulent fluid in an effusion may appear isoechoic on ultrasound.[1]
- In difficult subcostal evaluations, try having the patient hold his or her breath to obtain a subcostal 4-chamber view.[1]
- If unable to get a good IVC evaluation, ultrasound or visual examination of the jugular vein may also be used to estimate central venous pressure. This is not necessarily part of CLUE but can augment evaluation of the patient.[1]

Pitfalls

- When assessing for LV dysfunction, remember that false-negative results can occur from acute LV dysfunction without symmetric dilation. This can occur in acute apical ischemia or stress-induced (Takotsubo) cardiomyopathy. These may be better assessed with apical views not included in CLUE.
- Abnormal anterior mitral valve leaflet motion from eccentric aortic insufficiency or leaflet calcification/mitral stenosis can lead to false-positive results for LV dysfunction.
- Although the anterior–posterior diameter has been shown to be a good evaluation of LA size/enlargement, limitations in space caused by skeletal deformities like pectus excavatum, or overall enlargement of the right heart, can cause false negatives through asymmetric dilation of the left atrium.[1,13,17,18]
- Aortic root aneurysms will cause false-negative results in assessment of the left atrium.
- Comet tails can be chronic secondary to pulmonary fibrosis, as opposed to acute inflammation or edema.[1,31]
- Small pleural effusions can be missed at the lung bases if the probe is not posterior enough.
- When looking for pleural effusions at the lung bases, do not mistake ascites or gastric fluid for pleural effusions. Be sure that the fluid is cephalad to the diaphragm.[1]
- When evaluating the IVC, identify both the IVC and the aorta to be sure to avoid confusing the two. The aorta is to the patient's left, has no connection to hepatic veins, and is pulsatile.[1,13]

BILLING

CPT Code	Description	Global Payment	Professional Component	Technical Component
93308	Echocardiography, transthoracic, real time with image documentation (2D) includes M-mode recording when performed; follow-up or limited study	$126.03	$26.14	$99.89

CPT codes and average national reimbursement for Medicare in 2016. Payment data are from https://www.cms.gov/apps/physician-fee-schedule/search/search-criteria.aspx. See Chapter 2 for details on ultrasound billing.

References

1. Kimura BJ, Shaw D, Amundson S, Phan J, Blanchard D, DeMaria A. Cardiac limited ultrasound examination techniques to augment the bedside cardiac physical examination. *J Ultrasound Med*. 2015;34(9):1683-1690.

2. Kajimoto K, Madeen K, Nakayama T, Tsudo H, Tadahide K, Abe T. Rapid evaluation by lung-cardiac-inferior vena cava (LCI) integrated ultrasound for differentiating heart failure from pulmonary disease as the cause of acute dyspnea in the emergency setting. *Cardiovasc Ultrasound*. 2012;10:49.

3. Oren-Gringberg A, Talmor D, Brown SM. Concise definitive review: focused critical care echocardiography in the ICU. *Crit Care Med*. 2013;41(11):2618-2626.

4. Benjamin E, Griffin K, Leibowitz AB, et al. Goal-directed transesophageal echocardiography performed by intensivists to assess left ventricular function: comparison with pulmonary artery catheterization. *J Cardiothorac Vasc Anesth*. 1998;12(1):10-15.

5. Kimura BJ, Shaw DJ, Agan DL, Amundson SA, Ping AC, DeMaria AN. Value of a cardiovascular limited ultrasound examination using a hand-carried ultrasound device on clinical management in an outpatient clinic. *Am J Cardiol*. 2007;100:321-325.

6. Shah SP, Shah SP, Fils-Aime R, et al. Focused cardiopulmonary ultrasound for assessment of dyspnea in a resource-limited setting. *Crit Ultrasound J*. 2016;8:7.

7. Croft LB, Duvall WL, Goldman ME. A pilot study of the clinical impact of hand-carried cardiac ultrasound in the medical clinic. *Echocardiography*. 2006;23(6):439-446.

8. Jensen MB, Sloth E, Larsen KM, Schmidt MB. Transthoracic echocardiography for cardiopulmonary monitoring in intensive care. *Eur J Anaesthiol*. 2004;21(9):700-707.

9. Jones AE, Craddock PA, Tayal VS, Kline JA. Diagnostic accuracy of left ventricular function for identifying sepsis among emergency department patient with nontraumatic symptomatic undifferentiated hypotension. *Shock*. 2005;24(6):513-517.

10. Moore CL, Rose GA, Tayal VS, Sullivan M, Arrowood JA, Kline JA. Determination of left ventricular function of emergency physician echocardiography of hypotensive patients. *Acad Emerg Med*. 2002;9(3):186-193.

11. Lucas BP, Candotti C, Margeta B, et al. Diagnostic accuracy of hospitalist-performed hand-carried ultrasound echocardiography after a brief training program. *J Hosp Med*. 2009;4(6):340-349.

12. Kimura BJ, Amundson SA, Phan JN, Agan DL, Shaw DJ. Observations during development of an internal medicine residency training program in cardiovascular limited ultrasound examination. *J Hosp Med*. 2012;7(7):537-542.

13. Kimura BJ, Yogo N, O'Connell CW, Phan JN, Showalter BK, Wolfson T. Cardiopulmonary limited ultrasound examination for "Quick-Look" bedside application. *Am J Cardiol*. 2011;108(4):586-590.

14. Lew W, Henning H, Schelbert H, Karliner JS. Assessment of mitral valve E-point septal separation as an index of left ventricular performance in patients with acute and previous myocardial infarction. *Am J Cardiol*. 1978;41: 836-845.

15. Silverstein JR, Laffely NH, Ritkin RD. Quantitative estimation of left ventricular ejection fraction from mitral valve E-point septal separation and comparison to magnetic resonance imaging. *Am J Cardiol*. 2006;97:137-140.

16. Martin LD, Howell EE, Ziegelstein RC, et al. Hand-carried ultrasound performed by hospitalists: does is improve the cardiac physical examination? *Am J Med*. 2009;122(1):35-41.

17. Kimura BJ, Fowler SJ, Fergus TS, et al. Detection of left atrial enlargement using hand-carried ultrasound devices to screen for cardiac abnormalities. *Am J Med.* 2005;118:912-916.

18. Kimura BJ, Kedar E, Weiss DE, Wahlstrom CL, Agan DL. A hand-carried ultrasound sign of cardiac disease: the left-atrium-to-aorta diastolic ratio. *Am J Emerg Med.* 2010;28:203-207.

19. Kimura BJ, Gilcrease GW 3rd, Showalter BK, Phan JN, Wolfson T. Diagnostic performance of a pocket-sized ultrasound device for quick-look cardiac imaging. *Am J Emerg Med.* 2012;30(1):32-36.

20. Volpicelli G, Elbarbary M, Blaivas M, et al; International Liason Committee on Lung Ultrasound (ILC-LUS) for International Consensus Conference on Lung Ultrasound (ICC-LUS). International evidence-based recommendations for point-of-care lung ultrasound. *Intensive Care Med.* 2012;38(4):577-591.

21. Picano E, Frassi F, Agricola E, Gilgorova S, Gargani L, Mottola G. Ultrasound lung comets: a clinically useful sign of extravascular lung water. *J Am Soc Echocardiogr.* 2006;19(3):356-363.

22. Liteplo AS, Marill KA, Villen T, et al. Emergency thoracic ultrasound in the differentiation of the etiology of shortness of breath (ETUDES): sonographic B-lines and N-terminal pro-brain-type natriuretic peptide in diagnosing congestive heart failure. *Acad Emerg Med.* 2009;16(3):201-210.

23. Katoaka H, Takada S. The role of thoracic ultrasonography for evaluation of patients with decompensated chronic heart failure. *J Am Coll Cardiol.* 2000;35:1638-1646.

24. Wong CL, Holroyd-Leduc J, Straus SE. Does this patient have a pleural effusion? *JAMA.* 2009;301:309-317.

25. Roguin A, Behar D, Ben Ami H, et al. Long-term prognosis of acute pulmonary oedema—an ominous outcome. *Eur J Heart Fail.* 2000;2(2):137-144.

26. Ercan S, Davutoglu V, Altunbas G, et al. Prognostic role of incidental pleural effusion diagnosed during echocardiographic evaluation. *Clin Cardiol.* 2014;37(2):115-118.

27. Kimura BJ, Amundson SA, Willis CL, Gilpin EA, DeMaria AN. Usefulness of a hand-held ultrasound device for the bedside examination of left ventricular function. *Am J Cardiol.* 2002;90:1038-1039.

28. Frémont B, Pacouret G, Jacobi D, Puglsi R, Charbonnier B, de Labriolle A. Prognostic value of echocardiographic right/left ventricular end-diastolic diameter ratio in patients with acute pulmonary embolism: results from a monocenter registry of 1,416 patients. *Chest.* 2008;133(2):358-362.

29. Lainscak M, Pernat A. Importance of bedside echocardiography for detection of unsuspected isolated right ventricular infarction as a casue of cardiovascular collapse. *Am J Emerg Med.* 2007;25:110-114.

30. Goonewardena SN, Gemigani A, Ronan A, et al. Comparison of hand-carried ultrasound assessment of the inferior vena cava and N-terminal pro-brain natriuretic peptide for predicting readmission after hospitalization for acute decompensated heart failure. *JACC Cardiovasc Imaging.* 2008;1(5):595-601.

31. Bedetti G, Gargani L, Corbisiero A, Frassi F, Poggianti E, Mottola G. Evaluation of ultrasound lung comets by hand-held echocardiography. *Cardiovasc Ultrasound.* 2006;4:34.

32. Grimberg A, Shigueoka DC, Atallah AN, Ajzen S, Iared W. Diagnostic accuracy of sonography for pleural effusion: systematic review. *Sao Paulo Med J.* 2010;128(2):90-95.

33. Kasper W, Konstantinides S, Geibel A, Tiede N, Krause T, Just H. Prognostic significance of right ventricular afterload stress detected by echocardiography in patients with clinically suspected pulmonary embolism. *Heart.* 1997;77:346-349.

34. Brennan JM, Blair JE, Goonewardena S, et al. Reappraisal of the use of the inferior vena cava for estimating right atrial pressure. *J Am Soc Echocardiogr.* 2007;20(7):857-861.

Focused Ultrasonography in Trauma (FAST)

Caroline Brandon, MD and Tarina Lee Kang, MD, MHA, FACEP

● Clinical Vignette

A 19-year-old woman presents with acute-onset right lower quadrant abdominal pain. She recently took a home pregnancy test that came back positive. Her last menstrual period was 6 weeks ago. She denies nausea, vomiting, or vaginal bleeding. She had an appendectomy 3 years prior. Her only significant past medical history is an episode of pelvic inflammatory disease (PID) that was treated with oral antibiotics. Vitals sign are a heart rate of 90; blood pressure of 100/60; respiratory rate of 18; an oral temperature of 98.4°F; and an oxygen saturation of 99%. Her abdomen is moderately distended and diffusely tender in all quadrants. Labs are significant for a positive urine human chorionic gonadotropin (hCG) and a hemoglobin of 10. You are concerned for a ruptured ectopic pregnancy.

LITERATURE REVIEW

In the 1980s, several German papers cited the use of ultrasound (US) to evaluate patients with suspected blunt abdominal trauma (BAT). Using US at the bedside in this manner on BAT patients quickly gained momentum in Europe and Asia, but it did not make its way to the United States until the 1990s.[1] In 1992, Tso and his colleagues were one of the first to publish an article from the United States regarding the use of US on BAT patients.[2] This was a prospective study that took place over 8 consecutive months and that looked at the sensitivity and specificity of US to detect hemoperitoneum. Overall, 163 trauma patients with suspected BAT were enrolled; 20 of them underwent diagnostic peritoneal lavage (DPL) and 149 received computed tomography (CT) with intravenous contrast of the abdomen. US was performed on all 163 patients by a surgical trauma fellow (PGY6) after short training. Overall, the sensitivity was 69% and specificity was 99% for US as compared to a sensitivity of 75% and specificity of 100% for DPL in the ability to detect peritoneal bleeding. The authors concluded that US was both rapid and sensitive for detecting hemoperitoneum and could be a valuable screening tool to determine the need for additional testing.[2] These findings were profound because the gold standard for identifying hemoperitoneum at that time was DPL. However, DPL was thought to be invasive and oftentimes impractical given the need to decompress the stomach and bladder prior to procedure and the risk of abdominal vascular injury.

More Focused Ultrasonography in Trauma (FAST) validation studies soon followed. Chambers and Pilbrow concluded that the hepatorenal view in the right upper quadrant (RUQ) reliably showed the presence of peritoneal fluid and was a viable, noninvasive alternative to the DPL.[3] In 1997, however, Nordenholz et al. published a review article in the Annals of Emergency Medicine that compared the sensitivity of US versus CT and DPL in detecting hemoperitoneum in suspected BAT patients. Overall, DPL was found to be both sensitive and specific, but there were many contraindications, such as previous abdominal surgery, coagulopathy, pregnancy, and morbid obesity. Its usefulness was also limited by long lab waiting times for fluid interpretation in equivocal cases and the time required to perform the test.[4] CT was equally as sensitive and specific but was far less invasive. US had a sensitivity approaching 90% with appropriate US training. The authors concluded that one test was not superior to another.[4,5] Limitations of CT were substantial at the time, including the risk of contrast allergy, the need to transfer a potentially unstable patient outside the department, time, cost, variable radiologist experience with CT, and the need for additional personnel to perform the scan. CT imaging technology and experience continued to advance, however, such that the use of CT to assess patients with suspected BAT eventually became and continues to be the primary imaging modality in many hospitals.[5]

Although earlier studies proclaimed impressive performance of the FAST, more recent studies have exposed its limitations. Rothlin et al. conducted a prospective study that compared US to CT or laparotomy in the detection of intra-abdominal injury in 312 patients. The authors concluded that US was poorly sensitive in detecting solid organ injuries compared to CT, ultimately recommending that a CT scan be performed in stable patients with a positive FAST to determine the source of bleeding.[6,7] More recent studies continue to support the belief that the FAST should be used solely to look for the presence or absence of free abdominal and pleural fluid, and that its sensitivity increases in patients who are hemodynamically unstable with a compelling reason to have hemoperitoneum, such as a ruptured ectopic or a significant abdominal trauma, but is still poorly sensitive for diagnosing intra-abdominal injuries, especially in stable patients.

Accepting these limitations, the FAST continues to be an integral management tool for both trauma and nontrauma patients. In 2013, Sheng et al. looked at the use of US and CT over the past decade. The study showed an overall increase in the use of US and a decrease in the use of CT for certain blunt trauma patients.[8] The FAST not only continues to stand firmly as a resource tool in the Advanced Trauma Life Support (ATLS) protocol for trauma patients to help guide management, but also serves as an amenity for decision making for advanced imaging and procedures for nontrauma patients as well.

Because of the success of the FAST examination in the emergency medicine setting, several studies looked at whether US can be effectively used at the bedside by primary care physicians. Flick concluded in the Journal of Ultrasound Medicine that use of point-of-care US by primary care physicians to evaluate the abdomen is a cost-effective and safe way to evaluate patients in the nonemergent setting, using applications similar to that used in the emergent setting. He concluded that US implementation by primary care physicians

TABLE 50-1	Recommendations for Use of Point-of-Care Ultrasound in Clinical Practice		
Recommendation		**Rating**	**References**
FAST ultrasound, including views of the right and left upper quadrants as well as the suprapubic and cardiac views, has a high sensitivity for evaluating for hemoperitoneum and hemopericardium.		A	3-7
Point-of-care ultrasound for evaluation of peritoneal fluid can be performed effectively by practitioners with only brief training.		A	9-11

A = consistent, good-quality patient-oriented evidence; B = inconsistent or limited-quality patient-oriented evidence; C = consensus, disease-oriented evidence, usual practice, expert opinion, or case series. For information about the SORT evidence rating system, go to http://www.aafp.org/afpsort.

decreases cost and performance accuracy. It can be achieved with as little as 3 hours of didactic training followed by 5 hours of hands-on training.[9] Wong et al. published a pilot US training curriculum for family medicine practitioners. Wong concluded that accurate and effective clinical decision making based on US findings can occur once an educational curriculum and consistent US teaching regimen could be implemented into the program.[10] Hall et al. further exposed challenges of point-of-care US training, noting that 2.2% of family medicine residencies had an US curriculum and 11.2% of programs were in the process of starting the curriculum implementation process. Hall et al. concluded that the greatest barrier to training was not the curriculum implementation, but, rather, the lack of trained faculty in US and the perceived utility of point-of-care US for patients by attending physicians.[11]

Although the FAST examination was initially designed for the surgeon and emergency medicine physician, the rationale behind its incorporation into the primary care setting can be easily validated. It is common for patients with atraumatic free fluid in the abdomen to present to the primary care setting for evaluation. Additionally, the FAST examination can diagnose the presence of pleural fluid, hemothorax, and pericardial fluid. Patients presenting with correlative symptoms of these diagnoses can be expeditiously transferred to an emergent care setting for further treatment.

PERFORMING THE SCAN

1. **Prepare the patient.** Place the patient in the supine position on the gurney. Avoid having the patient sitting upright or semi-recumbent, as this allows peritoneal fluid to move into gravity dependent missed by the FAST. Cover the patient with drapes to expose only the abdomen and the lower thorax. Place the US machine to the patient's right. Make sure the US machine and patient bed are at the appropriate height for the examiner. Plug the machine in. Use a low-frequency probe 2-5 mHz. Select the "abdominal" examination setting on the US machine. A phased-array probe or curvilinear probe can be used (**Figure 50-1**).

2. **Evaluate the RUQ for free fluid in the abdomen and thorax.** Place the low-frequency probe in the RUQ in the mid-axillary line between the 8th and 11th intercostal space, with the probe indicator pointing toward the patient's head (**Figure 50-2**).

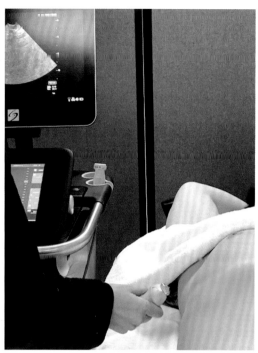

FIGURE 50-1. Ultrasound setup for FAST examination with the examiner and ultrasound machine to the patient's right side. Select the abdominal preset and select a low-frequency probe. Adjust the depth to approximately 16 to 19 cm.

Placing the probe in this position creates a coronal view of the hepatorenal space, also known as Morrison's pouch (**Figure 50-3**). Ensure that the liver tip is also visualized to rule out small fluid collections in this space. Fluid in Morrison's pouch will appear as an anechoic stripe (**Figure 50-4**). Next, move the probe cephalad

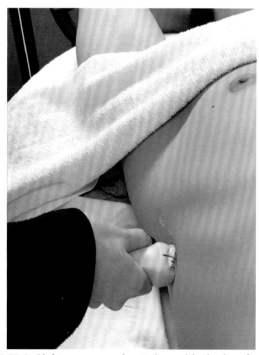

FIGURE 50-2. Right upper quadrant view with the low-frequency probe selected. Place the probe in the mid-axillary line between the 8th and 11th rib spaces.

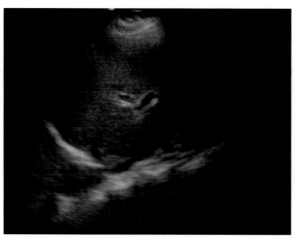

FIGURE 50-3. Normal right upper quadrant Focused Ultrasonography in Trauma views.

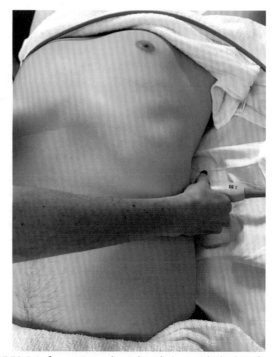

FIGURE 50-5. Right upper quadrant Focused Ultrasonography in Trauma views with positive thoracic fluid. Fluid appears as anechoic and will be above the diaphragm. You should see an extension of the spine into the thoracic cavity that is not present when there is no fluid present.

to evaluate the perihepatic space between the liver and the diaphragm. Fluid in the thoracic cavity will appear as an anechoic collection superior to the diaphragm (**Figure 50-5**). If fluid is visualized superior to the liver but inferior to the diaphragm, the

liver has detached from the diaphragm and peritoneal fluid has filled this space. Rib shadows are long, hypoechoic columns that run vertically across the screen and can obscure views. Rotate the probe counterclockwise such that the probe face is nestled in the intercostal space to clear the screen of rib shadows.

3. **Evaluate the left upper quadrant for free fluid.** Place the low-frequency probe in the left upper quadrant (LUQ) along the posterior axillary line between the 6th and 9th intercostal spaces, with the probe indicator pointing toward the patient's head (**Figure 50-6**). The LUQ view can be difficult to obtain

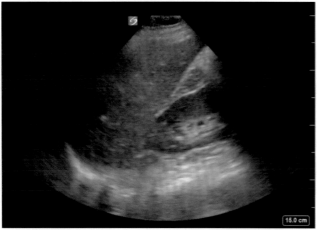

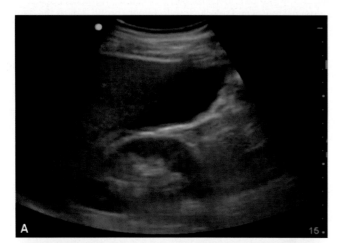

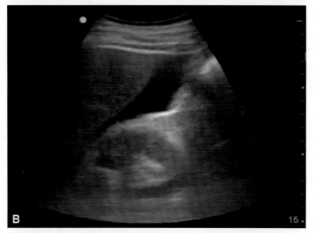

FIGURE 50-4. A and B, Positive right upper quadrant Focused Ultrasonography in Trauma view of Morrison's pouch. Fluid appears as an anechoic strip between the kidney and liver.

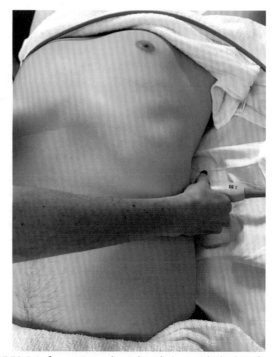

FIGURE 50-6. Left upper quadrant (LUQ) view with the low-frequency probe selected. Place the probe in the posterior axillary line between the 6th and 9th rib spaces.

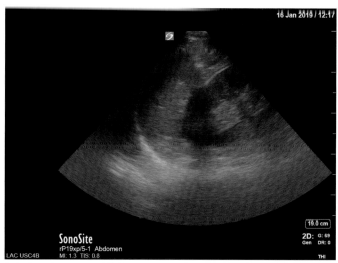

FIGURE 50-7. Normal left upper quadrant Focused Ultrasonography in Trauma view. Make sure to visualize both the entire spleen, paying close attention to the interface between the spleen and diaphragm where fluid collects first.

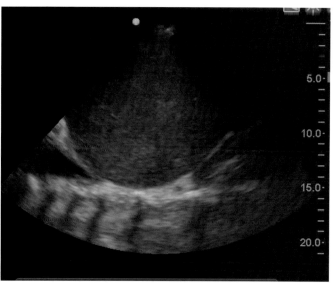

FIGURE 50-9. Left upper quadrant Focused Ultrasonography in Trauma view with positive thoracic fluid. Fluid appears as anechoic and will be above the diaphragm. Look for an extension of the spine into the thoracic cavity not normally seen if the lung is fully aerated.

because the spleen is located more posteriorly and has a much smaller acoustic window compared to the liver (**Figure 50-7**). Look for fluid between the kidney and spleen, in the subdiaphragmatic spaces of the spleen first and along the tip of the spleen (**Figure 50-8**). Again, this view can be obscured by rib shadows, so rotate the probe face such that it is in plane with the intercostal space between the ribs. If thoracic fluid is present, anechoic fluid will appear above the diaphragm. Additionally, fluid in the thorax allows vertebral bodies in the thoracic spine to be more radiodense, resulting in the visualization of the thoracic spine across the entire bottom screen (**Figure 50-9**).

4. **Evaluate the pelvis for free fluid.** While the patient is lying supine, place a low-frequency probe in the suprapubic region just above the public bone, with the probe indicator first pointing toward the patient's right in the transverse orientation (**Figure 50-10A**). Normal pelvic FAST view (**Figure 50-10B**). Fan through the bladder in this orientation by moving the probe face cephalad to caudad (**Figure 50-10C**). Next obtain a longitudinal view of the bladder by rotating the probe clockwise 90° so that the indicator on the probe points toward the patient's head (**Figure 50-11**). Peritoneal fluid will accumulate behind the bladder, which can be appreciated to the left of the bladder on the screen (**Figure 50-12**). In female patients, the uterus sits behind the bladder. Peritoneal fluid can accumulate both posterior to the uterus in the pouch of Douglas and in the potential spaces between the bladder and the uterus (**Figure 50-13**).

5. **Evaluate the subxiphoid 4-chamber view of the heart for pericardial fluid.** Have the patient lie supine. Place a low-frequency probe in the subxiphoid region under the xiphoid process, with the probe indicator pointing toward the patient's right. Lower the heel of the probe to approximately 30° to the patient's chest, with the face of the probe facing the patient's right shoulder (**Figure 50-14**). Slowly fan the probe toward the patient's left shoulder. The liver should be viewed on the left of the screen and the heart inferior and posterior to the liver (**Figure 50-15**). A pericardial effusion appears as an anechoic fluid collection within the pericardial sac (**Figure 50-16**). An alternative view of the heart is the parasternal long-axis view. Place the probe lateral to the patient's left of the sternum, between the 4th and 5th intercostal space with the probe indicator toward the patient's left hip (**Figure 50-17A**). In this view both the anterior and posterior sides of the pericardium can be seen. Look for fluid above the right ventricle (anterior) and deep to the left ventricle (posterior) (**Figure 50-17B**).

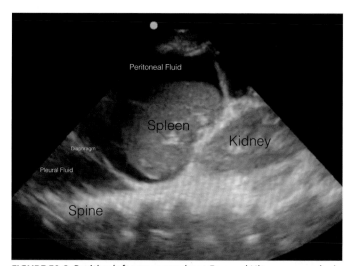

FIGURE 50-8. Positive left upper quadrant Focused Ultrasonography in Trauma view of perisplenic space. Fluid appears as an anechoic strip between the spleen and diaphragm.

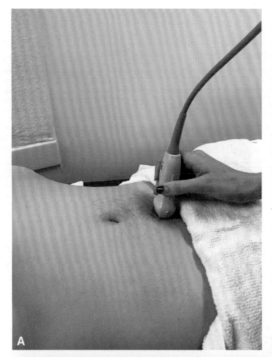

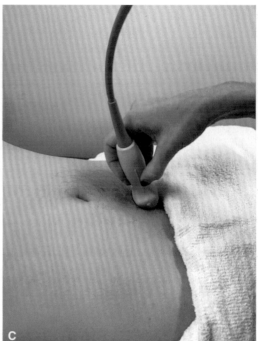

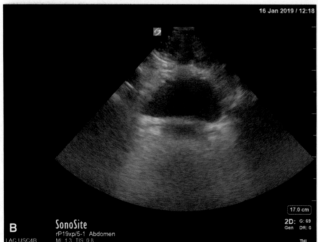

FIGURE 50-10. A and B, Suprapubic view with the low-frequency probe selected. Place the probe in the lower abdomen, in the midline, just above the pubic bone, with the indicator pointing toward the patient's right (A). Normal pelvic Focused Ultrasonography in Trauma view (B). Fan from cephalad to caudad to visualize the entire bladder (C).

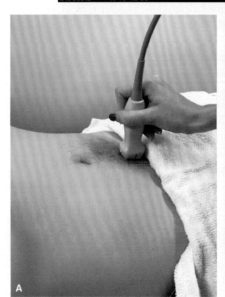

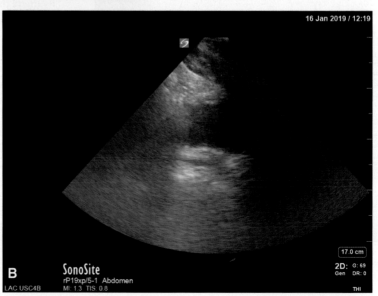

FIGURE 50-11. Normal suprapubic view in the longitudinal orientation. Make sure to visualize the entire bladder in both transverse and longitudinal orientation (A). Turn the gain down to decrease posterior acoustic enhancement from the bladder to allow better visualization of space posterior to bladder (B).

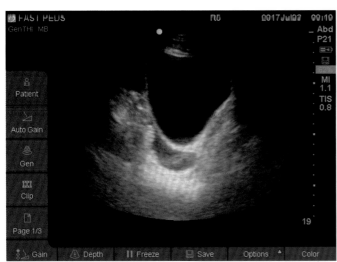

FIGURE 50-12. Positive suprapubic Focused Ultrasonography in Trauma view. Fluid appears as an anechoic strip posterior to the bladder.

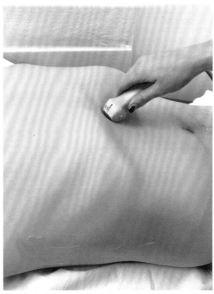

FIGURE 50-14. Subxiphoid cardiac view with the low-frequency probe selected. Place the probe in the subxiphoid space with the probe marker toward the patient's right. Angle the probe into the chest cavity using the liver as your acoustic window.

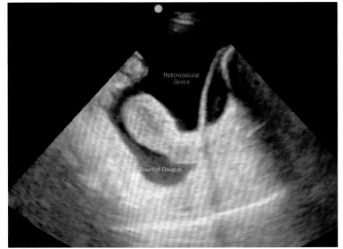

FIGURE 50-13. Positive suprapubic Focused Ultrasonography in Trauma view in the female. A small pocket of fluid appears as an anechoic collection posterior to the uterus, seen in the longitudinal orientation.

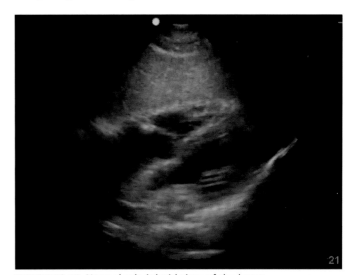

FIGURE 50-15. Normal subxiphoid view of the heart.

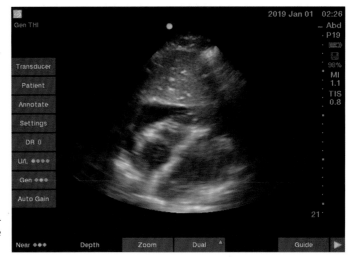

FIGURE 50-16. Subxiphoid views of the heart with circumferential anechoic strips of fluid in the pericardial sac, indicating the presence of a pericardial effusion.

PART 3

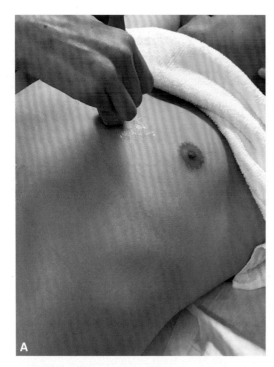

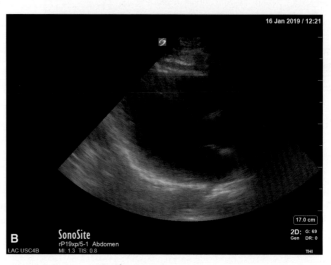

FIGURE 50-17. A and B, Parasternal long-axis view of the heart with the low-frequency probe selected. Place the probe to the left of the sternum at the level of the 4th or 5th intercostal space. Rotate the probe marker toward the patient's left hip to obtain a proper view (A). Normal parasternal long view of the heart (B).

PATIENT MANAGEMENT

In patients with suspected traumatic or atraumatic hemoperitoneum, the results of the FAST examination can help guide further management. In the setting of suspected BAT and a positive FAST examination, management would follow the ATLS Trauma Protocol, where stable patients would receive a CT with IV contrast of the abdomen and pelvis to determine the source of the hemoperitoneum. Unstable patients with a positive FAST may proceed directly to the operating room for an exploratory laparotomy or be kept in the trauma bay for resuscitation, depending on the team involved. In nontrauma patients with a positive FAST, the algorithm is similar depending on patient presentation and stability. For a patient with a positive hCG with abdominal pain who has a positive FAST, a ruptured ectopic pregnancy can be a life-threatening emergency. Bedside US exposing the hemoperitoneum can expedite resuscitation efforts by the treatment

team and accelerate a consult to the obstetric service for further operative management.

There are several times when fluid seen on FAST may not warrant immediate evaluation by CT or laparotomy. Patients with liver cirrhosis and ascites will almost always have free peritoneal fluid on the FAST. Patients on peritoneal dialysis will also likely have a positive FAST. Patients with other chronic diseases such as congestive heart failure or cancer may have chronic accumulation of fluid in the thorax, abdomen, or pericardium. It is not uncommon to find physiologic abdominopelvic fluid in women and pediatric patients.[12] The patient's history, presentation, and physical examination can help determine whether the free fluid warrants emergent management. Findings of the FAST in conjunction with vital signs and hemoglobin can help determine the best next step for the patient. When in doubt, refer the patient to the emergency department for further evaluation (**Figure 50-18**).

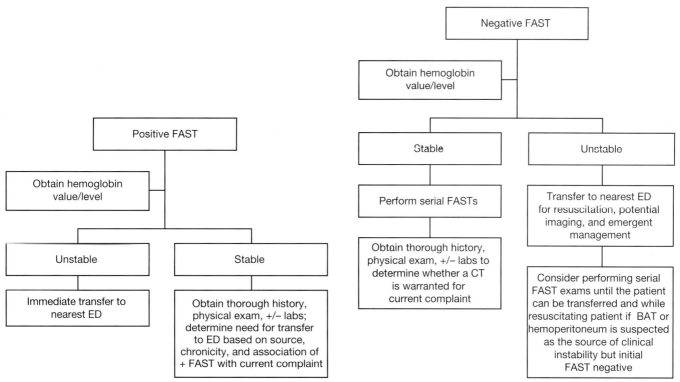

FIGURE 50-18. FAST management algorithm in the primary care setting. BAT, blunt abdominal trauma; CT, computed tomography; FAST, Focused Ultrasonography in Trauma.

PEARLS AND PITFALLS

Pearls

- Use a low-frequency phased-array probe. Lower frequency will allow adequate penetration into the abdomen. The phased array has a smaller footprint compared to the curvilinear probe so it is easier to get between rib spaces to evaluate the upper quadrants. Conversely, curvilinear probe provides more probe-to-skin contact on larger patients.
- Trendelenburg positioning uses gravity to allow pooling of fluid in the cavity seen on FAST.
- Make sure to control for adequate depth, usually 16 to 19 cm, so the entirety of each structure can be visualized clearly.
- Make sure to obtain view of the RUQ from the upper pole of the kidney to the liver tip in order to visualize the entire area where fluid may collect.
- When evaluating the RUQ and LUQ, make sure to look for the presence of free pleural fluid, denoted by the continuation of the spine across the lower screen past the diaphragm.
- Rib shadow can make obtaining RUQ and LUQ views difficult. Rotate the probe counterclockwise and aim more posteriorly with the probe, which allows for better views between rib spaces.
- Control the gain, particularly the far gain, when evaluating the pelvis to prevent overgain of acoustic enhancement posterior to the bladder.

Pitfalls

- Make sure to scan all the way through each view to increase your sensitivity of finding small pockets of free fluid and decrease the chance of false-negative scans.
- Males have seminal vesicles, which are posterior to the bladder and appear hypoechoic. These can easily be mistaken for free fluid. Scan through the bladder in two planes and take note of where the fluid outside the bladder is symmetric and contained. If it is, it is much more likely to be seminal vesicles.
- A focal hypoechoic or anechoic area along the anterior pericardium is likely to be a normal fat pad, whereas circumferential fluid is more likely to be a pericardial effusion.
- Focal posterior fluid along the pericardium in the parasternal long-axis view may be a pleural effusion (▶ **Video 50-1**). Remember if the fluid tracks anterior to the descending aorta it is a pericardial effusion; if it is posterior and lateral to the aorta, it is a pleural effusion.
- If the FAST is equivocal, consider performing serial examinations if suspicion is high, especially if advanced testing such as CT is not available.
- Don't mistake perinephric fat, which appears hypoechoic, for free fluid around the kidney. Look at both upper quadrants and compare.

BILLING

CPT Code	Description	Global Payment	Professional Component	Technical Component
76705	Ultrasound, abdominal, real time with image documentation limited	$93.31	$30.15	$63.16
76604	Ultrasound, chest, B-scan (includes mediastinum) and/or real time with image documentation	$90.08	$27.63	$62.45
93308	Echocardiography, transthoracic, real time with image documentation (2D) includes M-mode recording	$126.69	$26.20	$100.49

CPT codes and average national reimbursement for Medicare in 2016. Payment data are from https://www.cms.gov/apps/physician-fee-schedule/search/search-criteria.aspx. See Chapter 2 for details on ultrasound billing.

References

1. Scalea TM, Rodriguez A, Chiu WC, Brenneman FD, et al. Focused Assessment with Sonography for Trauma (FAST): results from an international consensus conference. *J Trauma*. 1999;46:466-472.
2. Tso P, Rodriguez A, Cooper C, et al. Sonography in blunt abdominal trauma: a preliminary progress report. *J Trauma*. 1992;33:39-44.
3. Chambers JA, Pilbrow WJ. Ultrasound in abdominal trauma: an alternative to peritoneal lavage. *Arch Emerg Med*. 1988;5:26-33.
4. Nordenholz K, Rubin M, Gularte G, et al. Ultrasound in the evaluation and management of blunt abdominal trauma. *Ann Emerg Med*. 1997;29:357-366.
5. Federle MP, Crass RA, Jeffrey RB, et al. Computed tomography in blunt abdominal trauma. *Arch Surg*. 1982;117:645-650.
6. Rothlin MA, Naf RN, Amgwerd M, et al. Ultrasound in blunt abdominal and thoracic trauma. *J Trauma*. 1993;34:488-495.
7. Huang MS, Liu M, Wu JK, et al. Ultrasonography for the evaluation of hemoperitoneum during resuscitation: a simple scoring system. *J Trauma*. 1994;36:173-177.
8. Sheng AY, Dalziel P, Liteplo AS, Fagenholz P, Noble VE. Focused assessment with sonography in trauma and abdominal computed tomography utilization in adult trauma patients: trends over the last decade. *Emerg Med Int*. 2013:678380. doi:10.1155/2013/678380.
9. Flick D. Bedside ultrasound education in primary care. *J Ultrasound Med*. 2016;35:1369-1371.
10. Wong F, Franco Z, Phelan MB, Lam C, David A. Development of a pilot family medicine hand-carried ultrasound course. *WMJ*. 2013;112:257-261.
11. Hall JW, Holman H, Bornemann P, et al. Point of care ultrasound in family medicine residency programs: a CERA study. *Fam Med*. 2015;47(9):706-711.
12. Rathaus V, Grunebaum M, Konen O, et al. Minimal pelvic fluid in asymptomatic children: the value of the sonographic findings. *J Ultrasound Med*. 2003;22(1):13-17.

CHAPTER 51

Rapid Ultrasound for Shock and Hypotension (RUSH)

Mena Ramos, MD

Clinical Vignette

A 45-year-old man with a history of hypertension presents with shortness of breath, chest pain, a nonproductive cough of 1 week duration, and dizziness. The patient is alert and oriented, though he appears distressed and diaphoretic. His vital signs are remarkable for a blood pressure of 85/60, heart rate of 120, respiratory rate of 30, and O_2 sat 95% on room air. On physical examination, his lungs are clear to auscultation, he does not appear to have jugular venous distention (JVD), he has no appreciable cardiac murmur, though he has 1+ pitting pretibial edema bilaterally. His electrocardiogram (ECG) showed no acute ischemic changes.

LITERATURE REVIEW

"*Choc*" was first used during the 18th century by the French surgeon Le Dran to describe severe traumatic injuries ultimately leading to circulatory collapse.[1] Today, shock is defined as a state of diffuse systemic tissue hypoperfusion, which if left untreated can often lead to irreversible multiorgan failure and death. Patients presenting to emergency departments with symptomatic hypotension are associated with more adverse outcomes.[2] The early detection and treatment of the cause of shock has the potential to lead to significant improvements in morbidity and mortality.[3] Bedside ultrasound facilitates a more rapid diagnosis of the cause of shock, which highlights its utility for front-line providers who may be at a considerable distance from the nearest intensive care unit (ICU) leading to delays in diagnosis and treatment.[4] In situations where front-line providers are at a substantial distance from the nearest hospital, a rapid stepwise approach to the critical patient is of considerable value.

The literature describes multiple sonographic approaches to patients with elements of shock summarized well by Seif et al.,[5] such as ACES,[6] FALLS,[7] Trinity,[8] SIMPLE,[9] CAUSE,[10] RUSH-HIMAP,[11] and RUSH—"Pump, Tank and Pipes,"[12] among others. They are all similar in the specific clinical questions they attempt to answer. The Rapid Ultrasound in Shock (RUSH) protocol was coined in 2006 by Weingart et al. and published in 2009 as a rapid sonographic approach to identify the etiology of shock using the acronym HIMAP (Heart, inferior vena cava [IVC], Morrison's, Aorta, Pneumothorax).[13,14] This chapter describes one physiology-based approach to the RUSH examination published in 2010 by Perera et al. (Pump, Tank, Pipes).

The benefits of goal-directed ultrasound protocols in patients with shock show a 30% greater accuracy among physicians in the initial diagnosis of the cause of shock from 50% to 80%.[15] In a recent study evaluating the accuracy of the RUSH protocol, ER physician- or radiologist-performed RUSH protocol suggested a negative predictive value (NPV) of 97% for hypovolemic, cardiogenic, and obstructive shock and a positive predictive value (PPV) of 100% though with a lower sensitivity for distributive and mixed etiology shock.[16] This study stresses the importance of ruling out certain etiologies of shock on the initial assessment. In a prospective study comparing the RUSH examination diagnosis and the final diagnosis, the overall sensitivity was found to be 88% with a specificity of 96%.[17] A meta-analysis from 2018 to determine the diagnostic accuracy of the RUSH protocol showed a high positive likelihood ratio of 19.19 and a low negative likelihood ratio of 0.23.[18] See Table 51-1 for clinical recommendations for the application of the RUSH protocol.[19]

TABLE 51-1 Recommendations for Use of Point-of-Care Ultrasound in Clinical Practice		
Recommendation	Rating	References
RUSH protocol should be performed in patients with undifferentiated shock referred to the emergency department because it has good ability to distinguish the causes of shock.	A	18
Core views focus on determining the category of shock, whether cardiogenic or noncardiogenic, consist of basic cardiac views (subxiphoid or parasternal long axis), lung views for pleural fluid and B-lines for filling status, and inferior vena cava (IVC) views for filling status.	C	19
Supplementary views should be performed if further information is required regarding pericardial fluid or cardiac form or function and include parasternal short and apical views.	C	19
Additional views including peritoneal fluid, aorta, and pelvic views, and proximal leg veins for deep vein thrombosis (DVT) should be performed when indicated.	C	19

A = consistent, good-quality patient-oriented evidence; B = inconsistent or limited-quality patient-oriented evidence; C = consensus, disease-oriented evidence, usual practice, expert opinion, or case series. For information about the SORT evidence rating system, go to http://www.aafp.org/afpsort.

PERFORMING THE SCAN

The protocol is performed in a stepwise approach addressing the pump (heart), the tank (IVC, pleural/peritoneal spaces, lungs), and the pipes (aorta, deep vein thrombosis [DVT]). The recommended probes are the phased array cardiac transducer (3.5-5 MHz) for scanning of the abdomen and thorax, and the linear/vascular transducer (7.5-10 MHz) for the venous examination and pneumothorax.

Step 1: **Evaluation of the pump.** Evaluate the heart for a pericardial effusion/tamponade, left ventricular (LV) contractility, and acute right heart strain using the parasternal long and short axis, apical 4-chamber, and subxiphoid views. Apply four views to answer the clinical question at hand because some views may be difficult to obtain (**Figure 51-1**).

Part A. *Evaluate for a pericardial effusion in the parasternal long and subxiphoid views.* Place the phased array probe in the 3rd to 5th intercostal space just left of the sternum with the probe marker facing the patient's right shoulder (**Figure 51-2**). More than trace pericardial fluid should raise suspicion for possible cardiac tamponade because the volume of fluid is not a direct indicator of tamponade but rather the rapidity of accumulation.[20] The cardiac probe is placed in the subxiphoid position with the probe marker facing the patient's left (**Figure 51-3**). A pericardial effusion is best visualized between the right ventricle (RV) and the liver (**Figure 51-4**). Signs of pericardial tamponade include right atrial (RA) and ventricular collapse appearing as a serpentine-like motion during diastole known as the "trampoline sign" as the pressure in the pericardial sac overcomes RV diastolic pressure (▶ **Video 51-1**). Pericardial tamponade can also be evaluated in the subxiphoid view (**Figure 51-5**). See Chapter 10 for details.

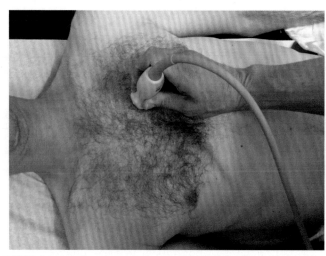
FIGURE 51-2. Probe placement: parasternal long axis.

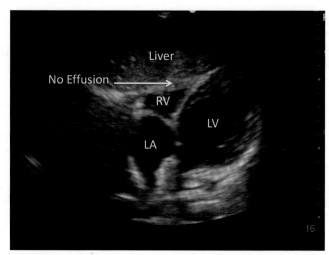
FIGURE 51-3. Probe placement: subxiphoid.

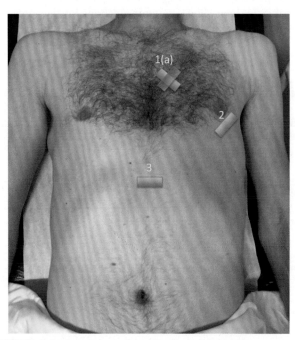
FIGURE 51-1. Probe placement: evaluation of the pump.

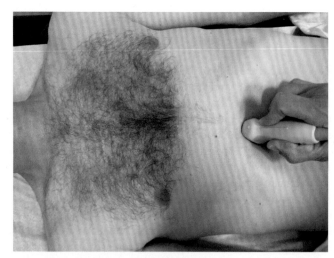
FIGURE 51-4. Subxiphoid normal. LA, left atrium; LV, left ventricle; RV, right ventricle.

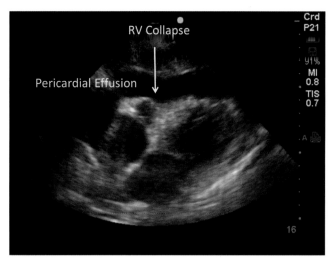

FIGURE 51-5. Cardiac tamponade: pericardial effusion with right ventricular collapse in diastole.

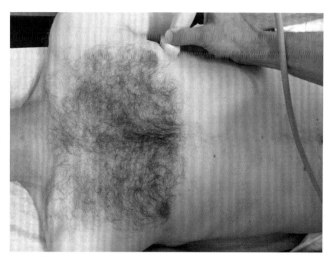

FIGURE 51-6. Probe position: apical 4-chamber.

Part B. *Evaluate LV contractility in the parasternal long (Figure 51-2) and apical 4-chamber views* **(Figure 51-6).** There are multiple techniques to estimate LV contractility/ejection fraction. Studies show that with adequate experience, a simple visual qualitative approach is a reliable estimate of ejection fraction.[21] The most rapid approach is a qualitative visual estimate, though this technique requires witnessing enough normal and abnormal examinations to group between normal, depressed, and severely depressed LV contractility. In general, if the anterior leaflet of the mitral valve touches the septum during diastolic filling, this corresponds with a normal ejection fraction. M-mode can be used to calculate the E-point septal separation (EPSS) to approximate ejection fraction **(Figures 51-7 and 51-8).** Another approach is by observing the LV myocardial thickening at the level of the papillary muscles. If there is a less than 30% size difference of the myocardial thickness between the end of diastole and the end of systole, this corresponds with a severely depressed ejection fraction. A fourth method

PART 3

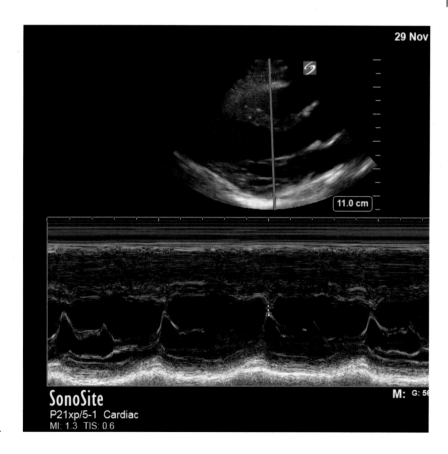

FIGURE 51-7. M-mode: normal ejection fraction.

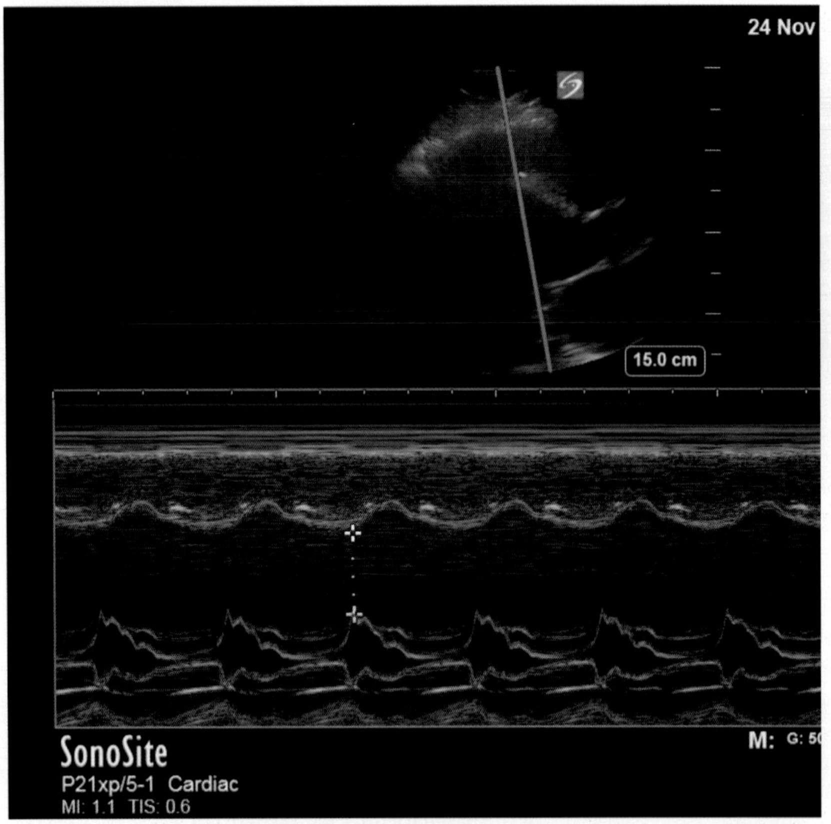

FIGURE 51-8. M-mode: severely depressed ejection fraction.

is to evaluate fractional shortening (FS) that refers to the % reduction of the LV diameter from diastole to systole. FS greater than 25% corresponds with a normal ejection fraction, whereas an FS less than 15% corresponds with a severely depressed EF. A depressed or severely depressed LV systolic function could be an indication of cardiogenic shock from ischemic cardiomyopathy or secondary to sepsis and toxins.

Conversely, if the LV walls touch at the end of systole and there appears to be a change greater than 90% between end diastole and end systole, this suggests

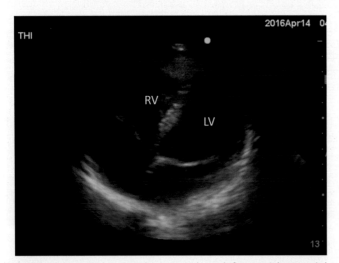

FIGURE 51-9. Apical 4-chamber normal. LV, left ventricle; RV, right ventricle.

a hyperdynamic heart likely from reduced preload because of distributive/septic shock, hypovolemic or hemorrhagic shock. See Chapter 8 for details.

Part C. *Evaluate for RV heart enlargement in the parasternal long, parasternal short, and apical 4-chamber views.* A better image is usually obtained in the left lateral decubitus position. Place the cardiac probe at the 5th intercostal space at the point of maximum impulse directed toward the left axilla (Figure 51-6). Decrease the angle of the probe to lie at approximately 30° to 45° angle from the anterior chest wall. Compare the size of the RV to LV. Under normal conditions, the RV is approximately 60% the size of the LV (**Figure 51-9**). If the RV is greater than or the same as the LV in an acutely unstable patient, strong consideration should be given to massive pulmonary embolism as the diagnosis and appropriate treatment initiated[22] (**Figure 51-10**). See Chapter 11 for details.

Step 2: Evaluate the pipes

Part A. *Evaluate the "fullness of the tank" by evaluating the IVC and jugular veins for size and collapse with inspiration.* Place the cardiac probe in the subxiphoid position with the heart in view (**Figure 51-11**). Slowly rotate the probe to the longitudinal position until the IVC is visualized entering the RA. Another technique is starting with the probe in the longitudinal position just beneath the xiphoid process and slowly sliding the probe to the patient's right. The hepatic vein will enter the IVC prior to entering the RA. Although

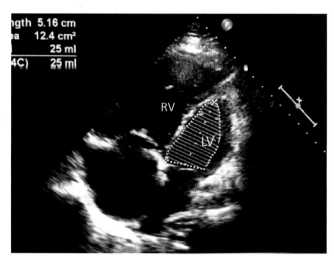

FIGURE 51-10. Acute right heart strain. LV, left ventricle; RV, right ventricle.

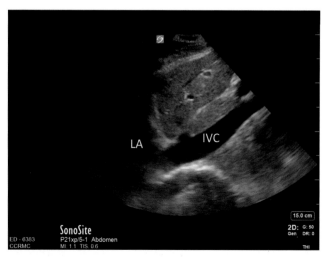

FIGURE 51-12. Inferior vena cava more than 50% inspiratory collapse. LA, left atrium; IVC, inferior vena cava

the IVC size and inspiratory collapse can be used to estimate CVP,[23] the IVC remains controversial as a predictor of volume responsiveness; nevertheless, the IVC is helpful in its extremes. An IVC measuring less than 2 c) with an inspiratory collapse greater than 50% correlates with a CVP less than 10 mm Hg, more likely suggesting distributive shock state (**Figure 51-12**), whereas a CVP greater than 2 cm with less than 50% inspiratory change suggests cardiogenic or obstructive state (**Figure 51-13**).[24] See Chapter 46 for details.

Part B. *The internal jugular veins can also be used to estimate intravascular volume similarly to the JVD on physical examination.* At a 30° position, place the linear transducer in the short axis position to identify the internal jugular, then turn the probe in the long axis to locate the closing meniscus at which point the walls of the vein touch. A closing meniscus higher in the neck corresponds with a higher CVP.[25]

Step 3:   Evaluate the tank

Part A. *Evaluate for "leakiness of the tank."* Perform the Focused Assessment with Sonography for Trauma (FAST) and inspect the peritoneal cavity for intra-abdominal fluid in both trauma and nontrauma states. Although the curvilinear probe is typically used for this examination, for the purposes of RUSH, use the phased array probe because it can also obtain the necessary images while saving time from switching probes. Evaluate the peritoneal cavity in the hepatorenal space, perisplenic space, and the suprapubic spaces for hemothorax or ascites. The same examination can be applied for women of child-bearing age to evaluate for signs of ruptured ectopic pregnancy. Then turn your attention to the pleural space by sliding the probe cephalad to the hepatorenal and perisplenic views to observe the area above the diaphragm for a pleural effusion or hemothorax. A pleural effusion will appear to be an anechoic space above the diaphragm with disappearance of the normal mirror artifact on

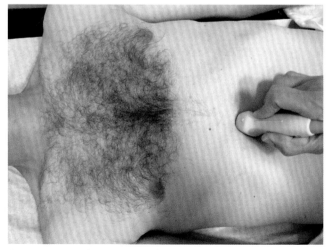

FIGURE 51-11. Probe position inferior vena cava.

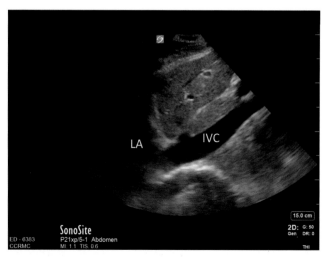

FIGURE 51-13. Inferior vena cava < 50% inspiratory collapse. LA, left atrium; IVC, inferior vena cava

the hepatic side as well as the presence of a spine sign. See Chapters 13 and 50 for details.

Part B. *Evaluate for "compromise" of the tank.* A tension pneumothorax can lead to mediastinal shifts obstructing venous inflow to the heart leading to obstructive shock. Several studies support an increased sensitivity (92%-98%) of ultrasound compared to portable upright chest x-ray (52%-57%) to detect pneumothorax.[26,27]

Evaluate for pneumothorax using either the high-frequency linear probe or the phased array probe at the midclavicular line at approximately the 3rd to 5th intercostal space **(Figure 51-14)**. Identify the pleural line as the hyperechoic horizontal line visible between the rib spaces. In normal lung, the visceral and parietal pleura slide against one another, creating a flickering appearing hyperechoic horizontal line that creates the image of "ants marching on a log." The presence of lung sliding effectively rules out pneumothorax though the absence of lung sliding can be present in other conditions including chronic obstructive pulmonary disease (COPD) and pneumonia.[28,29] A more specific (100%) but less sensitive (66%) sign for pneumothorax is the lung point sign characterized by the disappearance of the lung sliding at a particular location on the chest wall adjacent to lung sliding pattern.[30] Evaluation for pneumothorax can also be done via M-mode. The pneumothorax pattern creates a "stratosphere" or "barcode" sign that appears to be horizontal lines stacked across the screen because of lack of lung motion in comparison to the "sandy beach" or "seashore sign" in the presence of normal lung sliding. In the unstable patient with undifferentiated shock, a positive ultrasound for pneumothorax should warrant immediate consideration for needle decompression. See Chapter 14 for details.

Part C. *Evaluate for "tank overload."* Increased pressure in the pulmonary vasculature resulting from obstructive or cardiogenic shock leads to fluid extravasation and pulmonary edema. The vertical lung artifacts known

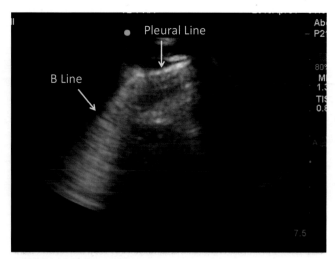

FIGURE 51-15. B-line artifact.

as B-line artifact (BLA) are created by reverberation of sound waves through fluid-filled lung, which was described by Lichtenstein in 1998 as a sign of pulmonary edema[31] **(Figure 51-15)**. Since then, BLA has been incorporated into multiple protocols including BLUE and FALLS to evaluate acute dyspnea and acute circulatory failure.[32] Although BLA is present in cardiogenic pulmonary edema, it is not specific and can also be found in other diseases such as pneumonia, diffuse or focal interstitial lung disease, malignancy, and acute respiratory distress syndrome (ARDS).[33] However, coupled with dilated minimally collapsing IVC and depressed LV contractility, it should raise the suspicion for cardiogenic shock.[34]

In the supine position, evaluate for BLA using the phased array probe in the anterolateral chest wall between the 2nd and 5th rib interspaces, the lateral mix axillary wall, and the posterior–inferior lateral wall. B-lines appear as hyperechoic lines extending from the pleural line vertically like a fan-like pattern deep into the lung. B-lines differ from comet-tail artifacts found in normal lung in that B-lines extend to the far lung field and are more visible. See Chapter 12 for details.

Step 4: Evaluate the pipes

Part A. *Evaluate for "rupture of the pipes" in the form of aortic aneurysm or dissection.* Literature supports emergency ultrasound with a sensitivity of 95% and specificity of 100% for detecting abdominal aortic aneurysm (AAA).[35] Place the phased array probe in the transverse orientation just beneath the xiphoid process perpendicular to the skin. Identify the aorta just above and to the right of the vertebral body **(Figure 51-16)**. Applying constant pressure, slide the probe caudally to the iliac bifurcation. An AAA is defined by external wall diameter greater than 3 cm for the abdominal aorta and iliac external wall diameter greater than 1.5 cm. Visualize the aorta in longitudinal axis to identify saccular and fusiform aneurysms **(Figure 51-17)**. Furthermore, measure the aorta from the outer to the outer wall to

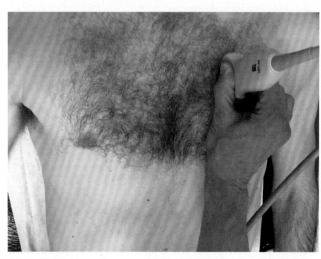

FIGURE 51-14. Lung ultrasound pneumothorax.

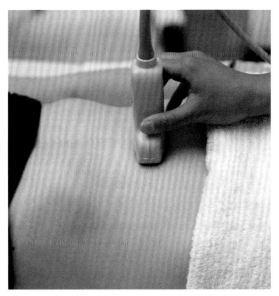

FIGURE 51-16. Probe position: aorta transverse.

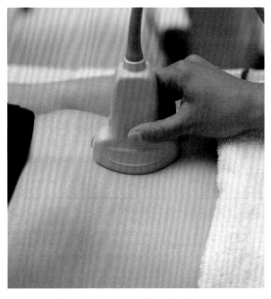

FIGURE 51-17. Probe position: aorta longitudinal.

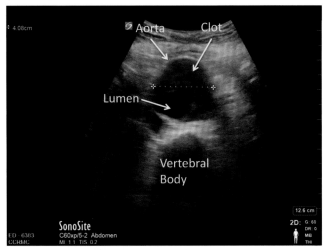

FIGURE 51-18. Aortic aneurysm.

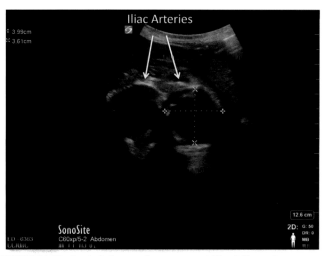

FIGURE 51-19. Aorta infrarenal aneurysm at iliac bifurcation.

avoid missing an AAA by only measuring the lumen of a clot (**Figures 51-18 and 51-19**). Be sure to evaluate the aorta to the iliac bifurcation because the majority of AAA are infrarenal. See Chapter 47 for details.

Part B. Evaluate for "clogging of the pipes" in the form of a DVT in the femoral and popliteal regions. ED-performed ultrasonography of lower extremity (LE) DVTs have been shown to have high sensitivity (100%) and specificity (99%) on 2-point compression testing.[36] Using the linear vascular transducer with the patient in supine position with the knee bent and externally rotated, identify the femoral vein at the saphenous junction, slide distally compressing at 1 cm intervals until the bifurcation of the femoral and deep femoral veins. Then continue to slide distally and identify the popliteal vein in the popliteal region just superficial to the popliteal artery. Compress the popliteal vein and slide distally until the level of the trifurcation and compress. Wall-to-wall compression of the femoral and popliteal veins rules out the presence of a DVT in those locations. See Chapter 45 for details.

PATIENT MANAGEMENT

Shock is a life-threatening condition that must be recognized and treated rapidly. Diagnosis of shock is based on clinical features, which may include any of the following: hypotension, tachycardia, tachypnea, oliguria, encephalopathy, decreased capillary refill, metabolic acidosis, and elevated serum lactate. By assessing the underlying physiology of shock, the RUSH protocol rapidly narrows down diagnostic possibilities for the underlying causes and allows for targeted empiric treatment. Targeting treatment to the type of shock is critical because certain treatments that could be beneficial in one type (such as intravenous [IV] fluid in hypovolemic or distributive shock) could be detrimental in another (such as IV fluids in cardiogenic shock).

Although ultrasound is a useful tool, diagnosis of underlying conditions should be geared first and foremost by the patient's clinical presentation and the most likely cause of the patient's shock.

PART 3

For example, in the patient with chest pain, shortness of breath, and unilateral leg pain and swelling, the evaluation of the heart should be succeeded by evaluation of the leg for DVT. Similarly, in a patient with tachycardia, dizziness, and severe abdominal pain with radiation to the back, examination of the heart should be followed by evaluation for AAA.

Obstructive Shock

Patients with obstructive shock will often have elevated jugular venous pressure, distant heart sounds, unilateral breath sounds, or known risk factors for cardiac tamponade, tension pneumothorax, or pulmonary embolism. Obstructive shock requires immediate resolution of the underlying cause of the obstruction. IV fluids are unlikely to be helpful and may be detrimental.

If the cardiac examination shows pericardial effusion, especially if there are signs of cardiac tamponade, urgent pericardiocentesis should be considered. Conversely, if the IVC is noted to be small and collapsing more than 50% with respiration, tamponade is not likely to be causing shock even if a pericardial effusion is present. If signs of acute RV strain are present, pulmonary embolism is likely and immediate thrombolysis should be considered if there are no contraindications.[37] This diagnosis is strengthened if DVT is also found on LE venous examination. If lack of lung sliding is noted unilaterally, then tension pneumothorax should be considered as the cause especially if a lung point is seen, and immediate needle thoracotomy and chest tube placement should be considered.

Cardiogenic Shock

Patients in cardiogenic shock will often have chest pain, ECG abnormalities, and risk factors for cardiac disease. A severely depressed ejection fraction is suggestive of cardiogenic shock and findings of pulmonary edema bilaterally or a dilated IVC support this diagnosis. As in obstructive shock, IV fluids are unlikely to be helpful and likely to be detrimental. If cardiogenic shock is suspected, the underlying cause must be identified and treated. Patients should be assessed for possible arrhythmia, acute valvular insufficiency, or acute coronary syndrome. If life-threatening arrhythmia is present, it should be treated per the Advanced Cardiac Life Support (ACLS) algorithms.[38] Inotropes can help stabilize undifferentiated cardiogenic shock while awaiting further investigation and treatment, which will often require cardiac specialist evaluation.[39]

Hypovolemic and Distributive Shock

In a patient with a hyperdynamic heart and small, collapsing IVC, hemorrhagic or distributive shock should be strongly considered. Initial treatment in hypovolemic or distributive shock should always include rapid resuscitation with IV fluids. Further testing should be geared toward determining the cause of the patient's hypovolemic or distributive shock.

If the FAST scan is positive or AAA is noted, then hemorrhagic shock should be considered. Emergent surgical consultation should be sought. If shock is stabilized, further testing such as a computed tomography scan should be considered. In patients with shock accompanied by fever or possible source of infection, sepsis should be considered. These patients should also have early administration of broad-spectrum antibiotics and control of any suspected source of infection.[40] Anaphylaxis should be considered in patients with inspiratory stridor, oral and facial edema, hives, or a history of recent exposure to common allergens. These patients should also receive rapid administration of intramuscular epinephrine (**Figure 51-20**).

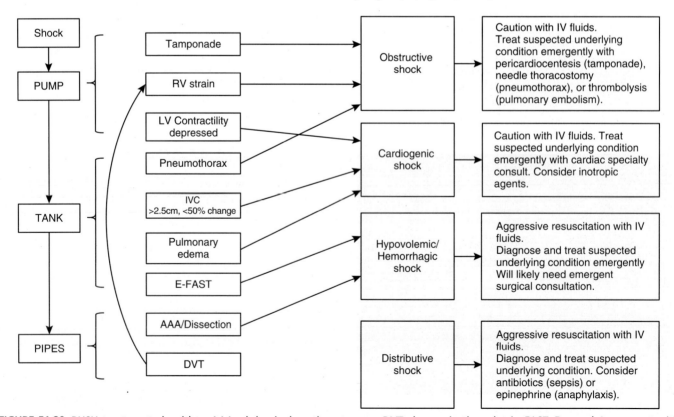

FIGURE 51-20. RUSH treatment algorithm. AAA, abdominal aortic aneurysm; DVT, deep vein thrombosis; FAST, Focused Assessment with Sonography for Trauma; IVC, inferior vena cava; LV, left ventricle; RUSH, Rapid Ultrasound for Shock and Hypotension; RV, right ventricle.

PEARLS AND PITFALLS

Pearls

- After the cardiac and IVC examinations, alter the components and sequence of the examination based on the clinical scenario presented, prioritizing the examinations that are highest on the differential diagnosis. For example, in a patient with shortness of breath and an echo with acute RV strain, proceed to look for DVT. In a patient with abdominal pain, proceed to the FAST and aorta examinations.
- Use different cardiac views to focus on specific clinical questions. If you are unable to obtain a view, proceed to the next view.
- Do not rely solely on the IVC to determine volume status but rather as an adjunct, useful in its extremes (dilated with no respiratory change vs. small and fully collapsible).
- When evaluating the aorta, apply constant pressure to the abdomen in order to disperse bowel gas to visualize the aorta.

Pitfalls

- Take care not to confuse pericardial effusion and pleural effusion in the parasternal long view. A pericardial effusion will be anterior to the descending thoracic aorta, whereas pleural effusion will be posterior to the aorta.
- An anterior cardiac fat pad can be confused for a pericardial effusion. Pericardial effusion tends to layer posteriorly and inferiorly and so will be visible around the heart.[41]
- Do not confuse the RV for the LV. Depending on the machine you use, some standard cardiac settings place the screen marker to the right of the screen, thereby slipping all images 180° and reversing the orientation of the LV and RV. The LV is always longer than the RV with the mitral annulus inserting.
- Incomplete visualization of the RV and LV chambers can lead to the impression of a falsely dilated RV. Be sure to fan through the image to see the ventricular wall borders and confirm with multiple views.
- When evaluating for DVT, be sure to release compression when sliding distally because constant pressure will often obscure the vein and make it difficult to trace.

BILLING

CPT Code	Description	Global Payment	Professional Component	Technical Component
93308	Limited cardiac echo	$100.19	$26.31	$73.88
76604	Limited chest (lung)	$90.46	$27.75	$62.71
76705	Limited abdominal (FAST)	$92.26	$29.91	$62.35
76775	Limited retroperitoneal (AAA)	$117.33	$29.38	$87.42
93971	Limited venous lower extremity (DVT)	$123.25	$23.07	$100.19

CPT codes and average national reimbursement for Medicare in 2016. Payment data are from https://www.cms.gov/apps/physician-fee-schedule/search/search-criteria.aspx. See Chapter 2 for details on ultrasound billing.

References

1. Strehlow M. Early identification of shock in critically ill patients. *Emerg Med Clin North Am.* 2010;28:57-66.
2. Jones AE, Abornk LS, Kline JA. Severity of emergency department hypotension predicts adverse hospital outcome. *Shock.* 2004;22(5):410-414.
3. Rivers E, Nguyen B, Haystad S, et al. Early goal directed therapy in the treatment of severe sepsis and septic shock. *N Engl J Med.* 2001;348:1368-1377.
4. Jones A, Tayal V, Sullivan M, Kline J. Randomized, controlled trial of immediate versus delayed goal-directed ultrasound to identify the cause of nontraumatic hypotension in emergency department patients. *Crit Care Med.* 2004;32(8):1703-1708.
5. Seif D, Perera P, Mailhot T, Riley D, Mandavia D. Bedside ultrasound in resuscitation and the rapid ultrasound in shock protocol. *Crit Care Res Pract.* 2012;2012:503254.
6. Atkinson PRT, McCauley DJ, Kendall RJ, et al. Abdominal and Cardiac Evaluation with Sonography in Shock (ACES): an approach by emergency physicians for the use of ultrasound in patients with undifferentiated hypotension. *Emerg Med J.* 2009;26(2):87-91.
7. Lichtenstein DA, Karakitsos D. Integrating ultrasound in the hemodynamic evaluation of acute circulatory failure (FALLS-the fluid administration limited by lung sonography protocol). *J Crit Care.* 2012;27(5):53.
8. Bahner DP. Trinity: a hypotensive ultrasound protocol. *J Diagn Med Sonogr.* 2002;18(4):193-198.
9. Mok KL. Make it SIMPLE: enhanced shock management by focused cardiac ultrasound. *J Intensive Care.* 2016;4:51. doi:10.1186/s40560-016-0176-x.
10. Hernandez C, Shuler K, Hannan H, Sonyika C, Likourezos A, Marshall J. C.A.U.S.E.: cardiac arrest ultra-sound exam—a better approach to managing patients in primary non-arrhythmogenic cardiac arrest. *Resuscitation.* 2008;76:198-206.
11. Weingart SD, Duque D, Nelson B. Rapid ultrasound for shock and hypotension (RUSH-HIMAPP). 2009. http://emedhome.com
12. Perera P, Mailhot T, Riley D, Mandavia D. The RUSH exam: rapid ultrasound in Shock in the evaluation of the critically ill. *Emerg Med Clin North Am.* 2010;28(1):29-56.
13. EMCrit Project. http://emcrit.org/rush-exam/original-rush-article/. Accessed 9 November, 2016.
14. Weingart SD, Duque D, Nelson B. Rapid ultrasound for shock and hypotension. 2009. http//emedhome.com/
15. Jones AE, Tayal VS, Sullivan DM, Kline JA. Randomized, controlled trial of immediate versus delayed goal-directed ultrasound to identify the cause of nontraumatic hypotension in emergency department patients. *Crit Care Med.* 2004;32(8):1703-1708.
16. Ghane M, Gharib M, Ebrahimi A, et al. Accuracy of Rapid Ultrasound in Shock (RUSH) exam for diagnosis of shock in critically ill patients. *Trauma Mon.* 2015;20(1).
17. Bagheri-Hariri S, Yekesadat M, Farahmand S, et al. The impact of using RUSH protocol for diagnosing the type of unknown shock in the emergency department. *Emerg Radiol.* 2015;22:517-520.
18. Keikha M, Salehi-Marzijarani M, Soldoozi Nejat R, Sheikh Motahar Vahidi H, Mirrezaie SM. Diagnostic Accuracy of Rapid Ultrasound in Shock (RUSH) exam: a systematic review and meta-analysis. *Bull Emerg Trauma.* 2018;6(4):271-278. doi:10.29252/beat-060402.

19. Atkinson P, Bowra J, Milne J, et al. Sonography in Hypotension and Cardiac Arrest (SHoC) protocol consensus statement. *CJEM*. 2017;19459-470. doi:10.117/cem.2016.394.

20. Walsh BM, Tibias LA. Low-pressure pericardial tamponade: case report and review of the literature. *J Emerg Med*. 2016. doi:10.1016/j.jemermed.2016.05.069.

21. Moore CL, Rose GA, Tayal VS, et al. Determination of left ventricular function by emergency physician echocardiography of hypotensive patients. *Acad Emerg Med*. 2002;9:186-193.

22. Rudski L, et al. Guidelines for the echocardiographic assessment of the right heart in adults: a report from the American Society of Echocardiography. *J Am Soc Echocardiogr*. 2010;23:685-713.

23. Kircher BJ, Himelman RB, Schiller NB. Noninvasive estimation of right atrial pressure from the inspiratory collapse of the inferior vena cava. *Am J. Cardiol*. 1990;66(4):493-496.

24. Perera P, Mailhot T, Riley D, Mandavia D. The RUSH exam: rapid ultrasound in Shock in the evaluation of the critically ill," *Emerg Med Clin North Am*. 2010;28(1):29-56.

25. Jang T, Aubin C, Naunheim R, et al. Ultrasonography of the internal jugular vein in patients with dyspnea without jugular venous distention on physical examination. *Ann Emerg Med*. 2004;44:160-168.

26. Blaivas M, Lyon M, Duggal S. A prospective comparison of supine chest radiography and bedside ultrasound for the diagnosis of traumatic pneumothorax. *Acad Emerg Med*. 2005;12:844-849.

27. Soldati G, Testa A, Sher S, Pignataro G, La Sala M, Silveri NG. Occult traumatic pneumothorax: diagnostic accuracy of lung Ultrasonography in emergency department. *Chest*. 2008;133:204-211.

28. Lichtenstein DA, Menu Y. A bedside ultrasound sign ruling out pneumothorax in the critically ill. Lung sliding. *Chest*. 1995;108(5);1345-1348.

29. Lichtenstein DA, Meziere GA. Relevance of lung ultrasound in the diagnosis of acute respiratory failure: the BLUE protocol. *Chest*. 2008;134:117-125.

30. Lichtenstein D, Meziere G, Biderman P, Gepner A. The "lung point": an ultrasound sign specific to pneumothorax. *Intensive Care Med*. 2000;26(10):1434-1440.

31. Lichtenstein D, Meziere G. A lung ultrasound sign allowing bedside distinction between pulmonary edema and COPD: the comet-tail artifact. *Intensive Care Med*. 1998;24(12):1331-1334.

32. Lichtenstein D. FALLS-protocol: lung ultrasound in hemodynamic assessment of shock. *Heart Lung Vessel*. 2013;5(3):142-147.

33. Dietrich CF, Mathis G, Blaivas M, et al. Lung B-line artefacts and their use. *J Thoracic Dis*. 2016;8(6):1356-1365.

34. Gaskamp M, Blubaugh M, McCarthy LH, Scheid DC. Can bedside ultrasound inferior vena cava measurements accurately diagnose congestive heart failure in the emergency department? A Clin-IQ. *J Patient Cent Res Rev*. 2016;3(4):230-234.

35. Dent B, Kendall RJ, Boyle AA, Atkinson PRT. Emergency ultrasound of the abdominal aorta by UK emergency physicians: a prospective cohort study. *Emerg Med J*. 2007;24:547-547.

36. Crisp J, Lovato L, Jang T. Compression ultrasonography of the lower extremity with portable vascular ultrasonography can accurately detect deep venous thrombosis in the emergency department. *Ann Emerg Med*. 2010;56:601-610.

37. Kearon C, Akl EA, Ornelas J, et al. Antithrombotic therapy for VTE disease: CHEST Guideline and Expert Panel Report. *Chest*. 2016;149(2):315-352. doi:10.1016/j.chest.2015.11.026. Erratum in: *Chest*. 2016 Oct;150(4):988.

38. Link MS, Berkow LC, Kudenchuk PJ, et al. Part 7: adult advanced cardiovascular life support: 2015 American Heart Association Guidelines update for cardiopulmonary resuscitation and emergency cardiovascular care. *Circulation*. 2015;132(18 suppl 2):S444-S464.

39. Yancy CW, Jessup M, Bozkurt B, et al. 2013 ACCF/AHA guideline for the management of heart failure: executive summary: a report of the American College of Cardiology Foundation/American Heart Association Task Force on practice guidelines. *Circulation*. 2013;128(16):1810-1852.

40. Rhodes A, Evans LE, Alhazzani W, et al. Surviving sepsis campaign: international guidelines for management of sepsis and septic shock: 2016. *Intensive Care Med*. 2017;43(3):304-377.

41. Blanco P, Volpicelli G. Common pitfalls in point-of-care ultrasound: a practical guide for emergency and critical care physicians. *Crit Ultrasound J*. 2016;8:15.

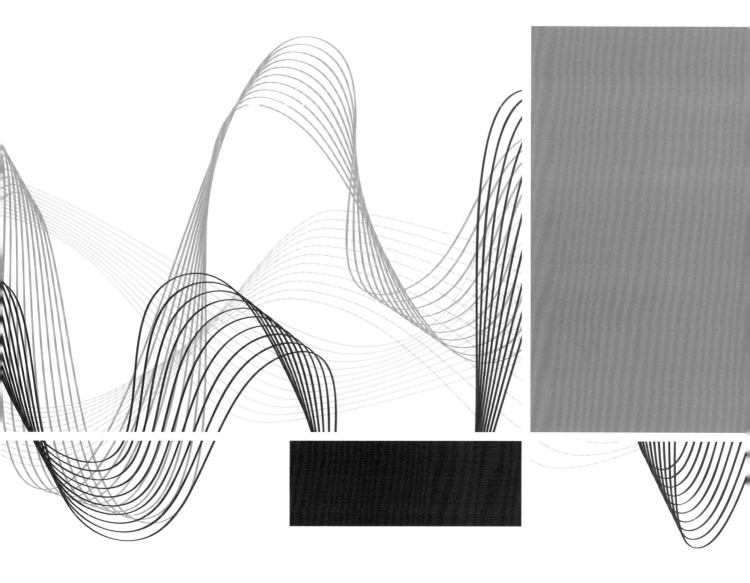

PART 4

PROCEDURES

Musculoskeletal Aspirations and Injections

Alexei O. DeCastro, MD, Dae Hyoun (David) Jeong, MD, and Jock Taylor, MD

LITERATURE REVIEW

Ultrasound-guided musculoskeletal injections have several benefits, such as real-time visualization and guidance. The most important benefit may be the ability to constantly visualize the needle throughout the procedure. This improves both outcome and safety, as important structures like blood vessels and nerves are avoided while the needle is accurately placed in any target. This assures high accuracy and minimizes complications and pain, as compared to landmark or palpation-guided injections.[1,2]

Ultrasound-guided procedures can be separated into either a direct or an indirect approach. In the indirect approach, ultrasound is only used to identify the target and determine depth. The skin overlying the area is marked accordingly. This works best for large superficial targets, because the needle is not visualized during the procedure. The direct approach is preferred, with the needle either in-plane or out-of-plane of the transducer. The direct approach can be performed with the needle in-plane with the ultrasound image or out-of-plane. The in-plane approach is the favored approach. It allows continuous, real-time correction of both angle and depth of the needle.

Ultrasound-guided knee injections and aspirations offer more accurate and better outcomes.[1,2] In studies comparing ultrasound-guided versus landmark-guided knee injections, ultrasound-guided procedures had 48% less procedural pain, 42% more pain reduction,107 more responders, and 52% less nonresponders. Ultrasound-guided knee injections also proved to be more cost effective, although with a higher upfront cost. It was shown to produce 13% less cost/patient/year and 58% less cost/responder/year.[3] Outcomes for knee aspirations showed 183% more fluid aspirated.[4] Also, it may be more imperative when injecting viscosupplementation to ensure that the medication is deposited accurately, which improves efficacy and avoids complications such as severe pain by mistakenly injecting it into the soft tissue.

The commonly performed anterior landmark-guided approach to a knee injection is not as effective because of the location of Hoffa's fat pad directly behind the patellar tendon.[1] In a clinical situation it is imperative to discern whether a knee effusion is septic arthritis because this would be a true knee emergency. In the above situation, it would also help differentiate gout and/or other causes of an inflammatory effusion.

Injection of the acromioclavicular (AC) joint may be considered for patients with recalcitrant pain resulting from an AC joint–associated pain generator that is unresponsive to appropriate activity modifications, oral or topical medications, therapeutic modalities, therapeutic exercises, and protection or bracing where indicated. In addition, AC joint injection may be used for diagnostic purposes if the primary pain generator is uncertain based on history, physical examination, or imaging.

Blind AC joint injection accuracy has been documented to be about 40% to 72%.[2] Ultrasound-guided AC joint injections have been shown to achieve an accuracy rate of 95% to 100%.[5] In two studies, AC joint injections were shown to be significantly more accurate using ultrasound guidance versus palpation guidance.[6] The clinical outcomes of palpation-guided versus ultrasound-guided AC joint injections have been reported as similar at up to 3 weeks postinjection in one study.[7]

Hip injections may help with the diagnosis as source of pain and also ultrasound guidance provide better accuracy.[8] Injections have shown to decrease pain and increase range of motion.[9] Because of decreased accuracy, landmark-guided injections of the hip have increased risk of damage or irritation to adjacent neurovascular structures.[10] Fluoroscopic and computed tomography (CT)-guided injections have radiation and increased cost when compared to ultrasound. In addition, fluoroscopic-guided injections do not have the benefits of visualizing the neurovascular bundle as ultrasound does.

TABLE 52-1. Recommendations for Use of Point-of-Care Ultrasound in Clinical Practice

Recommendation	Rating	References
Accurate injections are more efficacious than inaccurate injections.	A	11
Ultrasound-guided arthrocentesis is less painful and more efficacious than landmark-guided arthrocentesis.	B	11

A = consistent, good-quality patient-oriented evidence; B = inconsistent or limited-quality patient-oriented evidence; C = consensus, disease-oriented evidence, usual practice, expert opinion, or case series. For information about the SORT evidence rating system, go to http://www.aafp.org/afpsort.

EQUIPMENT

- Sterile probe covers
- 18 to 25 gauge, 1.5 to 2 in needle
- 5 to 25 mL syringe
- 0.5 to 5 mL lidocaine 1% without epinephrine and 0.5 to 2 mL injectable corticosteroid, or 2 to 6 mL hyaluronic acid, depending on size of the joint injected

INDICATIONS

- Knee
  - Osteoarthritis of the knee
  - Crystal-induced arthropathy of the knee (gout, pseudogout)
  - Aspiration of an effusion
  - Recurrent patellofemoral pain syndrome (if failed conservative management)
  - Degenerative meniscal tear
- AC joint
  - Chronic AC joint pain
  - AC joint arthritis Grade I or Grade II AC joint sprain (if the pain remains severe despite at least 2 weeks of conservative management)
- Hip
  - Osteoarthritis of the hip
  - Femoroacetabular impingement
  - Tear of the acetabular labrum of the hip
  - Diagnostic injection to rule out intra-articular pathology versus extra-articular pathology

CONTRAINDICATIONS

- Absolute contraindications
  - Overlying cellulitis
  - Bacteremia
  - Joint prosthesis
  - Acute fracture
  - Acute anterior cruciate ligament (ACL), posterior cruciate ligament (PCL), or medial collateral ligament (MCL) injury
- Relative contraindications
  - Severe coagulopathy
  - Anticoagulant therapy (especially international normalized ratio [INR] greater than 3.5-4.0)
  - Lack of response after two to four injections
  - Unstable joint (chronic instability)
  - Evidence of surrounding osteoporosis
  - Recent intra-articular joint osteoporosis
  - History of allergy or anaphylaxis to injectable pharmaceuticals

PERFORMING THE PROCEDURE

General Preparation Considerations for Arthrocentesis

Regardless of the anatomic location of the arthrocentesis, it is good practice to first scan the join and identify pertinent landmarks and pathology such as joint effusions.

Next, mark ideal probe location based on your initial scan. Prep the patient with betadine or chlorhexidine and ensure a clear wide area. Place a sterile drape and probe cover.

Anesthetize the skin by placing a wheal underneath the skin using a regular 25-gauge needle with 1% lidocaine at the site marked for the needle. With ultrasound guidance, place the 1% lidocaine deeper within the subcutaneous tissues then exchange a 25-gauge needle for a larger 18- to 22-gauge needle. If aspiration is not being performed, only a smaller 25-gauge needle is needed for injection. In these cases,

the skin anesthesia step can often be skipped. However, anytime a 22 gauge or larger needle is used, skin anesthesia is recommended.

Knee Arthrocentesis

Step 1. Place the patient in the supine position. This will help to make them more comfortable, reduce movement, and avoid potential vasovagal syncope. The superolateral approach is preferred using a freehand, in-plane technique (**Figure 52-1**).

Step 2. Place a towel roll under the posterior knee, which will put the knee in slight flexion to approximately 20°. This will help identify the suprapatellar recess and relax the quadriceps muscle. In this position, a joint effusion is most noticeable as the synovium bulges superiorly and laterally at the patellofemoral joint when the patient is lying supine. Sometimes, the patient can press the knee down posteriorly and the effusion may become more conspicuous.

Step 3. Use a linear array transducer placed over the quadriceps tendon as an initial landmark. Then, identify the joint effusion in both a longitudinal and transverse position. Mark this location and then prep the patient for the procedure as described earlier.

Step 4. Identify the point of entry for the needle. Keep the transducer in a transverse position on the knee (over the suprapatellar bursa). The best point of entry is at the soft spot between the iliotibial (IT) band and vastus lateralis. The recess is located between quadriceps tendon or quadriceps fat pat that is superficial and prefemoral fat that is deep. To help orient the needle, push with a gloved finger on the lateral aspect of the knee very close to the probe, and the deep fat pad will move underneath the bursa. Insert the needle at the lateral aspect of the knee directing the tip medially (**Figure 52-2**).

Step 5. Stop the needle insertion once the needle tip is visualized in the joint effusion (**Figure 52-3**).

Aspirate the superolateral aspect of the joint recess.

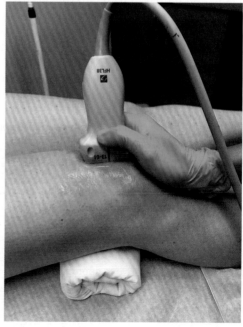

FIGURE 52-1. Patient is supine. Landmarks are identified first by orienting the probe with the probe marker toward the patient's head.

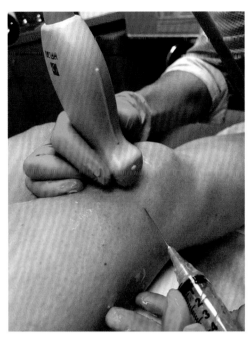

FIGURE 52-2. The probe is positioned for the superior lateral approach. The transducer will be in short axis to the quadriceps tendon overlying the superior knee recess.

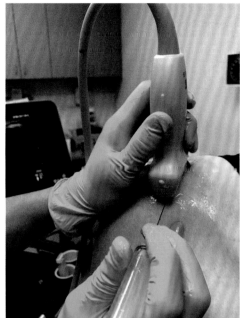

FIGURE 52-4. Transducer and needle positioning for an anterior in-plane approach for ultrasound-guided acromioclavicular joint injection.

Acromioclavicular Arthrocentesis

Step 1. Position the patient sitting upright in a chair or examination table. The ipsilateral arm is held adducted in a neutral position. Visualize the AC joint in a sagittal plane over the anterior aspect of the AC joint and subsequently in modified long axis view by rotating the transducer about 30° medially (**Figure 52-4**).

Step 2. Prep the patient for the procedure as described earlier.

Step 3. Insert the needle anterior to posterior, out-of-plane with the transducer. Stop the needle insertion once the tip is visualized in the joint. It will appear as a hyperechoic dot. Inject the contents of the syringe (**Figure 52-5**).

Hip Arthrocentesis

Step 1. Position patient laying supine on the table (**Figure 52-6**).

Step 2. Scan anteriorly, in the long axis of the femoral neck. Target the femoral head and neck junction and look for the overlying joint capsule (anterior synovial recess). The scan plane should be lateral to the femoral vessels (**Figure 52-7**).

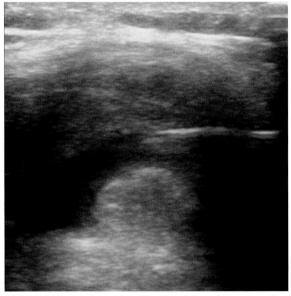

FIGURE 52-3. The needle is visualized in-plane while advancing into the synovium.

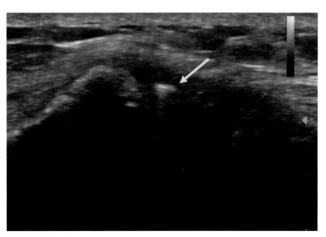

FIGURE 52-5. Ultrasound image of out-of-plane needle (arrow) during guided acromioclavicular joint injection.

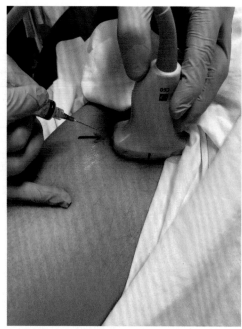

FIGURE 52-6. Anterior oblique approach to an ultrasound-guided hip injection. The transducer is placed in-plane with a cephalomedial approach.

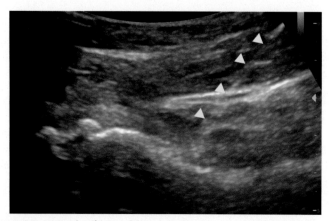

FIGURE 52-7. The femoral head and neck are visualized in long axis. The needle (arrowheads) is visualized in-plane going into the anterior synovial recess located between the femoral head and femoral neck.

Step 3. Prep the patient for the procedure as described earlier.

Step 4. Advance the spinal needle with ultrasound guidance to the level of the femoral head and neck junction.

Step 5. Test inject to see if there is easy flow. If there is no resistance and distention of the joint capsule is visualized, inject entire contents of syringe.

POSTPROCEDURE INSTRUCTIONS

After removing the needle, clean the skin with alcohol and place bandage if any bleeding is noted. Inform the patient that the area may be sore, throbbing or a little swollen for several days. Advise them to rest the area of the injection for 24 to 48 hours after the procedure. Ice may be applied to the area for 15 to 20 minutes every 1 to 2 hours for 1 to 2 days, which may help decrease the pain. The local anesthetic can last for 5 to 12 hours but the corticosteroid may take up to 2 to 5 days to take effect. Educate the patient about warning signs, such as worsening swelling, redness, rash, or even shortness of breath. If the patient has diabetes and is on insulin, blood sugars may be elevated for 1 to 5 days. Direct the diabetic patient to check their blood sugars periodically postprocedure and consider covering with sliding scale insulin to help control the elevated blood glucose level. Viscosupplementation may take up to a month to see an effect, and the duration of the effect is variable among patients.

COMPLICATIONS

- Postinjection flare
- Steroid arthropathy
- Tendon rupture
- Facial flushing
- Skin atrophy, depigmentation
- Iatrogenic infectious arthritis
- Transient paresis of injected extremity
- Hypersensitivity reaction
- Asymptomatic pericapsular calcification
- Acceleration of cartilage attrition

PATIENT MANAGEMENT

Steroid injections have been shown to decrease pain and increase range of motion.

Ultrasound can be used to accurately identify the joint effusions (Chapter 35). Arthrocentesis and subsequent synovial fluid analysis should be done in all cases of unexplained joint effusions.[11] The aspirated fluid should be analyzed for cell count, Gram stain, cultures, and crystal analysis. The synovial fluid aspirate should be analyzed for: complete blood count (CBC) with differential (white blood cell [WBC], polymorphonuclear leukocytes), crystal examination, culture and Gram stain, viscosity, glucose. The presence of crystals cannot exclude septic arthritis with certainty. Septic arthritis occurs concurrently with gout or pseudogout in less than 5% of cases (Table 52-2). If a septic knee effusion is proven, start intravenous (IV) antibiotics for the suspected infective agent. Orthopedic consult may be necessary because drainage of the joint is associated with rapid recovery and low morbidity. Arthroscopy allows visualization of the joint, provides the ability to lyse adhesions, drains any purulent pockets, and can facilitate debridement of necrotic material if needed.[11]

In patients with osteoarthritis, an intra-articular injection of lidocaine can help confirm the source of pain to be originating from the joint. Additionally, intra-articular injections of corticosteroids or viscosupplementation may provide therapeutic benefit; however, these benefits are often only temporary.

TABLE 52-2 **Synovial Fluid Analysis**

Arthritis diagnosis	Color	Transparency	Viscosity	WBC Count (per mm³)	PMN cell count (%)	Gram stain	Culture	Crystals
Normal	Clear	Transparent	High/thick	<200	<25	Negative	Negative	Negative
Noninflammatory	Straw	Translucent	High/thick	200-2000	<25	Negative	Negative	Negative
Inflammatory: crystalline disease	Yellow	Cloudy	Low/thin	2000-100 000	>50	Negative	Negative	Positive
Inflammatory: noncrystalline disease	Yellow	Cloudy	Low/thin	2000-100 000	>50	Negative	Negative	Negative
Infectious: Lyme disease	Yellow	Cloudy	Low	3000-100 000 (mean: 25 000)	>50	Negative	Negative	Negative
Infectious: gonococcal	Yellow	Cloudy-opaque	Low	34 000-68 000	>75	Variable (<50%)	Positive (25%-70%)	Negative
Infectious: nongonococcal	Yellow-green	Opaque	Very low	>50 000 (>100 000 is more specific)	>75	Positive (60%-80%)	Positive (>90%)	Negative[a]

[a]Crystalline disease can coexist with septic arthritis. A positive result does not exclude infection.

Abbreviation: PMN, polymorphonuclear.

Reprinted with permission from Horowitz DL, Katzap E, Horowitz S, et al. Approach to septic arthritis. *Am Fam Physician.* 2011;84(6):653-660. Copyright © 2011 by the American Academy of Family Physicians.

PEARLS AND PITFALLS

Pearls

- Know where the tip of the needle is at all times.
- Anchor the transducer against the patient by holding it near the skin with the nondominant hand and maintaining contact with the transducer and patient with that hand at all times. Use your dominant hand to advance the needle with your other hand.
- Do not move transducer and needle at the same time. Keep the needle still once it penetrates the skin and move the transducer to find the needle.
- "Jiggling" the tip or using a sewing machine maneuver, where the bevel of the needle is rotated, may help identify the tip as the needle is advanced.

Pitfalls

- Don't advance the needle if you can't see the tip.
- Penetrating the thickened part of the synovial membrane by needle may cause severe pain so try to advance the needle within the effusion or suprapatellar bursa.
- Be sure that the needle is long enough to reach the targeted joint. In deep joints such as the hip, a spinal needle is often needed.
- Avoid poly-injection syndrome. As a rule of thumb, do not perform more than three times per year or separate injections by less than 6 weeks.

BILLING

CPT Code	Description	Professional Component	Facility Fee
20604	Arthrocentesis, aspiration, and/or injection; small joint or bursa (e.g., fingers, toes) with ultrasound guidance, with permanent recording and reporting	$73.40	$47.26
20606	Arthrocentesis, aspiration, and/or injection; intermediate joint or bursa (e.g., temporomandibular, acromioclavicular, wrist, elbow or ankle, olecranon bursa) with ultrasound guidance, with permanent recording and reporting	$81.28	$54.06
20611	Arthrocentesis, aspiration and/or injection, major joint or bursa (e.g., shoulder, hip, knee, subacromial bursa); with ultrasound guidance, with permanent recording and reporting	$93.09	$63.37

CPT codes and average national reimbursement for Medicare in 2016. Payment data are from https://www.cms.gov/apps/physician-fee-schedule/search/search-criteria.aspx. See Chapter 2 for details on ultrasound billing.

References

1. Jackson D, Evans N, Thomas B. Accuracy of needle placement into the intra-articular space of the knee. *J Bone Joint Surg Am.* 2002;84:1522-1527.

2. Curtiss H, Finnoff J, Peck E. Accuracy of ultrasound guided and palpation-guided knee injections by an experienced and less-experienced injector using a supero-lateral approach: a cadaveric study. *PM R.* 2011;3:507-515.

3. Sibbitt WL Jr, Band PA, Kettwich LG, et al. A randomized controlled trial evaluating the cost-effectiveness of sonographic guidance for intra-articular injection of the osteoarthritic knee. *J Clin Rheumatol.* 2011;17(8):409-415.

4. Sibbitt WL Jr, Kettwich LG, Band PA, et al. Does ultrasound guidance improve the outcomes of arthrocentesis and corticosteroid injection of the knee? *Scand J Rheumatol.* 2012;41(1):66-72.

5. Bain GI, Van Riet RP, Gooi C, Ashwood N. The long-term efficacy of cortico-steroid injection into the acromioclavicular joint using a dynamic fluoroscopic method. *Int J Shoulder Surg.* 2007;1:104-107.

6. Sabeti-Aschraf M, Lemmerhofer B, Lang S, et al. Ultrasound guidance improves the accuracy of the acromioclavicular joint infiltration: a prospective randomized study. *Knee Surg Sports Traumatol Arthrosc.* 2011;19(2):292-295.

7. Sabeti-Aschraf M, Ochsner A, Schueller-Weidekamm C, et al. The infiltration of the AC joint performed by one specialist: ultrasound versus palpation a prospective randomized pilot study. *Eur J Radiol.* 2010;75(1):e37-e40.

8. Robinson R, Keenan AM, Conaghan PG. Clinical effectiveness and dose response of image-guided intra-articular corticosteroid injection for hip osteoarthritis. *Rheumatology (Oxford).* 2007;46(2):285-291.

9. Kullenberg B, Runneson R, Tuvhag R, et al. Intraarticular corticosteroid injection: pain relief in osteoarthritis of the hip? *J Rheumatol.* 2004;31(11):2265-2268.

10. Sofka CM, Saboeiro G, Adler RS. Ultrasound-guided hip injections. *J Vasc Interv Radiol.* 2005;16(8):1121-1123.

11. Gerena L, DeCastro A. *Knee Effusion.* StatPearls [Internet]. Treasure Island, FL: StatPearls Publishing; 2019.

Central Line Placement

Jilian R. Sansbury, MD, FACP

LITERATURE REVIEW

Central lines are appropriate for delivery of a wide variety of advanced medications and are used in a broad array of settings. Patients who require monitoring of central venous pressure or require a central line restricted medication will need a central line. Such medications include hypertonic saline, vasopressors, rapid infusions of intravenous electrolytes, or when multiple intravenous medications or solutions must be given simultaneously.[1]

Tunneled catheters are central lines that are tunneled under the skin to exit at a location away from the central vein. Tunneled catheters have lower long-term complications but are usually placed by specialists. Nontunneled catheters do not contain a cuff device and provide direct access into a central vein. They can be inserted and removed without a surgical procedure and typically have a dual or triple lumen. Quinton catheters are nontunneled devices that can be placed for short-term hemodialysis or apheresis. Nontunneled central lines can also be used for hemodynamic monitoring, typically with a Cordis or Swan–Ganz catheter.[2]

Central lines are referred to by their location of placement (internal jugular, subclavian, femoral). The subclavian vein location for central line placement, as it underlies the clavicle, is particularly difficult for utilization of the ultrasound probe. The internal jugular, as well as the femoral site, may be accessed easily with an ultrasound device. Femoral lines have fallen out of favor as the incidence of central line–associated blood stream infections (CLABSI) is significantly higher with femoral venous placement.[3]

For the purposes of this ultrasound-guided procedure, we will be utilizing the internal jugular vein. The internal jugular vein is located at the apex of the triangle formed by the sternal and clavicular heads of the sternocleidomastoid muscle located lateral to the carotid artery (**Figure 53-1**).

The medical literature is replete with information regarding the use of ultrasound to improve the safety and precision of central line placement. In one meta-analysis, authors illustrate that dynamic

2-D ultrasound significantly reduced inadvertent arterial puncture, pneumothorax, and hematoma formation.[4] A Cochrane review evidenced a reduction in the rate of overall central line placement–related complications by 71%.[5]

In addition to real-time guidance during placement, ultrasound can serve to confirm location of the catheter tip in the superior vena cava (SVC) as well as rule out pneumothorax once the procedure is complete. A meta-analysis found a pooled sensitivity and specificity of catheter malposition of 82% and 98%, respectively. Ultrasound was also found to decrease time to diagnosis of a mispositioned central line by 58.3 minutes compared to standard chest x-ray. The pooled sensitivity for ruling out a postprocedure pneumothorax was nearly 100%.[6]

EQUIPMENT

This is a sterile procedure and requires the individuals performing the procedure to don a gown and gloves in sterile fashion. There will be some variability in the central line kits used at different institutions, but the basic implements of a triple-lumen central line kit are outlined below:

1. Sterile gown, gloves, cap, mask, and face shield
2. Sterile ultrasound probe cover
3. Skin preparation solution—chlorhexidine is preferred
4. Sterile skin prep and drape or sterile towels
5. Lidocaine solution
6. Sterile gauze
7. Syringes
8. Scalpel
9. Suture and needle driver
10. Saline flushes—one for each lumen of the central line catheter
11. Caps—one for each lumen of the central line catheter
12. Catheter, dilator, needle, and guidewire—7F 15- or 20-cm triple-lumen catheters are most commonly used in adults. For fluid resuscitation or hemodialysis, larger bore catheters are preferable, typically 11.5F 20-cm double-lumen devices are used. The catheter of choice should be tested to ensure patency with saline flush via each lumen prior to accessing the vein with the device (**Figure 53-2**).

INDICATIONS

- Vasopressor administration
- Hypertonic saline administration
- Rapid infusion of IV electrolyte solutions
- Rapid transfusion of blood products
- Emergent hemodialysis or apheresis
- Central venous pressure monitoring
- Lack of peripheral IV access when additional modes of IV access are contraindicated

| TABLE 53-1 | Recommendations for Use of Point-of-Care Ultrasound in Clinical Practice |

Recommendation	Rating	References
Use of point-of-care ultrasound in the placement of central venous catheters	A	7
Use of point-of-care ultrasound in the verification of placement of central venous catheters	C	2

A = consistent, good-quality patient-oriented evidence; B = inconsistent or limited-quality patient-oriented evidence; C = consensus, disease-oriented evidence, usual practice, expert opinion, or case series. For information about the SORT evidence rating system, go to http://www.aafp.org/afpsort.

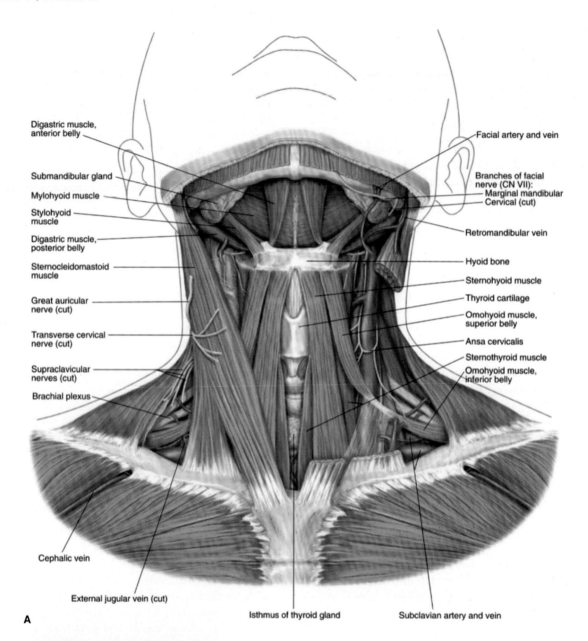

Digastric muscle, anterior belly

Submandibular gland

Mylohyoid muscle

Stylohyoid muscle

Digastric muscle, posterior belly

Sternocleidomastoid muscle

Great auricular nerve (cut)

Transverse cervical nerve (cut)

Supraclavicular nerves (cut)

Brachial plexus

Cephalic vein

External jugular vein (cut)

Facial artery and vein

Branches of facial nerve (CN VII):
Marginal mandibular
Cervical (cut)

Retromandibular vein

Hyoid bone

Sternohyoid muscle

Thyroid cartilage

Omohyoid muscle, superior belly

Ansa cervicalis

Sternothyroid muscle

Omohyoid muscle, inferior belly

Isthmus of thyroid gland

Subclavian artery and vein

A

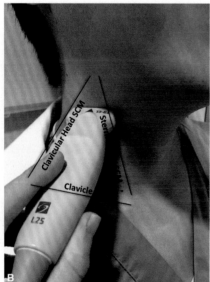

FIGURE 53-1. Anatomy of the line placement. SCM, sternocleidomastoid.

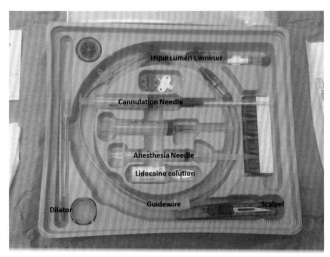

FIGURE 53-2. Typical central line kit contents.

CONTRAINDICATIONS

- Skin, soft tissue infection, cellulitis, or rash to the area overlying the target vessel
- Known venous thromboembolism to major vessel intended to be utilized for central line placement
- Known coagulopathy that would predispose the patient to excessive blood loss during a central line procedure

PERFORMING THE PROCEDURE

Some resources recommend a two-person approach for central line placement, which allows the practitioner to have both hands available for the procedure, while the second individual guides the ultrasound probe. With adequate practice, a single person can successfully complete the procedure while allowing for improved coordination between the ultrasound probe and needle placement. Typically, the nondominant hand holds the ultrasound probe while the dominant hand performs tasks necessary for the procedure. Use the high-frequency linear array probe for the procedure.

1. Adjust the bed to Trendelenburg 10° to 15°. This engorges the vein and decreases risk of air embolism. Typically, use of the *right* internal jugular vein is preferable as the SVC is in direct communication with this site. The patient's head should be facing toward the left (**Figure 53-3**).
2. Verify anatomy using ultrasound probe and mark a location on the skin beneath the center of the ultrasound probe. The internal jugular vein and carotid artery will be seen on the ultrasound image as black circles. The vein is the more compressible structure when gentle pressure is applied with the probe (**Figures 53-4 through 53-7**).
3. Prep and drape the patient in sterile fashion (**Figure 53-8**).
4. Open the central line kit and review all contents.
5. Flush all the lumens of the central line with saline to ensure patency of the lumens.
6. Test the guidewire through the center lumen of the central line to ensure that it passes smoothly and without resistance.

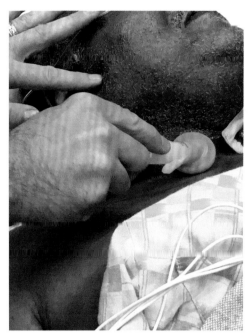

FIGURE 53-3. Preparation of the patient for internal jugular vein central line placement.

7. Prepare the ultrasound probe with sterile gel and a sterile probe cover.
8. A 25-gauge needle should be used to place a wheal under the skin with 1% lidocaine at the site previously marked. This may be done with or without ultrasound guidance.

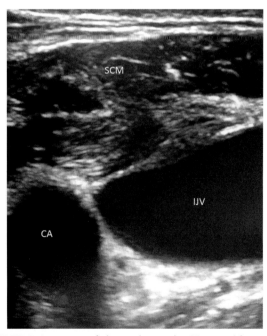

FIGURE 53-4. Anatomy of the neck vessels. CA, carotid artery; IJV, internal jugular vein; SCM, sternocleidomastoid.

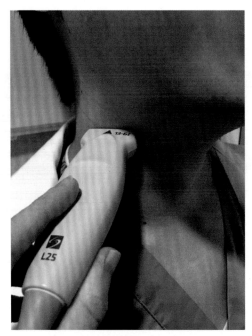

FIGURE 53-5. Proper probe placement.

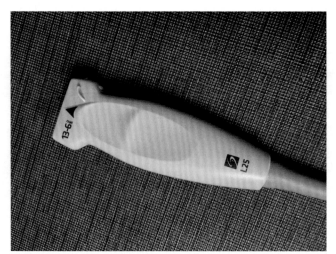

FIGURE 53-7. View of the ultrasound probe used for internal jugular vein central line placement.

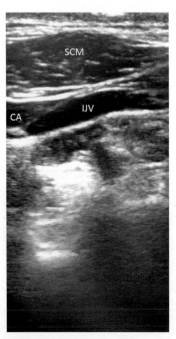

FIGURE 53-6. Compression of internal jugular vein venous structure with pressure applied to the ultrasound probe CA, carotid artery; IJV, internal jugular vein; SCM, sternocleidomastoid.

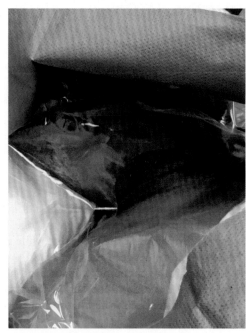

FIGURE 53-8. Sterile prep and drape placement.

9. Confirm needle insertion site with the ultrasound probe perpendicular to the skin.

10. Puncture the internal jugular vein with the needle while applying gentle negative pressure to the syringe—needle should be inserted at a 45° angle with the needle directed toward the midaxillary line on the ipsilateral side. You will see the shadow of the needle on the transverse ultrasound image, which can then be followed into the vessel for confirmation of placement. There will be a flash of dark red blood (nonpulsatile) in the needle when entry into the internal jugular vein is achieved. If the flow of venous blood is lost, gently pull back on the needle to reenter the vein, as the needle has likely just passed through the vein causing a flash to appear (**Figures 53-9 through 53-11**).

11. Remove the syringe and leave the needle in place with the nondominant hand on the needle at all times.

12. Once free flow of blood is achieved, the guidewire can be advanced into the needle using the introducer. The curved end of the guidewire should be advanced first (**Figure 53-12**).

13. Once the guidewire is in place, remove the needle while the guidewire remains in place. The nondominant hand should remain on the guidewire at all times (**Figure 53-13**).

a. A nurse or assistant should monitor the patient's telemetry while the guidewire is placed. If an arrhythmia occurs,

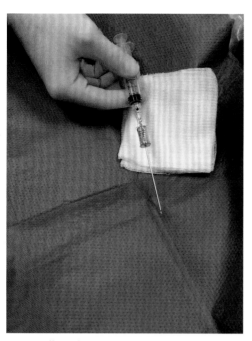

FIGURE 53-9. Needle utilized during aspiration technique while locating the internal jugular vein with ultrasound probe in place with sterile ultrasound probe cover.

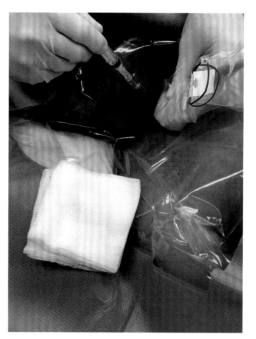

FIGURE 53-11. Aspiration of the internal jugular vein with negative pressure on the needle.

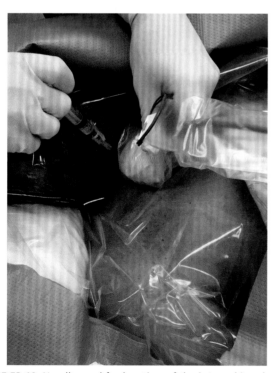

FIGURE 53-10. Needle used for location of the internal jugular vein.

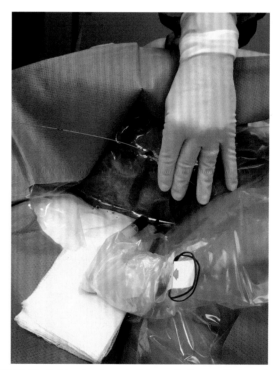

FIGURE 53-12. Guidewire threaded through the needle into the deep venous structures of the neck.

withdraw the guidewire back slightly until a normal heart rhythm returns.

b. Verify placement of the guidewire by turning the ultrasound probe longitudinally to follow its passage into the vessel. Obtain an image of the wire lying within the internal jugular vein and save it to the patient's chart to complete documentation

and illustrate correct placement within the vein for billing purposes (**Figures 53-14 and 53-15**).

14. Use a scalpel to create a small incision at the base of the guidewire at its insertion point in the skin of the neck. This will allow the dilator to advance through the skin. DO NOT CUT THE WIRE. To ensure safety with the scalpel step, use

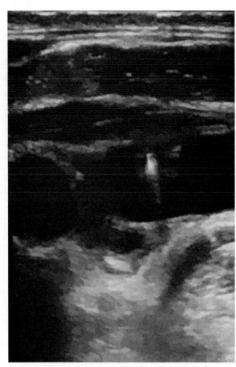

FIGURE 53-13. Verification of the needle and guidewire within the internal jugular vein with ultrasound.

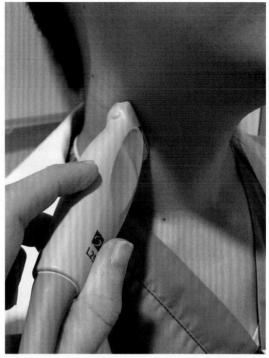

FIGURE 53-15. Parallel placement of the ultrasound probe on the neck.

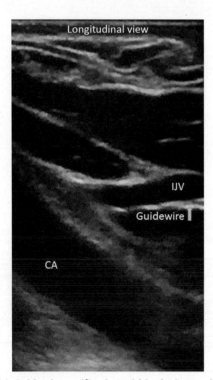

FIGURE 53-14. Guidewire verification within the internal jugular vein with ultrasound probe turned parallel to the track of the internal jugular vein within the neck. CA, carotid artery; IJV, internal jugular vein.

the blade facing outward away from the guidewire when making the incision in the skin.

   a. One hand should be on the guidewire at all times to prevent wire embolism or loss of wire within the body.

15. Advance the dilator over the guidewire gently until it is about halfway into the skin. The dilator does not need to be "hubbed," or fully advanced into the skin, for placement of an internal jugular central line.

   a. Advancement of the dilator is achieved most easily by holding the dilator close to the tip and rotating clockwise and then counterclockwise in a left to right motion until the dilator penetrates the skin and soft tissue.

   b. After the dilator is advanced halfway into the skin, it is removed over the guidewire while the guidewire remains in place (**Figure 53-16**).

16. Expose the external end of the wire and place the central venous catheter tip over the guidewire, through the skin, and advance to 17 to 20 cm length. Typically, the guidewire will have to be backed out of its location until it resurfaces at the distal end of the catheter (usually a brown hub among the three lumens at the distal end). Once the guidewire is seen at the distal end of the catheter, the catheter can be advanced over the catheter. Again, one hand should be on the guidewire at all times during this step.

   a. There will be a measurement marker on the catheter tip for distance approximation. The tip of the catheter should

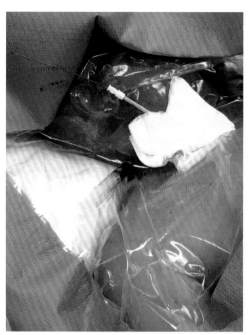

FIGURE 53-16. Dilator with guidewire in place during central line placement.

lie at the junction of the SVC and the right atrium (RA) (**Figure 53-17**).

17. The guidewire is removed by pulling it through the distal end of the catheter lumen.

18. Flush all of the ports with saline and apply caps to the hubs.

19. Place an antimicrobial gel pad directly over the skin at the catheter insertion site.

20. Secure the line with a suture to each side of the hub and apply sterile dressing to the site.

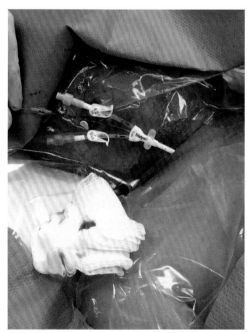

FIGURE 53-17. Catheter inserted over the guidewire and placed within the internal jugular vein at the right neck.

21. Assess proper placement of the line at the SVC-RA junction and assess for iatrogenic pneumothorax. This can be done with portable chest x-ray or with bedside ultrasound.

    a. If using bedside ultrasound, first use the linear probe to identify the pleural line on the anterior chest wall ipsilateral to the side of the neck in which the central line was placed. Visualized lung sliding would rule out an iatrogenic pneumothorax. Lack of lung sliding would require further assessment for a lung point to confirm pneumothorax. If there is no lung sliding and no lung point, advanced imaging may be needed to further evaluate (see Chapter 14 for details of assessment of pneumothorax).

    b. Next, use the linear probe to identify the internal jugular and subclavian vessels. Rapidly flush 10 mL normal saline into distal port of the central line. Assess for the presence or absence of echogenic bubbles. Repeat this for the contralateral neck vessels. Next, use the phased array probe to obtain the apical or subcostal four-chamber view and again rapidly flush 10 mL normal saline into the distal port. Please refer to Chapters 12 and 13 for details on acquiring these cardiac views. Normal catheter position would be indicated by lack of visualization of echogenic bubbles in the venous or arterial vessels and visualization of echogenic bubbles in the RA and ventricle. Abnormal catheter position would be indicated by visualization of echogenic bubbles in the venous or arterial vessels and by lack of visualization of echogenic bubbles in the RA and ventricle (▶ **Video 53-1**).

POSTPROCEDURE INSTRUCTIONS

Following the procedure, the site will be dressed with sterile clear dressing and the central line will be sutured to the skin. The patient should be instructed not to tamper with the suture site. This line is a temporary measure and should be removed as soon as the immediate indication for central line placement has been addressed.

COMPLICATIONS

- Bleeding at central line location
- Infection involving central line catheter that may lead to bacteremia or sepsis
- Infection involving skin surrounding central line site including cellulitis or rash
- Skin breakdown involving area surrounding central line location

PATIENT MANAGEMENT

The information obtained by the ultrasound-guided placement of a central venous catheter can assist the primary care practitioner in many situations. These include, but are not limited to, vasopressor or hypertonic saline administration, rapid infusion of IV electrolyte solution or transfusion of blood products, emergent hemodialysis or apheresis, or central venous pressure monitoring.

PEARLS AND PITFALLS

Pearls

- Central line placement is usually technically less difficult when performed on a well-hydrated patient. Encourage patient has adequate oral fluid intake prior to placement of the central venous catheter.
- Ensure correct placement of the guidewire by turning the probe longitudinally over the vessel. A picture of this placement may be saved to the ultrasound machine or printed for the patient's chart. An assistant should monitor the patient's heart rhythm during the procedure to watch for any arrhythmia, which means that the guidewire has reached the heart. Withdraw the guidewire slightly until the heart rhythm returns to normal. Frequent premature ventricular contractions (PVCs) are the telltale sign that the guidewire has been advanced beyond the junction of the SVC and the RA of the heart.
- Many practitioners will repeatedly press the needle up and down in a spring-like motion while watching the ultrasound

screen. This helps ensure alignment of the needle tip to its insertion target within the vessel. The tip of the needle will be seen as a "ring-down artifact" as it passes through the tissues on its way to the vessel wall.

Pitfalls

- Avoid breaking sterility to obtain needed materials. Ensure all materials are gathered prior to starting the procedure. There should be at least one assistant available for the entirety of the procedure.
- Avoid ergonomic complications from the procedure. Ensure that the patient's bed is at a comfortable height for you to work without bending over.
- Avoid placing a central line in a location where the artery lies deep to the vein, as this could result in unintentional puncture of the artery and potential bleeding complications.

BILLING

CPT Code	Description	Professional Component	Facility Fee
36555-36557	Insertion of nontunneled centrally inserted central venous catheters		$110-115
76937[a]	"Add-on" for ultrasound guidance used either for gaining access to venous entry site or for manipulating the catheter into final central position		$14-39

CPT codes and average national reimbursement for Medicare in 2016. Payment data are from https://www.cms.gov/apps/physician-fee-schedule/search/search-criteria.aspx. See Chapter 2 for details on ultrasound billing.

[a]Code 76937 requires an image be saved that documents the needle, guidewire, or catheter in the vein.

ACKNOWLEDGMENT

Special thanks to Dr. Thad Golden and Dr. Steven Allen for participating in photography sessions.

References

1. Agency for Healthcare Research and Quality. AHRQ patient safety indicators for central line placement. http://www.ahrq.gov/sites/default/files/wysiwyg/professionals/systems/hospital/qitoolkit/d4a-crbsi-bestpractices.pdf. Accessed November 14, 2016.
2. Institute for Healthcare Improvement. Implement the central line bundle. Cambridge, MA. http://www.ihi.org/IHI/topics/CriticalCare/IntensiveCare/Changes/ImplementtheCentralLineBundle.htm. Accessed November 14, 2016.
3. O'Grady NP, Alexander M, Burns LA, et al. Guidelines for the prevention of intravascular catheter-related infections. *Clin Infect Dis.* 2011;52(a):1087-1099.
4. Lalu MM, Fayad A, Ahmed O, et al. Ultrasound-guided subclavian vein catheterization. *Crit Care Med.* 2015;43(7):1498-1507. doi:10.1097/CCM.0000000000000973.
5. Smith AF, Kolodziej L, Schick G, Hellmich M, Brass P. Ultrasound guidance versus anatomical landmarks for internal jugular vein catheterization. *Cochrane Database Syst Rev.* 2017(1). doi:10.1002/14651858.cd006962.
6. Ablordeppey EA, Drewry AM, Beyer AB. Diagnostic accuracy of central venous catheter confirmation by bedside ultrasound versus chest radiography in critically ill patients: a systematic review and meta-analysis. *Crit Care Med.* 2017;45(4):715-724. doi:10.1097/CCM.0000000000002188.
7. Practice guidelines for central venous access: a report by the American Society of Anesthesiologists Task Force on Central Venous Access. http://www.google.com/url?sa=t&rct=j&q=&esrc=s&source=web&cd=1&ved=0ahUKEwiUp8vShKnQAhWBJCYKHQcsCLwQFggdMAA&url=http%3A%2F%2Fwww.asahq.org%2F~%2Fmedia%2Fsites%2Fasahq%2Ffiles%2Fpublic%2Fresources%2Fstandards-guidelines%2Fpractice-guidelines-for-central-venous-access.pdf&usg=AFQjCNFG99gtLzAA7tHcWD1cvWtIDfCLUA. Accessed November 13, 2016.

Diagnostic and Therapeutic Thoracentesis Using Point-of-Care Ultrasound

Wynn Traylor Harvey, II, MD, Sergio Urcuyo, MD, and Claire Hartung, MD

LITERATURE REVIEW

"Never let the sun set on a parapneumonic effusion" is the adage taught in medical schools across the United States. As it turns out, many medical societies including Thorax and The British Thoracic Society still recommend the sampling of pleural fluid in most cases when the procedure can be performed safely because of the diagnostic utility of fluid analysis.[1] However, despite how common this procedure is in medical practice, there are relatively few randomized controlled trials evaluating its technique and efficacy. Furthermore, the limited high-quality data that do exist have been gathered at larger inpatient centers with a high volume of procedures performed weekly. Because of this, it is difficult to cleanly extrapolate the existing data to outpatient settings where this procedure is not done as frequently except with a generally healthier population.

Early techniques used to perform thoracentesis involved chest radiographs (including decubitus films) or computed tomography (CT) to diagnose and localize pleural effusions. Chest x-rays are only 65% sensitive for the diagnosis of a pleural effusion, whereas ultrasound has been shown to have a sensitivity and specificity of up to 100%.[2] Chest CT is associated with a high radiation load to the patient and, while it can assist with diagnosing and estimating the size of the effusion, does not offer guidance on needle insertion for the procedure itself.

Ultrasound, however, has been demonstrated to be a safe and reliable method for choosing a needle insertion site for the procedure and results in fewer complications.[3,4] Localization techniques for thoracentesis had relied on manual percussion to localize the area of an effusion—this is a skill that requires experience and comes with a higher rate of failed attempts and pneumothoraces.[5] Ultrasound has the benefit of allowing the operator to directly visualize the effusion in the correct procedural position prior to inserting a needle. It also offers the comparable advantage of allowing the operator to define the depth of the effusion and whether lung enters the proposed needle insertion path during maximal inspiration (a contraindication to the procedure).[6] Ultrasound-guided thoracentesis has been shown to decrease pneumothorax rate by up to 52% and improve the rate of success by 25%. Additionally, it has been shown to decrease the cost of hospitalization by 20%.[7,8]

In short, point-of-care ultrasonography (POCUS) has become the standard of care for inpatient thoracentesis because of the clear benefits over traditional localization and procedural techniques. Although there are no robust randomized controlled trials to suggest that this is also true in the outpatient setting, the evidence cited earlier for improved safety with ultrasonography suggests that outpatient proceduralists should strongly consider using POCUS for confirmation of physical examination–based localization techniques.

TABLE 54-1	Recommendations for Use of Point-of-Care Ultrasound in Clinical Practice		
Recommendation		Rating	References
Thoracentesis should be performed with ultrasound guidance.		A	5, 6, 9
Routine postprocedure chest x-ray is not needed, and ultrasound is an effective alternative examination to evaluate for pneumothorax if suspected.		B	2, 5, 6

A = consistent, good-quality patient-oriented evidence; B = inconsistent or limited-quality patient-oriented evidence; C = consensus, disease-oriented evidence, usual practice, expert opinion, or case series. For information about the SORT evidence rating system, go to http://www.aafp.org/afpsort.

EQUIPMENT

- Phased array or curvilinear transducer
- Linear array transducer
- Thoracentesis catheter (usually 8 Fr over 18 gauge guide needle with attached 3-way stopcock)
- 22 gauge × 1½" needle (for drawing up lidocaine)
- 25 gauge × 1" needle (for injecting lidocaine)
- 10 mL syringe
- 60 mL syringe
- 1% lidocaine
- ChloraPrep
- Fenestrated sterile drape
- Scalpel #11 blade
- Gauze pads 4" × 4"
- Adhesive dressing
- Collection tubes for analysis
- Vacuum containers and tubing for collection of fluid if large volume removal is expected

INDICATIONS

- Pleural effusion is noted to be greater than 1 cm in depth above the diaphragm at the point of maximal exhalation AND one of the following.
- The cause of the effusion is unknown and diagnosis of exudative versus transudative processes would change management.
- The patient is symptomatic from the effusion and removing of the fluid would provide relief of those symptoms.

CONTRAINDICATIONS

- Absolute contraindications
  - Depth of effusion less than 1 cm during maximal exhalation
  - Signs of infection over the proposed puncture site
  - Known long-standing loculated effusions
- Relative contraindications
  - International normalized ratio (INR) is above 1.5.
  - Patient is on anticoagulation.
  - Platelets are less than 50,000 or you suspect the patient has clinical evidence of thrombocytopenia.[9]
  - Loculations are identified on ultrasound (these patients are more likely to need surgical exploration to address the loculations).[4]
  - Clinical suspicion is that the effusion is secondary to heart failure (in these cases the physician can opt to give a trial of 2 to 3 days of diuresis and reimage the effusion with ongoing medical management if the effusion improves over that period).
  - Patients with known poor lung reserves
  - Patients with severe lung disease of the contralateral lung (complications would be less tolerated)

PERFORMING THE PROCEDURE

1. **Position the patient for the procedure.** Place the patient in a seated position with a slight forward tilt over a mayo stand or some other rigid object (**Figure 54-1**). Ensure that the patient is comfortable because too much movement will alter anatomic landmarks.

2. **Start with a phased array or curvilinear transducer.** A low-frequency transducer will allow deep penetration and this will help evaluate the nature of the effusion. It is easier to visualize loculations and changes in echogenicity when using this technique (**Figure 54-2**).

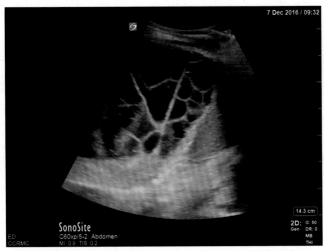

FIGURE 54-2. Loculated pleural effusion.

3. **Assess the effusion with ultrasound.** Start with the probe marker pointing cephalad in the 12th rib space in the midscapular line. Move sequentially upward through each rib space until a white linear diaphragm moving up and down is seen on the screen. Take note of any loculations, hyperechoic fluid (concerning for blood), or any other anatomic obstructions that could jeopardize the safety of the patient during the procedure. Ideal findings are a black fluid against a white, textured lung (see **Figure 54-3**). Take close mental note of the distance between the patient's skin and the effusion, the depth of the effusion, and the angle of the transducer relative to the skin.

4. **Mark the location for thoracentesis catheter insertion.** Once the appropriate intercostal space is identified, make a mark along the superior aspect of that rib space. Remember that the neurovascular bundle generally runs underneath the rib, so the safest point of entry will be above the lower rib (**Figures 54-4 and 54-5**).

5. **Assess for vasculature at insertion site.** Consider applying color flow just prior to performing the procedure, as there may be blood flow underneath the proposed puncture point. This step is best performed with the high-frequency linear array transducer.

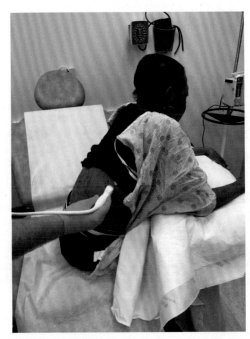

FIGURE 54-1. Correct positioning of patient and probe.

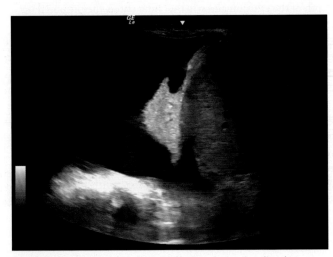

FIGURE 54-3. Diaphragm, pleural effusion, lung visualized.

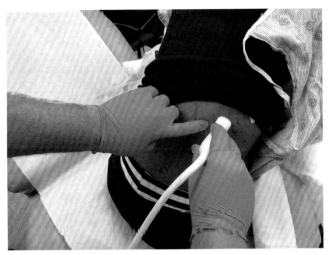

FIGURE 54-4. Curvilinear probe, identifying target.

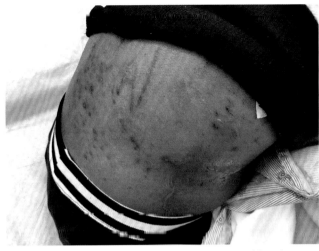

FIGURE 54-6. Indentation in skin made by pen cap marking the target.

Of note, the course of costal arteries is less predictable closer to the patient's spine.[10] Thus, if any approach other than midscapular line is chosen, strongly consider applying color flow to ensure there is no vascularity between you and the pocket of fluid.[6]

6. **Prep and drape the patient.** Use ChloraPrep or Betadine to clean the skin at the site marked for puncture and the surrounding 10 cm of skin. Apply the drape with adhesive side down and fenestration over the location marked for puncture (**Figure 54-6**).

7. **Anesthetize the track between the skin and the pleural space using sterile lidocaine (Figures 54-7 to 54-9).** Inject a wheal of lidocaine to numb the epidermis. Advance the lidocaine needle 5 to 10 mm at a time. Withdraw the needle, then deliver a small amount of lidocaine and repeat until pleural fluid is withdrawn. Retract the needle just far enough and inject a bolus of 2 to 3 mL of lidocaine just superficial to the pleura. Withdraw the needle while injecting a small amount of lidocaine on the way out.

8. **Prepare the collection tubes and equipment.** Lidocaine takes 45 to 90 seconds to take effect. Use this time to prepare collection tubes and the rest of the equipment (**Figure 54-10**). Test the anesthesia of the epidermis before proceeding and introduce more lidocaine if needed.

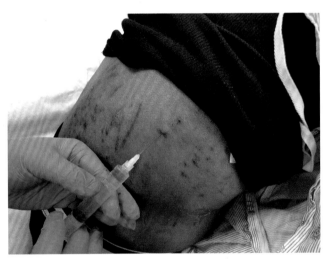

FIGURE 54-7. Wheal occurring with intradermal injection of lidocaine.

9. **Make an incision in the skin to the subcutaneous tissue.** Use an #11 blade and insert three-fourths of the depth of the blade (**Figure 54-11**). This will allow for easy insertion of the paracentesis catheter.

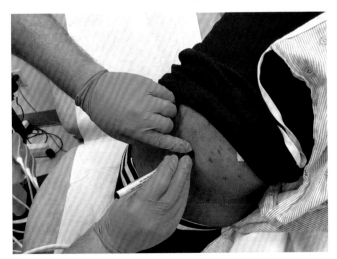

FIGURE 54-5. Marking target using pen cap.

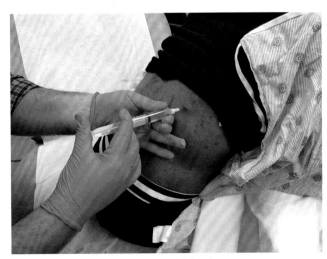

FIGURE 54-8. Subdermal injection of lidocaine.

PART 4

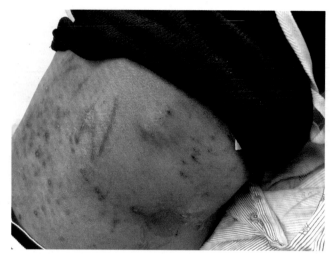

FIGURE 54-9. Target site after local anesthesia.

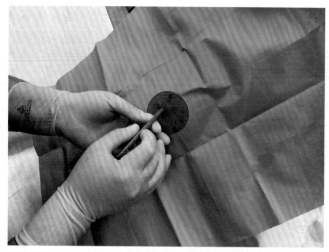

FIGURE 54-11. Create incision with a #11 blade scalpel.

10. **Mark the insertion depth on the thoracentesis catheter.** The insertion depth will be the distance from the epidermis to the pleura that was noted earlier. Many kits have cm markings on the needle itself, which makes this process more straightforward. Otherwise, simply hold the needle at a distance equal to the skin-to-effusion depth noted on ultrasound (**Figure 54-12**).

11. **Insert the thoracentesis catheter into the pleural space.** Be sure a syringe is attached to the guide needle and that the thoracentesis catheter is in place over the guide needle. Insert the thoracentesis catheter through the skin incision at the angle noted earlier during ultrasound. Insert above the lower rib but avoid contact with the periosteum as this can cause significant pain. Apply negative pressure to the syringe. Some resistance will be felt when the catheter tip reaches the pleura. "Pop" through the pleura by applying more pressure with a twisting or "screwing" motion of the catheter tip. Pleural fluid will drain into the syringe when the correct location has been cannulated (**Figure 54-13**).

12. **Advance the thoracentesis catheter over the guide needle.** As soon as pleural fluid is aspirated, stop advancing the guide needle. Maintain the guide needle in a fixed position and gently

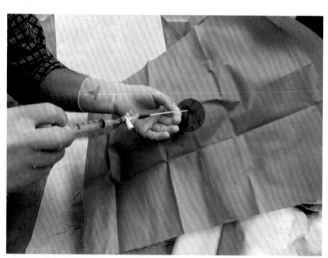

FIGURE 54-12. Insertion of catheter.

advance the thoracentesis catheter over the guide needle. Be sure not to withdraw or advance the guide needle while advancing the catheter. Once the catheter is fully advanced, withdraw the guide needle.

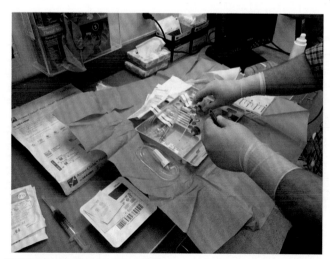

FIGURE 54-10. Thoracentesis kit.

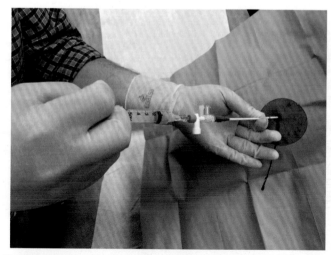

FIGURE 54-13. Apply negative pressure to syringe to allow for pleural fluid to drain into catheter.

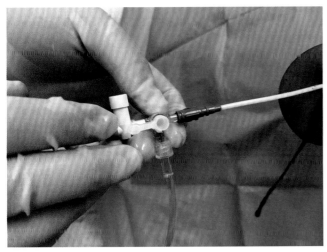

FIGURE 54-14. Three-way stopcock attached to syringe, catheter, and collection tubing.

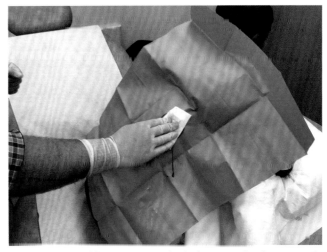

FIGURE 54-16. Hold pressure to obtain hemostasis after removing catheter.

13. **Attach the drainage system to the thoracentesis catheter.** Most kit types utilize a 3-way stopcock to connect the catheter to the syringe and to the collection container (**Figure 54-14**). Typically, an included bag and syringe system or a vacuum bottle is used. If using a vacuum bottle, attach via tubing to the vacuum bottle, as shown in **Figure 54-15**.

14. **Drain the pleural fluid.** The amount of fluid drained depends on whether the procedure is being done for a diagnostic or therapeutic indication. If the procedure is being performed for diagnostic evaluation, then only enough fluid to fill the collection vials is needed. If the procedure is being performed as a therapeutic maneuver, then the maximum volume of up to 1.5 to 2 L should be removed. No more than this amount should be removed because of the risk of reexpansion pulmonary edema.[11]

15. **Carefully withdraw the thoracentesis catheter.** Quickly pull out the catheter in one smooth movement. Ask the patient to bear down or cough to increase intrathoracic pressure and avoid air entering the pleural space (**Figure 54-16**).

16. **Cover with a Band-Aid or a plastic adhesive dressing** (**Figure 54-17**).

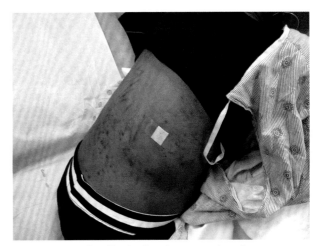

FIGURE 54-17. Apply adhesive bandage over site of entry.

17. **Lay the patient down in a reclined position and reassure him or her that the procedure is complete** (**Figure 54-18**).

18. **Strongly consider performing pneumothorax evaluation as described in Chapter 14 and documenting this as part of the procedure** (**Figure 54-19**).

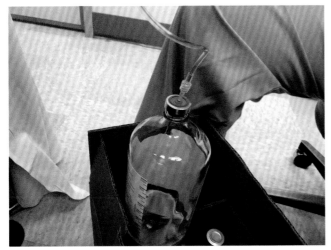

FIGURE 54-15. Example of vacuum bottle collection container.

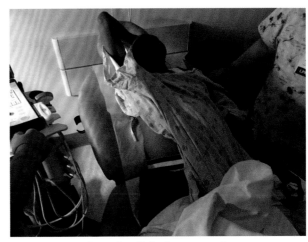

FIGURE 54-18. Have the patient lie back postprocedure.

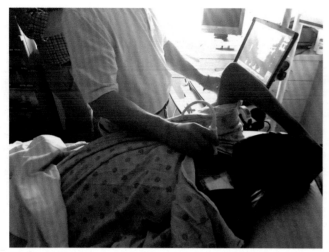

FIGURE 54-19. Checking for pneumothorax postprocedure.

POSTPROCEDURE INSTRUCTIONS

- Patient should lie in place for a brief 5-minute postprocedure period for monitoring.
- Patient should leave the Band-Aid or occlusive plastic dressing in place for 1 day.
- Patient should not participate in strenuous activity for 24 to 48 hours following the procedure.
- Patient should seek medical attention for hemoptysis, new chest pain, new dyspnea, new fever, pain not improved with over-the-counter (OTC) pain medications, signs of infection at the puncture site, or signs of fluid drainage from the puncture site.

COMPLICATIONS

- Pain during and after the procedure (common)
- Light-headedness
- Bleeding externally through puncture site that stops with simple pressure and simple bandage (common)
- Infection at the puncture site
- Pneumothorax (uncommon, below 2% with POCUS use in some studies)[11]—reason for ambulance transfer to an Emergency Department
- Hemothorax (rare)—reason for ambulance transfer to an Emergency Department
- Puncture of liver or spleen (rare)—reason for ambulance transfer to an Emergency Department
- Reexpansion pulmonary edema (rare)—reason for ambulance transfer to an Emergency Department

PATIENT MANAGEMENT

For information on diagnosing a pleural effusion, please refer to Chapter 35. Once pleural effusion is diagnosed, thoracentesis should be performed for the indications described earlier. The procedure can be both diagnostic and therapeutic. Fluid analysis can provide crucial insight to the cause of the pleural effusion. Routine testing of the fluid should include gross inspection, protein and lactate dehydrogenase (LDH) levels (fluid and serum), Gram stain,

TABLE 54-2	Examples of Transudates and Exudates	
Transudate	**Exudate**
Left ventricular failure	Malignant effusion
Cirrhosis	Parapneumonic effusions
Hypoalbuminemia	Tuberculosis
Peritoneal dialysis	Pulmonary embolism
Hypothyroid	Rheumatoid arthritis
Nephrotic syndrome	Benign asbestos effusion
Mitral stenosis	Pancreatitis
Constrictive pericarditis	Post–myocardial infarction
Meigs syndrome	Post–coronary artery bypass graft
Urinothorax	Fungal infections

Derived from Hooper C, Lee YCG, Maskell N. Investigation of a unilateral pleural effusion in adults: British Thoracic Society pleural disease guideline 2010. *Thorax*. 2010;65(suppl 2):ii4-ii17. doi:10.1136/thx.2010.136978.

culture, acid-fast bacillus (AFB, mycobacterial if indicated), and cytology. Upon gross inspection, evaluate for any blood suggesting a hemothorax, bile staining suggesting biliary fistula, milky white coloration suggesting a chylothorax, or food particles that could be present in esophageal rupture.

An important step in fluid analysis is to determine whether the fluid is transudative or exudative using Light's criteria. Fluid must meet one of the following criteria to be considered exudative:

- Pleural fluid protein divided by serum protein is greater than 0.5.
- Pleural fluid LDH divided by serum LDH is greater than 0.6.
- Pleural fluid LDH is more than two-thirds the upper limit of laboratory normal value for serum LDH.

The causes of both transudative and exudative effusions are listed in Table 54-2. Cytology can be helpful to diagnose malignant pleural effusion as atypical or malignant cells can be identified and evaluated with immunohistochemistry to differentiate further the type of malignancy. Additional tests that can be helpful include a pleural fluid hematocrit that if more than 50% of serum hematocrit suggests hemothorax, amylase that can support the pancreatitis as a cause, triglycerides and cholesterol to differentiate between chylothorax and pseudochylothorax. Finally, a pleural fluid pH (obtained in blood gas analyzer) can be obtained, and a pH less than 7.2 suggests a complicated pleural infection and likely need for a chest tube (**Figure 54-20**).[12] See ⏺ **Videos 54.1 to 54.8** for additional content.

PEARLS AND PITFALLS

Pearls

- The site of puncture can be marked by applying pressure to the skin with a pen cap. This will provide a mark on the skin that will not be cleaned away in the skin prep process like ink from a marking pen could be.
- The epidermis and pleura are the two most sensitive locations encountered during thoracentesis. Providing adequate anesthesia to both locations can allow for a nearly pain-free procedure.
- Malignant effusions are often bloody and can be quite unsettling to see. If you are concerned that you might be withdrawing

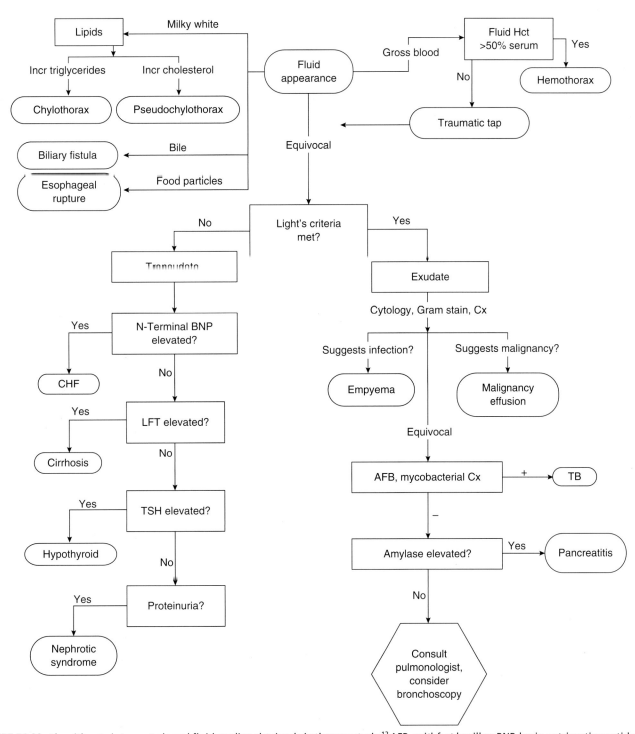

FIGURE 54-20. Algorithm to interpret pleural fluid studies obtained via thoracentesis.[12] AFB, acid-fast bacillus; BNP, brain natriuretic peptide; CHF, congestive heart failure; Cx, culture; Hct, hematocrit; Incr, increased; LFT, liver function test; TB, tuberculosis; TSH, thyroid-stimulating hormone.

Pearls and Pitfalls, Continued

blood and not a bloody effusion, place some of the fluid in a clean receptacle and allow it to sit for 1 minute. If there is no coagulation, then it is unlikely to be frank blood and more likely to be a bloody effusion.

- A patient will usually begin coughing when the pleural effusion is completely drained because of irritation of the pleura. This is an indication to remove the catheter.

Pitfalls

- If the catheter is not advanced after pleural fluid is initially withdrawn, then fluid will not easily be aspirated once the guide needle is removed. Thus, it is important to advance the catheter and not just simply pull out the guide needle.
- It is critical to be sure that a patient does not move in the time between marking the puncture site with ultrasound and performing the puncture.

PART 4

BILLING

CPT Code	Description	Professional Fee	Facility Fee
32554	Thoracentesis, needle or catheter, aspiration of the pleural space; without imaging guidance	$216.59	$92.98
32555	Thoracentesis, needle or catheter, aspiration of the pleural space; with imaging guidance	$306.69	$116.05

CPT codes and average national reimbursement for Medicare in 2016. Payment data are from https://www.cms.gov/apps/physician-fee-schedule/search/search-criteria.aspx. See Chapter 2 for details on ultrasound billing.

References

1. Havelock T, Teoh R, Laws D, Gleeson F. Pleural procedures and thoracic ultrasound: British Thoracic Society pleural disease guideline 2010. *Thorax.* 2010;65(suppl 2):i61-i76. doi:10.1136/thx.2010.137026.

2. Xirouchaki N, Magkanas E, Vaporidi K, et al. Lung ultrasound in critically ill patients: comparison with bedside chest radiography. *Intensive Care Med.* 2011;37(9):1488-1493. doi:10.1007/s00134-011-2317-y.

3. Hibbert RM, Atwell TD, Lekah A, et al. Safety of ultrasound-guided thoracentesis in patients with abnormal preprocedural coagulation parameters. *Chest.* 2013;144(2):456-463. doi:10.1378/chest.12-2374.

4. Sikora K, Perera P, Mailhot T, Mandavia D. Ultrasound for the detection of pleural effusions and guidance of the thoracentesis procedure. *ISRN Emerg Med.* 2012;2012:1-10. doi:10.5402/2012/676524.

5. Gordon CE. Pneumothorax following thoracentesis. *Arch Intern Med.* 2010;170(4):332. doi:10.1001/archinternmed.2009.548.

6. Kanai M, Sekiguchi H. Avoiding vessel laceration in thoracentesis. *Chest.* 2015;147(1). doi:10.1378/chest.14-0814

7. Barnes TW, Morgenthaler TI, Olson EJ, Hesley GK, Decker PA, Ryu JH. Sonographically guided thoracentesis and rate of pneumothorax. *J Clin Ultrasound.* 2005;22(9):442-446.

8. Diacon AH, Brutsche MH, Solèr M. Accuracy of pleural puncture sites: prospective comparison of clinical examination with ultrasound. *Chest.* 2003;123(2):436-441.

9. Mohammed I, Maddirala S, Khan A. Evaluating clinical predictors of complications of thoracentesis. *Chest.* 2010;138(4). doi:10.1378/chest.10230.

10. Yoneyama H, Arahata M, Temaru R, Ishizaka S, Minami S. Evaluation of the risk of intercostal artery laceration during thoracentesis in elderly patients by using 3D-CT angiography. *Intern Med.* 2010;49(4):289-292. doi:10.2169/internalmedicine.49.2618.

11. Ault MJ, Rosen BT, Scher J, Feinglass J, Barsuk JH. Thoracentesis outcomes: a 12-year experience. *Thorax.* 2014;70(2):127-132. doi:10.1136/thoraxjnl-2014-206114.

12. Hooper C, Lee YCG, Maskell N. Investigation of a unilateral pleural effusion in adults: British Thoracic Society pleural disease guideline 2010. *Thorax.* 2010;65(suppl 2):ii4-ii17. doi:10.1136/thx.2010.136978.

Paracentesis

Andrew D. Vaughan, MD and Daniel P. Dewey, MD

LITERATURE REVIEW

Ascites is defined as fluid within the peritoneal cavity. Portal hypertension, from a variety of processes, is the most common etiology,[1] Those pathologic processes include cirrhosis, alcoholic hepatitis, hepatic veno-occlusive disease, heart failure, pericarditis, and nephrogenic ascites. It can also be caused by hypoalbuminemic states such as nephrotic syndrome, peritoneal disease of malignant or infectious origin, or pancreatic disease among many other etiologies. Patients typically present with symptoms of abdominal distention, early satiety, dyspnea, and symptoms related to the underlying etiology of the ascites.[2]

Ultrasound has been used for procedural guidance for more than 30 years. The availability, accessibility, increasing quality, and improved affordability of machines have helped make point-of-care ultrasound for procedural guidance in paracentesis the standard of care over the traditional landmark-based technique.

Paracentesis has well-known risks including bowel or other organ/structure perforation, bleeding from inadvertent vascular puncture, introducing infectious agents and pain. Using either static or dynamic ultrasound guidance during the procedure can minimize those risks.[3] Ultrasound guidance also improves the diagnostic accuracy of ascites prior to performing paracentesis (see Chapter 21). A distended abdomen on examination is obviously not always ascites.[4] Confirming ascites, using ultrasound, is straightforward and can rule out other causes for abdominal distention, such as increasing obesity, bowel obstruction, bladder outlet obstruction, solid masses, pregnancy, and large cysts.

Studies show ultrasound improves the safety, accuracy, and first-attempt success while reducing overall cost.[5] Postprocedure bleeding, using the landmark-based technique, is more common given the great variability in vascular anatomy among individuals. In particular, perforating the inferior epigastric vessels is a hazard using the traditional technique. Point-of-care ultrasound using color flow can identify any blood vessels in the intended path of the paracentesis needle. This improves safety of the procedure and avoids bleeding complications and hospitalization, therefore reducing the overall cost.[6] First-pass success rate likely reduces infection rates given the additive effects of skin puncture for introducing an infection when multiple punctures are required. In addition, the patient will experience greater comfort during the procedure if ultrasound guidance helps prevent multiple skin punctures and puncture of abdominal organs or bowel.[3]

TABLE 55-1 Recommendations for Use of Point-of-Care Ultrasound in Clinical Practice

Recommendation	Rating	References
The use of ultrasound guidance for abdominal paracentesis is associated with lower costs and better patient outcomes including: fewer adverse reactions, fewer complications, more successful first attempts	A	3, 5, 6

A = consistent, good-quality patient-oriented evidence; B = inconsistent or limited-quality patient-oriented evidence; C = consensus, disease-oriented evidence, usual practice, expert opinion, or case series. For information about the SORT evidence rating system, go to http://www.aafp.org/afpsort.

EQUIPMENT

- **Preparation**
  - Chlorhexidine or iodine, topical antiseptic
  - Sterile and nonsterile gloves
  - Sterile drape
- **Local anesthesia**
  - Lidocaine 1% without epinephrine
  - 25- to 27-gauge needle at least 1.5 in.
  - Sterile syringe, 3 to 5 mL
- **Paracentesis**
  - Sterile 4 × 4 gauze pads
  - Paracentesis needle/catheter (needs could vary depending on therapeutic vs. diagnosis paracentesis; 16 to 18 gauge should be used for therapeutic paracentesis while 22 gauge or smaller could be appropriate for diagnostic paracentesis when only small volumes are needed). Length of preferred needle/catheter will also vary based on location of abdomen and habitus of patient.
  - 11-blade (typically only required if using large-bore needle/catheter for therapeutic procedure)
  - Adhesive bandage
- **Collection**
  - Large-volume vacuum bottles (as much a 8 L of fluid can be removed during a therapeutic paracentesis)
  - Appropriate specimen tubes for culture, Gram stain, cell count, etc. (not always necessary if only performing a therapeutic paracentesis)

INDICATIONS

- New-onset ascites
- Hospitalization of a patient with ascites[7]
- Management of tense ascites or ascites that is not responsive to diuretics
- Patient with ascites and new or worsening symptoms of
  - Fever
  - Abdominal pain
  - Abdominal tenderness
  - Leukocytosis
  - Worsening renal function
  - Acidosis

CONTRAINDICATIONS

- Absolute
  - None
- Relative
  - Severe bleeding disorder (disseminated intravascular coagulation [DIC], primary fibrinolysis)
  - Most patients undergoing paracentesis have an abnormal prothrombin time, but the actual risk of bleeding is very low (<1%).[8,9]
  - Exceptions are clinically apparent DIC or hyper-fibrinolysis. Correct bleeding disorder (if able) prior to procedure. Ultrasound can be used to help prevent large-vessel injury.
  - Ileus or bowel obstruction
  - Increases risk of bowel perforation. If paracentesis is performed, ultrasound can help to ensure that the bowel is not perforated.
- Previous abdominal surgery
  - Often evidenced by abdominal surgical scars. This increases the risk of peritoneal bowel adhesions and increases the chance of bowel perforation. If paracentesis is performed, ultrasound can help to ensure that the bowel is not perforated.

PERFORMING THE PROCEDURE

1. Have the patient empty their bladder or place a Foley catheter prior to the procedure in order to decompress the bladder. The patient should be in the supine position or semi-upright position (**Figure 55-1**). This allows gas-filled bowel to float in the ascetic

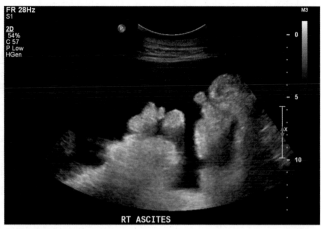

FIGURE 55-2. Ascitic fluid as seen with curvilinear low-frequency transducer.

fluid anteriorly toward the midline, creating pockets of ascites typically most prominent in the right and left lower quadrant.

2. Using the curvilinear ultrasound transducer or another low-frequency/high-penetration transducer, scan all four quadrants of the abdomen to confirm the presence of ascites and rule out other pathologic processes. Ascites is a hypoechoic collection most prominent in the right lower quadrant and left lower quadrant with the patient in the supine position (**Figure 55-2**). Identify the area of most prominent fluid collection with least amount of bowel, blood vessels, or other anatomy obscuring access to the fluid. The left lower quadrant is preferred over the right because of the fact that the cecum is relatively fixed in the abdomen compared to the more mobile sigmoid colon. If the right lower quadrant has a deeper collection of ascites than the left lower quadrant, then the practitioner may prefer to access the right lower quadrant. Once the location is chosen, place the patient partially in the lateral decubitus position (partially rolled to the left or right) to the side with largest most accessible pocket of fluid.

3. Use color flow to identify any blood vessels to be avoided prior to the procedure (**Figure 55-3**). With large-volume ascites, static ultrasound guidance can be used rather than dynamic. With the patient in the partial lateral decubitus position, using a skin marker, mark the site of preferred skin puncture. For more on the diagnosis of ascites, see Chapter 21.

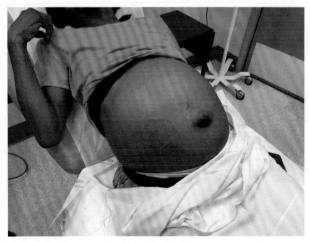

FIGURE 55-1. Proper patient positioning for paracentesis.

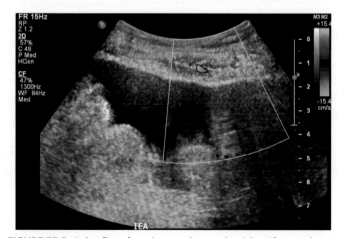

FIGURE 55-3. Color flow function can be used to identify vasculature in the overlying abdominal wall in order to avoid vascular injury.

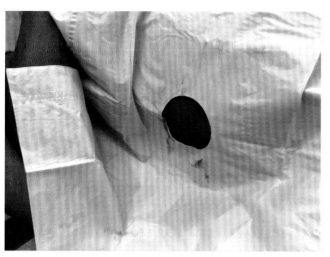

FIGURE 55-4. Prep the patient with antiseptic (iodine or chlorhexidine) and drape the patient in sterile fashion.

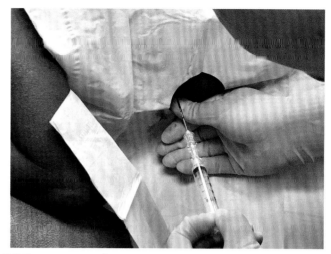

FIGURE 55-6. Insert the paracentesis catheter at the predetermined ultrasound-guided insertion site.

4. Prepare, drape, and cleanse the skin using universal sterile precautions. Keep the patient in the partial lateral decubitus position. Perform the procedure in usual fashion using either static or dynamic ultrasound guidance as explained in the next section (**Figure 55-4**).

5. Using a local anesthetic, infiltrate the skin down to the peritoneum.

6. If performing the procedure for therapeutic indications, a large gauge paracentesis catheter (16-18 gauge) is preferred; therefore, it is recommend to make a small incision using an 11-blade at the site of entry (**Figure 55-5**).

7. Direct the paracentesis angiocatheter needle perpendicular to the skin toward the previously identified ascetic pocket. Use Z-track technique to avoid postprocedure ascites leak in large-volume ascites. To perform the Z-track technique, the skin is gently pulled down while advancing the needle while aspirating. This skin traction causes self-sealing when the needle or catheter is finally removed. While drawing back on the connected syringe, advance the angiocatheter needle forward until fluid enters the syringe, then push the catheter forward into the peritoneal space and withdraw the needle (**Figure 55-6**).

8. Use the fluid collected in the syringe for any diagnostic studies desired. Attach the hub of the catheter to a 3-way stopcock or straight to the tubing and vacuum bottles or containers and vacuum system used by your facility for therapeutic removal of the ascites (**Figure 55-7**).

9. After flow stops, turn off the vacuum suction and perform an ultrasound on the patient once more to confirm the desired amount of fluid has been removed.

10. If fluid still remains, turn off suction and use ultrasound to reposition the tip of the catheter by turning the catheter 180°, repositioning the patient, and/or partially withdrawing the catheter before attempting to suction more fluid. Once the procedure is complete, turn off the suction and remove the catheter.

11. Observe for any persistent leakage and place a bandage on the puncture site.

Note: the above procedure may also be performed using the standard Seldinger technique using a guidewire for placement of the angiocatheter.

PART 4

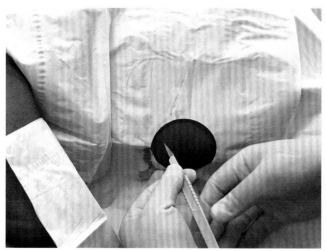

FIGURE 55-5. For therapeutic paracentesis, use an 11-blade to create incision for large-bore catheter placement.

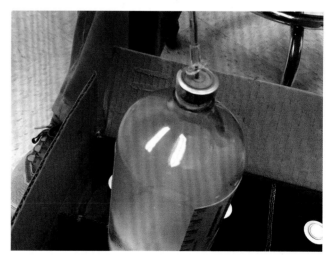

FIGURE 55-7. Vacuum canisters can be used to collect the ascitic fluid. In therapeutic paracentesis, as much as 8 L can be obtained.

Static Versus Dynamic Ultrasound for Procedural Guidance

Some practitioners prefer dynamic ultrasound guidance for all paracenteses, but most use the static technique for large-volume paracentesis and the dynamic approach for small volume, diagnostic paracentesis. Using the static technique, the desired pocket is identified using ultrasound; the site marked using a sterile marking pen and the ultrasound is not used during the procedure itself. Using dynamic guidance, after the initial scan (Step 2), the probe is covered in a sterile probe cover sheath and sterile gel is used. Set up the ultrasound machine on the opposite side of the patient from where the procedure is being performed. This allows direct visualization of the dynamic imaging without turning around to look at the ultrasound machine. Then the path of the angiocatheter needle is followed and guided into the peritoneum. This can be performed using either the in-plane or out-of-plane approach. The in-plane approach is preferred but this is dependent upon practitioner skill and experience. During this part of the procedure either the curvilinear or the linear probe can be used. It is often easier to see the needle using the linear probe while utilizing the in-plane approach. The procedure is then performed as described in Step 3 once the catheter is introduced into the fluid via ultrasound guidance.

POSTPROCEDURE INSTRUCTIONS

Following the procedure it is reasonable to observe the patient in the clinic or department for 30 to 60 minutes, monitoring vital signs and symptoms. If the patient is discharged home, they should undergo an ambulation trial to ensure no dizziness, hypotension, or concerns for falls and home safety, as fluid shifts can occur with large-volume paracentesis. Depending on the indication for the paracentesis and the findings, the patient may require admission to the hospital pending the diagnostic studies, such as is often the case for spontaneous bacterial peritonitis (SBP). For therapeutic paracentesis or outpatient diagnostic purposes, arrangements for follow-up should be made with the patient. The patient should be educated on the potential complications and return precautions such as hypotension, vomiting, fever, increasing abdominal distention/pain, bleeding, or significant leaking fluid. The patient should also be counseled on basic wound care and bandage changes. If a large-volume (greater than 5 L) paracentesis is performed, albumin can be administered in an attempt to prevent hypovolemia. Typically, this is administered when 6 to 8 g/L of fluid is removed.[10-12]

COMPLICATIONS

- Ascitic fluid leak
  - Most common complication, occurring in ~5% of cases[13]
  - Decrease risk by removing as much volume as possible during the procedure to decrease intra-abdominal pressure.
  - Z-track can also be used in order to decrease the risk of leakage.
- Hypovolemia
- More common with large-volume paracentesis, postprocedural albumin infusion may be considered.[10]
- Bleeding
  - Rare but can be severe and fatal[8,13]
  - Ultrasound improves safety by visualizing the underlying vasculature.

- Infection
  - Rare unless associated with bowel perforation
  - Bowel perforation by the paracentesis needle occurs in approximately 6/1000 taps.[14]

PATIENT MANAGEMENT

If the paracentesis is performed in order to diagnose the etiology of ascites, a complete cell count, albumin level, Gram stain, lactate dehydrogenase (LDH), and culture are typically obtained. A serum albumin level drawn at approximately the same time as the procedure is necessary in order to calculate a serum–ascites album gradient (SAAG). A SAAG ≥ 1.1 indicates that the ascitic fluid is present because of portal hypertension in the settings of cirrhosis, heart failure, or renal failure.

The number of polymorphonuclear neutrophils (PMNs) can be calculated by dividing the number of white blood cells detected (or total nucleated cell count) by the percentage of PMNs in the differential. If the number of PMNs is greater than 250 cells/mm^3, concern for bacterial infection (primary or secondary) should be high.

A SAAG ≥ 1.1 with concomitant PMN ≥ 250 should indicate high concern for SBP and is typically associated with cirrhosis.

If there is also concern for pancreatic ascites or for mycobacterium infection, an amylase level and mycobacterium testing should also be performed, respectively. See **Figure 55-8**.

PEARLS AND PITFALLS

Pearls

- Position the patient in the supine or semi-upright position to identify the largest most accessible pocket of fluid using the curvilinear probe.
- Always have the patient empty their bladder or place a Foley catheter to avoid puncturing a full bladder inadvertently.
- Always use color flow to identify and avoid any blood vessels during the procedure.
- Place the patient in the partial lateral decubitus position during the procedure.
- For small volume paracentesis, use in-plane dynamic ultrasound guidance.

Pitfalls

- Small blood vessels in the near field are easily missed when focusing on the deeper structures. Scan the near field using color flow for any blood vessels in order to avoid laceration of vessels. Be particularly wary of the inferior epigastric vessels.
- Urine in the bladder and simple ovarian cysts can be the same echogenicity as ascites. Use caution and diligence when identifying the ascites.
- During large-volume paracentesis, persistent leak is common if incomplete removal of fluid and/or Z-track method is not used. Postprocedural ultrasonography can be utilized to determine how much ascites remains.
- Losing visualization of the needle tip during dynamic ultrasound guidance in small volume paracentesis can lead to inadvertent organ puncture. Practice and become proficient at needle visualization during dynamic ultrasound-guided procedures.
- Do not allow the patient to move after marking the site and before the procedure as the fluid will shift and alter the anatomy.

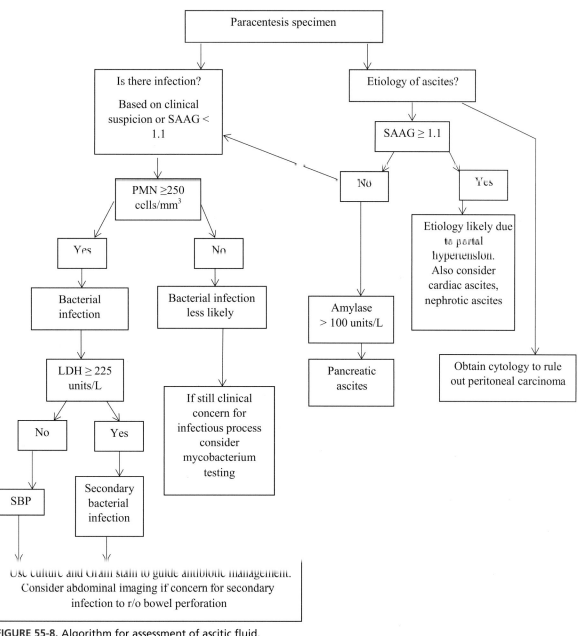

FIGURE 55-8. Algorithm for assessment of ascitic fluid.

BILLING

CPT Code	Description	Facility Fee	Nonfacility Fee
49082	Abdominal paracentesis	$76.40	$204.34
49083	Abdominal paracentesis with imaging	$112.08	$304.17

CPT codes and average national reimbursement for Medicare in 2016. Payment data are from https://www.cms.gov/apps/physician-fee-schedule/search/search-criteria.aspx. See Chapter 2 for details on ultrasound billing.

References

1. Runyon BA. Management of adult patients with ascites caused by cirrhosis. *Hepatology.* 1998;27:264.
2. Runyon BA. Care of patients with ascites. *N Engl J Med.* 1994;330:337.
3. Nazeer SR, Dewbre H, Miller AH. Ultrasound-assisted paracentesis performed by emergency physicians vs the traditional technique. *Am J Emerg Med.* 2005;23(3):363-367.
4. Cattau EL Jr, Benjamin SB, Knuff TE, Castell DO. The accuracy of the physical examination in the diagnosis of suspected ascites. *JAMA.* 1982;247:1164.
5. Patel PA, Ernst FR, Gunnarsson CL. Evaluation of hospital complications and costs associated with using ultrasound guidance during abdominal paracentesis procedures. *J Med Econ.* 2012;15(1):1-7.
6. Mercaldi CJ, Lanes SF. Ultrasound guidance decreases complications and improves the cost of care among patients undergoing thoracentesis and paracentesis. *Chest.* 2013;143(2):532-538.
7. Orman ES, Hayashi PH, Bataller R, Barritt AS IV. Paracentesis is associated with reduced mortality in patients hospitalized with cirrhosis and ascites. *Clin Gastroenterol Hepatol.* 2014;12:496.

8. Runyon BA. Paracentesis of ascitic fluid. A safe procedure. *Arch Intern Med.* 1986;146:2259.

9. McVay PA, Toy PT. Lack of increased bleeding after paracentesis and thoracentesis in patients with mild coagulation abnormalities. *Transfusion.* 1991;31:164.

10. Peltekian KM, Wong F, Liu PP, et al. Cardiovascular, renal, and neurohumoral responses to single large-volume paracentesis in patients with cirrhosis and diuretic-resistant ascites. *Am J Gastroenterol.* 1997;92:394.

11. Runyon BA; AASLD. Introduction to the revised American Association for the Study of Liver Diseases Practice Guideline management of adult patients with ascites due to cirrhosis 2012. *Hepatology.* 2013;57:1651.

12. Runyon BA. Patient selection is important in studying the impact of large-volume paracentesis on intravascular volume. *Am J Gastroenterol.* 1997;92:371.

13. De Gottardi A, Thévenot T, Spahr L, et al. Risk of complications after abdominal paracentesis in cirrhotic patients: a prospective study. *Clin Gastroenterol Hepatol.* 2009;7:906.

14. Runyon BA, Hoefs JC, Canawati HN. Polymicrobial bacterascites. A unique entity in the spectrum of infected ascitic fluid. *Arch Intern Med.* 1986;146:2173.

Lumbar Puncture

Naushad Amin, MD, FAAFP

LITERATURE REVIEW

Heinrich Quincke, a German physician, first described the basic lumbar puncture (LP), a procedure where a needle is introduced into the lumbar spine to obtain cerebrospinal fluid (CSF) using conventional surface landmarking technique.[1] Since the early days, the procedure has been performed for both diagnostic and therapeutic purposes. It has been used for diagnosing diseases such as meningitis, multiple sclerosis, Guillain–Barré syndrome, and normal-pressure hydrocephalus. It is a useful technique but is not without risk. Complications include unsuccessful or multiple attempts, resulting in tissue damage and pain, discomfort, headache, and CSF leak.[2] This is true especially in patients with known lumbar arthropathies, history of spinal surgeries, or obesity. A BMI greater than 35 can decrease the success rate dramatically to a low of 58%.[3] Alternate to the traditional landmarking technique, fluoroscopic-guided LP may not be readily available or practical due to time constraints.

The use of ultrasonography in LP was first described in 1971 in Russian anesthesia literature.[4] A recent meta-analysis showed that, in adults, ultrasound-guided LP is successful 90% of the time, whereas landmark-based methods are only successful 81.4%. Also, significant reduction in procedure time, attempts, traumatic outcome, and pain has been observed.[5-7] In the pediatric population, ultrasound-guided LP has shown superior outcomes in identification of optimal body position and landmarks, confirmation of intrathecal injection, and avoiding radiation.[8,9]

EQUIPMENT

You will need the following equipment. These are included in a typical LP tray.
- Sterile gloves and dressing
- Antiseptic solution and applicator
- Sterile drape
- A 23- to 25-gauge needle

TABLE 56-1	Recommendations for Use of Point-of-Care Ultrasound in Clinical Practice

Recommendation	Rating	References
When readily available, ultrasound-guided lumbar puncture should be performed to significantly minimize the risk of traumatic procedure and number of insertion attempts.	A	5, 6

A = consistent, good-quality patient-oriented evidence; B = inconsistent or limited-quality patient-oriented evidence; C = consensus, disease-oriented evidence, usual practice, expert opinion, or case series. For information about the SORT evidence rating system, go to http://www.aafp.org/afpsort.

- A 3 to 5 mL syringe
- Local anesthetic, usually 1% lidocaine without epinephrine
- Spinal needle, preferable an atraumatic one
- Manometer and three-way stopcock
- Four numbered CSF collection tubes
- Sterile ultrasound probe sleeve (optional)

INDICATIONS

- Diagnosis or evaluation of suspected:
- Meningitis, encephalitis, or brain abscess
- Central nervous system (CNS) malignancy
- Vasculitis involving the CNS
- Guillain–Barré syndrome and demyelinating diseases
- Normal-pressure hydrocephalus

Therapy
- Pseudotumor cerebri
- Administering intrathecal antibiotics, antifungals, and chemotherapy
- Spinal anesthesia

CONTRAINDICATIONS

Although there is no contraindication to using ultrasonography while performing LP, one must be aware of the contraindications of LP in general. These may include

- Increase in intracranial pressure
- Intracranial mass or abscess
- Bleeding diathesis including coagulopathies or thrombocytopenia. Avoid LP if platelet counts are less than 50 000/μL or international normalized ratio (INR) less than 1.5. In patients on warfarin therapy, LP should be postponed till INR is lesser than 1.5. In case LP is considered urgent, reversal agents may be considered. For patients on new oral anticoagulants (NOACs), LP should be postponed for 24 hours in normal renal function and 60 hours in case of impaired renal function. For patients on warfarin or NOAC, and considered high risk for thromboembolism, consider bridging therapy.
- Skin or soft tissue infection at the LP site

PERFORMING THE SCAN

1. **Place your patient in either a lateral recumbent position with the hips flexed or sitting position with the lower back arched** (**Figure 56-1**). Studies have shown better success rates with patients in a sitting position. This position widens the intraosseous space

413

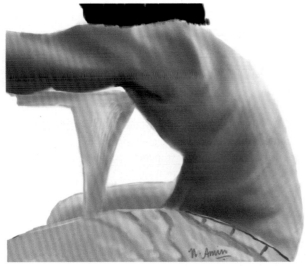

FIGURE 56-1. Illustration showing the proper sitting position of a patient for a lumbar puncture.

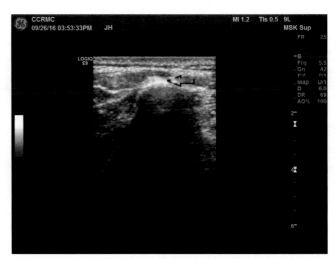

FIGURE 56-3. The spinous process appears as a hyperechoic crescent (hollow arrow) with a trailing anechoic shadow.

in both pediatric and adult patients, providing easier access to the subarachnoid space; however, patient comfort must be taken into consideration.[10] Ensure that the patient is comfortable and willing to maintain the desired position.

2. **Select the probe.** In most cases, the use of a high-frequency linear probe (5-10 MHz) is appropriate. However, in an obese patient, a curvilinear probe may be used.

3. **Place the probe in a transverse position in the midline over the L4 spinous process.** The probe marker points to the patients' left. This position usually corresponds to a line drawn between the two iliac crests (**Figure 56-2**).

4. **Find the spinous processes that appear as hyperechoic crescents with trailing anechoic shadow (Figure 56-3).** Adjust the probe placement to bring the spinous process into the center of the screen.

5. **Mark the skin at the center of the probe using a permanent surgery pen.** Repeat this process to mark the spinous process

cephalad. Draw a straight line parallel to the spinal column connecting the markings (**Figure 56-4**).

6. **Locate the interspinous space.** Turn the probe longitudinal, with the probe marker facing cephalad. Identify the interspinous space between two adjacent spinous processes as shown in **Figure 56-5**.

7. **Adjust the probe placement to bring the interspinous space in the center of the image on the screen.** Mark the skin at the center of either side of the probe as shown in **Figure 56-6**.

8. **Draw a straight line perpendicular to the spine, connecting the markings just made.** The intersection of the resultant cross will be the usual site of entry for the LP needle at the L3-L4 interspace as shown in **Figure 56-7**.

9. **Identify the ligamentum flavum and its distance to the skin using the probe in the longitudinal axis.** This provides a useful estimation of the distance the needle tip has to travel to access the CSF (**Figure 56-8**).

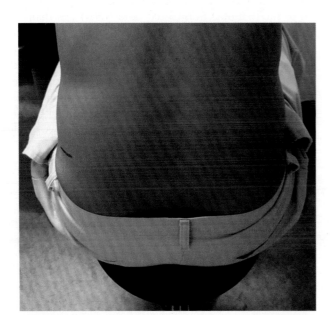

FIGURE 56-2. Bilateral iliac crest with Tuffier's line markings.

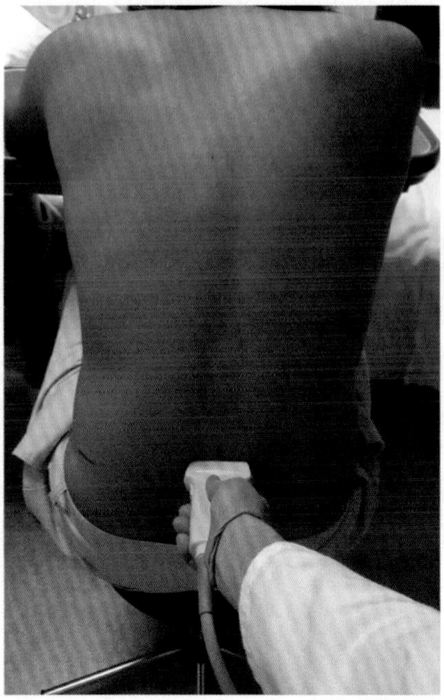

FIGURE 56-4. Probe positioning and marking of the spinous process.

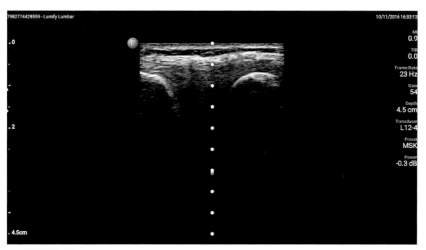

FIGURE 56-5. Dotted line demonstrates the centering of the intervertebral space.

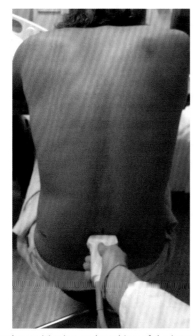

FIGURE 56-6. Probe positioning and marking of the interspinous process.

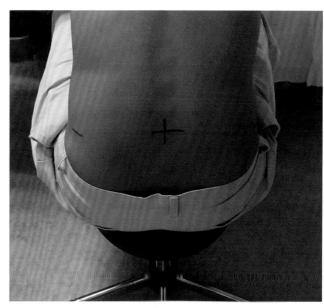

FIGURE 56-7. The cross center reflects the point of entry of the lumbar puncture needle.

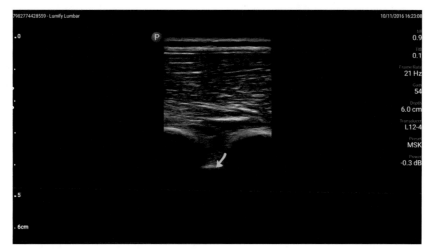

FIGURE 56-8. Arrow pointing to the ligamentum flavum. This image is obtained off-axis from the center line of the spinous processes and is centered above the lamina. Note the depth of the bony prominences (lamina) and the overlying paraspinal muscles. This plane is useful for measuring depth to the ligamentum flavum, but should not be used to mark the midline for needle entry.

PART 4

PERFORMING THE PROCEDURE

Once the landmarks have been identified using the ultrasound, the LP is performed in the usual sterile manner without the need for holding the probe at this time. However, having the ultrasound probe with a sterile sleeve covering the probe and the wire may be useful if reverification of landmarks is needed.

1. First set up the CSF collecting vials in numeric order in the given slots on the sterile spinal trap. Attach the three-way stopcock to the barometer column assembly provided in the LP kit.

2. Clean and sterilize the skin around the landmark site with the provided aseptic solution.

3. Use a 23- to 25-gauge needle to inject local anesthetic, first creating a subcutaneous wheel, then injecting into the deeper tissues (**Figure 56-9**).

4. Use an atraumatic needle to prevent headaches, although this technique makes it harder to obtain opening pressures.[11,12]

5. If a traditional cutting needle is used, ensure the bevel of the needle is parallel to the vertebral column when passing through the ligamentum flavum to avoid CSF leak.

6. Insert and advance the LP needle using the locations marked via ultrasound. Usually, the needle will point toward the umbilicus. The needle depth should correspond to the distance obtained from the skin to the ligamentum flavum using the ultrasound in the earlier steps.

7. When the needle tip is 1 cm away from the targeted depth, stop and pull the stylus out and check for the CSF flow. If no CSF flows, place the stylus back completely and advance the needle 1 to 2 mm and again check for CSF flow. Repeat this process until CSF flow is obtained. It is not unusual to feel a pop as the needle traverses the dura.

8. Attach the manometry assembly to the hub of the spinal needle and measure the opening pressure. Advise the patient to relax if possible, to obtain an accurate measure. Although a sitting position increases the overall success rate of performing LP, an accurate opening pressure recording requires patients to be in a lateral decubitus position (**Figure 56-10**).[13]

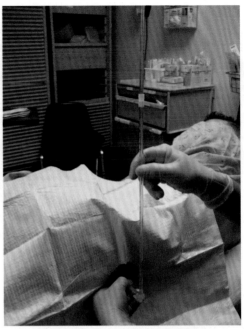

FIGURE 56-10. A manometry catheter is used to measure the cerebrospinal fluid pressure with the patient in the decubitus position. From Mayeaux EJ Jr. The Essential Guide to Primary Care Procedures. 2nd ed. Philadelphia, PA: Wolters Kluwer; 2015. Copyright Dr. EJ Mayeaux, Jr., used with permission.

9. Now turn the stopcock and collect 1 to 2 mL of the fluid in the given tubes, one by one, recapping and placing the tubes back onto the trap in a numbered fashion (**Figure 56-11**).

10. Finally replace the stylus completely prior to removing the spinal needle. Place a small sterile dressing at the puncture site.

POSTPROCEDURE INSTRUCTIONS

Despite common practice, prophylactic bed rest after LP has not shown additional benefits.[14-16] Patients can shower in 24 hours and let the adhesive bandage fall off on its own. Encourage extra fluid

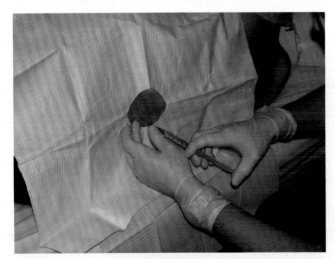

FIGURE 56-9. Local anesthesia is administered prior to the procedure. From Mayeaux EJ Jr. The Essential Guide to Primary Care Procedures. 2nd ed. Philadelphia, PA: Wolters Kluwer; 2015. Copyright Dr. EJ Mayeaux, Jr., used with permission.

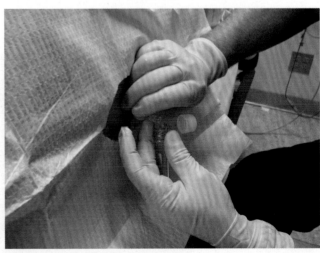

FIGURE 56-11. Spinal fluid is collected in vials. From Mayeaux EJ Jr. The Essential Guide to Primary Care Procedures. 2nd ed. Philadelphia, PA: Wolters Kluwer; 2015. Copyright Dr. EJ Mayeaux, Jr., used with permission.

intake. Monitor for excessive discomfort, vomiting, headache, neck stiffness, puncture site pain, redness, swelling, and discharge. Also, request patients to check for fever and notify their provider or seek immediate medical attention if one develops.

COMPLICATIONS

Although ultrasound-guided LP minimizes the related complications, the practitioners should be aware of the following complications:

- Postprocedure headaches
- Infections including puncture site cellulitis, epidural or spinal abscesses, discitis, and meningitis
- Puncture site hematoma
- Epidural, subdural, or subarachnoid hemorrhage, although rare, may occur. It is best to correct coagulopathies, thrombocytopenia, and other bleeding diathesis before performing LP if possible.
- Cerebral herniation is a serious complication that may occur post-LP. This can be avoided by ensuring normal intracranial pressure.

PATIENT MANAGEMENT

LP has both diagnostic and therapeutic indications in the management of neurologic illness. Sonogram-guided LP has shown to decrease the number of attempts, pain, traumatic outcomes and increase success rate, especially in patients with increased BMI. A generalized approach for use of LP in cases of suspected bacterial meningitis is described below.

Once the need of the LP is identified, blood and CSF cultures should be obtained prior to starting antibiotics if possible (**Figure 56-12**). However, because of the risk of cerebral herniation, any patient with risk factors or signs of increased intracranial pressure will need to have a CT scan done prior to LP. These include history of immunocompromise, history of CNS disease, new-onset seizure, papilledema, altered consciousness, or focal neurologic deficit. These patients should have blood cultures drawn immediately and then have IV antibiotics started while awaiting CT scan. Additionally, if any other delay in performance of diagnostic LP occurs, blood cultures should be drawn and initiation of IV antibiotic therapy should not be delayed. Intravenous steroids should also be considered

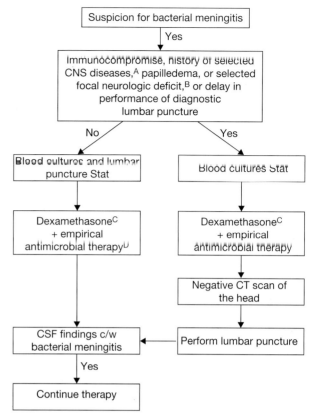

FIGURE 56-12. Treatment algorithm for suspected bacterial meningitis. "Stat" indicates that the intervention should be done emergently. c/w, consistent with. A, Includes those associated with cerebrospinal fluid (CSF) shunts, hydrocephalus, or trauma; those occurring after neurosurgery; or various space-occupying lesions. B, Palsy of cranial nerve VI or VII is not an indication to delay lumbar puncture. C, See text for recommendations for use of adjunctive dexamethasone in bacterial meningitis. D, Dexamethasone and antimicrobial therapy should be administered immediately after CSF is obtained. From Tunkel AR, Hartman BJ, Kaplan SL, et al. Practice guidelines for the management of bacterial meningitis. *Clin Infect Dis.* 2004;39(9):1267-1284. Reproduced by permission of Infectious Diseases Society of America.

in suspected bacterial meningitis with unknown source, or if the source is known and is *Streptococcus pneumoniae*. Table 56-2 shows typical CSF findings in different conditions.

PART 4

TABLE 56-2 | Typical CSF Findings in Different Conditions

Characteristic	Normal	Bacterial	Viral	Pseudotumor Cerebri	Subarachnoid Hemorrhage
Opening Pressure (cm H_2O)	5-20	>20	Normal to increased	Increased	Increased
White blood cell count (cells/mm³)	<5	>500	6-1000	Normal	Bloody sample
Differential	–	Polymorphonuclear predominance	Lymphocyte predominance	–	–
Glucose (mg/dL)	50-100 (or 60%-70% of blood glucose)	Decreased (0-40)	Normal	Normal	Normal
Protein (mg/dL)	15-45	>50	Normal to increased	Normal to decreased	Increased
Other	–	Lactate > 3.5 mmol/L, cerebrospinal fluid blood glucose ratio ≤ 0.4	–	–	Xanthochromia

From Mayeaux EJ Jr. The Essential Guide to Primary Care Procedures. 2nd ed. Philadelphia, PA: Wolters Kluwer; 2015. Copyright Dr. EJ Mayeaux, Jr., used with permission.

PEARLS AND PITFALLS

Pearls

- Plug the ultrasound to the wall supply to avoid running out of battery in the middle of the procedure.
- When obtaining the landmarks, note the angle of the probe, as this will be a useful guide while inserting the needle.
- While performing the LP, keep the sterile ultrasound probe ready, as the patient may move leading to shift in the landmarks. If this happens, the landmarks can be remarked.
- The distance from the skin to ligamentum flavum is crucial in choosing the size of the spinal needle. This is especially true while performing the LP in an obese patient.

Pitfalls

- Even though ultrasound-guided LP is superior to traditional landmarking, in patients with a BMI greater than 30, it may still be difficult. If body habitus delays LP, be sure to collect blood cultures and administer IV antibiotics if bacterial meningitis is suspected.
- Be careful not to mistake the lamina for the spinous processes when marking the midline. The spinous process will be seen just below the skin with no overlying muscle. The lamina will be seen deep with overlying paraspinal muscles. See Figure 56-8.

BILLING

CPT Code	Description	Global Payment	Professional Component	Technical Component
76942	Ultrasound-guided needle placement including lumbar puncture	$61.58	$34.01	$27.57
62270	Diagnostic lumbar spinal puncture	$162.55	–	–
62260	Therapeutic spinal puncture for drainage of cerebrospinal fluid	$206.23	–	–

CPT codes and average national reimbursement for Medicare in 2016. Payment data are from https://www.cms.gov/apps/physician-fee-schedule/search/search-criteria.aspx. See Chapter 2 for details on ultrasound billing.

References

1. Pearce JM. Walter Essex Wynter, Quincke, and lumbar puncture. *J Neurol Neurosurg Psychiatry*. 1994;57(2):179.
2. Armon C, Evans RW. Addendum to assessment: prevention of post LP headaches: report of the Therapeutics and Technology Assessment Subcommittee of the American Academy of Neurology. *Neurology*. 2005;65(4):510-512.
3. Edwards C, Leira EC, Gonzalez-Alegre P. Residency training: a failed LP is more about obesity than lack of ability. *Neurology*. 2015;84(10). doi:10.1212/wnl.0000000000001335.
4. Bogin IN, Stulin ID. Application of the method of 2-dimensional echospondylography for determining landmarks in LPs. *Zh Nevropatol Psikhiatr Im S Korsakova*. 1971;71(12):1810-1811.
5. Shaikh F, Brzezinski J, Alexander S, et al. Ultrasound imaging for LPs and epidural catheterisations: systematic review and meta-analysis. *BMJ*. 2013; 346:f1600.
6. Mofidi M, Mohammadi M, Saidi H, et al. Ultrasound guided lumber puncture in emergency department: time saving and less complication. *J Res Med Sci*. 2013;18(4):303-307.
7. Gottlieb M, Holladay D, Peksa GD. Ultrasound-assisted lumbar punctures: a systematic review and meta-analysis. *Acad Emerg Med*. 2019;26(1):85-96.
8. Wang PI, Wang AC, Naidu JO, et al. Sonographically guided LP in pediatric patients. *J Ultrasound Med*. 2013;32(12):2191-2197.
9. Neal JT, Kaplan SL, Woodford AL, et al. The effect of bedside ultrasonographic skin marking on infant LP success: a randomized controlled trial. *Ann Emerg Med*. 2017;69(5):610.e.1-619.e1.
10. Sandoval M, Shestak W, Sturmann K, Hsu C. Optimal patient position for LP, measured by ultrasonography. *Emerg Radiol*. 2004;10(4):179-181.
11. Lavi R, Yarnitsky D, Yernitzky D, et al. Standard vs atraumatic Whitacre needle for diagnostic LP: a randomized trial. *Neurology*. 2006;67(8):1492-1494.
12. Lavi R, Rowe JM, Avivi I. Traumatic vs. atraumatic 22 G needle for therapeutic and diagnostic LP in the hematologic patient: a prospective clinical trial. *Haematologica*. 2007;92(7):1007, 1008.
13. Doherty CM, Forbes RB. Diagnostic LP. *Ulster Med J*. 2014;83(2):93-102.
14. Spriggs DA, Burn DJ, French J, et al. Is bed rest useful after diagnostic LP? *Postgrad Med J*. 1992;68(801):581-583.
15. Ebinger F, Kosel C, Pietz J, Rating D. Strict bed rest following LP in children and adolescents is of no benefit. *Neurology*. 2004;62(6):1003-1005.
16. Teece S, Crawford I. Towards evidence based emergency medicine: best BETs from the Manchester Royal Infirmary. Bed rest after LP. *Emerg Med J*. 2002;19(5):432-433.

Peripheral Intravenous Catheter Placement

David Schrift, MD, RDMS, Carol Choe, MD, and Darien B. Davda, MD

LITERATURE REVIEW

Ultrasound use is considered standard of care when placing central venous catheters (CVCs). Recently, the role of ultrasound has expanded to include the placement of peripheral intravenous (PIV) catheters in patients who have poorly accessible veins. Ultrasound-guided peripheral intravenous (USGPIV) line placement has been shown to improve success rates, reduce complications, and increase patient satisfaction in individuals with difficult intravenous (IV) access. Venous access is required to obtain blood samples and to provide parenteral medications, IV fluids, and electrolytes.[1,2] As our population ages and demographics change, an increasing proportion of patients will have difficult IV access. Congestive heart failure, chronic kidney disease, and obesity are all factors that increase the difficulty in obtaining venous access and are expected to increase in the future.[3-5] For example, the prevalence of obesity (body mass index ≥ 30 kg/m^2) has risen from 13% to 38% between 1962 and 2014, according to the Centers for Disease Control.[6] Witting et al found providers had difficulty starting an IV catheter in 39% of emergency medicine patients, and 22% of patients required three or more punctures to establish an IV catheter.[7] These trends are a major reason why interest in the use of USGPIV lines has accelerated in recent years. Multiple studies have demonstrated that USGPIV line placement in patients with difficult IV access results in higher success rates, faster completion times, increased patient satisfaction, and better outcomes than landmark-based methods[8-14].

A common rescue method when providers have been unable to establish PIV access is to insert a CVC or peripherally inserted central catheter (PICC). This approach is suboptimal and results in unnecessary harm and cost to the patient. Millions of CVCs are placed in the United States annually, and their associated complications can increase the morbidity of the patient. Major complications include central line–associated bloodstream infections (CLABSIs), deep venous thromboses (DVTs), and pneumothoraces. A meta-analysis conducted by Marik et al found that CLABSIs occurred in 1.4% of 16 370 CVCs.[15] More recently, Parienti et al published a multicenter, randomized controlled trial that evaluated how the rate of CLABSIs varied by CVC insertion site and found a similar 1% CLABSI rate.[16] A single CLABSI may increase hospital length of stay by up to 20 days and increase health care costs by $56 000.[17] Additionally, DVTs and pneumothoraces have been shown to occur in up to 33% and 4.9% of CVC placements, respectively, although this depends on the insertion site and the use of ultrasound.[18,19] The potential morbidity from a catheter-related DVT includes the development of a pulmonary embolism, prolonged hospital stay,

need for thrombolytic medications, prolonged anticoagulation, and, rarely, superior vena cava syndrome. A pneumothorax can be life-threatening if not identified in a timely fashion; however, the most common morbidity is associated with the cost and discomfort of a tube thoracostomy that is often required to resolve the pneumothorax. Furthermore, many of these complications are no longer reimbursed by major insurance programs.[20]

USGPIV lines can drastically reduce the need for CVCs and PICCs, thereby reducing all of the aforementioned complications. Shokoohi et al found an 80% reduction in CVCs in emergency medicine patients after the implementation of a USGPIV program.[21] Au et al found a similar 85% reduction in the need for CVCs after failed PIV patients were referred for a USGPIV line instead of the usual CVC.[22] In patients who already have CVCs or PICCs, the use of USGPIV lines has been shown to hasten their removal.[11]

An oft-cited concern is that the placement of a USGPIV line is a difficult procedure to learn. Physicians, nurses, and other health care personnel have become proficient in USGPIV line placement with minimal training. Emergency department technicians can become proficient following a 2-hour training session, with 1 hour dedicated to didactics and the second hour used for hands-on instruction.[23] Nurses become competent with USGPIV lines after a 45-minute presentation followed by practice on an inanimate model.[9] Although training programs vary, a 3-hour program consisting of a combination of didactics, simulation, and hands-on training is recommended.

We recommend the routine use of USGPIV placement in patients with difficult IV access. This will improve cannulation success rates, reduce time to completion, increase patient satisfaction, and reduce complications, especially those associated with CVC or PICC placement. Additionally, this skill can be easily learned after just a few hours of training (Table 57-1).

Equipment

- Tourniquet
- Extension tubing
- Saline syringe
- Standard ultrasound gel
- Sterile lubrication gel
- Gauze
- Alcohol swab
- Chlorhexidine prep
- Adhesive tape
- An 18 to 20-gauge catheter for IV access. Catheters shorter than 1.75 in length should be avoided as they are not suitable for the deeper veins targeted with the USGPIV method (Figures 57-1 and 57-2).

TABLE 57-1 Studies Assessing USGPIV Line Success Rates Compared with Landmark-Based Technique

Study	Patient Population	USGPIV Line Success Rate	Landmark-Based Success Rate
Keyes et al[8]	101 difficult IV access patients in the ED	91%	0%*
Brannam et al[9]	321 difficult IV access patients in the ED	87%	0%*
Costantino et al[10]	60 difficult IV access patients in the ED	97%	33%
Gregg et al[11]	77 difficult IV access patients in the intensive care unit	99%	0%*
Ismailoğlu et al[12]	60 difficult IV access patients in the ED	70%	30%
Costantino et al[13]	60 difficult IV access patients in the ED	89%	55%
Bauman et al[14]	75 difficult IV access patients in the ED	81%	44%

*Studies in which USGPIV lines were placed in patients who failed the landmark-based technique previously.

Abbreviations: ED, emergency department; IV, intravenous; USGPIV, ultrasound-guided peripheral intravenous.

TABLE 57-2 Recommendations for Use of Point-of-Care Ultrasound in Clinical Practice

Recommendation	Rating	References
An ultrasound-guided peripheral intravenous catheter is recommended for difficult access patients.	A	8-14

A = consistent, good-quality patient-oriented evidence; B = inconsistent or limited-quality patient-oriented evidence; C = consensus, disease-oriented evidence, usual practice, expert opinion, or case series. For information about the SORT evidence rating system, go to http://www.aafp.org/afpsort.

Indications

- No easily visualized vessels on physical examination
- BMI $\geq$ 30 kg/m² or $\leq$18.5 kg/m²
- History of IV drug use
- History of difficult PIV access
- Landmark-based PIV failure

Contraindications

- There are no absolute contraindications to USGPIV access.

PERFORMING THE PROCEDURE

1. **Position the patient.** The patient can be either sitting or recumbent. The clinician can be sitting or standing during the procedure; however, the patient's arm should be positioned to maximize the ultrasonographer's comfort and exposure to the target vessel. This typically results in raising the bed/chair to an appropriate position, and abducting and externally rotating the patient's arm. Sometimes, the patient may not be able to support the arm in this position. In this case, his or her arm may need to be taped to a nearby structure to maintain optimal positioning. The clinician should arrange the ultrasound machine, so that the provider's view of the ultrasound screen is in line with the view of the procedure. Having to look over one's shoulder while performing the procedure will increase the difficulty of the procedure and minimize success (**Figures 57-3**).

2. **Selecting a vein.** Turn on the ultrasound machine and apply standard gel to the linear transducer. Set the probe to the venous or vascular preset and make sure the indicator on the ultrasound screen correlates with the indicator on the transducer. The easiest way to do this is by touching the surface on the far left side of the ultrasound probe (the side with the indicator). If the orientation is correct, there will be a shifting of the gel noted on the far left side of the ultrasound screen. The depth of the ultrasound machine should not be set below 2 cm because any vein identified below this depth cannot be cannulated with routine USGPIV placement. Place a tourniquet around the patient's arm near the axilla to engorge the extremity's blood vessels, thereby making them easier to locate. Scan the patient's arm in an out-of-plane (short axis) orientation to survey the venous

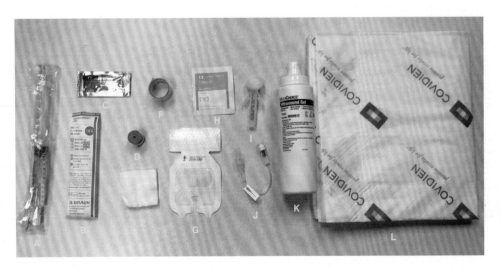

FIGURE 57-1. All items required for the procedure. A, saline prep; B, catheters; C, sterile gel packet; D, tourniquet; E, gauze; F, tape; G, Tegaderm; H, alcohol wipes; I, chlorhexidine prep; J, extension tubing; K, ultrasound gel; L, mattress pad.

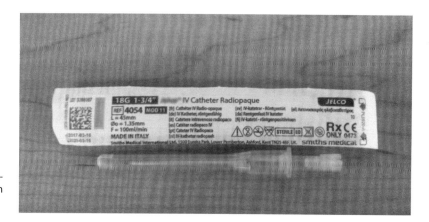

FIGURE 57-2. Close-up of an 18-gauge catheter for peripheral IV access. Note the catheter length is ≥1.75 in, which is the recommended length for this procedure.

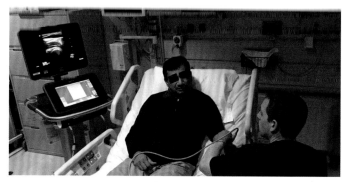

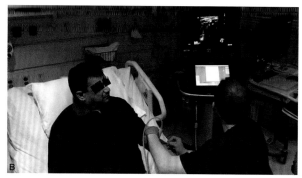

FIGURE 57-3. A, The ultrasound is correctly positioned because the procedural area and ultrasound screen are in the same line of sight. B, The ultrasound is incorrectly positioned because the provider must divert his attention away from the procedural area to view the ultrasound screen.

anatomy. The ideal vein will be superficial, straight, large, and sufficiently far from vital structures, such as arteries and nerves. Any vein that meets these criteria is suitable for cannulation. In patients with difficult IV access, these characteristics are most likely to be found within the basilic or cephalic veins because they are relatively superficial, do not have adjacent arteries or nerves, and are usually preserved in obese patients and IV drug users.[21] When 1.88 inch catheters are used, success rates fall dramatically when veins are less than 0.4 cm in diameter or more than 1.5 cm in depth. Alternatives should be sought prior to any cannulation attempt of veins with these characteristics.[25] When an appropriate vessel has been found, compress it gently with the transducer. A vessel that does not collapse with gentle pressure is either an artery or a thrombosed vein and should be avoided (**Figures 57-4 and 57-5**).

3. **Catheter insertion.** Once an appropriate vein has been selected, wipe off any remaining ultrasound gel from the skin and disinfect the site with an alcohol swab or chlorhexidine prep. Next, disinfect the ultrasound transducer in accordance with the manufacturer's instructions. Using disinfectant solutions that are not approved by the manufacturer may damage the probe and void the warranty. Apply sterile lubrication gel to the skin. Some providers prefer to place a Tegaderm over the transducer to keep it clean, but this is an optional step. Remove the selected catheter from its package and familiarize yourself with it. Hold the ultrasound probe in your nondominant hand to allow easy IV insertion with the dominant hand. The insertion aspect

of the procedure is typically performed in an out-of-plane or in-plane orientation.

a. **Out-of-plane (short-axis) method.** The transducer orientation should be perpendicular relative to the target vessel, so that the vein appears as a dark circle on the ultrasound screen. Prior to the start of the procedure, confirm that your orientation is correct. Ensure that the vein is centered on the screen before inserting the needle directly under the middle of the ultrasound probe. This step is critical because it ensures that the catheter and the vein will be appropriately aligned and will allow the catheter tip to be seen immediately upon skin entry. The catheter tip will be seen as a bright white dot. Once the catheter tip is identified, move the transducer proximally until the catheter tip just disappears. Advance the catheter until the catheter tip is again visualized. Repeat this process until the catheter tip cannulates the vein. This meticulous attention to catheter tip location is important because both the catheter tip and the shaft of the catheter will appear identical as a bright dot on the ultrasound screen. A common mistake is to erroneously identify the bright dot of the catheter shaft as the catheter tip and continuing to advance the catheter. This results in the actual catheter tip being unwittingly advanced into deeper or surrounding structures, leading to complications (**Figure 57-6** and ▶ **Video 57-1**).

b. **In-plane (long-axis) method.** Place the ultrasound probe parallel to the target vessel. When seen onscreen, the vein's anterior and posterior walls are two white lines running

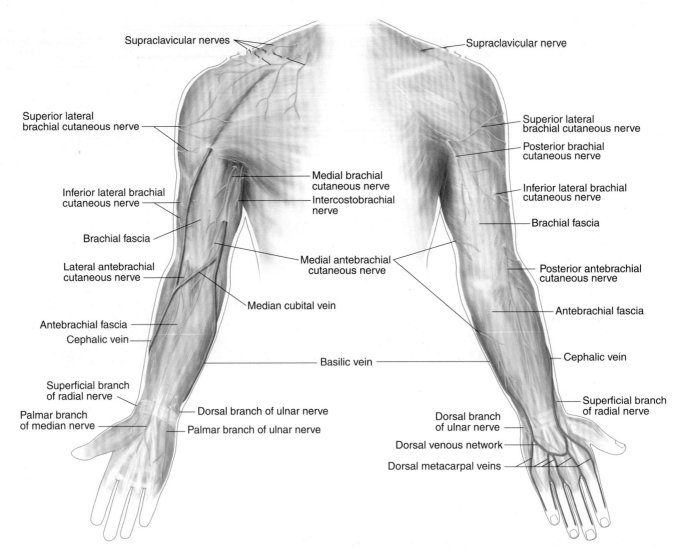

A. Anterior view

B. Posterior view

FIGURE 57-4. Diagram of venous anatomy of the arm. Reprinted with permission from Gest TR. *Lippincott Atlas of Anatomy*. 2nd ed. Philadelphia, PA: Wolters Kluwer; 2020:36. Plate 2-2.

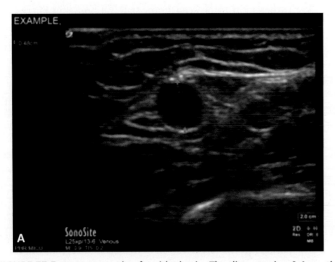
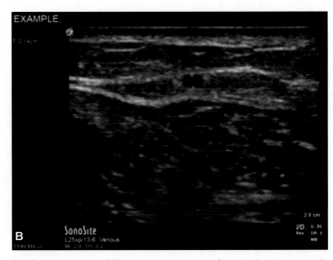

FIGURE 57-5. A, An example of an ideal vein. The diameter is >0.4 cm, the depth is <1.5 cm and there are not any nearby arteries or nerves. B, An example of a suboptimal vein. The diameter is <0.4 cm and the probability for a successful cannulation would be low. C, An example of a suboptimal vein. Although the diameter and depth are ideal, note the adjacent location of the median nerve (N) to the brachial vein (BV). Also, the brachial artery (BA) lies immediately posterior to the BV. The risk of an injury to one of these surrounding structures is high, and this vein should be avoided.

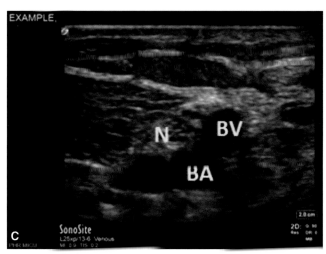

FIGURE 57-5. (continued)

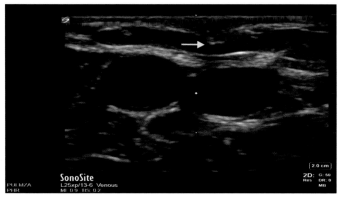

FIGURE 57-6. Catheter inserted through skin in out-of-plane orientation. The yellow arrow indicates the needle tip.

across the screen with a black center. Prior to the start of the procedure, confirm that your orientation is correct. Ensure that the vein is centered on the screen. This is achieved when the walls of the vein appear crisp and the lumen appears very black. As the transducer is moved from side to side to visualize the lateral aspects of the vein, the walls will become hazy and the lumen will appear smaller and less black. Now, insert the catheter directly under the center of the foot of the probe, so that the catheter travels under and parallel to the transducer. Once the catheter has punctured the skin, identify the catheter tip on the screen before advancing toward the vein. An advantage of the in-plane technique is that the entire catheter from tip to shaft can be seen throughout the procedure. When the catheter tip and vein are seen together on the screen, the catheter can be advanced until it enters the vein. Make sure the catheter tip is constantly visualized throughout the procedure until it cannulates the vein to optimize success and avoid complications. If at any time the catheter tip and vein are not seen together on the screen, they are no longer in the same plane and the catheter should not be advanced. To correct this, move the transducer laterally (left or right) until the middle of the vein is identified. Then, move the

transducer laterally to find the catheter tip. Once both have been located, you will be able to determine which direction the catheter should be guided to complete the procedure. As you redirect the catheter toward the vein, both should start to appear together on the ultrasound screen. If not, their locations will need to be reassessed as previously described and a larger redirection may be required. If too large a redirection is required, the procedure is unlikely to be successful and the catheter should be withdrawn and reinserted (🎥 **Video 57-2**).

c. **For both methods.** Be careful not to apply too much pressure with the transducer during the procedure as this will compress the vein, increasing the difficulty for successful cannulation and increasing the likelihood of a posterior wall puncture.

The angle of catheter entry should vary on the basis of the depth of the vessel. Superficial veins demand more shallow entry angles to avoid inadvertently advancing the catheter through the posterior wall. Deeper veins require steeper angles to avoid losing the entire length of the catheter in the subcutaneous tissue prior to reaching the vein. If enough catheter is not intraluminal, the life span of the USGPIV line will be shortened.[26] In general, catheters inserted at shallower angles will be more visible on ultrasound. If vessel depth allows, a ≤30° angle is recommended. Immediately prior to vessel entry, the catheter tip will often compress the anterior wall of the vein toward the posterior wall. If care is not taken, the catheter may pass completely through the anterior and posterior walls without actually entering the vein's lumen. This can be avoided by taking a more superficial angle at the point of vessel entry, or giving the catheter a small "stab" to pop through the anterior wall and into the vessel lumen. Once in the vein, a flash of blood will be seen in the catheter's chamber. Drop the angle of the catheter slightly and advance the catheter so that the catheter tip is directly in the middle of the vessel lumen. This will ensure that enough of the catheter is intraluminal so it does not inadvertently become dislodged when setting down the ultrasound probe. Place the transducer down and advance the catheter over the needle and into the vein.

4. **Completing the procedure.** Withdraw the needle and activate the safety mechanism to avoid a needle stick injury. Expect blood to flow out of the catheter once the needle is withdrawn. Attach the extension tubing to the catheter. Pre-flush the extension tubing before attaching it to the catheter in order to avoid introducing air into the vein. Draw back to ensure good blood return, although this may not occur even with a successfully placed IV line. After the catheter has been successfully placed, release the tourniquet before flushing the catheter to avoid rupturing the vein. The catheter should flush easily; there should be no signs of infiltration and the patient should not experience pain with flushing. If any of these do not occur, reassess the catheter to ensure that it is intraluminal. This can be done by reimaging the target vessel to ensure that the catheter is intraluminal. The catheter can be flushed under ultrasound guidance and, if intraluminal, one will see the flush remain within the vessel (🎥 **Video 57-3**). If it is extraluminal, the

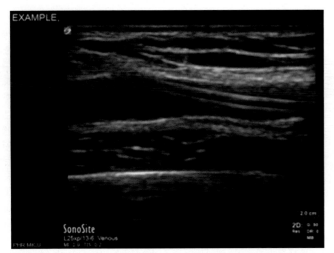

FIGURE 57-7. In-plane view of the catheter cannula inside a vessel. Upon completing the procedure, image the catheter in-plane to verify if the catheter is intraluminal.

flush will be seen expanding the surrounding soft tissue areas (▶ **Video 57-4**). Once IV access is confirmed, wipe any residual blood, gel, or debris from the IV site using an alcohol swab and gauze. Secure the catheter with adhesive tape, a Tegaderm, or both (**Figure 57-7**).

Complications

- A common cause of USGPIV failure occurs when the catheter is advanced over the needle the moment venous blood return is noted. If the catheter is barely within the vein, any subtle movement of the operator's hand may cause dislodgement.
- If an artery is accidentally cannulated instead of a vein, the patient can develop a local hematoma.
- Complications from traditional PIV placement can also occur with USGPIV placement (superficial skin infections, phlebitis, infiltration).[27] One study found no significant difference between infection rates in USGPIV lines versus traditional placement.[28]

PATIENT MANAGEMENT

Recognition of risk factors for difficult vascular access can allow a clinician to prepare ahead for those needing an ultrasound-guided intervention. Identifying a proper vessel with characteristics, as discussed previously, will increase cannulation success rates. By utilizing USGPIV lines appropriate care is not delayed in patients with difficult vascular characteristics, and more invasive, unnecessary procedures that could harm patients are avoided. **Figure 57-8** illustrates how to manage patients who require PIV access.

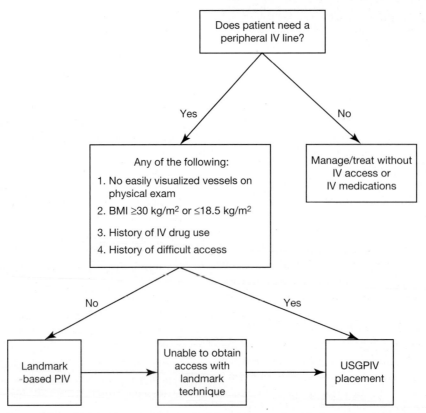

FIGURE 57-8 Algorithm for determining which patients are best suited for ultrasound-guided peripheral IVs (USGPIVs).

PEARLS AND PITFALLS

Pearls

- Reduce the angle of the catheter once venous return is obtained and continue to guide it using ultrasound into the center of the vein. This will ensure that the catheter tip and catheter are within the vein and the catheter is much less likely to become accidentally dislodged.
- Always apply a tourniquet before searching for veins to avoid missing suitable candidates, as the tourniquet increases the diameter of veins by 30% to 40%.[29]
- Once the appropriate vein has been identified, disinfect the overlying skin and use sterile ultrasound gel instead of the standard gel for the rest of the procedure. This has been shown to reduce unnecessary infection.[30] Individual sterile lubrication packets serve this function well (**Figure 57-9**).
- To avoid inadvertently placing a catheter into an artery or thrombosed vein, use the transducer to apply mild compression to the vessel. The compressible vessel is a suitable vein. Arteries require greater pressure to collapse and will appear pulsatile. Thrombosed veins are noncompressible and do not pulsate.
- For best results, choose a vein that is larger than 0.4 cm in diameter and less than 1.5 cm in depth.
- When 1.88 in catheters are used, success rates fall dramatically when veins are greater than 0.4 cm in diameter or less than 1.5 cm in depth.
- Use the ultrasound in an in-plane orientation to find where the catheter tip terminates. Retract slightly if it abuts the posterior wall or a valve.

- If it has penetrated the posterior wall, attach a saline-filled syringe to the catheter and, with gentle aspiration, withdraw the catheter tip until venous blood is obtained. Then gently flush while cautiously advancing the catheter.

Pitfalls

- A very common pitfall with USGPIV placement is failure to identify the needle tip, which can lead to failed USGPIV placement or injury to surrounding structures. The in-plane orientation provides the best catheter tip visualization; convert to this alignment after an initial out-of-plane attempt.
- Be cautious not to apply too much pressure during the procedure. Beginners are often nervous and may compress the vein by applying too much force on the transducer. This will increase the difficulty of the procedure.

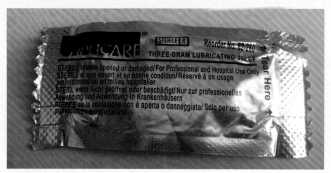

FIGURE 57-9. Sterile lubrication gel for ultrasound imaging.

BILLING

CPT Code	Description	Global Payment	Professional Component	Technical Component
76937	Placement of peripheral IV using ultrasound guidance	$29.71	$14.46	$15.24

CPT codes and average national reimbursement for Medicare in 2016. Payment data are from https://www.cms.gov/apps/physician-fee-schedule/search/search-criteria.aspx. See Chapter 2 for details on ultrasound billing.

References

1. Potter PA, Perry AG. *Fundamentals of Nursing: Concepts, Process, and Practice.* 4th ed. St Louis, MO: Mosby; 1997.
2. Crowley M, Brim C, Proehl J, et al. Emergency nursing resource: difficult intravenous access. *J Emerg Nurs.* 2012;38(4):335-343.
3. Finkelstein EA, Khavjou OA, Thompson H, et al. Obesity and severe obesity forecasts through 2030. *Am J Prev Med.* 2012;42(6):563-570.
4. Heidenreich PA, Albert NM, Allen LA, et al. Forecasting the impact of heart failure in the United States: a policy statement from the American Heart Association. *Circ Heart Fail.* 2013;6(3):606-619.
5. Hoerger TJ, Simpson SA, Yarnoff BO, et al. The future burden of CKD in the United States: a simulation model for the CDC CKD initiative. *Am J Kidney Dis.* 2015;65(3):403-411
6. Fryar CD, Carroll MD, Ogden CL, Division of Health and Nutrition Examination Surveys. Prevalence of overweight, obesity and extreme obesity among adults aged 20 and over: United States, 1960-1962 through 2013-2014. Hyattsville, MD: National Center for Health Statistics; 2016. https://www.cdc.gov/nchs/data/hestat/obesity_adult_13_14/obesity_adult_13_14.pdf.
7. Witting, MD. IV access difficulty: incidence and delays in an urban emergency department. *J Emerg Med.* 2012;42(4):483-487.
8. Keyes LE, Frazee BW, Snoey ER, Simon BC, Christy D. Ultrasound-guided brachial and basilic vein cannulation in emergency department patients with difficult intravenous access. *Ann Emerg Med.* 1999;34(6):711-714.
9. Brannam L, Blaivas M, Lyon M, Flake M. Emergency nurses' utilization of ultrasound guidance for placement of peripheral intravenous lines in difficult-access patients. *Acad Emerg Med.* 2004;11(5):583-584.
10. Costantino TG, Parikh AK, Satz WA, Fojtik JP. Ultrasonography-guided peripheral intravenous access versus traditional approaches in patients with difficult intravenous access. *Ann Emerg Med.* 2005;46(5):456-461.
11. Gregg SC, Murthi SB, Sisley AC, Stein DM, Scalea TM. Ultrasound-guided peripheral intravenous access in the intensive care unit. *J Crit Care.* 2010;25(3):514-519.
12. Ismailoğlu EG, Zaybak A, Akarca FK, Kıyan S. The effect of the use of ultrasound in the success of peripheral venous catheterization. *Int Emerg Nurs.* 2015;23(2):89-93.
13. Costantino TG, Kirtz JF, Satz WA. Ultrasound-guided peripheral venous access vs. the external jugular vein as the initial approach to the patient with difficult vascular access. *J Emerg Med.* 2010;39(4):462-467.

14. Bauman M, Braude D, Crandall C. Ultrasound-guidance vs. standard technique in difficult vascular access patients by ED technicians. *Am J Emerg Med.* 2009;27(2):135-140.

15. Marik PE, Flemmer M, Harrison W. The risk of catheter-related bloodstream infection with femoral venous catheters as compared to subclavian and internal jugular venous catheters: a systematic review of the literature and meta-analysis. *Crit Care Med.* 2012;40(8):2479-2485.

16. Parienti JJ, Mongardon N, Mégarbane B, et al. Intravascular complications of central venous catheterization by insertion site. *N Engl J Med.* 2015;373(13): 1220-1229.

17. Maki DG, Kluger DM, Crnich CJ. The risk of bloodstream infection in adults with different intravascular devices: a systematic review of 200 published prospective studies. *Mayo Clin Proc.* 2006;81(9):1159-1171.

18. Rao S, Badwaik G, Kujur R, Paraswani R. Thrombosis associated with right internal jugular central venous catheters: a prospective observational study. *Indian J Crit Care Med.* 2012;16(1):17-21.

19. Fragou M, Gravvanis A, Dimitriou V, et al. Real-time ultrasound-guided subclavian vein cannulation versus the landmark method in critical care patients: a prospective randomized study. *Crit Care Med.* 2011;39(7):1607-1612.

20. Firstenberg M, Kornbau C, Lee K, Hughes G. Central line complications. *Int J Crit Illn Inj Sci.* 2015;5(3):170-178.

21. Shokoohi H, Boniface K, Mccarthy M, et al. Peripheral intravenous access program is associated with a marked reduction in central venous catheter use in noncritically ill emergency department patients. *Ann Emerg Med.* 2013;61(2):198-203.

22. Au AK, Rotte MJ, Grzyboweki RJ, Ku BS, Fields JM. Disease in central venous catheter placement due to use of ultrasound guidance for peripheral intravenous catheters. *Am J Emerg Med.* 2012;30(9):1950-1954.

23. Schoenfeld E, Boniface K, Shokoohi H. ED technicians can successfully place ultrasound-guided intravenous catheters in patients with poor vascular access. *Am J Emerg Med.* 2011;29(5):496-501.

24. Sandhu NPS, Sidhu DS. Mid-arm approach to basilic and cephalic vein cannulation using ultrasound guidance. *Br J Anaesth.* 2004;93(2):292-294.

25. Witting MD, Schenkel SM, Lawner BJ, Euerle BD. Effects of vein width and depth on ultrasound-guided peripheral intravenous success rates. *J Emerg Med.* 2010;39(1):70-75.

26. Elia F, Ferrari G, Molino P, et al. Standard-length catheters vs long catheters in ultrasound-guided peripheral vein cannulation. *Am J Emerg Med.* 2012;l30:712-716.

27. Kagel EM, Rayan GM. Intravenous catheter complications in the hand and forearm. *J Trauma.* 2004;56(1):123-127.

28. Adhikari S, Blaivas M, Morrison D, Lander L. Comparison of infection rates among ultrasound-guided versus traditionally placed peripheral intravenous lines. *J Ultrasound Med.* 2010;29:741-747.

29. Lockhart ME, Robbin ML, Fineberg NS, Wells CG, Allon M. Cephalic vein measurement before forearm fistula creation: does use of a tourniquet to meet the venous diameter threshold increase the number of usable fistulas? *J Ultrasound Med.* 2006;25(12):1541-1545.

30. Safety Communication: Bacteria found in other-sonic generic ultrasound transmission gel poses risk of infection. Clinician Outreach and Communication Activity (COCA). CDC Emergency communication System. April 20, 2012.

Core Needle Biopsy/Fine Needle Aspiration

Paul Bornemann, MD, RMSK, RPVI and Mohamed Gad, MD, MPH(c)

LITERATURE REVIEW

Needle biopsy allows for collection of tissue cytology or histology that is less invasive than traditional surgical biopsy. Needle biopsies are generally either small caliber fine needle aspiration (FNA) or larger caliber core needle biopsy (CNB). FNA needles are typically 25 to 27 gauge, whereas CNB needles are typically 9 to 18 gauge. Because FNA uses a smaller needle, it tends to be associated with less pain and bleeding. However, it provides only a cytologic sample that is lacking in the details of histologic tissue architecture. CNB is performed with a spring-loaded cutting sheath around a needle with a side fenestration and provides a small tissue sample with histologic architecture. CNB has a slightly increased risk of complications over FNA; however, serious complications are very rare for both. Traditionally, needle biopsy was guided by palpation of target lesions; however, ultrasound guidance has quickly gained ground as the standard of care.[1] The use of real-time ultrasonography to guide needle biopsy has many advantages over unguided

biopsy. Ultrasonography allows for characterization of lesions prior to biopsy, localization of nonpalpable lesions, and real-time guidance of biopsy needles into the target lesion.

Ultrasound guidance may be done in-plane or out-of-plane. When done in-plane, the needle is aligned with the ultrasound beam and can be visualized in its entirety (see **Figure 58-1** and Video 58-1). When done out-of-plane, the needle is visualized in cross section. In-plane is generally preferred because it is easier to be certain of where the tip is at all times. Out of plane can also be beneficial when there is not enough space to perform guidance in-plane or when lateral corrections in the needle path to target need to be made (see **Figure 58-2**). If performing guidance out-of-plane, it is important to continually advance the ultrasound beam in front of the needle tip so that the location of the tip is known at all times. The beam can be swept in front of the needle until it is no longer visualized and then the needle can be advanced and stopped as soon as the tip is visualized (see an example of this in Video 58-2). Also, if the beam needs to remain stationary, such as when the target lesion is

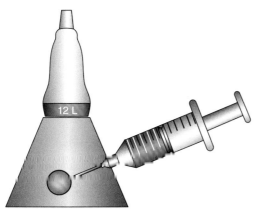
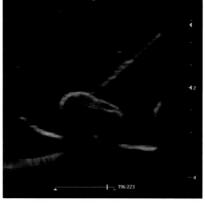

FIGURE 58-1. Ultrasound needle guidance using the in-plane technique. Note that the entire length of the needle is aligned with the ultrasound beam and can be visualized at all times.

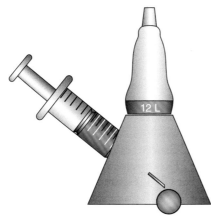
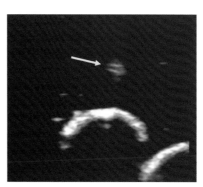

FIGURE 58-2. Ultrasound needle guidance using the out-of-plane technique. The tip of the needle is only visualized in cross section. Note the needle tip indicated by the yellow arrow.

427

small, the needle is advanced, stopping as soon as the tip is visualized, and then pulled back and advanced at a deeper angle again. This is repeated until the needle tip is visualized in the target.

Several common uses of needle biopsy are for sampling suspicious thyroid nodules, breast masses, or lymph nodes. The decision on when to biopsy a thyroid nodule is discussed in-depth in Chapter 5. FNA is reported to be an accurate and cost-effective initial testing modality when a nodule is selected for biopsy. It is recommended as the preferred technique by the American Thyroid Association guidelines.[2] FNA can be performed with negative pressure aspiration or through capillary action aspiration, and both methods are equally effective.[3] Ultrasound guidance has been shown to be more effective than palpation guidance in multiple randomized controlled trials.[4,5] Up to 20% of FNA biopsies of thyroid nodules can come back with indeterminate results (Bethesda Category III or IV). Underlying malignancy rates following these results range from 10% to 40%.[6] In these cases, follow-up with CNB has been shown to be helpful and safe.[7,8] Additionally, a sample for molecular testing can be obtained and held at the time of initial FNA. This testing can be run when cytology comes indeterminate and can help differentiate high- from low-risk lesions in these cases without the need for repeat biopsy.[9]

In addition to being studied for use in thyroid nodules, ultrasound-guided needle biopsies have also been studied for diagnosis of breast masses. The decision on when to biopsy a breast mass is discussed in-depth in Chapter 16. Needle biopsy is the preferred method in the evaluation of breast masses because it decreases the number of surgeries and overall cost of care compared to initial evaluation with surgical biopsy.[10,11] The Centers for Medicare and Medicaid Services (CMS) has established "needle biopsy to establish diagnosis of cancer precedes surgical excision" as a quality measure.[12] Although FNA can be an option if CNB is not available, FNA tends to lead to more inadequate samples than CNB, which can lead to delayed diagnosis.[13,14] The National Comprehensive Cancer Network's (NCCN) Guidelines for Breast Cancer Screening and Diagnosis recommend CNB as the preferred method for initial biopsy concerning breast masses.[15,16] Ultrasound guidance is recommended, even in palpable breast masses because it increases the sensitivity of biopsies.[17,18]

Vacuum-assisted biopsy (VAB) devices can be used in conjunction with needle biopsy. In essence, a VAB is a CNB that is done under negative pressure provided by an attached vacuum device. It can help to increase the sample size over CNB. It is unclear if this improves sensitivity over ultrasound-guided CNB, and this is especially unclear for palpable lesions. Additionally, VAB is more expensive than traditional CNB and is not routinely available in primary care. More evidence is needed to determine whether VAB is superior to CNB in any situation and whether it is cost-effective.[19]

Finally, needle biopsy can be useful in the evaluation of peripheral lymphadenopathy. The decision on when to biopsy a peripheral lymph node is discussed in-depth in Chapter 6. Surgical excisional biopsy has been considered the standard evaluation method for peripheral lymphadenopathy in the past because diagnosis of lymphoma will often require tissue histologic architecture. The NCCN guidelines on lymphoma recommend incisional or excisional lymph node biopsy as the preferred initial biopsy method.[20] However, CNB for assessment of lymph nodes concerning for malignancy has been shown to be an

acceptable alternative. It was demonstrated to have high diagnostic specificity (97.8%), sensitivity (94.4%), and accuracy (95.0%), with lower cost and less complications.[21] CNB does appear to be superior to FNA because it provides a higher sampling success rate as well as a higher positive predictive value.[22] Adjunctive studies, such as flow cytometry, can be run on CNB or FNA samples if appropriate collection tubes are used at the time of biopsy. However, there are limited data to suggest that this is helpful in improving the overall diagnostic rate.[23] FNA is most useful when metastatic disease is suspected because these lesions tend to be easily diagnosed from lymph node cytologic analysis with high accuracy.[24,25]

TABLE 58-1	Recommendations for Use of Point-of-Care Ultrasound in Clinical Practice		
Recommendation		**Rating**	**References**
Ultrasound-guided fine needle aspiration (FNA) is more accurate than palpation-guided FNA of thyroid nodules.		A	4, 5
Ultrasonography-guided core needle biopsy (CNB) should be considered before excisional biopsy to diagnose malignancy in women with suspicious breast lesions on imaging.		A	15
Ultrasonography-guided CNB is a reasonable first step in diagnosis of suspicious lymphadenopathy.		B	20

A = consistent, good-quality patient-oriented evidence; B = inconsistent or limited-quality patient-oriented evidence; C = consensus, disease-oriented evidence, usual practice, expert opinion, or case series. For information about the SORT evidence rating system, go to http://www.aafp.org/afpsort.

EQUIPMENT

- Alcohol swab for skin sterilization
- Chlorhexidine or iodine
- Sterile ultrasound gel
- 2 × 2 gauze
- Adhesive tape
- Ethyl chloride spray
- 2% lidocaine with epinephrine
- 18-gauge filter needle and 5 mL syringe (to draw up lidocaine)
- 25-gauge 1.5" needle (to administer lidocaine)
- For FNA (**Figure 58-3**):
  - 23 to 27-gauge needles most commonly used
  - 10 mL syringe
  - Intravenous catheter extension tubing
  - Glass slides
  - Fixative—either alcohol or formalin
  - Cytologic specimen preservative collection vial
  - Genetic testing collection vial (optional for thyroid nodules)
  - Flow cytometry collection vial (optional for lymph nodes)
- For CNB (**Figure 58-4**):
  - 9 to 18-gauge spring-loaded biopsy needle
  - 8 to 17-gauge coaxial guidance cannula with trocar
  - Formalin specimen container
  - Flow cytometry collection vial (optional for lymph nodes)

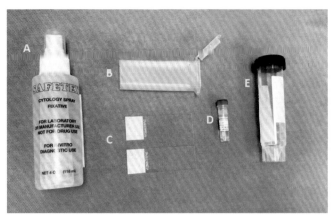

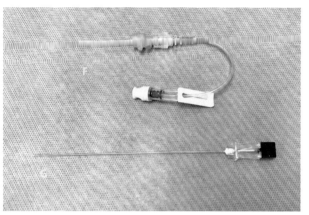

FIGURE 58-3. Equipment for fine needle aspiration. A, Spray fixative for slides. B, Slide holder. C, Glass slides. D, Genetic testing collection vial. E, Cytologic specimen preservative collection vial. F, 25 gauge 1.5" needle attached to extension tubing. G, 25 gauge 6" spinal needle.

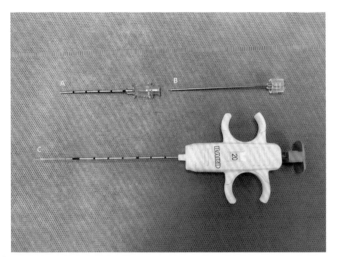

FIGURE 58-4. Equipment for core needle biopsy. A, 17 gauge coaxial guidance cannula. B, Trocar for guidance cannula. C, 18-gauge spring-loaded biopsy needle.

INDICATIONS

- Suspicious breast lesion
- Suspicious lymph nodes
- Suspicious thyroid nodules

CONTRAINDICATIONS

- There are no absolute contraindications
- Bleeding disorders and coagulopathy
- Skin infections over the biopsy site
- Neck mass suspicious for carotid body tumor

PERFORMING THE PROCEDURE

1. **Prepare equipment and position the patient.** Use a high-frequency linear array transducer for most biopsies. If a lesion is deeper than 4 to 6 cm, then a low-frequency curvilinear transducer may be needed. Apply a cover to the transducer to prevent any blood coming into contact with it. A transparent adhesive dressing, surgical glove, or manufactured transducer cover can work well.

    Position the patient directly in line between the provider performing the procedure and the ultrasound screen (**Figures 58-5 and 58-6**). There should be a direct line of vision so that the provider does not need to turn his or her head to view the patient or the ultrasound screen. Unless the lesion exists on the back, patients should lie in the supine position. Manipulation of the head position and rotation of the neck may help in obtaining easier access to thyroid nodules or cervical lymph nodes. Putting a pillow or rolled towel under the neck of the patient may help extend the spine and provide easier access to thyroid nodules. For breast lesions, the patient should lie with the ipsilateral arm extended above the head.

PART 4

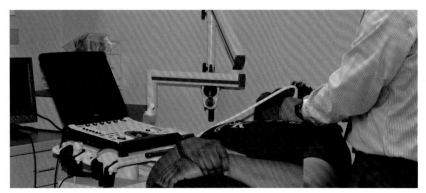

FIGURE 58-5. Correct positioning for a needle biopsy. The patient and ultrasound are all directly in the line of vision.

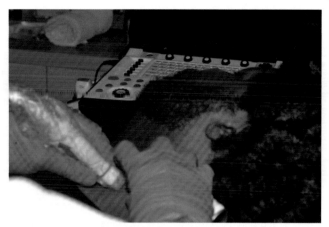

FIGURE 58-6. Correct positioning for a needle biopsy from the perspective of the provider performing the procedure. The patient and the ultrasound screen are visualized directly in line. A high-frequency linear array transducer with a cover is being used.

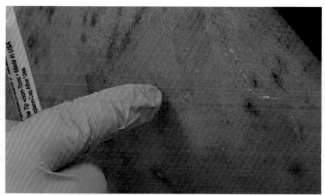

FIGURE 58-7. The area of planned needle insertion is marked on the skin with pressure from a pen cap.

2. **Find the lesion with ultrasound.** Position the ultrasound transducer above the lesion to be biopsied. Plan the approach to the biopsy. Determine the depth of the lesion. Plan to insert the needle a distance from the lesion in the horizontal plane that is equal to or larger than the depth. This will ensure an angle of needle insertion of 45° or less. Angles steeper than this will make the needle more difficult to visualize on ultrasound. Be mindful of the total distance from skin insertion to target lesion later when selecting needle length. Mark the area of planned skin insertion with a marking pen or by applying pressure to the skin with a needle cap (**Figure 58-7**).

3. **Provide local anesthesia to the skin and subcutaneous tissue surrounding the lesion.** Disinfect the marked area of skin with alcohol. If available, apply ethyl chloride spray to the marked area several seconds before administering lidocaine (**Figure 58-8A**). Use a 25-gauge needle to apply a wheal of lidocaine with epinephrine to the marked area of skin (**Figure 58-8B**). Next, numb the track of the planned needle insertion by advancing the needle, drawing back to confirm no blood is aspirated, and then injecting lidocaine as the needle is withdrawn slowly while

injecting. This can also be done under direct ultrasound guidance as will be described for the biopsy needle.

4. **Perform the needle biopsy.** Use the nondominant hand to hold the ultrasound transducer to visualize the target lesion in the same exact manner that was used in Step 2. Use a firm grip with several fingers or the base of the hand contacting the patient's skin to assure stability of the transducer. Be sure the transducer is aligned in a manner that the needle will enter the ultrasound screen from the expected side of the screen. It is generally preferable to have the needle enter the screen from the same side that the needle will be advanced to the transducer. For example, if the needle is advanced from the right side of the transducer, in-plane, it is best to have the transducer aligned so that the needle will enter the ultrasound screen from the right side as well. **Figure 58-9** shows the incorrect transducer orientation.

FINE NEEDLE ASPIRATION

Select needle gauge. For most solid lesions 25 or 27 gauge is preferred. Select a needle that is of appropriate length to reach the target lesion. In general, it will need to be at least 1.5″ but will depend on the depth of the lesion (see Step 2). Attach the intravenous catheter extension tubing to the needle. Insert the needle just into the dermis with the bevel pointing up (**Figure 58-10**).

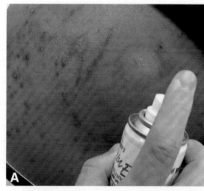
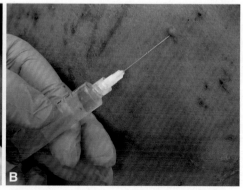

FIGURE 58-8. A, Ethyl chloride spray is applied to the marked area of skin. B, A wheal of lidocaine is administered to the area of planned needle insertion.

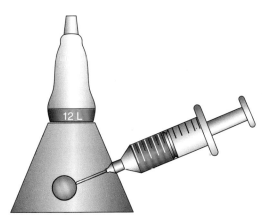

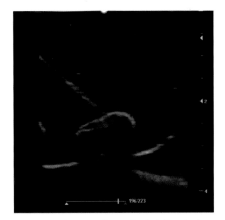

FIGURE 58-9. Incorrect transducer orientation. The needle is entering the ultrasound screen from the left but being passed to the target lesion from the right of the transducer. This can be fixed by twisting the transducer 180°. The correct orientation should appear as in Figure 58-1.

Adjust the ultrasound to be sure the needle tip is clearly visualized (**Figure 58-11** and ▶ **Video 58-3**). Advance the needle under direct ultrasound guidance into the lesion. Be sure to have the needle tip visualized at all times. When the tip of the needle is in the lesion, move the needle back and forth within the lesions rapidly, at a rate of about 3 times per second. The cellular sample will be collected via capillary action. Do this for 2 to 5 seconds and then withdraw the needle.

Fill a 10-mL syringe with air and then attach it to the extension tubing that is attached to the needle. Gently apply pressure to the syringe plunger to expel the aspirated sample on the glass slides (**Figure 58-12**).

Smear the sample on the slide using a second slide (**Figure 58-13** and ▶ **Video 58-4**). Repeat subsequent needle passes into the lesion as described earlier. Do this enough times to obtain at least four to six slides—half should be fixed with alcohol spray and half

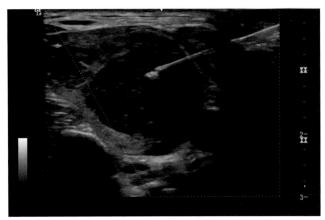

FIGURE 58-11. Fine needle aspiration needle is visualized in-plane. The tip is visualized inside of the target lesions. In this case it is a thyroid nodule.

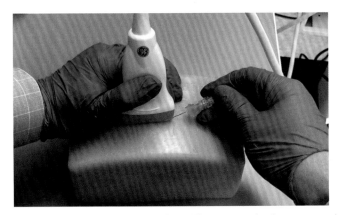

FIGURE 58-10. A linear array probe with correct grip demonstrated using several fingers and the base of the hand to contact the patient's skin to assure stability of the probe. A 25-gauge fine needle aspiration needle is attached to the extension tubing prior to ready insertion into skin.

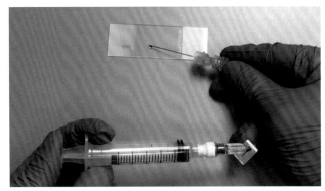

FIGURE 58-12. Fine needle aspiration needle contents are expressed onto a slide with pressure from a syringe that has been attached to the needle via extension tubing.

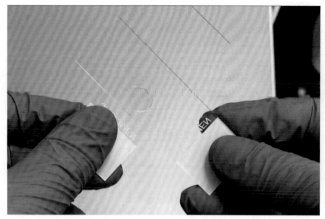

FIGURE 58-13. A smear is created from the contents of the fine needle aspiration after it is expressed onto a slide.

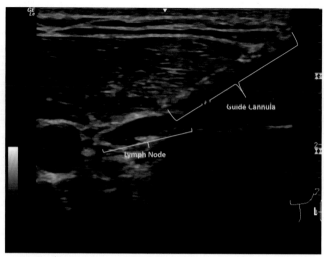

FIGURE 58-15. Ultrasound image of in-plane guide cannula next to lesion (a lymph node) that is to be biopsied.

unfixed. Label slides as fixed or unfixed. Also repeat for collection into the 30 mL cytologic specimen preservative collection vial and additional passes if desired for:
- Genetic testing collection vial (optional for thyroid nodules)
- Flow cytometry collection vial (optional for lymph nodes)

CORE NEEDLE BIOPSY

Select needle gauge. For most breast masses, larger gauge needles, such as 9 to 11 gauges, are preferred. For thyroid or lymph node, a smaller gauge such as 17 gauge is usually acceptable. Select a needle that is of appropriate length to reach the target lesion (see Step 2). Insert the trocar into the coaxial guide cannula. Insert the trocar tip just into the dermis with the bevel pointing up (**Figure 58-14**). Some larger gauge needles may require the skin to be punctured with an 11-blade scalpel first.

Adjust the ultrasound to be sure the cannula tip is clearly visualized. Guide the cannula so that it is visualized just next to the lesion to be biopsied. Be sure to have the tip visualized at all times (**Figure 58-15**).

Remove the trocar from the guide cannula. Prepare the biopsy needle system. Prime the instrument by pulling back on the plunger to withdraw the outer cannula and inner stylet and lock the outer

cannula in place (**Figure 58-16**). Most systems will allow for multiple depths of biopsy, for example, 10 or 20 mm. Choose the most appropriate depth for the lesion to be biopsied.

With the inner stylet fully retracted, so that the sample notch is covered by the cannula, insert the tip of the needle to the point to be biopsied. DO NOT advance the inner stylet by pressing on the plunger until the instrument is in position. Once in position press the plunger to advance the inner stylet into the lesion. The stylet will meet resistance when it is fully advanced. Confirm with ultrasound that the sample notch can be seen within the lesion (**Figures 58-17 and 58-18** and ▶ **Video 58-5**). Fire the cutting cannula by fully pressing the plunger.

Remove the needle from the patient and pull the plunger back to prime to the previous depth and then gently advance the plunger forward to expose the biopsy specimen (**Figure 58-19**). Be careful not to fire the cutting cannula at this point.

Place the small tissue sample into a formalin sample container.

Repeat the biopsy steps for as many cores as needed through the guide cannula.

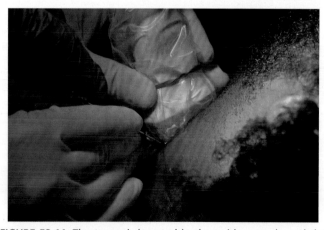

FIGURE 58-14. The trocar is inserted in the guide cannula and the cannula is directed to the lesion under ultrasound guidance.

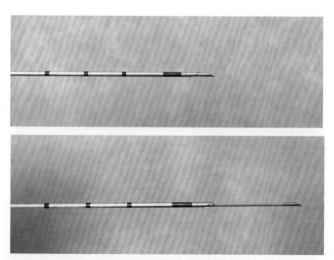

FIGURE 58-16. A core needle biopsy instrument before (top) and after (bottom) being primed to 20 mm. In the bottom image, the inner stylet has also been advanced out of the outer, cutting cannula to demonstrate the sample notch.

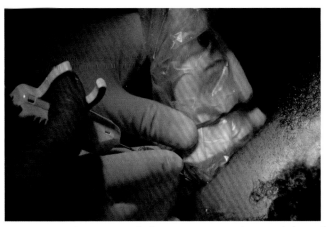

FIGURE 58-17. The core needle biopsy instrument is passed through the coaxial guide cannula.

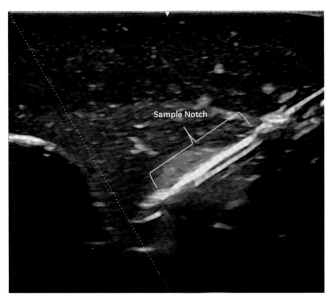

FIGURE 58-18. Ultrasound image of in-plane biopsy needle in a lesion (a simulated thyroid nodule). The sample notch of the stylet is visualized in the lesion.

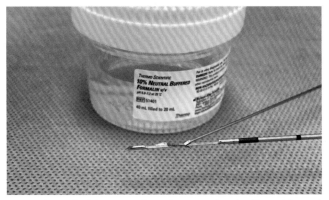

FIGURE 58-19. The biopsy specimen is exposed and collected from the core needle biopsy instrument prior to being placed in the formalin specimen container.

POSTPROCEDURE INSTRUCTIONS

- Patient is advised to apply slight pressure on the needle insertion site to minimize hematoma formation.
- Patient should avoid trauma to the aspiration site.
- Patient should be advised to consult with his or her physician if the skin becomes red, warm, and/or painful.

COMPLICATIONS

- Because of inadequate sample, repeat biopsy may be needed.
- Hematoma formation: a bruise or a hematoma may develop after removal of the needle because of injury of small vessels.
- Skin or subcutaneous tissue infection: Because of the invasive nature of the procedure, risk of infection exists. However, this can be minimized by the following aseptic techniques.
- Track seeding with tumor cells: A rare complication is seeding of the needle track with malignant cells.
- Injury to surrounding structures may occur.

PATIENT MANAGEMENT

The decision on whether to biopsy thyroid nodules, breast masses, and lymph nodes is discussed in previous chapters. Once the decision to perform a needle biopsy is made, FNA or CNB must be chosen. In general, FNA has lower complication rates with lower diagnostic yields. For most thyroid nodules, FNA will be the initial choice. For lymph nodes, generally CNB is performed initially. However, FNA may be performed initially if metastatic or recurrent cancer is highly suspected. For breast masses, CNB is the best initial biopsy option.

Thyroid nodule cytology results are reported using the Bethesda system.[26] Recommendations on management of different cytology classifications are from the American Thyroid Association guidelines.[2] Bethesda I is considered "nondiagnostic or unsatisfactory" and results when there is insufficient cellularity to make an assessment or when there is obscuring blood. This should be followed up with repeat FNA in 1 to 3 months. Bethesda II is considered "benign." This category has an overall low malignancy rate, but false negatives are possible. If the lesions originally appeared low risk on ultrasound and the patient does not have other risk factors, benign FNA lesions will usually not need follow-up. If the decision is made to follow up with repeat ultrasound, this can be done in 12 to 24 months. Repeat FNA should be considered if the lesion grows by more than 20% in at least two dimensions or if any new high-risk sonographic features are found (see Chapter 5). Bethesda III is considered "atypia of undetermined significance (AUS)" or "follicular lesion of undetermined significance (FLUS)". Bethesda IV is considered "follicular neoplasm." Bethesda III and IV are typically considered indeterminate because of intermediate rates of malignancy. If a vial was collected and held for genetic testing at the time of FNA, genetic testing can be run and can help to stratify into a low- or high-risk lesion. Low-risk lesions will typically be followed up with repeat ultrasound in 12 months, whereas high-risk lesions will be referred for surgical biopsy. Repeat FNA or CNB at that time or up to 3 months is another option. CNB has been shown

PART 4

Thyroid nodule cytology management

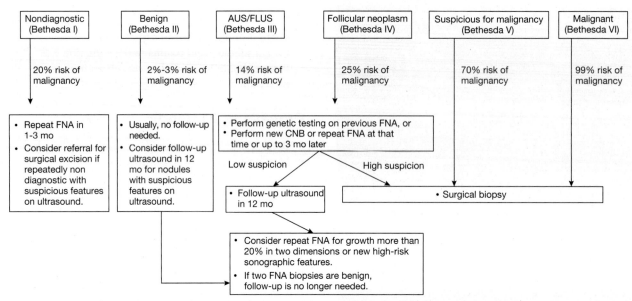

FIGURE 58-20. Algorithm for management of thyroid nodule FNA cytology. AUS, atypia of undetermined significance; CNB, core needle biopsy; FLUS, follicular lesion of undetermined significance; FNA, fine needle aspiration.

Derived from Haugen BR, Alexander EK, Bible KC, et al. 2015 American Thyroid Association Management Guidelines for Adult Patients with Thyroid Nodules and Differentiated Thyroid Cancer: The American Thyroid Association Guidelines Task Force on Thyroid Nodules and Differentiated Thyroid Cancer. *Thyroid.* 2016; 26:1.

to have higher diagnostic rates in these instances.[7] If a lesion continues to have indeterminate results on repeat FNA or CNB, surgical excisional biopsy is an option. Bethesda IV is considered "suspicious for malignancy" and Bethesda V is considered "malignant." Both should be referred for surgical excision. See **Figure 58-20** for a management algorithm.

Recommendations for management of breast masses are based on the NCCN Guidelines for Breast Cancer Screening and Diagnosis.[15] For most breast masses that are suspicious for malignancy in women over 30 years of age, bilateral screening mammogram should be performed to rule out other lesions, prior to CNB.

This can change management and CNB can create artifacts on mammography. Breast cysts are benign findings and usually only aspirated if they are symptomatic. Cyst contents do not need to be routinely sent for cytology. However, if contents appear frankly bloody, they should be sent for cytologic evaluation. Additionally, if any residual mass is seen after aspirating a cyst, CNB of the lesions should be considered. For most benign appearing lesions with benign pathology, follow-up imaging can be done at 12 months after biopsy.[27] Any solid lesion with initial imaging findings that were high risk (Breast Imaging, Reporting and Data System [BI-RADS] IV or V) and that result in benign pathology

Breast needle biopsy of palpable mass management

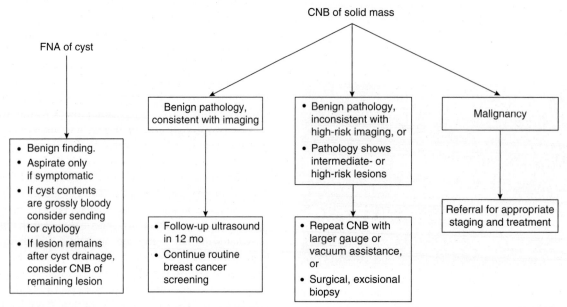

FIGURE 58-21. Algorithm for the management of breast needle biopsy results. CNB, core needle biopsy; FNA, fine needle aspiration.

on CNB should be assessed further. It is helpful to review with a pathologist. In most cases, these lesions should undergo repeat CNB with a larger gauge needle or with VAB. Referral for excisional biopsy should also be considered for high-risk breast lesions such as atypical ductal or lobular hyperplasia, lobular carcinoma in situ, or flat epithelial atypia. Further recommendations can be found from the American Society of Breast Surgeons.[28] Any cancerous lesions should be referred for appropriate treatment. See **Figure 58-21** for a management algorithm.

Lymph node biopsies will usually be done with CNB. If the lymph node is suspected to be from metastatic disease or malignancy recurrence, FNA can be an acceptable initial choice. In these cases, cytology consistent with metastatic malignancy should trigger workup for the underlying primary lesions. If lymphoma is suspected, CNB is the best initial assessment tool. Often the diagnosis of lymphoma can be made based on the histology from a CNB. Flow cytometry can be a useful adjunct and can be performed on FNA or CNB when the diagnosis is not clear.

PEARLS AND PITFALLS

Pearls

- CNB devices that will insert a marker clip at the location of the biopsy are available and are frequently used for breast biopsies. Different shapes or number of clips can be used. This can be especially useful when multiple breast masses are sampled to help surgeons differentiate them in the future.
- It is difficult to reposition horizontally if the needle is off target when using the in-plane technique. However, the ultrasound transducer can be twisted 90° to an out-of-plane technique. The needle can then be repositioned horizontally to align with the target and then the transducer can be twisted back to be in-plane with the needle.
- Several considerations should be in mind when repeating FNA after nondiagnostic cytology. If the result was because of scant cellularity, check if the lesion is partially cystic. If so, it should be drained by FNA first. A larger needle, such as a

23 gauge, usually works better in these instances. Negative pressure can be used by aspirating on a syringe attached to the extension tubing while the needle is in the cyst. This should be done before performing FNA as described earlier on the remaining solid component. If the sample was limited because of obscuring blood, be sure to use limited needle dwell time in the lesions because the longer time the needle is in, the more blood tends to be collected. Keep it in the lesion for less than 3 to 5 seconds per pass.

Pitfall

- When performing an FNA of solid lesions, larger caliber needles (23 gauge or larger) or long needle-in-lesion dwell times (greater than 5 seconds) can decrease the sensitivity of the biopsy by increasing the amount of blood in the sample that can obscure other cytology.

BILLING

CPT Code	Description	Professional Fee	Facility Fee
10022	Fine needle aspiration with imaging guidance	$143.22	$67.31
19000	Puncture aspiration of cyst of breast*	$114.93	$45.11
19083	Percutaneous breast biopsy with ultrasound guidance	$682.07	$164.34
38505	Core needle biopsy of lymph node(s)*	$129.61	$73.76
60100	Core needle biopsy of the thyroid*	$115.29	
76942	"Ultrasonic guidance for needle placement (eg, biopsy, aspiration, injection, localization device), imaging supervision, and interpretation"	$34.04	$27.95

* Nonbundled codes that can be billed in conjunction with 76942 when ultrasound guidance is used.
CPT codes and average national reimbursement for Medicare in 2016. Payment data are from https://www.cms.gov/apps/physician-fee-schedule/search/search-criteria.aspx. See Chapter 2 for details on ultrasound billing.

References

1. Gutwein L, Ang D, Liu H, et al. Utilization of minimally invasive breast biopsy for the evaluation of suspicious breast lesions. *Am J Surg*. 2011;202:127-132.
2. Haugen BR, Alexander EK, Bible KC, et al. 2015 American Thyroid Association Management Guidelines for adult patients with thyroid nodules and differentiated thyroid cancer: the American Thyroid Association Guidelines task force on thyroid nodules and differentiated thyroid cancer. *Thyroid*. 2016;26(1):1-133.
3. Lee J, Kim BK, Sul HJ, Kim JO, Lee J, Sun WY. Negative pressure is not necessary for using fine-needle aspiration biopsy to diagnose suspected thyroid nodules: a prospective randomized study. *Ann Surg Treat Res*. 2019;96(5):216-222.
4. Danese D, Sciacchitano S, Farsetti A, Andreoli M, Pontecorvi A. Diagnostic accuracy of conventional versus sonography-guided fine-needle aspiration biopsy of thyroid nodules. *Thyroid*. 1998;8(1):15-21.
5. Kumari K, Jadhav P, Prasad C, Smitha N, Jojo A, Manjula V. Diagnostic efficacy of ultrasound-guided fine needle aspiration combined with the Bethesda system of reporting. *J Cytol*. 2019;36(2):101-105.
6. Cibas ES, Ali SZ. The 2017 Bethesda system for reporting thyroid cytopathology. *Thyroid*. 2017;27:1341.
7. Yim Y, Baek JH. Core needle biopsy in the management of thyroid nodules with an indeterminate fine-needle aspiration report. *Gland Surg*. 2019;8(S2):S77-S85.
8. Ha EJ, Baek JH, Lee JH, et al. Complications following US-guided core-needle biopsy for thyroid lesions: a retrospective study of 6,169 consecutive patients with 6,687 thyroid nodules. *Eur Radiol*. 2017;27(3):1186-1194.
9. Patel KN, Angell TE, Babiarz J, et al. Performance of a genomic sequencing classifier for the preoperative diagnosis of cytologically indeterminate thyroid nodules. *JAMA Surg*. 2018;153(9):817-824.

10. Gutwein LG, Ang DN, Liu H, et al. Utilization of minimally invasive breast biopsy for the evaluation of suspicious breast lesions. *Am J Surg*. 2011;202(2):127-132.

11. Eberth JM, Xu Y, Smith GL, et al. Surgeon influence on use of needle biopsy in patients with breast cancer: a national Medicare study. *J Clin Oncol*. 2014;32(21):2206-2216.

12. Centers for Medicare and Medicaid Services. Needle biopsy to establish diagnosis of cancer precedes surgical excision/resection. https://cmit.cms.gov/CMIT_public/ViewMeasure?MeasureId=5436. Accessed October 20, 2019.

13. Wang M, He X, Chang Y, Sun G, Thabane L. A sensitivity and specificity comparison of fine needle aspiration cytology and core needle biopsy in evaluation of suspicious breast lesions: a systematic review and meta-analysis. *Breast*. 2017;31:157-166.

14. Tikku G, Umap P. Comparative study of core needle biopsy and fine needle aspiration cytology in palpable breast lumps: scenario in developing nations. *Turk J Pathol*. 2015;32:1-7.

15. Bevers TB, Helvie M, Bonaccio E, et al. Breast cancer screening and diagnosis, Version 3.2018, NCCN Clinical Practice Guidelines in Oncology. *J Natl Compr Canc Netw*. 2018;16(11):1362-1389.

16. Smith M, Heffron C, Rothwell J, Loftus B, Jeffers M, Geraghty J. Fine needle aspiration cytology in symptomatic breast lesions: still an important diagnostic modality? *Breast J*. 2012;18:103-110.

17. Lorenzen J, Welger J, Lisboa BW, Riethof L, Grzyska B, Adam G. Percutaneous core-needle biopsy of palpable breast tumors. Do we need ultrasound guidance? [in German]. *Rofo*. 2002;174(9):1142-1146.

18. Shah VI, Raju U, Chitale D, Deshpande V, Gregory N, Strand V. False-negative core needle biopsies of the breast: an analysis of clinical, radiologic, and pathologic findings in 27 consecutive cases of missed breast cancer. *Cancer*. 2003;97(8):1824-1831.

19. Huang XC, Hu XH, Wang XR, et al. A comparison of diagnostic performance of vacuum-assisted biopsy and core needle biopsy for breast microcalcification: a systematic review and meta-analysis. *Ir J Med Sci*. 2018;187(4):999-1008.

20. Zelenetz AD, Gordon LI, Abramson JS, et al. NCCN Guidelines Insights: B-cell lymphomas, Version 3, 2019. *J Natl Compr Canc Netw*. 2019;17(6):650-661.

21. Wilczynski A, Görg C, Timmesfeld N, et al. Value and diagnostic accuracy of ultrasound-guided full core needle biopsy in the diagnosis of lymphadenopathy: a retrospective evaluation of 793 cases. *J Ultrasound Med*. 2020;39:559-567.

22. Zhang WZ, Yang GY, Xu JP, Zhang L, Li J, Zhao D. Comparative study of core needle biopsy and fine needle aspiration cytology in the diagnosis of neck lymph node diseases with contrast-enhanced ultrasound. *Zhonghua Er Bi Yan Hou Tou Jing Wai Ke Za Zhi*. 2016;51:615-617.

23. Frederiksen JK, Sharma M, Casulo C, Burack WR. Systematic review of the effectiveness of fine-needle aspiration and/or core needle biopsy for subclassifying lymphoma. *Arch Pathol Lab Med*. 2015;139(2):245-251.

24. Prasad RR, Narasimhan R, Sankaran V, Veliath AJ. Fine-needle aspiration cytology in the diagnosis of superficial lymphadenopathy: an analysis of 2,418 cases. *Diagn Cytopathol*. 1996;15:382-386.

25. Nasuti JF, Yu G, Boudousquie A, Gupta P. Diagnostic value of lymph node fine needle aspiration cytology: an institutional experience of 387 cases observed over a 5-year period. *Cytopathology*. 2000;11(1):18-31.

26. Cibas ES, Ali SZ; NCI Thyroid FNA State of the Science Conference. The Bethesda System for reporting thyroid cytopathology. *Am J Clin Pathol*. 2009;132(5):658-665.

27. Johnson JM, Johnson AK, O'Meara ES, et al. Breast cancer detection with short-interval follow-up compared with return to annual screening in patients with benign stereotactic or US-guided breast biopsy results. *Radiology*. 2015;275(1):54-60.

28. The American Society of Breast Surgeons. Consensus guideline on concordance assessment of image-guided breast biopsies and management of borderline or high-risk lesions. https://www.breastsurgeons.org/docs/statements/Consensus-Guideline-on-Concordance-Assessment-of-Image-Guided-Breast-Biopsies.pdf. Accessed October 26, 2019.

Saline Infusion Sonography

Lauren Castleberry, MD, FACOG

LITERATURE REVIEW

Abnormal uterine bleeding can be further characterized by the acronym PALM-COEIN, a term coined by the International Federation of Gynecology and Obstetrics in 2011 to help standardize the nomenclature used to describe various forms of genital tract bleeding.[1] The first half of the acronym, "PALM" (Polyp, Adenomyosis, Leiomyoma, Malignancy and Hyperplasia), represents structural etiologies while the second half of the acronym, "COEIN" (Coagulopathy, Ovulatory disorder, Endometrium, Iatrogenic, and Not classified) represents nonstructural causes. In a study performed by Goyal et al. of 100 patients with abnormal uterine bleeding, polypoidal endometrium, polyps, or submucous fibroids were found at the time of hysteroscopy in 41.[2] Given that endometrial pathology may account for the etiology of a significant percentage of abnormal uterine bleeding, a workup would be incomplete without a thorough evaluation of the endometrial cavity.

Second to the physical examination, the pelvic ultrasound is a well-established and noninvasive modality to evaluate the female reproductive organs for structural etiologies of abnormal uterine bleeding. Although pelvic ultrasound allows for a global evaluation of the entire uterus, the gold standard for evaluation of the endometrial cavity is hysteroscopy. Unfortunately, hysteroscopy is not only invasive, but also costly and requires special training to perform. An alternative imaging modality, sonohysterography, is not only better tolerated by patients, but also affordable and more accessible. Sonohysterography is a modality that can be performed in the office setting to evaluate the endometrial lining and is performed by injecting sterile fluid through the cervix and into the uterus under ultrasound guidance.[3]

Over the past two decades, multiple studies comparing the efficacy of sonohysterography with hysteroscopy have been performed. A recent systematic review of diagnostic studies comparing 2D and/or 3D saline contrast sonohysterography (SCSH) with hysteroscopy and anatomopathology was conducted by Bittencourt et al.[4] A total of 1398 citations were identified but ultimately only 5 studies were included in the review and meta-analysis. From those five studies, and correlating 543 women, the sensitivity, specificity, and positive and negative likelihood ratios (LR+, LR–) were calculated. Sensitivity and specificity of 2D-SCSH for the detection of endometrial polyps were 93% and 81%, respectively, whereas for the detection of submucosal uterine leiomyomas, sensitivity and specificity were 94% and 81%, respectively. The LR+ and LR– were 5.41 and –0.10 for the detection of endometrial polyps and 4.25 and –0.11 for the detection of submucosal uterine leiomyomas, respectively. They concluded that 2-D SCSH has high diagnostic accuracy for the detection of endometrial polyps and submucosal

TABLE 59-1	Recommendations for Use of Point-of-Care Ultrasound in Clinical Practice		
Recommendation		Rating	References
Use 2D-SCSH as a first-line diagnostic method in the workup for women with abnormal uterine bleeding.		A	4

A = consistent, good-quality patient-oriented evidence; B = inconsistent or limited-quality patient-oriented evidence; C = consensus, disease-oriented evidence, usual practice, expert opinion, or case series. For information about the SORT evidence rating system, go to http://www.aafp.org/afpsort.

uterine leiomyomas in women of reproductive age with abnormal uterine bleeding. Given these findings, 2-D SCSH is an outpatient imaging modality that should be routinely utilized in the evaluation of patients with abnormal uterine bleeding.

EQUIPMENT

- Transvaginal ultrasound probe
- Patient bed that allows for lithotomy position
- Single-use disposable sterile probe cover
- Ultrasound gel
- Open-sided speculum
- Betadine or other cleansing solution
- Sonohysterography or hysterosalpingogram catheter
- 20 mL syringe
- Sterile saline
- Single-tooth tenaculum
- Cervical Os Finder

INDICATIONS

For the evaluation of:
- Abnormal uterine bleeding
- Uterine cavity
- Abnormalities detected on transvaginal ultrasonography—including focal or diffuse endometrial or intracavitary abnormalities
- Recurrent pregnancy loss
- Infertility
- Suboptimal visualization of the endometrium on transvaginal ultrasonography[3]

CONTRAINDICATIONS

- Confirmed or possible pregnancy
- Existing pelvic infection or unexplained pelvic tenderness

PERFORMING THE PROCEDURE

Steps

1. First, obtain informed consent from the patient.

   Explain the risks and benefits to the patient and obtain a consent form signed by both the patient and health care provider. Perform a pregnancy test to reliably exclude the chance of pregnancy.[5]

   A health care provider can be reasonably certain that a woman is not pregnant if she has no symptoms or signs of pregnancy and meets any one of the following criteria:

   - is ≤7 days after the start of normal menses
   - has not had sexual intercourse since the start of last normal menses
   - has been correctly and consistently using a reliable method of contraception
   - is ≤7 days after spontaneous or induced abortion
   - is within 4 weeks postpartum
   - is fully or nearly fully breastfeeding (exclusively breastfeeding or the vast majority [≥85%] of feeds are breastfeeds), amenorrheic, and <6 months postpartum

2. Second, place the patient in the lithotomy position (**Figure 59-1**).

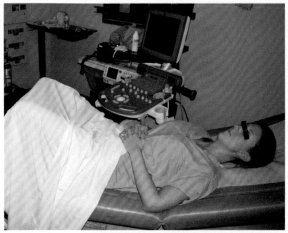

FIGURE 59-1. Patient in the lithotomy position.

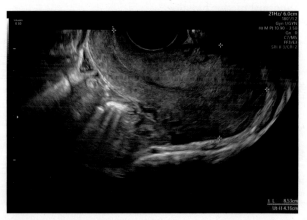

FIGURE 59-2. Preprocedural image of a retroverted uterus in the sagittal plane.

3. Obtain precatheterization images.

4. Obtain precatheterization images and measurements of the pelvic contents using the covered transvaginal probe. After obtaining these images and measurements, remove the probe (**Figure 59-2**).

5. Place a one-sided speculum in the patient's vagina (**Figure 59-3**).

6. After visualizing the cervix, clean the external cervical os with betadine or another appropriate cleansing solution (**Figure 59-4**).

7. Prepare the catheter for insertion.

8. Draw up approximately 20 mL of saline into the syringe and flush the catheter to not only ensure patency, but also to remove any air (**Figure 59-5**).

9. Place the catheter through the cervical os into the uterine cavity using sterile technique.

   The goal is to have the catheter tip at the level of the lower uterine segment. If using a catheter with a balloon, inflating the balloon is optional (**Figure 59-6**).

10. Carefully remove the speculum from the vagina, being sure to hold the catheter in place.

11. Insert the covered transvaginal probe into the vagina (**Figure 59-7**).

12. Instill the sterile saline into the uterine cavity slowly and perform real-time imaging.

    Perform imaging in both the sagittal and transverse planes so as to visualize the entire endometrial cavity. Obtain cine clips for later review. Additionally, if any abnormalities are detected, perform color Doppler and/or 3D imaging (**Figure 59-8** and ▶ **Video 59-1**).

13. Remove the catheter. After completion of the endometrial cavity assessment, remove the catheter slowly; if a catheter with an inflated balloon has been used, deflate the balloon and perform a final assessment with imaging of the cervical canal (**Figure 59-9**).

14. Remove the transducer.

15. Document the findings in a written report.

    The report should include standard patient identifiers, the indication for the procedure, the technique employed, precatheterization measurements, any abnormal findings, and interpretation of the results.[3]

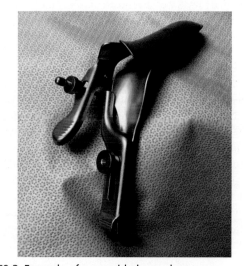

FIGURE 59-3. Example of a one-sided speculum.

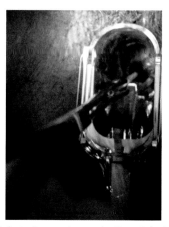

FIGURE 59-4. Apply betadine to the cervix. Copyright Dr. EJ Mayeaux, Jr., used with permission.

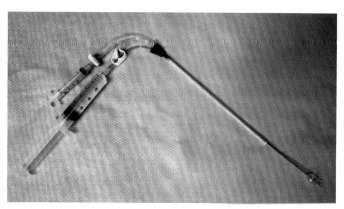

FIGURE 59-5. Example of an hysterosalpingogram catheter. Note the air-filled balloon at the tip of the catheter (filled to better demonstrate; balloon should be deflated upon insertion)

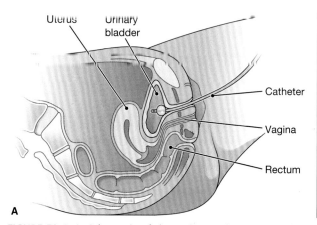

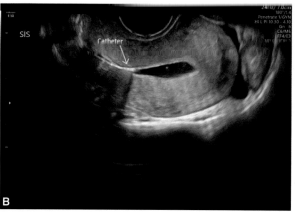

FIGURE 59-6. A, Schematic of the catheter placement within the lower uterine segment. From Cohen BJ. Ann DePetris A. *Medical Terminology: An Illustrated Guide.* 8th ed. Jones & Bartlett Learning: Burlington, MA; 2020. www.jblearning.com. Reprinted with permission. B, Catheter visible in the cervical canal on ultrasound.

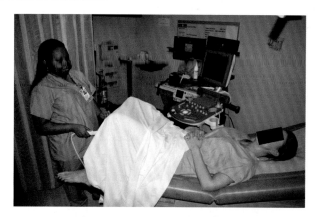

FIGURE 59-7. Insertion of the vaginal transducer.

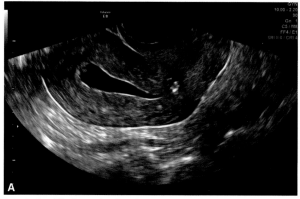

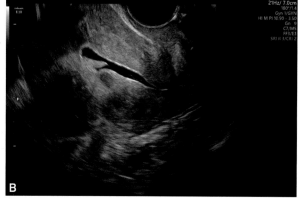

FIGURE 59-8. A, Instillation of saline into a normal uterine cavity. B, Focal endometrial lesion visible at the top of the uterine cavity.

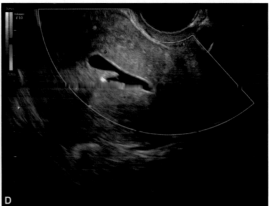

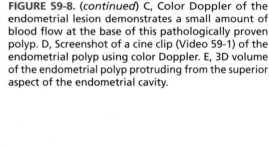

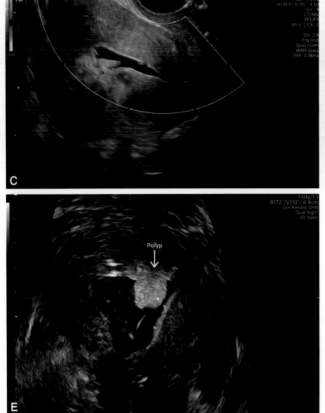

FIGURE 59-8. (*continued*) C, Color Doppler of the endometrial lesion demonstrates a small amount of blood flow at the base of this pathologically proven polyp. D, Screenshot of a cine clip (Video 59-1) of the endometrial polyp using color Doppler. E, 3D volume of the endometrial polyp protruding from the superior aspect of the endometrial cavity.

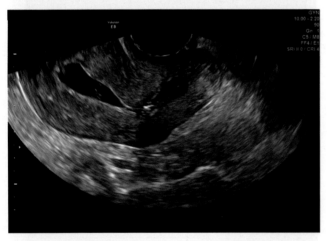

FIGURE 59-9. Removal of the catheter with continued instillation of saline illuminates the contour of the endocervical canal.

POSTPROCEDURE INSTRUCTIONS

Inform the patient that the fluid inserted during the procedure will leak from the vagina throughout the day. Provide a sanitary pad to use as needed. If the procedure was uncomplicated, the patient can return to her daily schedule without any restrictions. Tell the patient to notify the provider of any concerns, particularly if she develops fever, chills, pelvic pain, or foul-smelling vaginal discharge. Have her schedule a follow-up visit to discuss the results and management options.

COMPLICATIONS

- Infection
- Bleeding
- Uterine perforation
- Loss of pregnancy if present

PATIENT MANAGEMENT

Abnormal findings from SCSH can include endometrial polyps, submucosal leiomyoma, adhesions, congenital abnormalities, and endometrial lesions of undetermined significance. With regard to abnormal uterine bleeding, the most common abnormalities will be polyps, leiomyomas, and other lesions of undetermined significance. Once identified, management can range from medical management (for leiomyomas) to operative management (for polyps, leiomyomas, and all other lesions). If uterine conservation is desired, then operative management via hysteroscopy with dilation

and curettage is the next step. This allows for direct visualization of the pathology, as well as directed biopsy in the case of lesions with undetermined significance. Additionally, if the pathology involves a submucosal leiomyoma or polyp, hysteroscopic resection can be performed. If uterine conservation is not desired and surgical management is planned, then office biopsy should be performed if indicated and subsequent hysterectomy scheduled (**Figure 59-10**).

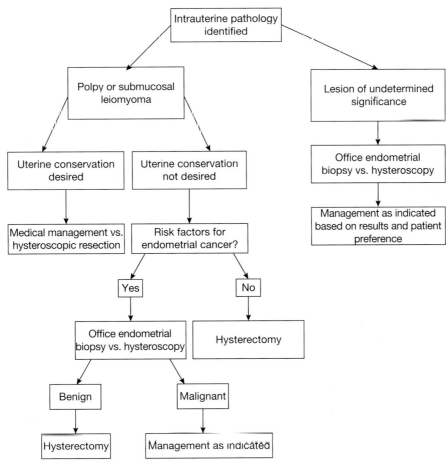

FIGURE 59-10. Flowchart of patient management algorithm.

PEARLS AND PITFALLS

Pearls

- Strive to position the speculum such that the cervical os is facing you at a direct angle instead of being tilted superiorly or inferiorly. This assists with placement of the catheter.
- Most procedures do not require the use of a tenaculum if the cervix is positioned as noted above.
- If cervical stenosis is encountered, first try to dilate the cervix using an Os Finder alone. If this is ineffective, place the tenaculum on the anterior lip of the cervix and try again with the Os Finder while maintaining counter-traction with the tenaculum.

- Inflating the balloon in a multiparous patient can help keep the catheter in place and fluid inside the cavity.

Pitfalls

- Only pass the catheter to the level of the lower uterine segment, that is, 3 to 4 cm. Uterine cramping is expected during placement of the catheter and procedure. Sharp pain may indicate you have advanced the catheter too far or perforated the uterus.
- Do not inject the saline quickly. A slow instillation works just as well, minimizing patient discomfort.

PART 4

BILLING

CPT Code	Description	Global Payment	Professional Fee	Technical Fee	Facility Fee
58340	Catheterization and introduction of saline or contrast material for saline infusion sonohysterography (SIS) or hysterosalpingography	N/A	N/A	N/A	59.76
74740	Hysterosalpingography, radiologic supervision and interpretation	75.96	19.44	56.52	75.96
76831	Saline infusion sonohysterography (SIS), including color flow Doppler, when performed	122.76	37.80	84.96	N/A

CPT codes and average national reimbursement for Medicare in 2016. Payment data are from https://www.cms.gov/apps/physician-fee-schedule/search/search-criteria.aspx. See Chapter 2 for details on ultrasound billing.

References

1. Munro MG, Critchley HO, Broder MS, Fraser IS. FIGO classification system (PALM-COEIN) for causes of abnormal uterine bleeding in nongravid women of reproductive age. FIGO Working Group on Menstrual Disorders. *Int J Gynaecol Obstet.* 2011;113:3-13 (Level III).
2. Goyal BK, Gaur I, Sharma S, Saha A, Das NK. Transvaginal sonography versus hysteroscopy in evaluation of abnormal uterine bleeding. *Med J Armed Forces India.* 2015;71:120-125.
3. Sonohysterography. Technology assessment no. 12. American College of Obstetricians and Gynecologists. *Obstet Gynecol.* 2016;128:e38-e42.
4. Bittencourt CA, Dos Santos Simoes R, Bernardo WM, et al. Accuracy of saline contrast sonohysterography in detection of endometrial polyps and submucosal leiomyomas in women of reproductive age with abnormal uterine bleeding: systematic review and meta-analysis. *Ultrasound Obstet Gynecol.* 2017;50(1):32-39.
5. Curtis KM, Jatlaoui TC, Tepper NK, et al. U.S. Selected practice recommendations for contraceptive use, 2016. *MMWR Recomm Rep.* 2016;65 (No. RR-4):1-66. doi:10.15585/mmwr.rr6504a1.

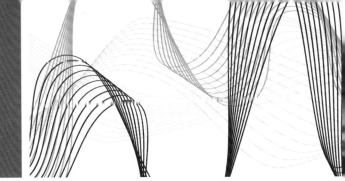

INDEX

Page numbers followed by "*f*" indicate figure and those followed by "*t*" indicate table